Clinical PET

Springer
New York
Berlin
Heidelberg
Hong Kong
London
Milan
Paris
Tokyo

Clinical PET
Principles and Applications

E. Edmund Kim, MD
The University of Texas M.D. Anderson Cancer Center, Houston, Texas, USA

Myung-Chul Lee, MD, PhD
Seoul National University College of Medicine
Seoul, Korea

Tomio Inoue, MD, PhD
Yokohama City University School of Medicine, Yokohama, Japan

Wai Hoi Wong, PhD
The University of Texas M.D. Anderson Cancer Center, Houston, Texas, USA

Editors

With 250 Illustrations

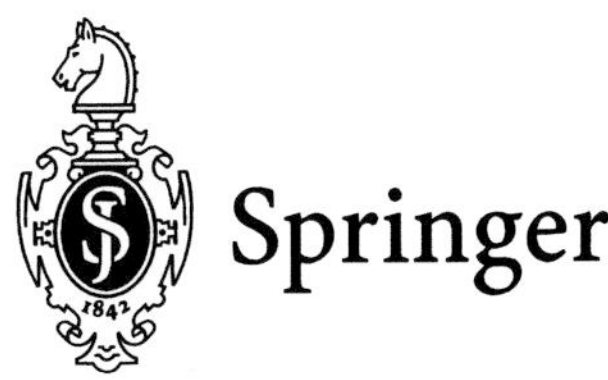

Springer

E. Edmund Kim, MD
Wai Hoi Wong, PhD
The University of Texas
M.D. Anderson Cancer Center
1515 Holcombe Blvd., Box 0059
Houston, TX 77030, USA

Myung-Chul Lee, MD, PhD
Seoul National University College of Medicine
Department of Nuclear Medicine
28 Yongon-dong, Chongno-gu
Seoul, 110-744 Korea

Tomio Inoue, MD, PhD
Yokohama City University
School of Medicine
3–9 Fukuura, Kanazawa-ku
Yokohama 236, Japan

Cover illustrations: (Background, Figure 9-1, see p. 148) Selected coronal whole-body PET images show a subcutaneous extravasation of FDG solution. (Foreground and back cover, Figure 10-3, see p. 168) Four cases of occipital lobe epilepsy.

Library of Congress Cataloging-in-Publication Data
Clinical PET: Principles and Applications / [edited by] E. Edmund Kim . . . [et al.].
p. ; cm.
Includes bibliographical references and index.
ISBN 0-387-40854-1 (alk. paper)
1. Tomography, Emission. 2. Diagnostic imaging. 3. Cancer—Tomography. I. Kim, E. Edmund.
[DNLM: 1. Tomography, Emission-Computed—methods. 2. Neoplasms—diagnosis. WN 206 T355 2003]
RC78.7.T62T465 2003
616.07′575—dc22 2003058705

ISBN 0-387-40854-1 Printed on acid-free paper.

Printed in the United States of America (MP/MVY)

9 8 7 6 5 4 3 2 1 SPIN 10942819

Springer-Verlag is a part of *Springer Science+Business Media*

springeronline.com

This book is dedicated to Thomas T. Haynie, MD, doctor-teacher-friend.

Foreword

Nuclear medicine contributes significantly to the initial diagnosis of disease, assessment of response to therapy, and exploration of the natural history of disease, and is beginning to have an expanded role in therapy. The techniques enable appraisal of anatomy and physiology. An area of the field of nuclear medicine with many applications and great potential is positron emission tomography (PET), which has evolved from a research tool to active clinical use in less than 30 years. The progression from the first experimental animal studies of ^{14}C-labeled deoxyglucose used to measure functional brain activity by means of postmortem autoradiography in the early 1970s to the application of ^{18}F-fluorodeoxyglucose (FDG)-PET on a routine clinical basis has been exhilarating. For many diseases and physiologic evaluations, PET has shown itself to be superior to other imaging techniques. This is especially true for such functions as the differentiation of recurrent tumor from radiation necrosis (brain tumors), and staging and following the effects of therapy for Hodgkin and non-Hodgkin lymphomas, head and neck tumors, breast cancer, melanoma, ovarian neoplasms, and others. In benign areas, PET helps in the assessment of tissue viability (myocardial infarction and stroke), infection, and inflammation.

Positron emission tomography imaging offers the opportunity and challenge of taking advantage of metabolic activity as well as anatomy. Cancer cells have a generally increased uptake of glucose. Hence, the ever-expanding role of ^{18}F-FDG PET in nuclear oncology. This metabolic difference is useful in evaluating whether pulmonary lesions are benign or malignant. The sensitivity and specificity of PET in Hodgkin and non-Hodgkin lymphomas continues to be expanded. Use of radioactive nitrogen, radiolabeled purines, pyrimidines, and amino acids offer diverse opportunities to apply PET to metabolic, anatomic, and functional oncologic clinical studies. Altered metabolic pathways imaged in real time can aid in predicting therapeutic efficiency. Functional studies may permit measurement of therapeutic response before anatomic changes are noted. An even more exciting potential is the possibility of using PET to detect early epithelial or tissue changes at the molecular level that may presage clinical cancer. Here early detection may provide opportunities for prevention or earlier therapeutic intervention.

PET interpretation requires knowledge of physics, pharmacy, anatomy, physiology, disease process, and artifacts. This book presents the current science, technology, and, where applicable, the art necessary to synthesize the complexities of PET. The diagnostic competence and acumen of the nuclear medicine physician/radiologist will be tested to make proper interpretations today and be prepared to move to incorporate new knowledge and techniques tomorrow. Future PET techniques and radiopharmaceuticals will emerge and be implemented. Expanded and exciting avenues are here now, and a universe of PET and related techniques are on the horizon.

Dr. Kim and his colleagues have provided us with a beacon and a path for this journey.

Armand B. Glassman, M.D.
Olla S. Stribling Distinguished Chair for Cancer Research
The University of Texas M.D. Anderson Cancer Center
Houston, Texas
December 2003

Preface

Positron emission tomography (PET) has been around long enough that it is hard to think of it as being anything special. It has been a valuable research tool in academic institutions since the 1970s, but its move into clinical practice in community hospitals has just begun.

Those who are now working with PET, or have made the decision to do so, understand just how different a perspective on disease this modality provides. In most patients for whom it is indicated, PET provides earlier and more sensitive detection. It is special, but not in ways that are immediately evident. It requires a shift in the diagnostic paradigm, and adjustments in patient management, to capture the advantages of early diagnosis.

Questions remain on how and when payment will be made for PET studies, but as with so much else in medicine, once patients and referring physicians know what PET can do for them, it will not be refused. Given time, it will eventually be documented that PET saves money overall by eliminating unnecessary and futile interventions in patients with advanced disease. That's the power of imaging the body's biochemistry.

The momentum toward the use of PET is expected to grow with the advent of molecular imaging. The sequencing of the genome and proteomes is establishing the fundamental molecular basis of how cells function. Molecules can now be designed to stop the disease or to prevent it from occurring. Imaging of gene expression could eventually provide the basis for developing therapeutic strategies individualized to a patient's genetic characteristics. Biology and genetics were merged with medicine to produce the new field of molecular medicine, and that created the need for an imaging technology that looks at the biology of a disease. As drug company research and molecular imaging converge, imaging probes will be used to select patients for treatment with specific drugs.

The main impact of PET in community practice now, and likely for several years to come, is in oncology. Whole-body PET in cancer patients enables clinicians to identify malignant diseases in their early stages, differentiate benign from malignant tumors, examine the entire body for metastases, and determine the effectiveness of cancer therapeutics.

It has been predicted that PET would undergo spectacular growth in the 21st century as molecular medicine becomes central to the analysis of disease. The burgeoning world of PET is reflected in recent scientific meetings including Radiological Society of North America (RSNA) and Society of Nuclear Medicine (SNM).

This book provides comprehensive information on the basic principles and clinical applications of PET. Emphasis is placed on the familiarization of normal distribution, artifacts, and pitfalls of common agents such as fluorodeoxyglucose (FDG) in conjunction with computed tomography (CT), magnetic resonance imaging (MRI), or ultrasound (US) to establish the clinical effectiveness of PET. Practical understanding of updated PET scanners, cyclotron, image process, and quantification is also stressed. This book is therefore divided into two parts: the first part discusses the basic principles of PET, such as instrumentation, image process, fusion, radiopharmaceuticals, radiosynthesis, safety and economics. The second part discusses the clinical applications of the technique in neurology, cardiology, infection, and oncology.

We hope this book meets the growing needs of diagnostic radiologists, nuclear physicians, and clinicians for understanding the basic principles and clinical applications of PET.

Acknowledgments

I am very appreciative of and indebted to Bonnie Schroeder for her tremendous efforts of typing and editing materials as well as communicating with contributors to make this book publishable. I am also deeply grateful to all contributors, whom I often harassed for their timely work, and also to Rob Albano at Springer–New York for his patience and support in creating and editing this book.

E. Edmund Kim
The University of Texas
M.D. Anderson Cancer Center
Houston, Texas
December 2003

Contents

Part II Clinical Applications

Contributor List

Ali Azhdarinia, PhD
Graduate Research Assistant
Department of Experimental Diagnostic Imaging
The University of Texas M.D. Anderson Cancer Center
1515 Holcombe Blvd., Unit 59
Houston, TX 77030, USA

Hossain Baghaei, PhD
Assistant Professor
Department of Experimental Diagnostic Imaging
The University of Texas M.D. Anderson Cancer Center
1100 Holcombe Blvd.
Box 217, HMB 15.529
Houston, TX 77030, USA

June-Key Chung, MD, PhD
Professor
Department of Nuclear Medicine
Seoul National University College of Medicine
Seoul National University Hospital
28 Yongon-dong, Chongno-gu
Seoul 110-744, Korea

Tetsuya Higuchi, MD, PhD
Research Associate
Department of Nuclear Medicine and Diagnostic Radiology
Gunma University School of Medicine
3-39-22 Showa-machi
Maebashi 371-8511, Japan

Tomio Inoue, MD
Professor
Department of Radiology
Yokohama City University Graduate School of Medicine and School of Medicine
3-9 Fukuura, Kanazawa-ku
Yokohama 236-0004, Japan

Byung-Tae Kim, MD, PhD
Professor
Department of Nuclear Medicine
Sung-Kyun-Kwan University
Samsung Medical Center
50 Ilwon-dong, Kangnam-ku
Seoul 135-710, Korea

E. Edmund Kim, MD
Professor
Departments of Nuclear Medicine and Diagnostic Radiology
The University of Texas M.D. Anderson Cancer Center
1515 Holcombe Blvd., Box 0059
Houston, TX 77030, USA

Sang-Eun Kim, MD, PhD
Associate Professor
Department of Nuclear Medicine
Sung-Kyun-Kwan University
300 Gumi-dong, Bundang-gu
Sungnam-shi, Gyeonggi-do 463-707, Korea

Sung-Eun Kim, MD
Chief
Department of Nuclear Medicine
Inha University College of Medicine
Korea Institute of Radiological & Medical Sciences
215-4 Gongneung-Dong, Nowon-Gu
Seoul 139-706, Korea

Carlos Gonzalez Lepera, PhD
Adjunct Professor
Department of Experimental Diagnostic Imaging
The University of Texas M.D. Anderson Cancer Center
1515 Holcombe Blvd.
Houston, TX 77030, USA

Dong-Soo Lee, MD, PhD
Associate Professor
Department of Nuclear Medicine
Seoul National University College of Medicine
Seoul National University Hospital
28 Yongon-dong, Chongno-gu
Seoul 110-744, Korea

Ho-Young Lee, MD
Department of Nuclear Medicine
Seoul National University College of Medicine
Seoul National University Hospital
28 Yongon-dong, Chongno-gu
Seoul 110-744, Korea

Kyung-Han Lee, MD, PhD
Associate Professor
Department of Nuclear Medicine
Sung-Kyun-Kwan University
Samsung Medical Center
50 Ilwon-dong, Kangnam-ku
Seoul 135-710, Korea

Myung-Chul Lee, MD, PhD
Professor
Department of Nuclear Medicine
Seoul National University College of Medicine
Seoul National University Hospital
28 Yongon-dong, Chongno-gu
Seoul 110-744, Korea

Osama Mawlawi, PhD
Assistant Professor
Department of Imaging Physics
The University of Texas M.D. Anderson Cancer Center
1515 Holcombe Blvd., Box 56
Houston, TX 77030, USA

Noboru Oriuchi, MD, PhD
Associate Professor
Department of Nuclear Medicine and Diagnostic Radiology
Gunma University School of Medicine
3-39-22 Showa-machi
Maebashi 371-8511, Japan

Jin-Chul Paeng, MD
Department of Nuclear Medicine
Seoul National University College of Medicine
Seoul National University Hospital
28 Yongon-dong, Chongno-gu
Seoul 110-744, Korea

Nobukazu Takahashi, MD, PhD
Department of Radiology
Yokohama City University School of Medicine
3-9 Fukuura
Kanazawa-ku, Yokohama 236-0004, Japan

Jorge Uribe, PhD
Assistant Professor
Department of Experimental Diagnostic Imaging
The University of Texas M.D. Anderson Cancer Center
1100 Holcombe Blvd.
Box 217, HMB 15.527
Houston, TX 77030, USA

Richard Wendt III, MD
Associate Professor
Department of Imaging Physics
The University of Texas M.D. Anderson Cancer
1515 Holcombe Blvd., Unit 056
Houston, TX 77030, USA

Franklin C.L. Wong, MD, PhD, JD
Associate Professor
Departments of Nuclear Medicine and Neuro-Oncology
The University of Texas M.D. Anderson Cancer Center
1515 Holcombe Blvd., Unit 59
Houston, TX 77030, USA

Wai-Hoi Wong, PhD
Professor
Department of Experimental Diagnostic Imaging
The University of Texas M.D. Anderson Cancer Center
1515 Holcombe Blvd., Box 217
Houston, Texas 77030, USA

David J. Yang, PhD
Associate Professor
Department of Experimental Diagnostic Imaging
The University of Texas M.D. Anderson Cancer Center
1515 Holcombe Blvd., Box 0059
Houston, TX 77030, USA

Massashi Yukihiro, MD, PhD
2500-1-30 G Nakanogou
Fujikawa-cho, Ihara Shizouka 421-3306, Japan

PART I

Basic Principles

1

Principles of Positron Emission Tomography Imaging

Hossain Baghaei, Wai-Hoi Wong, and Jorge Uribe

Positron emission tomography (PET) is a noninvasive medical imaging technology that can generate high-resolution images of human and animal physiologic functions. It is used for a variety of clinical applications in oncology, neurology, and cardiology, but the principal clinical application of PET is in oncology, where it is used to locate malignant tumors. It can be used not only to detect disease, but also to help in planning its treatment and monitoring the effectiveness of the treatment. The PET camera can detect therapeutic changes earlier than anatomic imaging modalities, because the structure being studied must significantly change in size and shape before it is detectable by anatomic imaging devices.

The PET camera measures the distribution of positron-emitting radionuclides (tracers) within an object. Positron-emitting radionuclides are used for imaging because of their unique tomographic capability and the availability of a group of metabolically important radionuclides. The unique tomographic capability comes from the simultaneous emission of two nearly back-to-back 511-keV gamma rays when a positron is annihilated by an electron, and from the ability to provide accurate quantitation of tracer uptakes with its attenuation-correction capability. The medical importance of PET imaging derives from the availability of many useful positron-emitting tracers, such as isotopes of carbon (^{11}C), nitrogen (^{13}N), and oxygen (^{15}O), which are basic elements of all living organisms and their physiologic processes. Hence, more tissue-specific and chemistry-specific tracers can be synthesized and injected into humans or animals for studying the physiologic functions of normal or pathologic tissues in vivo. Another important positron-emitting isotope, fluorine (^{18}F), is widely used to label a glucose analog, ^{18}F-fluorodeoxyglucose (FDG), which follows the glucose pathway in its transport from plasma to tissue cells. However, unlike glucose, FDG remains trapped in the cell, without undergoing further metabolism, which can be used for imaging purposes.

Imaging modalities are commonly categorized as functional or anatomic devices. These two different modalities provide complementary data that can be integrated for the purpose of diagnosis, and for planning, performing, and evaluating the effectiveness of therapy. Indeed, the interpretation of nuclear medicine functional images is improved when they are co-registered with anatomic images. Very recently, the PET camera has been combined with anatomic x-ray computed tomography (CT) to provide CT transmission scans for attenuation correction and for the co-registration of PET and CT data to facilitate the localization of tumors.

Basic Physics of PET

The atomic nucleus is made up of nucleons: protons and neutrons. The proton has a positive electric charge, and the neutron has no net electric charge. Inside the nucleus, the protons and neutrons are mainly subject to two kinds of forces: the short-range strong attractive nuclear force that acts between all nucleons to hold the nucleons together, and the repulsive electric force that acts between the charged protons. Unstable proton-rich nuclei may transform to a more stable state by reducing their excess positive electric charge. One of the allowed decay processes for a proton-rich nucleus is to have a proton decay into a neutron, a neutrino, and a positively charged particle called a positron. Because the mass of a proton is less than that of a neutron, this decay process can take place only inside the nucleus. The neutrino is a particle with no mass and no electric charge that leaves the surrounding tissue without any interaction. The positron (β^+) is the antiparticle of the electron (β^-) and has the same mass as an electron but the opposite charge. A proton-rich isotope can be made in an accelerator (e.g., cyclotron), which generates a beam of high-energy protons or deuterons to penetrate the target nuclei to implant the target nuclei with more protons.[1]

The kinetic energy released in the nucleus decay process is shared between the positron and the neutrino, so the actual energies of the emitted positrons are distributed in a continuous spectrum from almost zero to the full decay energy of the isotope. Table 1.1 shows the average kinetic energy of the emitted positrons for several commonly used radionuclides.[2–4] After a positron is produced, it travels a very short distance (0.2 to 2 mm for most commonly used tracers) until it loses almost all of its kinetic energy through scattering in the surrounding tissue, and then it combines with an electron in an annihila-

TABLE 1.1. Physical properties of some common positron-emitting isotopes

Positron isotopes	^{11}C	^{13}N	^{15}O	^{18}F	$^{68}Ga^*$
Half-life (min)	20.4	9.96	2.07	109.7	68.3
Average positron energy (MeV)	0.3	0.4	0.6	0.2	0.7
Average positioning error (mm)	0.28	—	—	0.22	1.35

*^{68}Ga is generated from a $^{68}Ga/^{68}Ge$ generator (the parent ^{68}Ge has a half-life of 275 days).

tion process. In this process, both the positron and electron are annihilated and their mass is converted to energy ($E = mc^2$) in the form of a pair of photons. Following the basic laws of physics, conservation of energy, and linear momentum, each gamma ray (photon) has energy of 511 keV, the energy equivalent to the mass of an electron or a positron. The two generated photons are emitted almost back-to-back (180 ± 0.6 degrees), so the net momentum of two gamma rays going in opposite directions is zero, as shown in Figure 1.1. It is this back-to-back emission of the gamma pair that provides the special tomographic and quantitative imaging properties of positron imaging. The annihilation radiations are detected externally and are used to determine both the quantity and the location of the positron emitter. In addition, PET scanners exploit the back-to-back emission property to "electronically collimate" the photon pairs and determine the path along which the annihilation occurred. Since no physical collimator is required for event localization, the PET camera has a 50 to 100 times higher sensitivity advantage over single photon imaging cameras. The lack of a collimator also contributes to higher image resolution.

The emitted positrons have to travel a short distance before generating the gamma-ray pair, which implies that the site of positron emission, that is, the site of the positron-labeled molecule and the site of gamma generation detected by the PET cameras, are slightly different. The distance that a positron travels before annihilation, called the "positron range," depends on its initial kinetic energy. The positron range and photon noncolinearity (the fact that the two gamma rays are

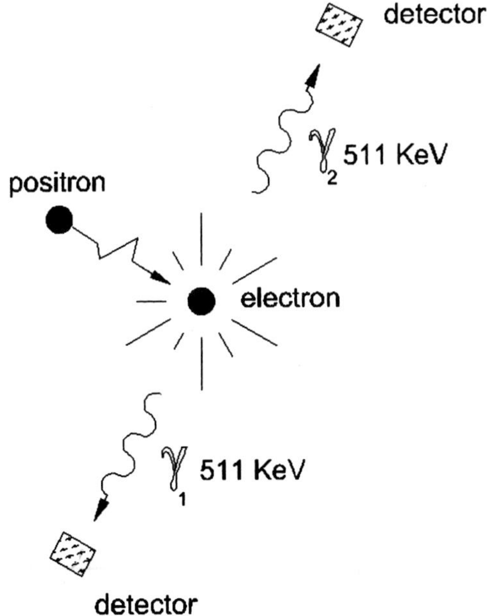

FIGURE 1.1. Schematic of positron emission and annihilation with an electron in tissue to generate two gamma rays traveling in opposite directions (180 degrees) that are detected in coincidence by two external scintillation detectors.

not exactly back-to-back) cause an uncertainty in positioning the event, and this contributes to the fundamental resolution limit of PET imaging (Table 1.1). However, in a conventional PET camera, used for clinical scan using FDG, the main spatial resolution limitation to PET imaging comes from the size of the individual small crystals used for detection.

Not all the emitted photons in the object (body) reach the surrounding detector system. These photons can either interact with the body tissue or pass through it without interaction. The interactions of photons with the body occur mainly in the form of photoelectric interaction or Compton scattering. The photons involved in photoelectric interaction are completely absorbed and so do not reach the detectors. The dominant form of interaction for photons at 511 keV in tissue is Compton scattering, which is caused by the collision of a photon with a loosely bound electron in an outer shell of an atom. When a photon interacts with an electron, it loses some energy and its path is deflected, thereby reducing the number of photons that would otherwise reach the detectors. The loss in photon flux due to interactions in a body (or any object) is called attenuation. In PET systems, the probability that the two photons generated in one event (a positron annihilation) "survive" the attenuation in the body is independent of the position of the annihilations along the line joining the two detectors. Therefore, it is possible to correct for the attenuation effect by performing a transmission scan using an external source.

Coincidence Detection

The PET camera takes advantage of the fact that the two photons generated from the positron annihilation are created simultaneously and therefore rejects all events that do not satisfy the time-coincidence condition. Two photons are considered to be in coincidence if they are detected within a specific time interval known as the coincidence window, which is typically 10 to 20 nanoseconds. If a detected gamma ray is not accompanied by a second gamma ray within this timing window, the event is discarded. Not every detected coincidence gamma pair necessarily originated from the same annihilation event. Events that are found in coincidence are classified as true coincidences, random coincidences, or scatter coincidences. True events are coincidence events that are originated from the same positron annihilation (Fig. 1.2, event 1). Random (or accidental) events are coincidence events in which two detected photons are originated from two different annihilation events but are found accidentally in coincidence because of the finite size of the coincidence window (Fig. 1.2, event 2). Scatter events are coincidence events that are originated from a single annihilation event, but one or both of the photons are scattered in the object (Fig. 1.2, event 3). The scatter process changes the direction and energy of the photon such that the position information on the event is lost. For many annihilation events, only one of the two photons will be detected, and these events are called "singles." There is no way for the detector to

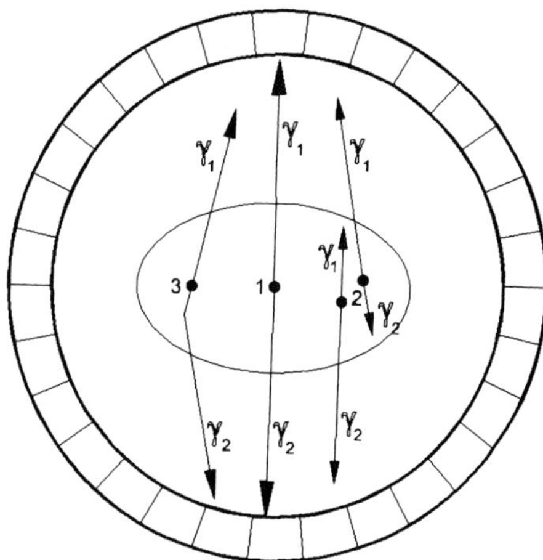

FIGURE 1.2. Coincidence events: (1) a true coincidence event, (2) a random coincidence event, and (3) a scatter coincidence event.

determine whether a particular coincidence event is a true, random, or scatter event. The good events are the true events; the other events (random and scatter) should be measured or estimated and removed from the total coincidence events.

In PET measurements, random and scatter events are the sources of background noise. They appear as a general blurring background in the reconstructed image of the tracer distribution, reducing the image quality. The magnitudes of the random and scatter coincidence events depend on the distribution of the tracer activity (inside and outside the field of view), the composition of the object under study, and the design of the PET scanner. While true and scatter rates are linearly proportional to the activity concentration, the random rate is proportional to the square of the activity concentration. Thus, the random events could constitute a large fraction of events, especially at high activity levels, and it is important to minimize them. Several techniques are used to reduce the number of random events, including adding lead-tungsten septa between detector rings in multi-ring PET systems and adding end-plate shielding to reduce the contribution of activity outside the field of view. In addition, because the random rate is linearly proportional to the coincidence window, minimizing the coincidence window is also important in reducing the number of random events. The random events' contribution can be measured directly by a second delayed coincidence window, or it can be estimated from the single rates. Scatter events could also constitute a significant fraction of the events detected by the scanner. However, because scattered photons lose some of their energy, the energy discrimination (energy threshold) can be used to reject a portion of the scatter events. For dedicated PET cameras operating in two-dimensional (2D) mode (with septa between detectors rings), scatter events typically constitute 10% to 20% of the total counts. In three-dimensional (3D) mode (no septa), scatter events typically constitute 30% to 60% of the total counts. Scatter events can result in a loss of resolution and an apparent migration of activity from hot to cold regions in images. Scatter correction methods generally fall into two groups: those that estimate the contribution of scatter events by measuring coincidences in one or more energy windows, in addition to the standard photopeak window, and those that model it using complex algorithms and Monte Carlo simulations.[5–7] Scatter correction (in addition to attenuation correction) must be applied when absolute quantitative imaging is required.

Radionuclides

A large number of radionuclides are used in PET imaging. Some of these PET tracer molecules contain isotopes of carbon (^{11}C), nitrogen (^{13}N), and oxygen (^{15}O) that can be used as biologically relevant substances for the human body, while other atoms can be substituted for use as analogs. For example, fluorine (^{18}F) can be substituted for hydrogen in the glucose analog deoxyglucose to form FDG. They usually have very short half-lives ranging from a few minutes to a few hours. The half-lives of the most often used positron isotopes in medical imaging are listed in Table 1.1.[2–4]

Because of the very short half-lives of ^{11}C, ^{13}N, and ^{15}O, they can be used only when a cyclotron is located near the imaging device. In addition, the fast decay of these radionuclides makes them less suitable for low count rate scans. In contrast, ^{18}F has a half-life of about 2 hours and can be distributed from a central site with a cyclotron. Although many types of positron-emitting radionuclides have been used to label hundreds of molecules to study basic physiology and disease processes, FDG is used in most clinical applications because every cell uses glucose. FDG, being an analog of glucose, follows the pathway of glucose as it is transported from blood to tissue cells. However, unlike glucose, the FDG, which is not a significant substrate for further metabolism, is trapped in cells and it is released slowly.

After the intravenous injection of FDG, patients are usually kept at rest for about 40 to 50 minutes to allow for the organ uptake of FDG. In the meantime, a large fraction of the free FDG in plasma is cleared because of tissue uptake and because of clearance through the kidneys to the bladder. When FDG is injected into a human, it is distributed to all tissues, but only those tissues metabolizing glucose will take up FDG. Thus, any metabolically active muscles will show increased uptake relative to the rest of the body. Many malignant tumors also accumulate FDG due to their glycolysis and proliferation rate. Benign tumors usually take up less FDG, so they can potentially be distinguished from malignant tumors. Therefore, coincidence detection can also be used to assess the presence of malignancy in patients with known or suspected metastatic disease. In addition, for the noninvasive evaluation of cardiac viability and the detection of lesions, FDG imaging with a dedicated whole-body PET scanner is a useful technique.

Because the most useful positron isotopes for biologic studies are ^{11}C, ^{13}N, ^{15}O, and ^{18}F, which have only six to nine protons in the nucleus, the electrostatic repulsive force encountered by the accelerated particles (protons/deuterons) on their way to penetrate the nucleus to initiate a nuclear reaction is small. Hence, a small cyclotron that can accelerate protons to the 10- to 17-MeV range is sufficient to overcome the nuclear electrostatic repulsion force to produce the nuclear reactions for biomedical positron imaging.[1] In recent years, small cyclotrons and chemical synthesis devices have been integrated into one unit to facilitate the synthesis of radiopharmaceuticals for clinical use. Small linear accelerators are also being developed to provide radionuclides.

Image Reconstruction

Tomographic images of the distribution of the positron-emitting radionuclides within the patient are reconstructed based on the assumption that the annihilation photons are emitted back to back (180 degrees) and that the line along which the two photons are detected (i.e., the line that joins the two detectors, also called the line of response) contains the location of the tracer molecule from which the positron originated. Therefore, the sum of all photon pairs emitted along a given direction represents the line integral of positron-emitting activity located on that line (or tube). The set of line integrals having the same angular direction through the tracer distribution comprises a parallel projection of the distribution at that angle.

The above assumption is correct only for the true coincidence events. Therefore, the measured projection data must be corrected for the contribution of random and scatter events. In addition, the effects of attenuation (the fact that some true coincidence events are absorbed or scattered out of the field of view), detector efficiency, and detector dead time must be considered.

From a complete set of line integrals measured at different angular views around the object, the images of positron-emitter distribution, within a slice or volume, can be reconstructed using various techniques. The reconstruction technique most commonly used in PET is the filtered back-projection method. If a point in space has a concentration of positron tracer, the emission of coincidence pairs will be uniformly distributed over all angles, because the emissions are random, with no preferential direction. If the uniformly distributed detection lines are drawn, a blurred image of the point will emerge. In other words, the parallel projections at each angle are projected back into the image grid, where they are superimposed to form an approximation image of the original object. To obtain a sharper image of the point, the spatial distribution of the coincidence data are filtered numerically before the back-projection process. This filtered back-projection image reconstruction method is also used in x-ray CT and single photon emission computed tomography (SPECT) cameras.[8–11] Because the object to be imaged can be considered as a collection of point sources with different activity levels, an image of the subject can be obtained with coincidence detection data and the filtered back-projection reconstruction algorithm. The derivation of filtered back-projection is based on noise-free ideal projection data. However, the acquired projection data are noisy, and the filtered back-projection technique amplifies this statistical noise. Windowing or reducing the cutoff frequency of the filter could reduce the amount of noise, but it also results in a loss of spatial resolution.[12–15] The most commonly used low-pass windows are the Hann, Hamming, and Butterworth window functions.[16,17]

Currently, most dedicated multi-ring PET cameras operate in 2D mode, with tungsten-lead septa separating the detector rings, to reduce single, random, and scatter events. These cameras use 2D reconstruction algorithms, which are reasonably fast. Modern PET cameras can also operate in 3D mode by removing the septa, or they do not have septa and operate only in 3D mode. The most widely used 3D reconstruction algorithm in volume PET imaging is the three-dimensional reprojection algorithm (3DRP), which is based on an extension of the standard 2D filtered back-projection into three dimensions.[18] The 3DRP algorithm incorporates a preliminary step in which projections that are partially measured in the 3D data acquisition are, because of the truncated cylindrical geometry of the scanner, completed by forward projection of an initial low-statistics image obtained from the completely measured (direct) projections. The forward-projected sinograms are less noisy than their measured counterparts and show some loss in spatial resolution.[19] Differences between measured sinograms and forward-projected sinograms have a differential effect on the final 3D reconstructed images, because proportionately more forward-projected data are used in the outer planes.

The 3D PET acquisition in comparison to 2D PET acquisition improves the sensitivity of the system and has the potential to reduce the data acquisition time compared to 2D PET. Whether 3D acquisition or 2D acquisition is better for conventional PET cameras in clinical applications is still an open question. Because the increase in sensitivity in 3D mode comes at the cost of an increase in random and scatter events, it does not necessarily translate into better image quality. However, it has been found that 3D acquisition may have advantages in lesion detection and noise characteristics in imaging the brain, small patients, and animals, especially at low activity levels.[20–23]

Because of large number of lines of response, the 3D image reconstruction is time-consuming, which makes it impractical for everyday clinical studies. As an alternative to the full 3D image reconstruction, the 3D projection data may be rebinned (sorted) into a stack of ordinary 2D sinogram data by making certain approximations and then using a 2D reconstruction algorithm; however, rebinning may result in loss of spatial resolution and degrade the image quality. The most widely used rebinning algorithms are the single-slice rebinning (SSRB), multislice rebinning (MSRB), and the Fourier rebinning (FORE) algorithms.[24–26] The SSRB algorithm assigns an oblique line of response to the mid-transaxial slice between the two detectors. This is a reasonable approximation when the tracer distribution is concentrated close to the axis of the scanner. In the MSRB method, an oblique line of response contributes to all transaxial slices that it intercepts within the limit of the transverse field of view. In the FORE algorithm, the 2D Fourier transform of each oblique sinogram is taken to produce a set of direct-plane and cross-plane data. The FORE method is still an approximation; however, it is more accurate than the other two rebinning methods.

The activity distribution images can be reconstructed from projection data with either analytic techniques (e.g., the 3DRP algorithm) or iterative algorithms. Iterative algorithms progressively improve the estimate of the distribution (image), which, in principle, converges toward a solution that maximizes an objective function. The iterative algorithms can model noise in emission data as well as other physical processes, such as attenuation correction, anatomic information, and detector response function and incorporate them into the reconstruction process to improve image quality. These algorithms are generally more time-consuming than filtered back-projection methods. The most widely used iterative algorithm is the maximum likelihood expectation maximization (ML-EM) algorithm and its accelerated variant, the ordered subsets expectation maximization (OSEM) method.[27,28] Iterative reconstruction appears to improve the quality of the image, especially for low-statistics data.[29] However, ML-EM and OSEM have some drawbacks, including a tendency to develop noise artifacts with the increasing number of iterations. To control noise artifacts and drive the image estimate sequence toward a smoother convergence, several methods have been used to regularize the image updating mechanism, including the addition of a smoothing step between iterations, and bayesian methods.[30,31]

Quality Control and Performance Measurements

Quality Control and Normalization

In PET imaging, standard algorithms for reconstruction of images, such as filtered back-projection, require that all lines of response (LORs) have the same sensitivity. However, there are several factors that cause nonuniformity of the response of the detectors. The efficiencies of coincidence detector pairs are inherently nonuniform due to the random and systematic variations in efficiencies of individual crystals and the inevitable drift in photomultiplier gains over time. In addition, due to circular design of the PET systems, there are geometric factors that affect the efficiencies of the LORs from the center to the edge of the field of view. Since sinograms are binned as parallel beam, the distance between detector pairs decreases with increasing distance from the center of the field of view, and the exposed face of the crystal decreases. In addition, the angle of incidence of the gamma ray changes. The ability of a scintillation crystal to detect a gamma ray depends not only on the energy of the gamma ray and the size and shape of the crystal, but also on the angle that the gamma ray hits it.

For dedicated multi-ring PET cameras with tens of thousands of crystals, hundreds of photomultiplier tubes (PMTs), and complicated electronics, the quality control measurements to check all detector components at the time of installation and thereafter at regular intervals are critical to ensure that the camera is operating within specifications and to detect changes over time before they become a serious problem. For example, for a scanner using block detectors, where generally a single PMT reads several crystals, the loss of one PMT can disable a large part of the system; even a small gain shift could cause mispositioning of data. Therefore, it is important to develop reproducible quality control procedures to detect a problem at an early stage before it affects the image quality and to schedule adjustments or replacement. The quality control procedures should at least check (1) the shift in PMTs amplification gains and electronics, (2) the stability of the system in terms of the efficiencies of the detectors, and (3) spatial resolution throughout the field of view.[32–34] Currently, performing all of these quality control tests on a daily basis is not practical due to the long data acquisition time. However, the daily performing of these tests, especially the recalibration of PMT gains and checking the electronics, could become a reality in the next generation of PET cameras.[35,36]

The stability of the system in terms of detector efficiencies is generally checked by performing a "blank" scan, in which a uniform cylindrical phantom, a uniform planar phantom, or attenuation-correction rotating rods are used to illuminate each LOR by the same activity level.[32,34] The planar source is regarded as the most favorable geometry due to the low level of scattered photons, but it is impractical to implement on a routine basis because it requires measurements at several source positions (e.g., six) extending the data acquisition time. A comparison study has shown that the uniformity obtained from cylinder-derived detector efficiencies is nearly identical to that obtained from planar source derived efficiencies.[37] In PET imaging, the detection of positron annihilations requires that two gamma rays be detected simultaneously. The ability of a detector pair to detect annihilation on its LOR is proportional to the product of the average detection efficiencies of the individual detectors and a geometric factor. Many PET systems allow the angular and axial compression of the data to minimize storage requirements and reconstruction time; in addition, some cameras rotate during the data acquisition.[38–40] These features complicate the normalization of the detector responses because an individual bin in a sinogram may be the combination of multiple detector pairs. The calibration of LORs, referred to as normalization, is what is important for image reconstruction. The correction factor for each LOR is referred to as the normalization coefficient. After the calibration, the individual normalized count rate of all detector pairs should be the same for a uniform source activity.

For modern PET cameras, the number of individual LORs is very large, and acquiring sufficient counts for reasonable statistical accuracy is very time-consuming and is not suitable for a daily control check. Usually, normalization coefficients for PET scanners are calculated using a component-based variance reduction method.[41–42] In this model, normalization coefficients are expressed as the product of intrinsic crystal efficiencies and some geometric factors. These coefficients are not all independent, and if the geometric factors are accurately known, the number of unknown factors is reduced from the number of LORs to the number of crystals.[33,42] Since the geometry of the scanner is unlikely to change significantly after initial installation, only occasional high-statistics acquisition needs to be performed to obtain the geometric factors, and routine normalization involves only the acquisition of data from which to calculate the intrinsic crystal efficiencies.

Performance Measurements

The PET camera performance is generally evaluated with the standard tests established by the National Electrical Manufacturers Association (NEMA).[43–46] The first PET performance tests were introduced in 1994 and referred to as NEMA NU 2-1994.[43,44] In 2001, these tests were updated, and the new standard was known as NEMA NU 2-2001.[45,46] The most significant change in the NU 2-2001 standard, compared with the NU 2-1994 standard, is the replacement of a 19-cm-long cylindrical phantom with a 70-cm-long cylindrical phantom for some of the tests as discussed below. While the 19-cm phantom still can be used to test the performance of scanners used for brain imaging, the 70-cm phantom is more appropriate for cameras used for whole-body studies.

The performance tests are divided into two groups. The first group includes tests for measuring the basic intrinsic characteristics of cameras: spatial resolution, sensitivity, scatter fraction, and count rate losses and random coincidences. In general, for a given activity concentration, achieving higher sensitivity and lower random and scattered events is more desirable. The second group includes measurements of the accuracy of corrections for physical effects such as uniformity correction, scatter correction, attenuation correction, and count rate linearity correction. In addition, NEMA NU 2-2001 included criteria for evaluating the overall image quality. The only radioisotope that is recommended for these tests is ^{18}F.

The spatial resolution is a measure of the camera's ability to distinguish between two points of radioactivity in a reconstructed image, and it is characterized by the width of the image of a point source (point spread function). The width of the point spread function is reported as the full width at half maximum (FWHM) and full width at tenth maximum (FWTM). It is recommended that a point source of ^{18}F, with dimensions of less than 1 mm in any direction, be imaged in air, and resolution be reported for six different locations of the point source. To avoid high count rate problems (dead-time and pileup effects), the data should be taken at low count rates. It is also recommended that data be reconstructed with filtered back-projection using a ramp filter, with a cutoff at the Nyquist frequency, and the image pixel size should be smaller than one third of the expected resolution.

The sensitivity of a scanner represents its ability to detect annihilation radiations. In the NEMA NU 2-1994 standard, the sensitivity is suggested to be measured using a standard cylindrical phantom (20 cm in diameter, 19 cm long) filled with uniform activity of low concentration, and the rate of coincidence events reported for a given activity concentration in that phantom. In the new NEMA NU 2-2001 standard, it is suggested to use a 70-cm-long plastic tube filled with a known amount of radioactivity, which is sufficiently low that count losses and randoms are negligible. The tubing is encased in metal sleeves of varying thickness and imaged twice: first with the tube in the center of the transverse field of view, and then with the tube off-set radially 10 cm from the transverse field of view.

The intrinsic scatter fraction is a measure of the system sensitivity to scattered events. The scatter fraction is defined as the ratio of scattered events to total events, which are measured at a sufficiently low counting rate so that random coincidences, dead-time effects, and pileup are negligible. Therefore, total events are the sum of unscattered events (true events) and scattered events. The suggested phantom, based on NEMA NU 2-20001, for this measurement is a 20-cm-diameter solid polyethylene cylinder with an overall length of 70 cm. Activity is placed in a line source (2.3-mm inner diameter) that is threaded through a hole in the cylinder at a radius of 4.5 cm and parallel to the central axis. To measure the scatter fraction for the 3D data, it is suggested to first rebin the 3D data into 2D sinograms using the single-slice rebinning algorithm. The transaxial field of view used for calculation of scatter is limited to 24 cm (4 cm larger than the phantom diameter). The sinogram profile is used to calculate the number of scatter events within the field of view and the number of true events within a 2-cm radius of the source. The scatter within the peak is estimated by assuming a constant background under the peak. The sinogram profile is analyzed as a function of the angle, and results are averaged. NEMA NU-2 2001 recommends that the scatter fraction for each slice and the average of the slice scatter fraction be reported.

Most PET scans are performed under conditions that count rate losses due to the dead time, and randoms are not negligible. So it is suggested that the system dead time and randoms for a wide range of activity levels be measured. Randoms can be determined by the delayed coincidence technique or estimated from single rates. Dead time is determined from the measured true rate at a given activity level and from the true rate extrapolated from the low count rate data.

The counting rate performance is measured as a function of activity using the same 70-cm polyethylene cylinder and the line source used for the scatter fraction. For this procedure, the line source is filled with a sufficiently high initial activity that allows both the peak true rate and peak noise equivalent count (NEC) rate to be measured. Data are taken until the randoms and dead-time losses are negligible. The total counting rate within the 24-cm transverse field of view is determined as the activity decays. The background, resulting from randoms and scatter, is estimated, and the true events rate is then determined by subtracting the background from the total rate. The total, true, random, scatter, and NEC rates are plotted against an effective activity concentration. From this plot, the peak true counting rate and peak NEC rate should be determined. The NEC rate, which defines an effective true count rate by accounting for additional noise from the randoms and scatter, is defined as

$$R_{NEC} = R_{trues}^2/(R_{trues} + R_{scatter} + kR_{randoms})$$

where R_{trues} is the true event rate, R_{scatter} is the scatter event rate, R_{randoms} is the random event rate, and $k = 2$ if the randoms are measured directly by delayed coincidence technique, and $k = 1$ if they are estimated (noise-free).

The image quality test is designed to produce images simulating those obtained in a whole-body study with both hot and cold lesions. It is suggested that spheres of different diameters placed in a simulated body phantom with nonuniform attenuation be imaged. It is also recommended that activity should be present outside the scanner. To quantitate the image quality, it is suggested that regions of interest on the spheres and throughout the background be drawn and that the coefficient of variations of the means in the background be calculated, along with the contrast recovery coefficient for the hot spheres and cold spheres. The diameters of the region of interest should be equal to the physical inner diameters of the spheres. To assess the accuracy of the corrections for attenuation and scatter, it is suggested that the ratio of the average counts in a region of interest in the lung area and the average counts in the background be calculated.

The Positron Camera

Any camera that can image a positron-emitting tracer can be called a positron camera. These cameras can range from the simple, less expensive thallium-doped sodium iodide [NaI(Tl)] gamma cameras to multimillion dollar dedicated multi-ring PET cameras. Positron cameras can be divided into six groups: (1) NaI(Tl) gamma cameras or SPECT cameras with lead collimators; (2) dual-head rotating NaI(Tl) cameras with modified electronics for coincidence detection and with the lead collimator removed[47]; (3) dedicated NaI(Tl) PET cameras with the detection system in the form of a ring[48,49]; (4) dedicated multi-ring PET cameras consisting of a large number of small detector elements made from high-sensitivity scintillation materials such as bismuth germinate (BGO)[50–52] or cerium-doped lutetium oxyorthosilicate (LSO)[53]; (5) dedicated small animal PET cameras[54]; and (6) hybrid systems such as SPECT/PET, SPECT/CT, and PET/CT systems.[55,56] Dedicated PET cameras can be further divided into two subgroups: cameras with full detection rings and cameras with partial detection rings. Three basic designs of PET cameras are shown in Figure 1.3.

Traditionally, gamma cameras have been used only for single photon studies (both planar and tomographic acquisitions), and the imaging of 511-keV photons has been performed with dedicated PET scanners. In recent years, despite significant differences between these two modalities, several products have been introduced to fill the gaps between these imaging techniques, including dual-purpose SPECT/PET gamma cameras. The low sensitivity and limited counting rate capability of gamma camera PET systems are partially offset by the larger field of view. In addition, using thicker NaI(Tl) crystals and removing the collimators also improve the sensitivity of these devices.

NaI(Tl) Gamma Cameras with Lead Collimators

The NaI(Tl) gamma cameras with lead collimators are the least expensive devices for imaging positron-emitting tracer distribution.

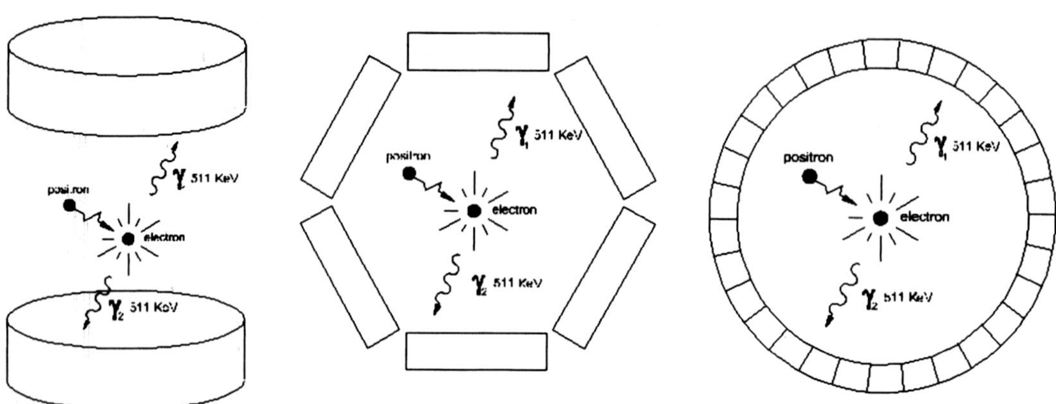

FIGURE 1.3. Schematic of three different designs of PET camera: (left) a dual-head single photon emission computed tomography (SPECT) with lead collimators removed and coincidence detection circuit added, (middle) a dedicated PET camera using large NaI(Tl) detectors, and (right) a dedicated PET camera using small bismuth germinate (BGO) detectors.

These cameras also have the lowest detection sensitivity for positron imaging. There are two reasons for their low sensitivity. First, the use of lead collimation to define the direction of the detected gamma ray is very inefficient, because the collimator can absorb 95% or more of the incoming gamma rays. Second, the thin NaI(Tl) detector is optimized for stopping the 140-keV gamma ray for technetium (^{99m}Tc) imaging, and so most of the higher energy (511-keV) gamma rays from positron annihilation penetrate this thin detector without any interaction (about a 70% escape fraction). Therefore, only a few percent of the positron gamma rays that hit the gamma camera detector are detected. The low-detection efficiency implies that only very large lesions (3 cm) can be detected. This group of cameras may provide a way to take advantage of the more tumor-specific positron tracers, such as breast cancer applications, without incurring the expense of buying and operating a dedicated PET camera.[57]

Coincidence Gamma Camera PET Systems

A gamma camera PET system is a modified dual-head rotating NaI(Tl) camera with coincidence electronics added and collimators removed.[47] With added coincidence detection capability, the direction of the two detected gamma rays is defined by two detected locations on opposite sides of the subject, and the inefficient lead collimators are no longer needed. Elimination of the lead collimator increases the detection sensitivity by 20 times or more over the regular single-head gamma cameras. However, the thin NaI(Tl) detector still has low sensitivity for detecting 511-keV gamma rays, because the probability of photon interaction (photoelectric and Compton) is about 0.3. Therefore, the probability of detecting both photons of positron annihilation, for coincidence detection, would be about 0.09. When compared with a dedicated BGO PET camera, which uses detectors made of BGO scintillation material, the sensitivity of this modified SPECT camera is still 9 to 10 times lower for identical detection areas. However, the detection sensitivity of this class of camera is a substantial improvement (5 to 10 times) over dual-head cameras with lead collimators. Studies have shown that this kind of camera can detect lesions as small as 1.5 to 2.0 cm.[58,59] Hence, this camera type is a better choice than the lead collimator gamma camera for taking advantage of the more tumor-specific positron tracers with a relatively small additional investment.

The removal of the lead collimator, which improves the detection efficiency, leads to a new problem. The head of each gamma camera is basically one large detector, and when a gamma ray is detected, the whole camera head is dead until all the stimulated scintillation light caused by that gamma detection is emitted. If there is a second incoming gamma ray, there will be a pileup of signals in the large detector, resulting in combining the two signals to yield erroneous energy and position. With the removal of the lead collimator, the flux of gamma rays incident onto the detector causes severe signal pileup in the NaI(Tl) detector, such that the tracer dose injected in the patient has to be lowered by roughly 80% compared with the dose used with a dedicated BGO PET camera to minimize the signal pileup artifacts in the image. Hence, the quality of the image is further reduced by the smaller tracer dose in addition to the lower detection efficiency. However, this reduction in injected dose may be eliminated by a newly developed detector signal processing electronic algorithm. This technique, called high-yield pileup event-recovery (HYPER), eliminates most pileups and recovers the correct energy and position of pileup events, thereby allowing the count rate to be increased by 10 times for NaI(Tl).[60]

Another deficiency of this camera design is that the coincidence detection efficiency in the transaxial field of view is geometrically dependent; the region near the center of rotation has the highest efficiency, and the coincidence efficiency goes to zero at the edge of the camera. Therefore, it is important for this camera type to be larger than the patient field of view to yield usable efficiency at the edge of the field of study.

Dedicated PET Camera with NaI(Tl) Detectors

The dedicated PET camera with a NaI(Tl) detector ring is similar to the dual-head NaI(Tl) gamma camera with coincidence detection electronics. It is a whole-body camera operating in 3D mode and has six planar or curved heads.[61] The six heads are configured to form a fixed ring around the patient. Because the camera is designed to be a dedicated PET camera instead of also performing ^{99m}Tc imaging, the thickness of the NaI(Tl) detector has been increased from 1 to 2.54 cm to increase its detection sensitivity. This increased detector thickness contributes to an almost fourfold increase in coincidence detection efficiency over a dual-head coincidence camera (with the same active detection area). Furthermore, with the detectors completely surrounding the patient, the detection efficiency is uniform in the transaxial field of view. However, because the detector design is basically that of a gamma camera, the signal pileup can still be a problem if the injected dose is not reduced. Even though these cameras generally use special hardware techniques (e.g., pulse clipping) to shorten the signal collection time and to reduce the detector dead time, the injected dose is still needed to be reduced by 60% to 80% from that used with a dedicated PET using BGO scintillation detectors. The HYPER processing method can also be used in this type of NaI(Tl) PET camera to allow higher dose injection to improve its imaging performance. Although the intrinsic resolution of this camera (about 4.6 mm for curved and 4.9 mm for planar heads) can rival that of the more expensive BGO camera, the more limited image counts collected cause the practical/clinical image resolution to be lower. On the other hand, the lower production cost of this dedicated PET makes it a viable option for imaging positron tracers.

Dedicated PET Camera with BGO Detector Rings

The multi-ring PET cameras using BGO crystals are more efficient than the three previously discussed cameras, because they can handle a higher count rate and also have higher image quality. These cameras are also the most expensive ones ($1.5 to $2 million). Unlike the three positron camera types discussed above, which are based on gamma camera technology using a single, large NaI(Tl) detector, the BGO camera uses tens of thousands of discrete BGO detectors.[50–52] The discrete BGO detectors are packed into many detector rings circumscribing the patient, eliminating the need to rotate the detection system. The elimination of camera rotation during imaging may be important for imaging tracers that change rapidly with time, such as ^{15}O and ^{13}N, which have short half-lives. For FDG imaging, camera rotation is generally acceptable.

The multiplicity of detectors in this kind of camera allows the cameras to operate at much higher count rates, which translates to a higher injected dose to provide a higher quality image. Furthermore, BGO crystals have about two times higher density and about 1.5 times higher atomic number than NaI(Tl), and also have substantially higher detection sensitivity for the higher energy gamma rays generated by positron annihilation. Hence, the detected counts-per-unit injected dose is also higher with the dedicated BGO PET than with the other three camera types using NaI(Tl) detectors, enabling this camera to provide a further improvement in image quality. Practical resolution and image quality are highest with this kind of camera. Currently, the highest intrinsic spatial resolution of dedicated BGO PET cameras is about 4.5 mm. The practical image resolution is lower depending on the number of counts collected. Under optimal conditions, such as brain imaging with FDG, the practical image resolution may reach 6 mm. For whole-body imaging, the image resolution will be worse because of severe gamma ray attenuation by the body. For FDG cancer imaging, the smallest detectable lesion size also depends on the ratio of tumor uptake to normal tissue uptake. With this camera type, smaller tumors (6 to 10 mm) are detectable.

In recent years, LSO crystals have also been used in multi-ring PET cameras.[53] Both BGO and LSO have excellent physical properties. They both have high densities and atomic numbers that result in efficient detection of gamma rays. In addition, they are rugged and nonhygroscopic, which makes the detector fabrication less problematic. Table 1.2 compares some of the physical properties of BGO and LSO crystals to NaI(Tl).[62] The BGO and LSO crystals each have some advantages and disadvantages. The BGO has a slightly higher linear attenuation coefficient and a higher probability that the first gamma interaction within the crystal will be a photoelectric interaction, and it is cheaper. The LSO has a shorter decay constant, which is good for coincidence timing and handling higher detection rates. In addition, the LSO's higher light output allows the use of more small crystals per photomultiplier tube. However, the LSO has a low level of natural radioactivity as a result of the presence of ^{176}Lu, which generates some undesirable background. This background generates a relatively negligible coincidence background event rate; however, it can have a significant effect on the single transmission measurement used for attenuation correction.[63]

Dual-Modality PET/CT System

Imaging modalities used in medical imaging are generally differentiated as functional or anatomic devices. These two complementary modalities provide valuable information that can be used for early diagnosis and more accurate tumor detection and localization, and they facilitate the planning, performance, and better assessment of patient responses to radiation therapy and chemotherapy.

Interpretation of nuclear medicine functional images is improved when they are co-registered with anatomic images, especially in the abdomen, because of the absence of identifiable anatomic structures in PET images. This is achieved either by visual comparison of the two separate data sets or by the fusion of images. Until the recent introduction of combined PET/CT systems, the anatomic and functional images used to be acquired on different and separated scanners and at different times, and then fused using software procedures. However, such procedures were not widely used for studies outside the brain be-

TABLE 1.2. Comparison of physical properties of some common scintillator crystals

Crystal	Density (g/cm^3)	Effective atomic number	Attenuation coefficient (cm^{-1})	Light output [NaI(Tl) = 100]	Decay time (ns)
BGO	7.13	75	0.96	15	300
GSO	6.71	59	0.67	41	65
LSO	7.40	65	0.87	75	40
NaI(Tl)	3.67	51	0.35	100	230

BGO, bismuth germinate; GSO, cerium-doped gadolinium oxyorthosilicate; LSO, cerium-doped lutetium oxyorthosilicate; NaI(Tl), thallium-doped sodium iodide.

cause of the technical difficulties of implementation on a routine basis. The dual-modality PET/CT system can overcome some difficulties associated with the software approaches by acquiring both anatomic and functional images in a single scanning session. In addition, CT images can provide attenuation correction information and anatomic information to the model-based scatter correction algorithms.

Even with combined PET/CT there are some motions that could affect the accuracy of the co-registration of two sets of data. Some of these motions are patient breathing, cardiac motion, and patient movements between the PET and CT studies. Patient motion may be avoidable, but respiratory motion is not and may require some correction by, for example, respiratory gating of PET data.[64] The quality of images will be compromised if co-registration errors occur. Such errors could not only deteriorate the image quality but also lead to the wrong anatomic positioning. In a study of patients with lung tumors using a combined PET/CT camera, a maximum 5- to 6-mm misalignment of the PET and CT images for tumors in the anterior region of the lungs was observed; however, such a mismatch did not affect the diagnostic accuracy of the fused image.[65] In another study, it was found that the accuracy of PET/CT image co-registration for lung lesions is better in patients who underwent CT scanning during normal expiration than in patients who performed shallow breathing during CT scanning, and it is better in the upper and central parts of the lung.[66] In a more recent study of lesion mislocalization on PET/CT studies, it was found that when CT data were used for both fusion and attenuation correction, of 300 patients who were scanned, 2% (six patients) had lesion mislocalization, likely due to respiratory motion differences between PET and CT.[67]

Future Developments in Positron Emission Tomography

Recent trends in the development of positron cameras have concentrated on several issues: (1) lowering the production cost of the cameras, (2) using new scintillation materials, (3) improving spatial resolution, and (4) combining the functional and anatomic modalities.

For the current dedicated PET cameras with BGO detectors, the detection system often accounts for more than 50% of the total production cost. Hence, some of the developmental efforts have focused on lowering the detection system cost. In recent years, a new PET detector design has been introduced based on a photomultiplier-quadrant sharing technique.[68] This technique can substantially reduce detector cost by reducing the number of photomultipliers. A prototype camera, based on this design, has been constructed and has achieved a spatial resolution of about 3 mm.[69,70] Another way to save in detector costs is to build partially populated detector rings and rotate them during the scan. A rotating BGO multi-ring PET camera has been built with two thirds of the detectors removed from the ring so that only two opposing sectors of the detection system remain.[71] This reduces the camera cost by 50%, but it also reduces the camera sensitivity by about 66% for smaller objects and 80% for large objects. This kind of camera requires detector rotation during the data acquisition to cover all the angular views.

Another effort is the development of a SPECT/PET camera based on a rotating dual-head tomograph using two layers of pixelated NaI(Tl) and LSO scintillators.[55] This dual-purpose camera is basically a conventional SPECT with two major modifications: (1) the adoption of the lower cost, discrete detector design of the photomultiplier quadrant-sharing detector design used in the prototype camera mentioned in the previous section; and (2) the use of a second layer of LSO crystals, which has higher sensitivity than NaI(Tl) for detecting the 511-keV positron gamma rays. The NaI(Tl) detector layer, the front layer, is for the conventional SPECT imaging, and the LSO detector layer, behind the NaI(Tl) detectors, is for positron coincidence-detection PET imaging. The reason that LSO is not used for single photon or SPECT imaging is that it has a natural gamma radiation background covering the energy range of SPECT tracers. The LSO detector not only is more sensitive than NaI(Tl), but also is capable of counting six times faster than NaI(Tl), due to its shorter decay time. Therefore, it allows the camera to detect the 511-keV gamma rays at a much higher rate than a regular dual-head SPECT. In addition, since small detectors are used instead of single large-area detectors, significant gains in counting-rate capability can be obtained. A prototype camera is being developed using this design.[55] Using two layers of detectors with different pulse decay time has the potential to provide information on depth of interaction that can be utilized to improve spatial resolution further.

Another development in positron imaging is the construction of small dedicated breast cameras and dedicated brain PET cameras. The dedicated breast cameras are generally small, lower-cost cameras with two opposing detector heads that have high resolution.[72,73] These cameras are generally designed to image the compressed breast in the projection mode similar to x-ray mammography instead of the tomography mode. This camera type takes advantage of the higher diagnostic accuracy of positron imaging than of x-ray mammography. The disadvantage is that very small lesions or lesions with lower contrast may not be detected because of the overlapping of cancer signals with the normal breast signal in this projection or nontomographic imaging mode. The first clinical results for a dedicated breast camera show that the camera has 80% sensitivity, 100% specificity, and 86% accuracy, and it can detect breast tumors of 2 mm or even smaller size.[73]

The proposed dedicated brain cameras are generally multi-ring PET cameras with a smaller detector ring (smaller transaxial field of view) to increase the detection sensitivity over the whole-body scanners and also to reduce the production cost.[53] However, this kind of camera will also have higher scatter fraction, and random count rate, compared to whole-body cameras for the same activity concentration, which could compromise the performance of the camera and may require operating the camera with lower activity.[74] A prototype BGO PET camera with convertible geometry that can operate in both whole-body mode and brain/breast mode has shown promising results in breast and brain lesion detectability when scanning phantoms.[70,75]

Another development has been the use of a cerium-doped gadolinium oxyorthosilicate (GSO) scintillator for PET detector. In Table 1.2, the physical properties of GSO are compared to the other common scintillator crystals. The GSO crystal has short decay time (about 60 ns) and high light output and relatively high density (but lower than that of LSO and BGO). A prototype dedicated brain camera made of GSO crystals has been constructed.[76]

With improved instrumentation in the future, positron cameras will be more cost effective, and image quality will be improved. The intrinsic image resolution can be improved from the current industrial standard of 4.5 mm to 3 mm or lower. An experimental, multislice, whole-body PET camera using BGO detectors has demonstrated an intrinsic image resolution of 3 mm.[69,70] Some small experimental cameras designed for rat/mouse animal models have already demonstrated 1- to 2-mm resolution[77,78] for imaging with ^{18}F, which has the lowest positron-range blurring effect.

Quantitation and Parametric Imaging

In PET imaging the tracer uptake and dynamic can be accurately qualified, in principle, from the image data because of PET attenuation-correction capability. This information can help to expand the observer's ability in interpreting images. PET imaging with FDG, the most clinically useful cancer imaging tracer today, can benefit from using quantitative measures of uptake to determine the likelihood that a tumor is malignant, from its level of metabolic activity, and to assess tumor response to therapy.

There are several ways to approach quantitation, from visual assessment to complex kinetic analysis with dynamic data acquisition and blood sampling.[79] The simplest assessment is visual assessment of images. A slightly better method is graded visual assessment where the abnormality is classified relative to normal structures on a 5- to 10-point scale using pseudo-color representation of the tissue uptake. The tumor to normal tissue activity ratio is the next level of quantitation. It requires attenuation-corrected images, but no other calibration. This approach is more objective but has significant limitations. Values derived depend on the placement of regions of interest (ROIs), the definition of normal tissue, the reconstruction algorithm, the image resolution, and whether maximum or average counts are used. The tumor-to–normal tissue count density ratio method can be useful but should be implemented with explicit attention to these issues.

The most widely used quantitative method for assessing FDG uptake is the standardized uptake value (SUV), which estimates fractional FDG uptake by tumor.[80,81] This measure is also referred to as the dose uptake ratio or differential uptake ratio (DUR). The SUV is often used as a measure to characterize the malignancy versus benignancy of lesions. The SUV can be defined as the tissue concentration of tracer as measured by a PET camera divided by the activity injected divided by body weight:

$$SUV = [\text{Tissue Activity in } \mu Ci/gr] \,/\, [\text{Injected Dose in } \mu Ci \text{ per g Body Weight}].$$

The use of SUV requires, in addition to attenuation correction, that the administered dose be accurately determined, corrected for residual activity in the syringe and tubing, and that the dose must be decay corrected to the time of imaging. For FDG, the tissue activity used is generally the tracer uptake between 30 and 60 minutes after injection. However, to achieve a model independent assessment of glucose metabolism, the SUV should be measured after the tissue concentration of FDG has reached a plateau. There is much variability in this measurement depending on the exact implementation in each clinical site. To minimize variability for comparison purposes, all the studies in the same site should follow the same quality control parameters, such as the waiting time after injection, the duration of imaging, and fasting protocols. To further minimize variability, plasma glucose level correction[82,83] should also be applied:

$$SUV\ (Corrected) = SUV \times [Plasma\ Glucose/100]$$

In addition, there should be a body-fat correction term[84,85] to account for the reduced uptake of FDG in body fat. The SUV can be extracted either as the peak value in an ROI or by displaying the SUV pixel by pixel as a pseudo-color quantitation SUV image.

The SUV quantitation is not as accurate as the compartmental analysis, but it is very simple to implement and requires no blood sampling, which may be more practical in a clinical environment. There are more reliable, but also more complex, quantitation methods, including simplified kinetic analysis, Patlak graphical analysis, and kinetic analysis with parameter optimization; however, because of practical constraints, these methods are usually not used except in research studies.

With tracer-transport modeling and multiple scans over a time period (dynamic imaging), functional parameters can be quantified. Some common physiologic parameters generated by PET are blood flow,[86–88] metabolic rates,[89] blood volume,[90,91] and receptor densities. These quantified parameters may be more useful than a simple tracer uptake image. For example, a region with a high relative uptake of FDG may be either an area of high-blood volume/perfusion, especially if the images are taken right after injection, or an area of high-glucose metabolism; quantified parameters of glucose metabolic-rate and blood space would differentiate such an important ambiguity. The quantitation can be carried out in two different ways, depending on the complexity of the tracer transport model and the quality of the raw image data: (1) if the model is complex, involving many parameters coupled with noisy image data, it would be better to draw an ROI in the image data, for example, on a suspected tumor site, and compute the average functional parameters within the region; and (2) if the model is simple (one or two parameters) and the image quality is high, it may be more useful to generate a parametric image set that is equivalent to perform an ROI parametric calculation on a pixel-by-pixel basis for the whole image set. A set of parametric images displaying separately the metabolic-rate distribution and the blood volume distribution can be more useful clinically for cancer detection and treatment monitoring. Quantitation is especially useful for accurately monitoring the efficacy of therapy if a similar quantitation is performed before treatment.

Tracer modeling and parametric quantitation techniques for FDG have been studied extensively with different degrees of refinement and simplification, resulting in a compromise between practicality and accuracy.[89,92] Most FDG methods are based on the three-compartment model as shown in Figure 1.4. The physiologic parameters to be deduced are the rate constants k_1, k_2, k_3, and k_4: k_1 and k_2 are the rate of FDG transport from plasma into tissue and from tissue back into plasma; k_3 is the rate of FDG phosphorylation; and k_4 the rate of FDG dephosphorylation. One way to find the rate constants of a lesion is by drawing an ROI in the image set and extracting the time-activity data within the ROI. The ROI time-activity data are then combined with the time-activity data of the blood plasma tracer activity levels as inputs to a curve-fitting computer program for the three-compartment model. The curve-fitting program would output the rate constants.[93] This procedure generates the average rate constants in the ROI instead of a set of parametric images of the rate constants. Conceptually, the same method can be applied pixel by pixel to generate a set of parametric images of the rate constants. However, such an image processing procedure requires the image quality of the original uptake data to be very high so that the statistical errors for all the pixels are small. Furthermore, the curve-fitting time for all the image pixels may be impractically lengthy compared with the present computing technology.

A more practical method of generating an FDG metabolic image is based on the unidirectional flow model,[90,91] also called the Patlak-plot method, which is basically a three-compartment model, as shown in Figure 1.4, except that k_4 is assumed to be insignificantly small. A negligible k_4 implies that there is no leakage of the tracer from the trapped cell space. This simplifies the model from four parameters (k_1, k_2, k_3, and k_4) to two parameters (Ki, and Vd), where Ki is the macro metabolic rate constant and Vd is the blood distribution volume and vascular space. Mathematically, the macro metabolic rate constant Ki of the tissue-bound compartment is equivalent to $k_1 k_3 / [k_2 + k_3]$ in the three-compartment model. This method is computationally fast and less demanding on the quality of the raw image data. However, even this simplified method still requires the measurement of the tracer input function, the blood-time activity curve. Parametric imaging methods require the measurement of the tracer input function. The extrac-

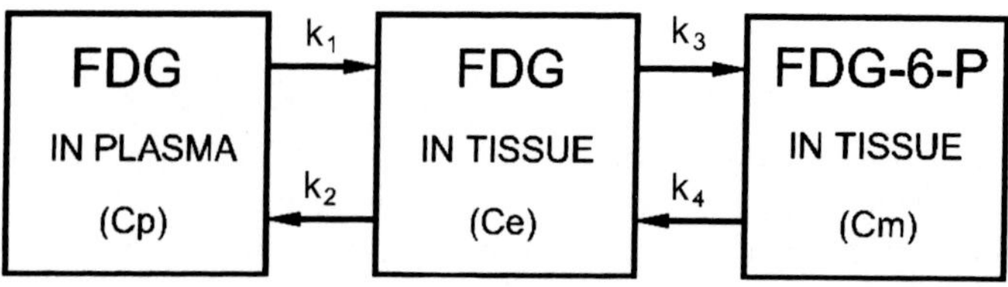

FIGURE 1.4. The fluorodeoxyglucose (FDG) three-compartment system consisting of reaction in blood, tissue, and product in tissue.

tion of 30 blood samples over the imaging time and the effort to measure the blood activity information of these samples are rather demanding, especially for clinical studies. As PET imaging moves into the clinics, many different ways of reducing the amount of blood sampling have been proposed, but the most accurate and simple way is with the use of an automated blood sampling system.[94,95]

References

1. Fowler JS, Wolf AP. Positron emitter-labeled compounds: priorities and problems. In: Phelps M, Mazziotta J, Schelbert H, eds. Positron Emission Tomography and Autoradiography: Principles and Applications for the Brain and Heart. New York: Raven Press, 1986:391–450.
2. Derenzo SE. Precision measurement of annihilation point spread distributions for medically important positron emitters. Proceedings of the 5th International Conference on Positron Annihilation, Sendai, Japan, 1979, pp. 819–824.
3. Phelps ME, Mazziotta JC, Schelbert HR, eds. Positron Emission Tomography and Autoradiography: Principles and Applications for the Brain and Heart. New York: Raven Press, 1986.
4. Sorenson JA, Phelps ME. Physics in Nuclear Medicine, 2nd ed. Philadelphia: WB Saunders, 1987.
5. King MA, Hademenos G, Glick SJ. A dual photopeak window method for scatter correction. J Nucl Med 1992;33:605–612.
6. Bentourkia M, Msaki P, Cadorette J, Lecomte R. Assessment of scatter components in high-resolution PET: correction by nonstationary convolution subtraction. J Nucl Med 36: 121–130.
7. Watson CC, Newport D, Casey ME, et al. Evaluation of simulation-based scatter correction for 3-D PET cardiac imaging. J Nucl Med 1997;44:90–97.
8. Defrise M, Kinahan PE. Data acquisition and image reconstruction for 3D PET. In: Bendriem B, Townsend DW, eds. The Theory and Practice of 3D PET. Dordrecht, Netherlands: Kluwer Academic Publishers, 1998:11–50.
9. Brooks RA, DiChiro G. Theory of image reconstruction in computed tomography. Radiology 1975;117:561–572.
10. Brownell GL, Burnham CA, Chesler CA, et al. Transverse section imaging of radionuclide distribution in heart, lung and brain. In: Ter-Pogossian MM, Phelps ME, Brownell GL, eds. Reconstruction Tomography in Diagnostic Radiology and Nuclear Medicine. Baltimore: University Park Press, 1977:293–307.
11. Shepp LA, Logan BF. The fourier reconstruction of a head section. IEEE Trans Nucl Sci 1974;NS-21:21–43.
12. Gilland DR, Tsui BMW, McCartney WH, et al. Determination of the optimum filter function for SPECT imaging. J Nucl Med 1988;29:643–650.
13. Beis JS, Celler A, Barney JS. An automatic method to determine cutoff frequency based on image power spectrum. IEEE Trans Nucl Sci 1995;42: 2250–2254.
14. Farquhar TH, Chatziioannou A, Chinn G, et al. An investigation of filter choice for filtered back-projection reconstruction in PET. IEEE Trans Nucl Sci 1998;45:1133–1137.
15. Baghaei H, Wong WH, Li H, et al. Evaluation of the effect of filter apodization for volume PET imaging using the 3-D RP algorithm. IEEE Trans Nucl Sci 2003;50:3–8.
16. Chesler DA, Riederer SJ. Ripple suppression during reconstruction in transverse tomography. Phys Med Biol 1995;20:632–636.

17. Huesman RH, Gullberg GT, Greenberg WL, Budinger TF. RECLBL Library Users Manual: Donnar Algorithms for Reconstruction Tomography. Publication 214. Berkeley, Lawrence Berkeley Laboratory, University of California, 1977:49–58.
18. Kinahan PE, Rogers JG. Analytic 3D image reconstruction using all detected events. IEEE Trans Nucl Sci 1989;46:964–968.
19. Cherry SR, Dahlbom M, Hoffman EJ. Evaluation of a 3D reconstruction algorithm for multi-slice PET scanners. Phys Med Biol 1992;37:779–790.
20. Kadrmas DJ, Christian PE, Wollenweber SD, et al. Comparative evaluation of 2D and 3D lesion detectability on a full-ring BGO PET scanner. J Nucl Med 2002;43(5):56P.
21. Pajevic S, Daube-Witherspoon ME, Bacharach SL, Carson RE. Noise characteristics of 3-D and 2-D PET images. IEEE Trans Med Imag 1998;17:9–23.
22. Bailey DL, Jones T, Spinks TJ, Gilardi MC, Townsend DW. Noise equivalent count measurements in a neuro-PET scanner with retractable septa. IEEE Trans Med Imag 1991;10:256–260.
23. Stearns CW, Cherry SR, Thompson CJ. NECR analysis of 3D brain PET scanner designs. IEEE Trans Nucl Sci 1994;42:1075–1079.
24. Daube-Witherspoon ME, Muehllehner G. Treatment of axial data in three-dimensional PET. J Nucl Med 1997;28:1717–1724.
25. Lewitt RM, Muehllehner G, Karp JS. Three-dimensional reconstruction for PET by multi-slice rebinning and axial image filtering. Phys Med Biol 1994;39:321–339.
26. Defrise M, Kinahan PE, Townsend DW, Michel C, Sibomana M, Newport DF. Exact and approximation rebinning algorithms for 3-D PET data. IEEE Trans Nucl Sci 1997;16:145–158.
27. Shepp LA, Vardi Y. Maximum likelihood reconstruction for emission tomography. IEEE Trans Med Imag 1982;MI-1:113–122.
28. Hudson HM, Larkin RS. Accelerated image reconstruction using ordered subsets of projection data. IEEE Trans Nucl Sci 1994;13:601–609.
29. Reader AJ, Visvikis D, Erlandsson K, Ott RJ, Flower MA. Intercomparison of four reconstruction techniques for positron volume imaging with rotating planar detectors. Phys Med Biol 1998;43:823–834.
30. Jacobson M, Levkovitz R, Ben-Tal A, et al. Enhanced 3D PET OSEM reconstruction using inter-update Metz filtering. Phys Med Biol 2000;45:2417–2439.
31. Herbert TJ, Leahy RM. A generalized EM algorithm for 3-D bayesian reconstruction from Poisson data using Gibs priors. IEEE Trans Med Imag 1989;8:194–202.
32. Daghighian F, Hoffman EJ, Huang SC. Quality control in PET systems employing 2-D modular detectors. IEEE Trans Nucl Sci 1989;36:1034–1037.
33. Hoffman EJ, Guerrero TM, Germano G, et al. PET system calibrations and corrections for quanitative and spatially accurate images. IEEE Trans Nucl Sci 1989;36:1108–1112.
34. Defrise M, Townsend DW, Bailey D, et al. A normalization technique for 3D PET data. Phys Med Biol 1991;36:939–952.
35. Wang Y, Wong W-H, Aykac M, et al. An iterative energy-centroid method for recalibration of PMT gain in PET or gamma camera. IEEE Trans Nucl Sci 2002;49:2047–2050.
36. Knoess C, Gremillion T, Schmand M, et al. Development of a daily quality check procedure for the high-resolution research tomograph (HRRT) using natural LSO background radioactivity. IEEE Trans Nucl Sci 2002;49:2074–2078.

37. Oakes, TR, Sossi V, Ruth TJ. Normalization in 3D PET: comparison of detector efficiencies obtained from uniform planar and cylindrical sources. IEEE Nucl Sci Symp 1997;2:1625–1629.
38. Adam LE, Zaers J, Ostertag H, et al. Performance evaluation of the whole-body PET scanner ECAT EXACT HR+ following the IEC standard. IEEE Trans Nucl Sci 1997;44:1172–1179.
39. Townsend DW, Wensveen M, Byars LG, et al. A rotating PET camera using BGO block detectors: design, performance and applications. J Nucl Med 1993;34:1367–1993.
40. Baghaei H, Wong W-H, Uribe J, et al. Correction factors for a high resolution variable field of view PET. J Nucl Med 2000;40:279.
41. Casey ME, Gadagkar H, Newport D. A component based method for normalisation in volume PET. Proceedings of the 3rd International meeting on Fully Three-Dimensional Image Reconstruction in Radiology and Nuclear Medicine, Aix-les-Bains, France, 1995, pp. 67–71.
42. Badawi RD, Lodge MA, Marsden PK. Algorithms for calculating detector efficiency normalization coefficients for true coincidences in 3D PET. Phys Med Biol 1998;43:189–205.
43. National Electrical Manufacturers Association. NEMA Standards Publication NU 2-1994: Performance Measurements of Positron Emission Tomographs. Washington, DC: National Electrical Manufacturers Association, 1994.
44. Karp JS, Daube-Witherspoon ME, Hoffman EJ, et al. Performance standards in positron emission tomography. J Nucl Med 1991;32:2342–2350.
45. National Electrical Manufacturers Association. NEMA Standards Publication NU 2-2001: Performance Measurements of Positron Emission Tomographs. Rosslyn, VA: National Electrical Manufacturers Association, 2001.
46. Daube-Witherspoon ME, Karp JS, Casey ME, et al. PET Performance measurements using the NEMA NU 2-2001 standard. J Nucl Med 2002;43:1398–1409.
47. Patton JA, Turkington TG. Coincidence imaging with a dual-head scintillation camera. J Nucl Med 1999;40:432–441.
48. Karp JS, Muehllehner G, Mankoff D, et al. Continuous-slice PENN-PET: a positron tomograph with volume imaging capability. J Nucl Med 1990;31: 617–627.
49. Adam LE, Karp JS, Daube-Witherspoon ME, et al. Performance of a whole-body PET scanner using curve-plate NaI(Tl) detectors. J Nucl Med 2001;42: 1821–1830.
50. Brix G, Zaers J, Adam LE, et al. Performance evaluation of a whole-body PET scanner using the NEMA protocol. National Electrical Manufacturers Association. J Nucl Med 1997;38:1614–1623.
51. DeGrado T, Turkington T, Williams J, Stearns C, Hoffman J. Performance characteristics of a whole-body PET scanner. J Nucl Med 1994;35:1398–1406.
52. Lewellen TK, Kohlmyer SG, Miyaoka RS, et al. Investigation of the performance of the General Electric ADVANCE positron emission tomograph in 3D mode. IEEE Trans Nucl Sci 1996;43:2199–2206.
53. Eriksson L, Wienhard K, Eriksson K, et al. The ECAT HRRT: NEMA NEC evaluation of the HRRT system, the new high-resolution research tomograph. IEEE Trans Nucl Sci 2002;49:2085–2088.
54. Chatziioannou AF, Cherry SR, Shao Y, et al. Performance evaluation of microPET: a high-resolution lutetium oxyorthosilicate PET scanner for animal imaging. J Nucl Med 1999;40:1164–1175.

55. Jones WF, Casey ME, van Lingen A, et al. LSO PET/SPECT spatial resolution: critical on-line DOI rebinning methods and results. 2000 IEEE Nucl Sci Symposium Conference Record 2000;3:16/54–16/58.
56. Beyer T, Townsend DW, Brun T, et al. A combined PET/CT scanner for clinical oncology. J Nucl Med 2000;41:1369–1379.
57. Holle LH, Trampert L, Lung-Kurt S, et al. Investigations of breast tumors with fluorine-18-fluorodeoxyglucose and SPECT. J Nucl Med 1996;36:615–622.
58. Yutani K, Tatsumi M, Shiba E, et al. Comparison of dual-head coincidence gamma camera FDG imaging with FDG PET in detection of breast cancer and axillary lymph node metastasis. J Nucl Med 1999;40:1003–1008.
59. Gerbaudo VH, Sugarbaker DJ, Britz-Cunningham S, et al. Assessment of malignant pleural mesothelioma with 18F-FDG dual-head gamma-camera coincidence imaging: comparison with histopathology. J Nucl Med 2002;43:1144–1149.
60. Wong WH, Li H, Uribe J, Baghaei H, Wang Y, Yokoyam S. Feasibility of a high speed gamma camera design using the high-yield-pileup-event-recovery (HYPER) method. J Nucl Med 2001;42:624–632.
61. Adam LE, Karp JS, Daube-Witherspoon ME, Smith RJ. Performance of a whole-body PET scanner using curve-plate NaI(Tl) detectors. J Nucl Med 2001;42:1821–1830.
62. Melcher CL. Scintillation crystals for PET. J Nucl Med 2000;41:1051–1055.
63. Huber S, Moses WW, Jones WF, Watson CC. Effect of ^{176}Lu background on singles transmission for LSO-based PET cameras. Phys Med Biol 2002;47:3535–3541.
64. Nehmeh S, Erdi Y, Ling C, et al. Effect of respiratory gating on reducing lung motion artifacts in PET imaging of lung cancer. Med Phys 2002;29:366–371.
65. Townsend DW. A combined PET/CT scanner: the choices. J Nucl Med 2001;42:533–534.
66. Goerres GW, Kamel E, Seifert B, et al. Accuracy of image coregistration of pulmonary lesions in patients with non-small cell lung cancer using an integrated PET/CT system. J Nucl Med 2002;43:1469–1475.
67. Osman MM, Cohade C, Nakamoto Y, et al. Clinically significant inaccurate localization of lesions with PET/CT: frequency in 300 patients. J Nucl Med 2003;44:240–243.
68. Wong W-H, Uribe J, Hicks K, Zambelli M. A 2-dimensional detector decoding study on BGO arrays with quadrant sharing photomultipliers. IEEE Trans Nucl Sci 1994;41:1453–1457.
69. Uribe J, Baghaei H, Li H, et al. Basic imaging characteristics of a variable field of view PET camera using quadrant sharing detector design. IEEE Trans Nucl Sci 1999;46:491–497.
70. Baghaei H, Wong W-H, Uribe J, et al. Breast cancer studies with a variable field of view PET camera. IEEE Trans Nucl Sci 2000;47:1080–1084.
71. Townsend DW, Wensveen M, Byars LG, et al. A rotating PET camera using BGO block detectors: design, performance and applications. J Nucl Med 1993;34:1367–1993.
72. Freifelder R, Karp JS. Dedicated PET scanners for breast imaging. Phys Med Biol 1997;42:2463–2480.
73. Murthy K, Aznar M, Thompson CJ, et al. Results of preliminary clinical trials of the positron emission mammography system PEM-I: a dedicated breast imaging system producing glucose metabolic images using FDG. J Nucl 2000;41:1851–1858.
74. Stearns CW, Cherry SR, Thompson CJ. NECR analysis of 3D brain PET

scanner designs. Nuclear Science Symposium and Medical Imaging Conference. IEEE Conference Record 1994;4:1657–1661.
75. Baghaei H, Uribe J, Li H, et al. An evaluation of the effect of filtering in 3-D OSEM reconstruction by using data from a high-resolution pet scanner. IEEE Trans Nucl Sci 2002;49:238–2386.
76. Karp JS, Surti S, Freifelder R, et al. Performance of a GSO brain PET camera. IEEE Nucl Sci Symposium Conference Record 2000;3:1711.
77. Chatziioannou AF, Cherry SR, Shao Y, et al. Performance evaluation of microPET: a high-resolution lutetium oxyorthosilicate PET scanner for animal imaging. J Nucl Med 1999;40:1164–1175.
78. Chatziioannou A, Tai Y, Shao Y, et al. Coincidence measurements on detectors for microPET II: a 1 mm^3 resolution PET scanner for small animal imaging. IEEE Nucl Sci Symposium Conference Record 2000;3:21/1.
79. Graham MM, Peterson LM, Hayward RM. Comparison of simplified quantitative analyses of FDG uptake. Nucl Med Biol 2000;27:647–655.
80. Keyes JW Jr. SUV: standard uptake or silly useless value? J Nucl Med 1995;36:1836–1839.
81. Hamberg LM, Hunter GJ, Alpert NM, et al. The dose uptake ratio as an index of glucose metabolism: useful parameter or oversimplification? J Nucl Med 1994;35:1308–1312.
82. Lindholm P, Minn H, Leskinen-Kallio S, et al. Influence of the blood glucose concentration on FDG uptake in cancer—a PET study. J Nucl Med 1993;34:1–6.
83. Langen K-J, Braun U, Kops ER, et al. The influence of plasma glucose levels on fluorine-18-fluorodeoxyglucose uptake in bronchial carcinomas. J Nucl Med 1993;34:355–359.
84. Zasadny KR, Wahl RL. Standardized uptake values of normal tissues at PET with 2-[fluorine-18-]-fluoro-2-deoxy-D-glucose: variations with body weight and a method for correction. Radiology 1993;189:847–850.
85. Kim CK, Gupta NC, Chandramouli B, Alavi A. Standardized uptake values of FDG: body surface area correction is preferable to body weight correction. J Nucl Med 1994;35:164–167.
86. Frackowiak RSJ, Lenzi G-L, Jones T, Heather JD. Quantitative measurement of emission tomography: theory, procedure and normal values. J Comput Assist Tomogr 1980;4:727–736.
87. Huang S-C, Carson RE, Hoffman EJ, et al. Quantitative measurement of local cerebral blood flow in humans by positron computed tomography and ^{15}O-water. J Cereb Blood Flow Metab 1983;3:141–153.
88. Ruotsalainen U, Raitakari M, Nuutila P, et al. Quantitative blood flow measurement of skeletal muscle using oxygen-15-water and PET. J Nucl Med 1997;38:314–319.
89. Phelps ME, Huang SC, Hoffman EJ, et al. Tomographic measurements of local cerebral glucose metabolic rate in humans with [^{18}F]2-fluro-2-deoxy-D-glucose: validation of method. Ann Neurol 1979;6:371–388.
90. Patlak C, Blasberg R, Fenstermacher J. Graphical evaluation of blood-to-brain transfer constants from multiple-time uptake data. J Cereb Blood Flow Metab 1983;3:1–7.
91. Gjedde A. Calculation of cerebral glucose phosphorylation from brain uptake of glucose analogs in vivo: a re-examination. Brain Res Rev 1982;4: 237–274.
92. Sokoloff L, Reivich M, Kennedy C, et al. The (^{14}C)-deoxyglucose method for the measurement of local cerebral glucose utilization: theory, procedure and normal values in the conscious and anesthetized albino rat. J Neurochem 1977;28:897–916.

93. Carson RE. Parameter estimation in positron emission tomography. In: Phelps M, Mazziotta J, Schelbert H, eds. Positron Emission Tomography and Autoradiography: Principles and Applications for the Brain and Heart. New York: Raven Press, 1986:347–390.
94. Hutchins GD, Hichwa RD, Koeppe RA. A continuous flow input function detector for $H_2{}^{15}O$ blood flow studies in positron emission tomography. IEEE Trans Nucl Sci 1986;NS-33:546–549.
95. Eriksson L, Holte S, Bohm C, et al. Automated blood sampling systems for positron emission tomography. IEEE Trans Nucl Sci 1988;Ns-35:703–707.

2

Production of Isotopes

Carlos Gonzalez Lepera and Wai-Hoi Wong

The rapid development and increasing interest in the use of metabolic imaging techniques has created a steady demand for on-site or regional production of radioisotopes. This chapter presents some basic concepts associated with radioisotope production, in particular, those aspects related to cyclotron production of positron-emitting radionuclide.

Concepts

Nuclear Reactions

The force experienced between two charged particles is described by Coulomb's law according to the relation (we have omitted some constant factors from the equations to simplify their expression):

$$F(r) = Q_1 Q_2 / r^2 \tag{1}$$

The potential associated with Coulomb's force described in equation 1 is

$$V(r) = Q_1 / r \tag{2}$$

where Q_1 and Q_2 are the electric charges of particles 1 and 2, respectively, and r is the distance between them. In the case of atomic nuclei this potential barrier can be represented as in Figure 2.1, where the potential energy of the particles inside the nucleus (radius R) $\boldsymbol{U_0}$, is assumed to be much lower than the barrier height $\boldsymbol{B}$, that is $\boldsymbol{U_0} << \boldsymbol{B}$. Experimental evidence strongly supports this assumption.

In a simplified picture to describe a nuclear reaction, an incoming positively charged projectile (proton or deuteron) needs to surmount this repulsive positively charged barrier presented by the target nucleus. In other words, the projectile has to approach the target nucleus at a minimum distance of the order of the nuclear radius for a nuclear reaction to occur. This minimum energy is therefore

$$E_B = Z_1 Z_2 e^2 / R \tag{3}$$

with $Q_1 = Z_1 e$, $Q_2 = Z_2 e$, and where Z_1 and Z_2 are the atomic number of projectile and target, respectively, e is the electron charge, and R is the nuclear radius. For protons incident on carbon this value is $E_B =$

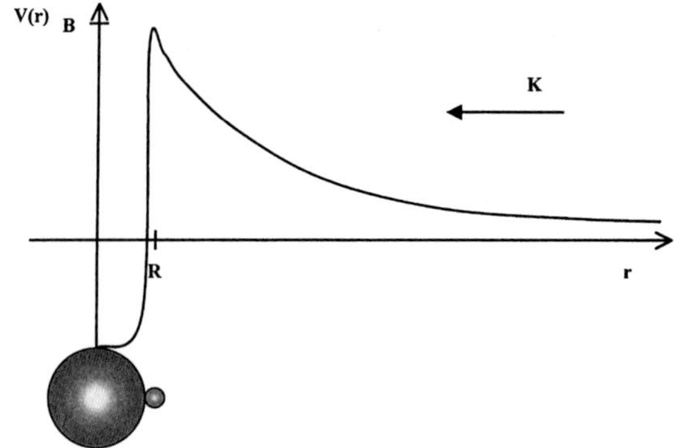

FIGURE 2.1. Coulomb potential $V(r)$ between two charged nuclides as a function of their distance r. The barrier height B represents the minimum energy that the projectile has to carry to penetrate the target when it reaches the target outer radius R. A projectile with kinetic energy K as shown would not be able to penetrate the target nucleus.

2.3 MeV, and for aluminum $E_B = 4.4$ MeV. From equation 3, a higher projectile energy is needed to penetrate the nucleus of a heavier target to produce a nuclear reaction.

The so-called compound nucleus model for nuclear reactions was first proposed by Bohr in 1936. It assumes that when some target T is bombarded by an incident nuclear particle i, the two may combine to form a compound nucleus $(T + i)$. This new compound nucleus possesses an excitation energy directly related to the incident projectile energy. The identity of the incoming particle is lost, and the total energy of the excited compound nucleus is shared in a complicated manner by all the nucleons. The same compound nucleus in the same excited state can also be formed starting from a different combination of projectile/target; that is, it is possible to have $(T + i) = (T' + i')$. The properties of the compound nucleus are independent of the reaction. As an example, the compound nucleus $^{30}Zn^{64}$ can be formed according to the following scheme:

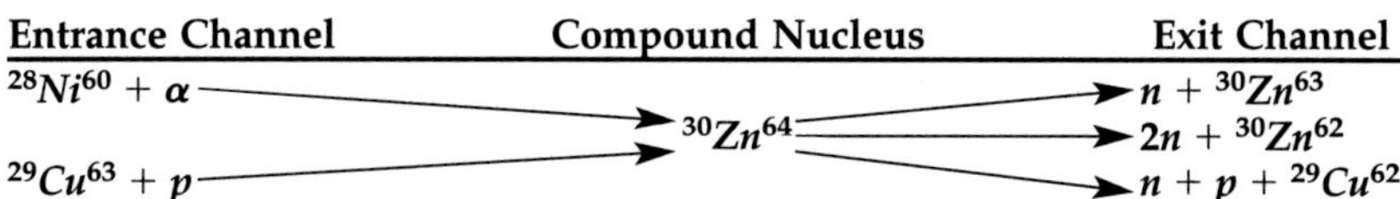

Cross Section for Nuclear Reactions

The cross section for production of a certain final nuclear product reaction channel can be expressed as the probability of formation of the compound nucleus (intermediate state) times the probability of decaying into that channel. It is expressed in units of area (1 mbarn = 10^{-3} barn = 10^{-27} cm^2). It can be interpreted as the *effective surface per nucleus presented by the target to the incoming projectile*. Due to quantum mechanical effects, the cross section for production of the compound nucleus is nonzero even for incident projectile energies lower than the

Coulomb barrier. Figures 2.2 through 2.5 present experimental cross sections for the production of some short-lived radioisotopes (^{11}C, ^{13}N, ^{15}O, ^{18}F).

Particle Accelerators

The force experienced by a particle with electric charge q in the presence of an electromagnetic field is described by the Lorentz force according to

$$\vec{F} = q(\vec{E} + \vec{\nu} \times \vec{B}) \quad (4)$$

where $\vec{E}$ is the electric field, $\vec{B}$ is the magnetic field, and $\vec{\nu}$ is the particle velocity. The vectorial nature of equation 4 requires intensity and spatial orientation to be considered for the magnitudes involved. The second term within the parentheses, defined as $\vec{\nu} \times \vec{B} = |\nu||B|\sin(\nu\angle B)$, shows that the magnetic field affects only the velocity component perpendicular to it. The electric field $\vec{E}$ is described as the difference in electric potential V per unit distance (gradient).

In the absence of magnetic fields, a particle exposed to a potential difference V will be accelerated to a final energy given by

$$E = E_0 + qV \quad (5)$$

where E_0 is the initial energy (not to be confused with electric field E). Equation 5 represents the basic accelerating mechanism behind any particle accelerator.

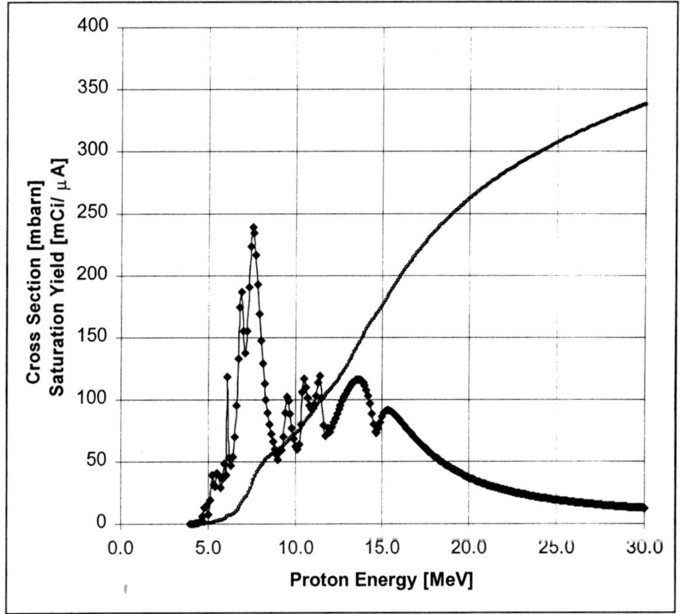

FIGURE 2.2. Experimental cross section and theoretical saturation activity shown as a continuous line (equation 20) for the reaction $^{18}O(p,n)^{18}F$.

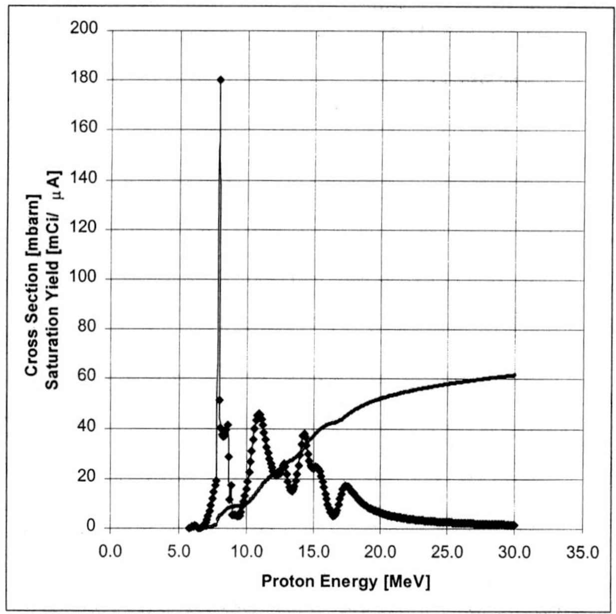

FIGURE 2.3. Experimental cross section and theoretical saturation activity shown as a continuous line (equation 20) for the reaction $^{16}O(p,\alpha)^{13}N$.

Static and alternating electric fields from a few volts up to tens of megavolts (MV) are currently used for charged particle acceleration. For example, on an early Van de Graaff accelerator an ion source is located inside a high-voltage terminal. Ions produced at this high voltage potential are accelerated toward ground potential, where the target is located. The acceleration takes place in an evacuated tube to avoid

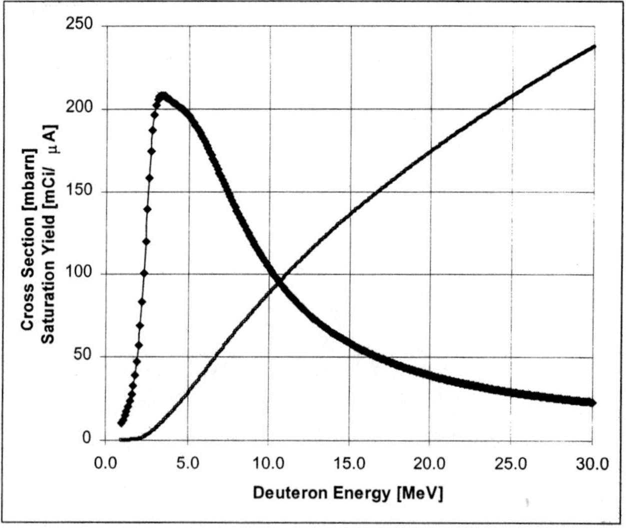

FIGURE 2.4. Experimental cross section and theoretical saturation activity shown as a continuous line (equation 20) for the reaction $^{14}N(d,n)^{15}O$.

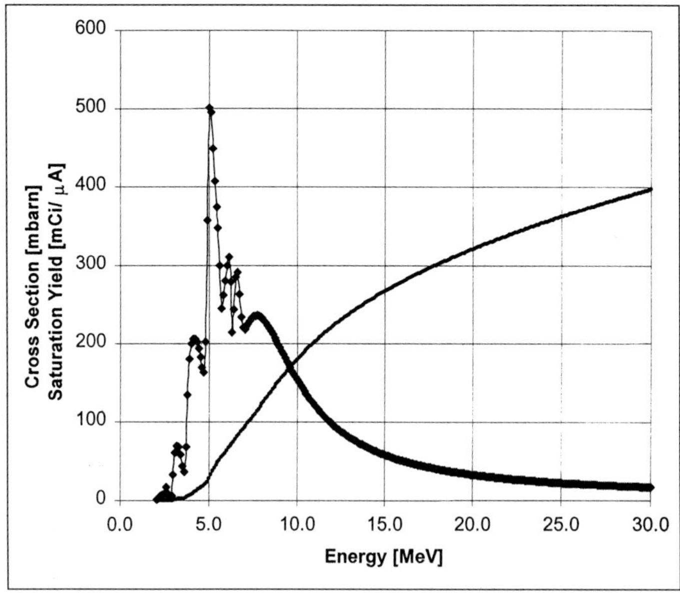

FIGURE 2.5. Experimental cross section and theoretical saturation activity shown as a continuous line (equation 20) for the reaction $^{14}N(p,\alpha)^{11}C$.

collisions between the ions and air molecules. Maximum attainable voltage at the terminal is limited by practical considerations, and it is close to 25 MV for state-of-the-art, large installations.

From equation 4 it follows that an alternative method to increase the ion's final energy, for a given potential difference, is to increase the ion's charge state (higher q). To take advantage of this mechanism, Van de Graaff accelerators have been modified to operate in a tandem geometry. In this mode, the high-voltage terminal (dome) is kept at a positive potential respect to ground. Negative ions are produced instead, at the ion source outside the accelerator, and injected into the accelerator tube. The negative ions are attracted, and hence accelerated by the positive dome. After acceleration toward the positive dome, electrons are stripped off the negative ions by collisions with gas molecules or a micron-thin carbon foil. Projectiles thus converted into positive ions are accelerated by repulsion again toward ground potential (target). This configuration is very effective to achieve higher energies, especially for heavy ions, since the final energy is a function of the ion final charge state. For protons, the maximum attainable energy can only be twice the value of the dome potential. Another limitation of the tandem configuration is that not all species can be produced as negative ions in usable amounts.

Alternating electric fields are also employed for charged particle acceleration. In this way extremely high energies have been achieved. Again, positive ions are produced and accelerated toward a series of electrodes where an alternating electric field is applied. When the ions exit the first electrode, the electric field has already changed polarity, further accelerating the ions. Bunches of ions are then accelerated in this fashion. These linear structures, commonly known as linear accelerators (LINACs), which are up to several kilometers in length, have successfully been employed to accelerate ions to velocities approaching the speed of light. The applied electric fields amount to several hundred kilovolts at frequencies from tens of Hz to GHz.

The Cyclotron

First conceived by Lawrence in 1929 and successfully demonstrated in 1930 with important contributions from Livingston, the cyclotron was and still is one of the primary sources for medical radioisotope production. According to equation 4, in the presence of a magnetic field the total force experienced by the charged particle will have an additional component perpendicular to the plane defined by the particle velocity and magnetic field, thereby restraining the moving particles into circular orbits. These kinds of accelerators are known as *circular accelerators* (betatron, cyclotron, synchrotron), due to the approximately circular orbits described by the particles.

The introduction of negative ion cyclotrons over the past two decades has significantly improved exit projectile flux, which increases the amount of radioisotope produced. The main components of the cyclotron are the following:

1. Vacuum chamber: To minimize collisions between ions and air molecules and thus minimize beam loss, the acceleration process takes place in areas where air density has been reduced to approximately 10^{-9} times that of atmospheric pressure. A short aluminum cylinder provides an airtight seal between the magnet polar pieces. Vacuum pumps remove the air from this chamber.
2. Ion source: Positive ions are typically produced by collisions between gas molecules (hydrogen in the case of protons) and accelerated electrons emitted from a cathode. Source geometry and applied electric fields facilitate the extraction of produced ions into the main accelerating field. Negative ions are created by exposing desired gas molecules to an intense plasma discharge and again using favorable geometries and electric and magnetic fields to extract hydrogen (or deuterium) atoms that have an extra electron attached.
3. Magnet: A strong ($\sim$1.5 tesla) magnetic field is applied across the magnet pole pieces defining the vacuum region. The effect of the magnetic field on the ions trajectories is to maintain them in circular orbits and to constrain the orbits near a plane perpendicular to the applied magnetic field as determined by equation 4.
4. Radiofrequency (RF) field: Ions are extracted from the source and injected into the vacuum chamber by a high-voltage alternating electric field applied to the accelerating structures, also known as *dees* due to the original shape proposed by Lawrence. While inside these hollow structures, ions continue to travel in an approximately circular orbit. When the ions reach the transition region between dees, the electric field has reversed polarity so that the distal dee has a higher potential than the proximal dee to accelerate the particles in the transitional gap. The particles are not accelerated inside the dees.

Tens of kiloelectron volts (keV) are gained during each transition. As the ion energy increases, its orbital radius becomes larger. Near the outer radius, where the magnetic field sharply decreases, ions have reached their maximum energy.

5. Extraction: When the ions reach the outer region of the vacuum chamber, the extraction mechanism varies depending on the polarity of the ions as injected from the ion source. In the case of positive ions, a negative voltage is applied to a plate placed around the outer radius, pulling the positive ions from the trapping magnetic field and directing them to proper targets or through a beam line for further transport. During this process between 10% and 50% of the beam is lost. When negatively charged ions are accelerated, a thin foil, typically a few micrometers thick carbon, is placed on the ions path. At several million electron volt (MeV) energies, the beam will traverse the foil with insignificant energy loss. Electrons from the negative ions are lost by interaction (stripping) with the solid foil, thereby converting them into positive ions. This sudden reversal of charge polarity reverses the Lorentz force direction (see equation 4) and the ions are pushed out of the machine by the same magnetic field that was keeping them inside. Extraction efficiencies close to 100% are currently achieved using this mechanism.
6. Targets: Although the main purpose of the cyclotron is to accelerate a particle beam to fairly high energies, targets for radioisotope production should be considered an integral part of the machine. Liquid, gaseous, or solid targets for production of radioisotopes need to be tailored to the particular characteristics of a given cyclotron to optimize use of beam energy, intensity, and profile. They can be located in close proximity to the cyclotron, or the beam can be transported through evacuated tubes (beam lines) under the guidance of focusing magnets (quadrupoles) to a distal location or a different room.

Cyclotrons for medical radioisotope production are commercially available from several manufacturers (Table 2.1). Typical beam energies ranging from 8 or 9 MeV up to 30 MeV are considered standard. Single-energy proton-only machines are widely used for production of positron emission tomography (PET) tracers. The energy range between 8 and 19 MeV can supply most PET radioisotopes. Cyclotrons with energies of 30 MeV and higher can also be used for production of single photon emission computed tomography (SPECT) tracers (T1 201, Ga 67, In 111, etc.). The other parameter defining radioisotope production rate is available beam current from the machine. The higher the beam current tolerated by the target, the higher the amount of isotope that can be expected from a production run.

Production of PET Isotopes

Radioisotopes for PET

The physical properties of the four radioisotopes most widely used for PET studies are given in Table 2.2. These "organic" radioisotopes are particularly well suited for labeling biomolecules. Their short half-life

TABLE 2.1. Commercially available cyclotrons

Manufacturer	Model	Energy	Standard features	Options
CTI Molecular Imaging Knoxville, TN (www.ctimi.com)	RDS 111	11-MeV protons	50-μA beam single port 40-μA per target in dual-port mode (80-μA total); self-shielded	RDS Eclipse; higher beam current and higher yield; ^{18}F targets
EBCO Technologies Richmond, BC, Canada (www.ebcotech.com)	TR13–19	13- to 19-MeV protons	100-μA protons; dual-port irradiations; fix energy or field upgradable to 19 MeV	Vault or self-shielded; 9-MeV deuterons on TR-19; 300-μA protons; multiple beam lines on one or both ports
GE Medical Systems (www.gemedicalsystems.com)	PETtrace	16.5-MeV protons 8.4-MeV deuterons;	75-μA protons; six ports for targets	Vault or self-shielded
	MINItrace	9.6-MeV protons	Self-shielded	Dual-port irradiations
IBA Louvain-la-Neuve, Belgium (www.iba.be)	CYCLONE 10/5	10-MeV protons; 5-MeV deuterons	60-μA protons 35-μA deuterons	Dual-port irradiations standard on both models; multiple beam lines on one or both ports
	CYCLONE 18/9	18-MeV protons; 5-MeV deuterons	80-μA protons 35-μA deuterons	

Note: Stated machine characteristics were extracted from brochures and/or Web sites provided by manufacturers. For latest features, contact cyclotron manufacturers.

TABLE 2.2. Characteristics of commonly used PET isotopes

Isotope	Half-life (minutes)	Mode of decay (%)	End-point energy of β^+ groups (keV)	Maximum β^+ range in water (mm)	Principal nuclear reactions (energy range MeV)
^{11}C	20.3	β^+ (99.8), EC (0.2)	960	4.1	$^{14}N(p,\alpha)^{11}C$ (15–4)
^{13}N	9.96	β^+ (100)	1190	5.1	$^{16}O(p,\alpha)^{13}N$ (20–5)
^{15}O	2.03	β^+ (99.9), EC (0.1)	1723	7.3	$^{14}N(d,n)^{15}O$ (6–0) $^{15}N(p,n)^{15}O$ (15–5)
^{18}F	109.7	β^+ (96.9), EC (3.1)	635	2.4	$^{18}O(p,n)^{18}F$ (15–3) $^{20}Ne(d,\alpha)^{18}F$ (30–0)

EC, electron capture.

provides the benefit of fast clearing from the patient's body, but it requires the on-site or nearby production of the radioisotope. Another important advantage of these radioisotopes is their high branching ratio for positron emission. The number of potentially useful positron emitters is certainly not limited to the ones included in Table 2.2. Several others have been successfully employed for PET studies. Depending on the desired radioisotope, a combination of highly enriched target material or higher cyclotron energy or both may be necessary.

Production Cross Section

The concept of *cross section* for some event (σ_A) can be defined as the effective area per target atom presented to the projectile. Consider a target with area S, thickness Δx (small), and containing N atoms per unit volume. The probability P_A for a projectile to interact with a target atom producing an event A is given by the ratio of effective to total area:

$$P_A = n\sigma_A/S = N\Delta x\sigma_A \tag{6}$$

where $n = NS\Delta x$ is the total number of target atoms.

If the beam has a current density $J = I/S$, where I is the beam current, the average number of events A per unit time is given by

$$JSP_A = Jn\sigma_A \tag{7}$$

Equation 7 is valid only for single charged projectiles. Since we are dealing with number of events, the important quantity is the actual number of incident projectiles and not their charge state. For projectiles with charge state different from unity, for example; α particles, equation 7 needs to be divided by the projectile charge state.

Radioactive Decay

The total number of atoms $A(t)$ at time t remaining from the radioactive decay of A_0 atoms at time t_0 is

$$A(t) - A_0e^{-\lambda(t-t_0)} \tag{8}$$

where λ is the radioactive decay rate and $T = \ln 2/\lambda = 0.693/\lambda$ is the half-life of the radionuclide.

The total radioactive decay rate at any time is equal to the product of the total number of atoms A times the probability for radioactive decay λ_A, i.e., $A\lambda_A$.

Differential Equation for a Daughter Product

The radioactive decay of a nuclide A into a nuclide B, which is also radioactive, can be represented by

$$A \xrightarrow{\lambda_A} B \xrightarrow{\lambda_B} C$$

At any time the activity of A is $A\lambda_A$ and of B is $B\lambda_B$. The rate of change dB/dt in the number of atoms of type B is then equal to the balance between supply due to the decay of A minus the rate of loss of B through its own decay:

$$\frac{dB}{dt} = A\lambda_A - B\lambda_B \tag{9}$$

Replacing the number of atoms of type A at any given time using equation 9, we have

$$\frac{dB}{dt} = A_0\lambda_A e^{-\lambda_A t} - B\lambda_B \tag{10}$$

and solving the differential equation we obtain

$$B = A_0 \frac{\lambda_A}{\lambda_B - \lambda_A}\left(e^{-\lambda_A t} - e^{-\lambda_B t}\right) \tag{11}$$

The activity of B is $B\lambda_B$ or

$$B\lambda_B = A_0\lambda_A \frac{\lambda_B}{\lambda_B - \lambda_A}\left(e^{-\lambda_A t} - e^{-\lambda_B t}\right) \tag{12}$$

and since the activity of A at time t is $A\lambda_A = A_0\lambda_A e^{-\lambda_A t}$, we can replace into equation 12 to obtain

$$B\lambda_B = (A\lambda_A)\frac{\lambda_B}{\lambda_B - \lambda_A}\left(1 - e^{-(\lambda_B - \lambda_A)t}\right) \tag{13}$$

Production Yield

The process of radioisotope production by nuclear bombardment is mathematically analogous to the process of radioactive decay into a daughter product. The number of target atoms that are exposed to the beam during irradiation can be called A_0. The probability of transforming one of these atoms into nuclei B per unit of time can be called λ_A. Then, $A_0\lambda_A$ is the rate at which new atoms of B are produced. The target is equivalent to a radionuclide with activity $A_0\lambda_A$ producing the radioactive substance B. The probability λ_A is very small, but the product $A_0\lambda_A$ can be significant since A_0 is very large and can be taken as constant during irradiation ($A \equiv A_0$). Assuming that $\lambda_A << \lambda_B$, equation 13 can be approximated by

$$B\lambda_B = A\lambda_A(1 - e^{-\lambda_B t}) \tag{14}$$

The net activity accumulated during time t is therefore

$$B\lambda_B = A_0\lambda_A(1 - e^{-\lambda_B t}) \tag{15}$$

The interaction rate of time λ_A can be calculated as the product of the current I of incident projectiles and the cross section, summed over the projectile trajectory, that is,

$$\lambda_A = I \int_{x_1}^{x_2} \sigma(x)dx \tag{16}$$

and by replacing and $dx = \dfrac{dE}{(dE/dX)}$ and $\sigma(x) \equiv \sigma(E)$ we obtain

$$\lambda_A = I \int_{E_i}^{E_{Th}} \frac{\sigma(E)}{(dE/dx)} dE \tag{17}$$

where E_i is the incident projectile energy, E_{Th} is the threshold energy for the given nuclear reaction, $\sigma(E)$ is the cross section, and dE/dx is the projectile energy loss per unit of path length. Both magnitudes, $\sigma(E)$ and dE/dx, are experimentally obtained and readily available from the literature.

Rewriting equation 16 in a more practical way, we obtain

$$B\lambda_B = \frac{N_A\rho}{M} I(1 - e^{-\lambda_B t}) \int_{E_i}^{E_{Th}} \frac{\sigma(E)}{(dE/dx)} dE \tag{18}$$

with $A_0 = \dfrac{N_A\rho}{M}$, and N_A the Avogadro's number, M the atomic mass, and ρ the target density.

Equation 18 contains all the information necessary to calculate production yield for a given radioisotope. The number of new radioactive atoms being produced is proportional to the integral term, while the buildup of activity is described by the term inside the parentheses, which is a function of decay rate as well as the duration of irradiation. The exponential nature of the term within parentheses shows that 50% of the maximum attainable activity is produced in one-half life of the isotope. Extending irradiation another half-life produces only an extra 25%.

Those terms in equation 18 that are independent of beam current and irradiation time describe a quantity commonly known as *saturation activity*:

$$S_a = \frac{N_A\rho}{M} \cdot \int_{E_i}^{E_{Th}} \frac{\sigma(E)}{(dE/dx)} dE \tag{19}$$

This magnitude is a function of projectile incident energy and is usually expressed in units of [mCi/μA]. It includes all the necessary information to calculate production yields for any given projectile/target combination. Another commonly used magnitude that describes the production process is the *yield* Y, representing the slope at the origin from equation 18 and is defined as

$$Y = S_a \cdot \lambda_B \tag{20}$$

Production of Radiopharmaceuticals

The higher resolution and sensitivity provided by PET as compared to SPECT as a consequence of the collinearity of the two 511-keV photons after an annihilation event are not the only advantageous characteristics of this technique. The short half-life of the radioisotopes being used results in lower overall radiation doses to the patient. Simultaneously, it allows the use of labeled drugs in concentrations so small so as not to overwhelm the biologic systems or compete with the normal metabolic function while remaining well below any toxic levels. As an example, a typical 15-mCi dose of ^{13}N-labeled ammonia as routinely used for myocardial perfusion studies represents 13 pg of product, many orders of magnitude below what is considered a permissible safety level.

Since the introduction of PET as a research and clinical tool, ^{18}F has been the radioisotope most widely used because of its practical half-life of nearly 2 hours as compared to other tracers with half-lives of just a few minutes. The reaction of choice for the production of ^{18}F during the early stages of development was ^{20}Ne(d,α) ^{18}F. After the introduction in the mid-1980s by Hamacher et al[1] of the no-carrier added synthesis for 2-[^{18}F]-Fluoro-2-Deoxy-D-Glucose (FDG), the production of ^{18}F using the reaction ^{18}O(p,n)^{18}F with highly enriched ^{18}O-water targets became the method of choice. Furthermore, it permitted proton-only machines with energies as low as 10 MeV to produce considerable amounts of ^{18}F. This rapid and highly efficient conversion method motivated equipment manufacturers to offer remote and automated equipment for the synthesis of FDG. Second- or even third-generation synthesis boxes can produce single, double, or up to four batches of FDG with a single setup. Decay-corrected radiochemical yields (conversion efficiency from ^{18}F into FDG) as high as 75% to 80% are routinely achieved. Preventive maintenance programs combined with proper personnel training have improved equipment reliability to better than 98%. Some FDG production equipment permits, through software reconfiguration, modifying the system to process other compounds.

^{15}O demands the location of the camera facility not more than a few hundred meters from the production facility. Proton-only machines require use of the enriched isotope ^{15}N as target material through the reaction ^{15}N(p,n)^{15}O. Given the high cost of the starting material, provisions to recover the enriched isotope should be implemented if not supplied by the cyclotron manufacturer. Facilities where deuterons are available can take advantage of the reaction ^{14}N(d,n)^{15}O without recycling the target. Rapid processing of the radioisotope transforms the target product into ^{15}O-water, ^{15}O-O_2, or C^{15}O depending on the application.

Production of ^{13}N and simultaneous conversion to ^{13}N-ammonia is commonly done inside the target followed by a quick and efficient purification step through a disposable cartridge to remove potential contaminants (mainly traces of ^{18}F and metal ions from the target foil). Use of this tracer is limited to in-house production or distribution from a production facility within a relatively short distance.

Large amounts of C 11 can be produced even with modest energy cyclotrons through the reaction $^{14}N(p,\alpha)$ C 11. Several commercial units permit rapid and efficient methylation of the target product (typically in the form of $^{11}CO_2$) as the precursor step for radiolabeling of any number of compounds.

In general, a good number of other PET tracers can also be produced using enriched target materials at the low-energy end of commercial cyclotrons, with the option of using natural targets in some cases as the cyclotron energy is increased or when deuterons are available. Depending on the specific program requirements for one or several radioisotopes, a detailed analysis of different production routes, cost analysis of recovery processes in the case of enriched target materials, and an analysis of potential by-product impurities should be conducted prior to deciding on a particular cyclotron.

Facility Design

During planning and design of a particular facility, local and federal regulations for production of radiopharmaceuticals should be considered to ensure compliance and also to minimize the risk of potentially expensive upgrades or retrofit of the facility at a later time. Furthermore, cyclic guanosine monophosphate (cGMP) guidelines and regulations should be firmly implemented together with a strong training and enforcement program to assure product safety and quality as well as adherence to the ALARA concept (as low as reasonably achievable) to minimize radiation exposure to production personnel and the public in general. Cyclotron manufacturers provide assistance with facility design and planning, but their responsibility is typically limited to issues related to machine installation and commissioning. In the case of self-shielded cyclotrons, radiation levels outside the shields and within some distance as promised by the manufacturer should be incorporated as part of the machine acceptance criteria. This acceptance test should be conducted at maximum machine output during irradiation conditions that maximize production of γ-rays and neutrons.

A health or medical physicist or other qualified professional should be consulted during design stages to address the decision whether or not to install the cyclotron in a vault to evaluate the overall radiation shielding issues, fire and air conditioning, ventilation, air flow patterns, and exhaust monitoring. Personnel access and circulation through restricted areas should also be considered. Most facilities have adopted the criteria of keeping the vault or room where the cyclotron is located at negative pressure relative to the room where radioisotope processing takes place. This isotope production room, where the hot cells are typically installed, is also kept at negative pressure from the surrounding area for radiation safety reasons.

Reference

1. Hamacher K, Coenen HH, Stöcklin G. Efficient stereospecific synthesis of no-carrier-added 2-[^{18}F]-Fluoro-2-Deoxy-D-Glucose using aminopolyether supported nucleophilic substitution. J Nucl Med 1986;27:235–238.

3

Principles of PET/CT

Osama Mawlawi, Richard Wendt, III, and Wai-Hoi Wong

In recent years positron emission tomography (PET) has emerged as a unique imaging modality with applications in cardiology, neurology, oncology, and psychiatry due to its ability to produce accurately quantifiable images of physiologic information instead of anatomic structures. This ability, coupled with the extended PET reimbursement by major insurance carriers in the United States for a range of PET oncology studies, has further fueled the rapid increase in the clinical demand for this imaging modality. Research groups and industry strive to optimize this imaging technique. One of the very recent developments in PET imaging has been the introduction of a combined PET/computed tomography (CT) scanner. This chapter presents the reasons for this development, and discusses the advantages and artifacts presented by such imaging systems, and the impact of PET/CT on patient management as well as its applications in other areas, such as radiation treatment planning.

Why PET/CT?

There are three main reasons behind the merging of PET and CT in a combined scanner: (1) the need for a noise-free transmission scan for the attenuation correction of PET emission data; (2) the need to perform this correction in a rapid manner, thereby reducing the duration of a PET imaging session; and (3) the need for image fusion, whereby an anatomic framework is correlated with the physiologic information provided by PET.

PET Imaging and Its Disadvantages

PET is a noninvasive, diagnostic imaging technique for measuring the metabolic activity of cells in the human body. The majority of PET imaging has been concentrated in the field of oncology, in which a whole-body PET scan using the radiolabeled glucose analog fluorodeoxyglucose (FDG) plays an important role in the diagnosis and management of cancer. FDG accumulation detected by PET has been shown to be a reliable method for accessing the glucose metabolic rate of human cells.[1,2] Given that many malignant cells exhibit elevated glucose metabolism,[3] FDG-PET has been used in the primary staging and therapeutic monitoring of cancer. The high sensitivity, specificity, and accuracy of FDG-PET in detecting cancer in different regions of the body have been the driving forces behind its widening use.[4,5]

Transmission Scan and Attenuation Correction

In a whole-body FDG scan, the patient is injected with the radiopharmaceutical and is then asked to wait for about 1 hour during which the FDG distributes in the body. Following this waiting time, the patient is moved to the scanner and asked to lie supine on the patient couch. The patient is then positioned in the field of view of the scanner and the imaging session is initiated. A PET scan is composed of an emission and a transmission scan. The emission scan is used to depict the distribution of the radiopharmaceutical in the body (Fig. 3.1A), while

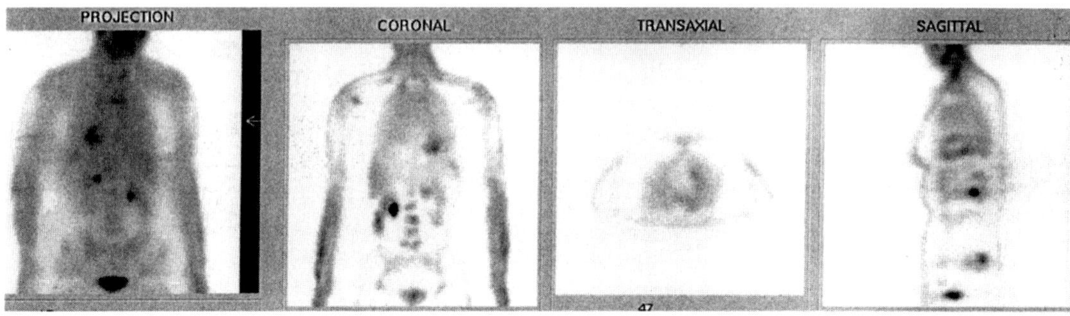

A

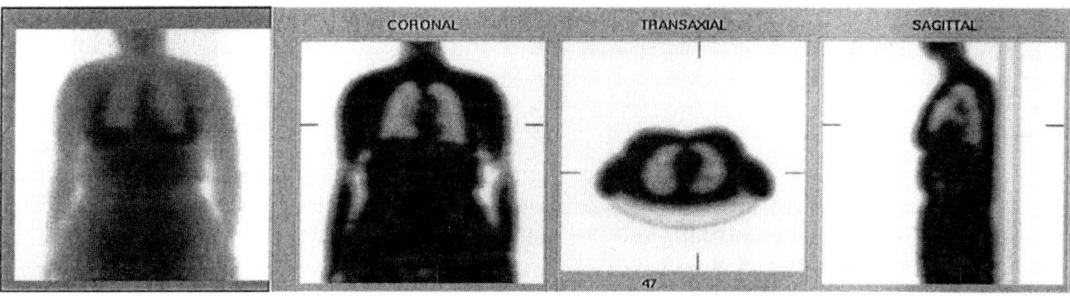

B

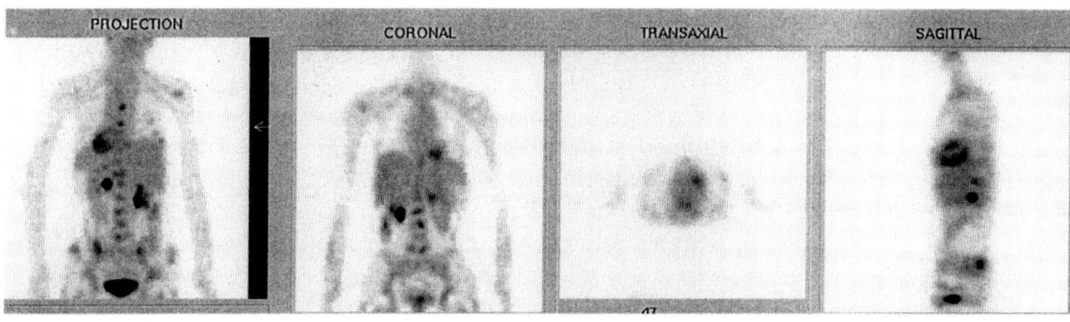

C

FIGURE 3.1. A: Nonattenuation corrected PET images. B: Reconstructed attenuation PET images. C: Attenuation corrected PET images.

the transmission scan is used for attenuation correction for the emission data. Attenuation correction is performed by rotating radioactive sources around the patient while the detectors that surround the patient collect the transmitted gamma rays—hence the term *transmission scan*. The transmission scan is used to generate a map representing the linear attenuation coefficients of different tissue types at the corresponding anatomic locations in a manner similar to CT imaging but at much poorer image resolution and quality (Fig. 3.1B). Multiplying the emission scan by the attenuation correction map generates the final corrected PET image (Fig. 3.1C). Attenuation correction is one of the major advantages of PET over other nuclear medicine imaging techniques due to its ability to accurately make up for the lost gamma rays stopped by the body. This correction produces PET images that depict an accurate distribution of the injected activity with minimal distortion in the shape, size, and location of a lesion. Hence, these data should be acquired in a reliable and accurate manner without inconveniencing the patient.[6]

Historically, transmission scans were done before the acquisition of emission data. The time it takes for the FDG to distribute in the patient (about 1 hour) and the requirement for exact patient positioning between emission and transmission data necessitated the emission and transmission data to be acquired consecutively without any time lapse 1 hour following the patient's injection with the radiopharmaceutical. However, this has resulted in transmission scans that are inherently contaminated by emission data and ultimately resulted in underestimated attenuation coefficients that led to inaccurate quantification of PET images.[7] In addition, transmission scans using a rotating radioactive source are noisy due to the low gamma-ray flux of the radioactive source. The noisy data result in inaccurate attenuation coefficients, which ultimately lead to a decrease in the apparent lesion contrast and small lesion detectability.

Several techniques have been proposed and implemented in routine clinical settings to correct for these transmission scanning drawbacks.[7] For emission contamination, transmission windowing and/or transmission image segmentation are currently being used. Windowing narrows the accepted coincident events only to those compatible with the instantaneous location of the radioactive source as it is rotating around the patient, and rejects the emission data from the rest of the field of view. This reduces the amount of potential emission contamination in the acquired transmission data. Transmission segmentation, on the other hand, refers to segmenting the reconstructed transmission scan to a predefined number of tissue types (air, water, bone) based on a preset range of attenuation values. Each segment is then filled with a constant attenuation value corresponding to that tissue type.[8,9] Transmission segmentation also significantly reduces the noise in the attenuation correction, thereby yielding higher quality final images. Although these techniques have minimized the effects of emission contamination and noise, transmission segmentation results in an attenuation map composed of only the predetermined number of segments. Rather than having a unique attenuation coefficient representing the corresponding tissue type at each voxel in the reconstructed image, the attenuation map is composed of clusters of attenuation coefficients representing the predetermined segments in the image and not reflecting the intermediate tissue densities in the patient.[10] Noise in the transmission scan can also be reduced by acquiring transmission data over a longer period of time or using higher radioactivity transmission sources. Both of these techniques, however, have disadvantages. A longer transmission scanning time results in a higher probability of patient motion during the scanning session and increases the inconvenience to the patient, while a higher radioactivity source results in larger detector dead-time.

PET Scan Duration

The acquisition of a transmission and emission scan to generate a PET image requires a relatively long imaging session, particularly when whole-body scans are performed. Since the axial field of view of current PET scanners is 15 to 17 cm only, several emission/transmission scans (five to seven) are needed to cover the whole body of a patient. Clinical studies have shown that the optimum scan duration per axial field of view (bed position) is in the range of 3 to 5 and 2 to 3 minutes for emission and transmission data, respectively, depending on the scanner and patient size. This translates to a total scanning time of 25 to 60 minutes (10 to 20 minutes of transmission data), during which the patient should remain motionless to minimize the mismatch between the emission and transmission data as well as to reduce image blurring. Such a scanning paradigm is inconvenient and uncomfortable for the patient. Furthermore, such long scan durations impose a restriction on the patient throughput of the scanner and thus limits its use.

The challenge lies in the compromise among the accuracy of attenuation correction, the noise propagation introduced by this process, the possibility of mismatch between the true and measured attenuation maps, and the scanning time reflected in patient throughput. Ideally, attenuation correction would add very little to the scanner time imposed by the emission image acquisitions, thereby leading to increased patient throughput, and there would be essentially no noise and no segmentation errors propagated in the final attenuation corrected image. These requirements, contrasted with the current state of attenuation correction, have led some institutions to skip transmission scanning altogether and rely on nonattenuation corrected images for their clinical evaluation of patients. This reduces the time spent on transmission scanning, with its inherent patient inconvenience, the risk of patient movement, as well as the loss of further income from scanning a second patient during the time spent on transmission scans, which by far outweigh the gain from accurate depiction of activity concentration.[11,12]

Image Registration and Fusion

Following the acquisition, attenuation correction, and reconstruction of PET data, the images are displayed for clinical evaluation. Regions of interest are usually drawn around areas of enhancing FDG activity, and an outcome measure such as the standard uptake value (SUV) is reported. A major difficulty for the interpretation of FDG-PET scans is the absence of anatomic structures. PET images are characterized by lower resolution, and are less accurate in their anatomic localization of foci of abnormal uptake, especially for less experienced PET physicians. The accurate anatomic localization of a lesion coupled with its metabolic activity can be important for the diagnosis, staging, and treatment of patients. The usefulness of fusing functional PET data with anatomic information from CT or magnetic resonance imaging (MRI) has been recognized in oncology.[13–16] It has been shown that the visual correlation of PET with CT can improve the accuracy of PET alone.[17] Traditionally image registration and fusion have been performed through the use of computer algorithms. Two image sets acquired from two different imaging modalities at two different times are read by the registration algorithms, and a transformation aligning one image set into the space of the other is generated. One of the major difficulties with the registration process is the different patient positioning between the two image sets. Although this difficulty has been circumvented in registering images of rigid bodies such as the brain,[18] its effect on aligning whole-body images, where the internal organs are nonstationary and deformable, has resulted in less satisfactory registrations. For whole-body images, nonlinear image warping algorithms are needed; however, these algorithms require longer converging time and are not always successful at aligning the two images, making their use less attractive in routine clinical PET imaging. Mental registration between PET and CT/MRI images is usually performed by image readers. Such mental image registrations are often adequate for experienced readers.

Advantages of PET/CT

To further improve PET imaging, a combined PET/CT scanner has been proposed. Computed tomography images are actually attenuation maps of the object being imaged, albeit at different electromagnetic energy from that used in PET. Mapping the CT attenuation coefficients corresponding to the different tissue types obtained at the CT equivalent energy to that of PET (511 KeV) generates an attenuation correction map without the need to acquire a separate transmission scan.[19] The CT images acquired post–FDG injection are less contaminated by emission data due to the large difference in flux between the CT x-rays and emission gamma rays. In addition, CT images are characterized by short acquisition time and low noise content. This latter characteristic is dependent on the x-ray current setting of the CT scanner. The short duration of CT scans allows higher patient throughput while maximizing patient comfort and minimizing patient motion. Finally, CT images provide high-resolution anatomic information, which, when combined with PET images, can improve diagnostic accuracy and patient management.[20–25] Other areas positively impacted by this combined imaging modality include patient scheduling and radiation treatment planning. Most patients who are scheduled for a PET scan also receive a diagnostic CT scan prior to their PET imaging session.[26] These separate scans could be performed on the same PET/CT scanner, thus facilitating patient scheduling and eliminating the need for transport from one imaging suite to the other. Patient waiting time would be reduced and throughput would improve. For radiation treatment planning, it has been shown that incorporating PET data with CT for treatment planning has the potential for improving the accuracy for delineating the primary target volume.[27–29] Obtaining the PET and the CT data at the same anatomic location greatly facilitates the incorporation of the PET data in the treatment plan.

Challenges of PET/CT Imaging

Although combining a PET and a CT scanner has many advantages, this hybrid imaging system also presents a new set of difficulties, most of which are centered on the use of CT for attenuation correction of the PET data. One of the major areas of difficulty is the presence of dense material such as dental filling, metallic prosthetics, and contrast agents in the CT image. In the case of dental fillings and metallic prosthetics, the resulting CT images are characterized by pronounced streaking artifacts due to the very high attenuation values. These artifacts are propagated to the PET image upon mapping the CT attenuation values to those corresponding to PET at 511 KeV.[30] The propagated artifacts are manifested as high attenuation correction factors, which result in an apparent increase in tracer concentration in the PET image.[31] For contrast agents whether oral (barium sulfate) or intravenous (iodine), the overestimation in the attenuation correction factor presents an even more complicated challenge since the overestimation is dependent on the concentration of the administered contrast agent. The concentration of contrast agents in the body is not a fixed amount, causing the overestimation in the attenuation correction factor to vary depending on several factors such as patient size, clearance, blood flow, and most importantly, the time between contrast administration and CT data acquisition time. It has been shown that both oral and intravascular contrast agents affect the quantitative and qualitative accuracy of PET images depending on the contrast concentration.[32–36]

Another area of major difficulty presented by PET/CT imaging is the attenuation artifact induced by the variation in the patient respiration during the CT scan as compared to the PET scan. The CT scans are characterized by short duration and are acquired during any stage of the patient's respiratory cycle. The PET scans, on the other hand, require longer imaging times and therefore are acquired over multiple breathing cycles. As such, images from the two scanning modalities show discrepancies in the anatomic localization of various organs, particularly evident in areas such as the dome of the liver and the base of the lungs. Since the CT images are used for attenuation correction of the PET emission data, the mismatch between the two image sets results in large quantitative and qualitative errors.[37–40] It has been shown, however, that by standardizing the CT acquisition to normal expiration breath holding, the CT images would best represent the resultant PET images, thereby largely reducing the magnitude of this effect.[38,41]

Another problem with PET/CT imaging is the difference in the size of the field of view (FOV) between the CT and PET scanners, resulting in truncation artifacts between the two corresponding image sets. Truncation artifact encompasses two forms of error. The first is due to large patients whose cross section extends beyond the FOV of the CT scan (50 cm), thus producing severe truncation at the edges of the CT images (Fig. 3.2). The second is due to truncated attenuation data resulting from the difference in the FOV size between the PET (70 cm) and CT images. The first error is manifested as streaking artifacts at the edge of the CT image, thus causing an artificial overestimation of the attenuation coefficients used in PET as well as degrading the quality of the CT image. The second error results in nonattenuated corrected PET data located at the periphery of the PET FOV. These two errors have been shown to affect the quantitative and qualitative accuracy of PET images.[42,43] One way of minimizing these errors is by scanning the patient, in both the CT and PET positions, with the arms above the head, thereby reducing the cross-sectional dimension of the patient. This scanning position, however, is very uncomfortable for most patients and results in involuntary movement during the relatively long PET imaging session. Furthermore, scanning the patients with their arms up strains their shoulder muscles and might interfere with the FDG accumulation in this region.

The challenges that PET/CT imaging introduces, as presented here, mainly fall within the realm of imaging physics and instrumentation concerns. The solution to these challenges is currently being investigated, and before long proper solutions should be presented. The advantages of PET/CT by far outweigh its disadvantages. The convinc-

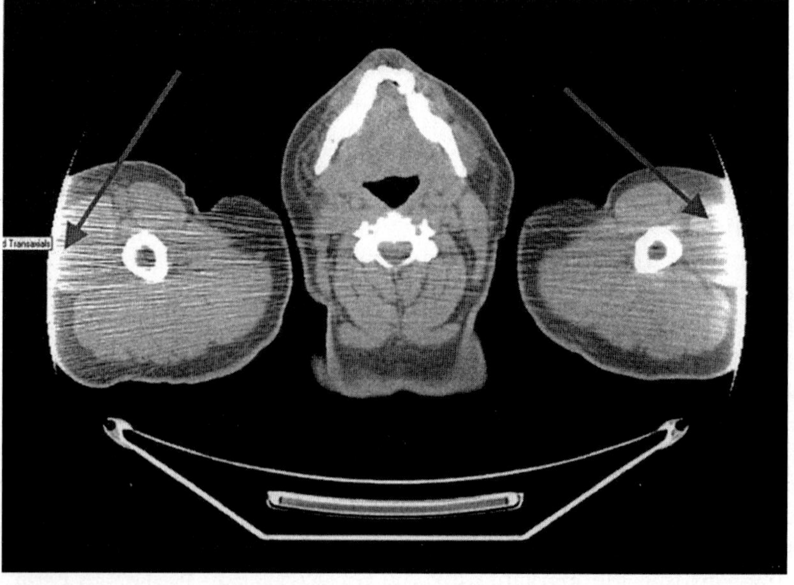

FIGURE 3.2. A 145-kg man scanned with arms up. Arrows show truncation artifacts.

ing evidence is seen in the instantaneous spread of PET/CT across the imaging community. It has already revolutionized the job of the nuclear physician. No longer will PET imaging be considered a specialized imaging technique; through the use of PET/CT, PET imaging will be part of the mainstream of radiology. It will become the road map for the best interpretation of CT, and CT will add the anatomic detail that PET lacks. The application of PET/CT in radiation treatment planning, with its unique advantages over CT only, will further bolster its widespread use and establish PET/CT as the standard in the evaluation and management of cancer.

The remainder of this chapter discusses the design specifications of PET/CT scanners in general, and those that are commercially available in particular.

PET/CT Scanner Design

PET/CT scanners are composed of a PET scanner attached to a CT scanner back to back. The combined structure is housed in a single gantry. The CT scanner is usually in the front, and the PET device is located behind the CT. The center of the two tomographs are separated by 60 to 70 cm axially to allow space for the CT and PET electronics and minimize crosstalk between the CT and PET detectors. This distance is also important to minimize the temperature variations—critical for the PET detectors—inside the gantry due to turning on and off the CT x-ray tube. The patient couch is located in front of the scanner and is used to advance the patient from the CT to the PET FOV. Since the center of the two tomographs is separated by a large distance, the whole patient couch assembly is translated in the axial direction rather than just translating the patient pallet. This is done to minimize the deflection of the pallet due to patient weight as it is extending from the CT to the PET FOV.

Depending on the manufacturer, the individual CT and PET scanner designs can vary considerably. The CT can be single or multislice, helical or axial, and with different rotation speeds, whereas the PET can be 2D and/or 3D capable, use bismuth germinate (BGO), cerium-doped gadolinium oxyorthosilicate (GSO), or cerium-doped lutetium oxyorthosilicate (LSO) detectors, and have a different number of slices per axial FOV. The functionality of PET/CT scanners, however, is the same regardless of manufacturer. Typically, a CT localizer is acquired to ensure proper patient positioning. This is followed by the CT scan, which is used to generate anatomic images and attenuation maps. At the end of the CT scan, the patient couch assembly is advanced from the CT to the PET FOV, where the PET acquisition is initiated. Following the data acquisition and reconstruction, the PET and CT images can be displayed side by side or fused together, assuming that the patient did not move between the two imaging sessions. Sophisticated image processing algorithms allow the PET and CT data to be displayed at the same anatomic location even though the PET and CT slices have different thicknesses.

The first prototype PET/CT scanner was developed by David Townsend at the University of Pittsburgh in joint collaboration with CTI Inc. (Knoxville, TN). The initial design work began with a grant from the National Cancer Institute in 1995, and the prototype became operational in 1998. The prototype PET/CT scanner was based on a spiral CT scanner, the single slice Somatom AR.SP (Siemens; Iselin, NJ), mated with a rotating partial-ring PET tomograph, the Emission Computed Axial Tomography (ECAT), Advanced Rotating Tomograph (ART) scanner. Both the PET and CT components were mounted on the same assembly with the PET components on the reverse side of the rotating support of the CT scanner. Both scanners were housed inside a single gantry with the centers of the two tomographs offset by 60 cm in the axial direction, allowing a dual-modality examination range of 100 cm only. The design specifics and first PET/CT images produced on this prototype scanner can be found elsewhere.[44] However, the widespread recognition of the importance of imaging anatomy and function together, led by the studies performed on this prototype PET/CT scanner, created a demand for combined PET/CT scanners for imaging cancer in the medical community and stimulated intense commercial activity.

Currently there are only three manufacturers of PET/CT scanners: GE Medical Systems, CTI Inc./Siemens Medical Solutions, and Philips Medical Systems. As of this writing, Philips, the newest vendor in the commercial PET/CT market, has just introduced its first PET/CT product, the Gemini. Siemens and CTI have a joint venture in a company called CPS Innovations that manufactures PET/CT scanners. Each company, however, markets the CPS product under a different name. There are currently nine PET/CT scanners available on the market. From GE we have the Discovery LS and Discovery ST. From CTI we have the Reveal HD, Reveal RT, and Reveal XVI. From Siemens we have the Biograph, the Biograph LSO, and the Biograph Sensation 16. From Philips we have the Gemini PET/CT system.

GE PET/CT Scanners

Discovery LS

This scanner is based on the GE Advance Nxi dedicated PET scanner combined with the GE LightSpeed Plus CT scanner, hence the name LS (Fig. 3.3). Major design considerations of this scanner are the following: (1) Four- or eight-slice CT scanner options with 0.5 second/rotation allow a marked reduction of the CT imaging time, with lower overall dose to the patient. (2) The PET scanner has BGO detectors. (3) PET can image in 2D and 3D modes. (4) PET generates 35 slices covering a 15.2-cm axial FOV. (5) The PET scanner has a transmission source for attenuation correction in addition to using the CT data for that purpose. This allows the comparison of attenuation performed on using the CT data and the transmission source. (6) The PET and CT scanners are air-cooled. (7) The patient port diameter changes from 70 to 59 cm as the patient is traversed from the CT to the PET FOV.

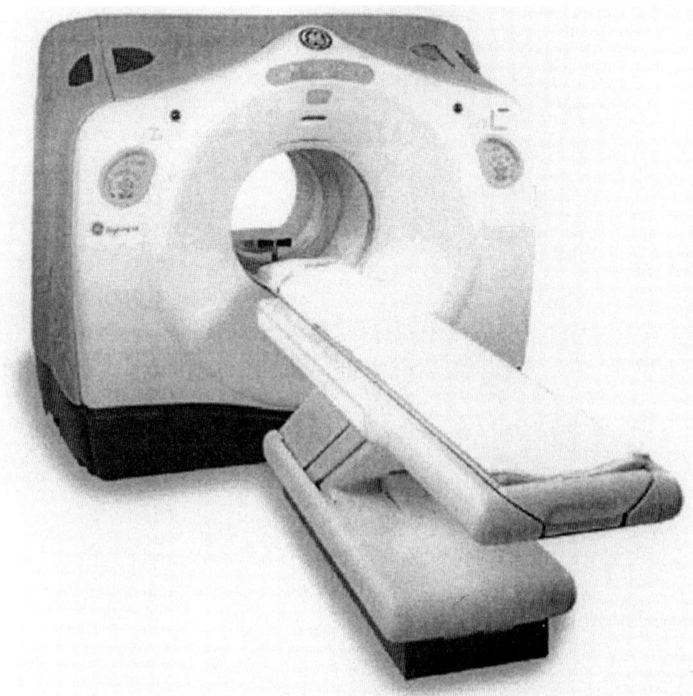

FIGURE 3.3. GE Discovery LS PET/CT scanner.

(8) The distance between the centers of both scanners is 70, thus limiting the patient imaging range to 150 cm. (9) The weight of the scanner, including the couch, is 5200 kg, and its dimensions are 235 cm (W), 205 cm (D), and 208 cm (H). Performance characteristics of the PET Advance Nxi can be found elsewhere.[45,46]

Discovery ST

This is the most recent entry of PET/CT products to the market (Fig. 3.4). As of this writing only two such systems have been installed. The Discovery ST (sensitivity and throughput) is based on a new PET design specifically engineered for a combined PET/CT scanner. The design has been optimized to mate with the GE LightSpeed CT product line while minimizing its size and footprint. Major design considerations of this scanner are the following: (1) Four (Light Speed Plus) or eight (Ultra) slice CT options with 0.5 second/rotation are available. (2) The PET scanner is based on BGO detectors. (3) PET is capable of 2D and 3D imaging modes. (4) PET generates 47 slices in a 15.5-cm axial FOV. (5) Attenuation correction is entirely CT based. (6) The PET and CT scanners are air-cooled. (7) The uniform patient port is 70 cm from the CT to PET FOV. (8) The 70-cm distance between the center of the CT and PET FOVs allows an examination range of 150 cm. (9) The weight of the scanner including the couch is 4200 kg, and its dimensions are 210 cm (W), 153 cm (D), and 185 (H) cm. Performance characteristics of the PET scanner can be found elsewhere.[47]

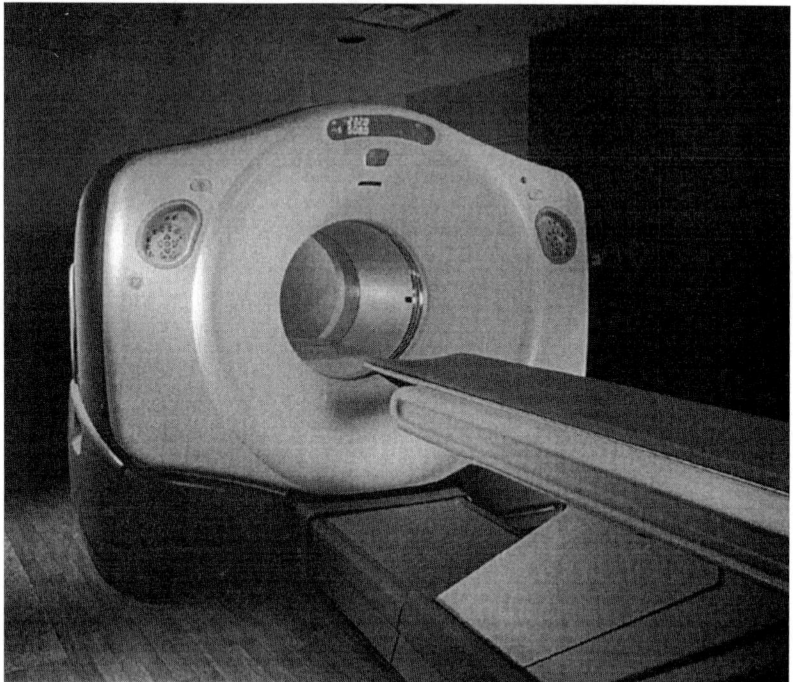

FIGURE 3.4. GE Discovery ST PET/CT scanner.

CTI PET/CT Scanners

Reveal HD

This scanner is the latest in the ECAT family of PET scanners and the first PET/CT scanner from CTI Inc. The ECAT Reveal HD (high-definition) scanner is based on the ECAT HR+ PET scanner combined with the Somatom Emotion CT scanner from Siemens. The major design considerations of this scanner are the following: (1) Single- or dual-slice CT with 0.8 second/rotation is available. (2) The PET scanner uses BGO detectors. (3) PET data are acquired in 3D mode only. (4) PET generates 63 slices in an axial FOV of 15.5 cm. (5) Attenuation correction is entirely CT based. (6) The PET scanner is water-cooled while the CT is air-cooled. (7) The uniform patient port is 70 cm from CT to PET FOVs. This was made possible without redesigning the HR+ scanner by removing the septa and allowing 3D data acquisition only. (8) The center of the FOV of the CT and PET scanners is offset by 80 cm axially, thus allowing 160 to 180 cm of dual-modality examination range. (9) The patient couch was completely redesigned to minimize the relative deflection between the CT and PET image planes. The new design features a fully cantilevered carbon fiber pallet, which is supported on a pedestal moving on a floor-mounted high-precision rail system driven by a linear motor. (10) The weight of the Reveal HD including the couch is 3200 kg. Its dimensions are 228 cm (W), 160 cm (D), and 189 cm (H). The detector size is 4.05 inplane and 4.39 axial, thereby providing a detector voxel of 0.072 mL. The performance characteristics of the HR+ scanner can be found elsewhere.[48] This scanner has been superseded by the Reveal RT product, although it is still available from the manufacturer upon request.

Reveal RT

This scanner is exactly similar in design to the Reveal HD, except that the PET scanner used in this PET/CT product is based on the ECAT Accel (recently renamed Reveal XL). The ECAT Accel in turn is based on the ECAT EXAC 47 PET scanner (47 slices per axial FOV of 16.2 cm), but with LSO detectors it is economical, since LSO is more expensive than BGO. The Reveal RT (rapid throughput) (Fig. 3.5) is one of the fastest PET/CT imaging products on the market. Through the use of LSO detectors, the emission acquisition time can be reduced to 3 minutes (instead of 4 to 5 minutes) per bed position, resulting in a total whole-body scan in 20 minutes. The weight of the Reveal RT including the couch is 3200 kg. The dimensions of the gantry are 228 cm (W), 160 cm (D), and 189 cm (H). The detector size is 6.45 × 6.45 mm, providing a detector voxel of 0.268 mL. The performance characteristics of the ECAT Accel scanner can be found elsewhere.[49]

Reveal XVI

This scanner (Fig. 3.6) is exactly similar to the Reveal RT, except that the CT product is the Somatom Sensation 16. The Sensation 16 is capable of producing 16 slices per rotation at 0.4 second per rotation. All other design features are similar to those of the REVEAL RT.

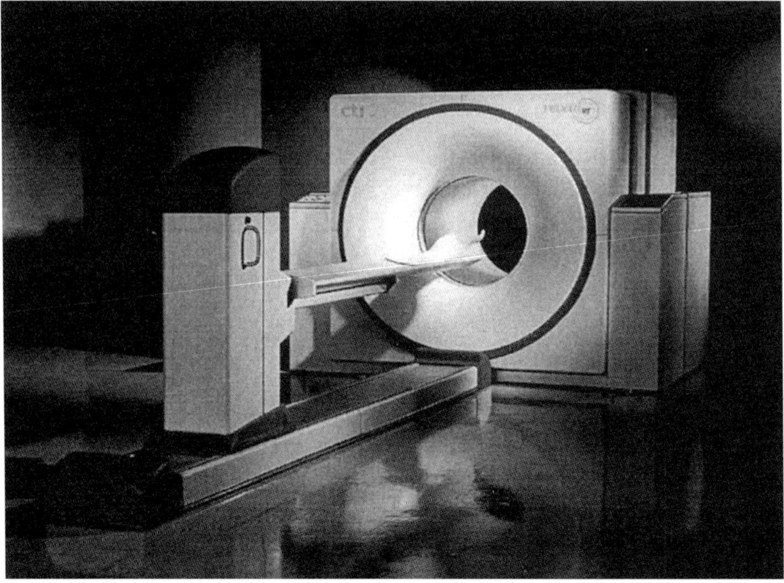

FIGURE 3.5. CTI Reveal RT PET/CT scanner.

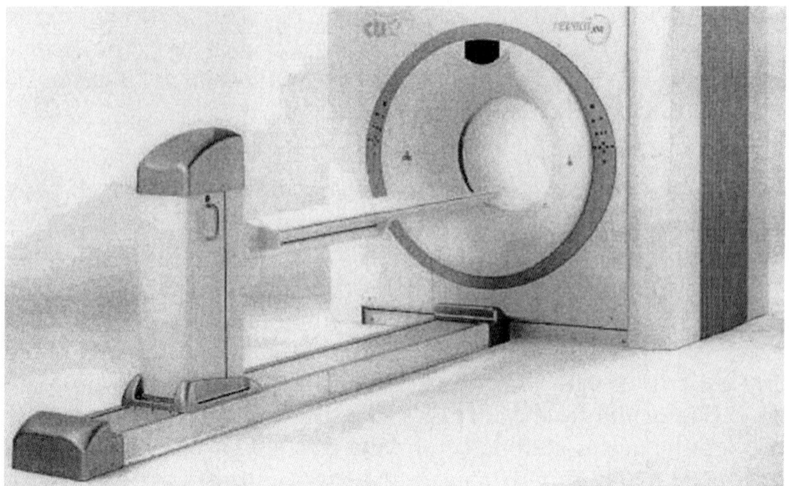

FIGURE 3.6. CTI Reveal XVI PET/CT scanner.

Siemens PET/CT Scanners

There are three PET/CT products from Siemens Medical Solutions: the Biograph, the Biograph LSO, and Biograph Sensation 16 (Fig. 3.7). These three scanners are the same as the Reveal HD, Reveal RT, and Reveal XVI from CTI but marketed under different names.

Philips PET/CT Scanners

Gemini

This is the first open design of a PET/CT scanner (Fig. 3.8). This design feature maximizes patient acceptance and comfort and allows easy

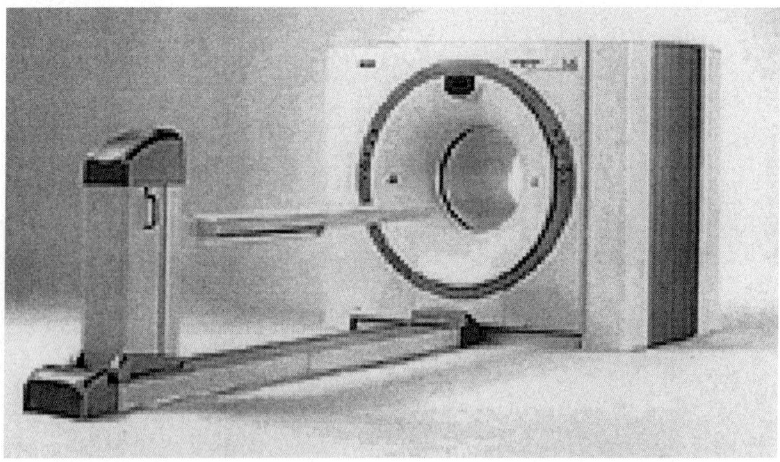

FIGURE 3.7. Siemens Biograph Sensation 16 PET/CT scanner.

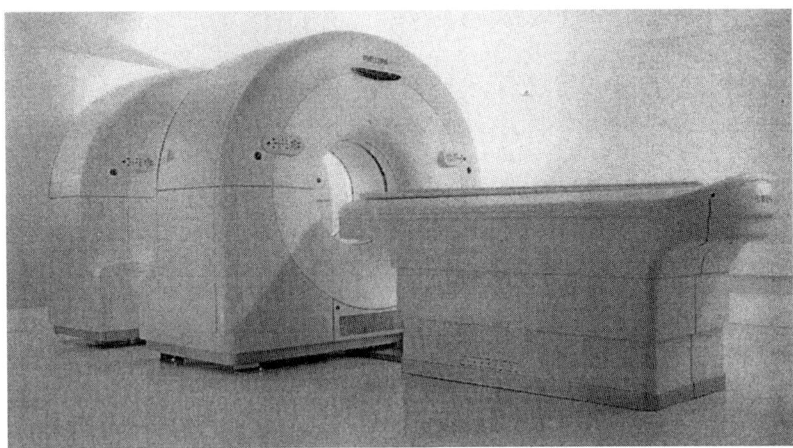

FIGURE 3.8. Philips Gemini PET/CT scanner.

access to the patient during the exam time. The Gemini also has the largest PET axial FOV on the market, allowing the largest patient coverage per bed position. This feature reduces the scan duration by minimizing the number of bed positions required to cover the whole body. The Gemini is composed of the Allegro PET scanner and the MX8000 multislice CT scanner from Philips. The major design considerations of this scanner are the following: (1) Dual-slice CT with 0.5 second/rotation is available. (2) The PET scanner uses GSO pixelated detectors. (3) PET data are acquired in 3D mode only. (4) PET generates 90 slices in an axial FOV of 18 cm. (5) Attenuation correction is done with a

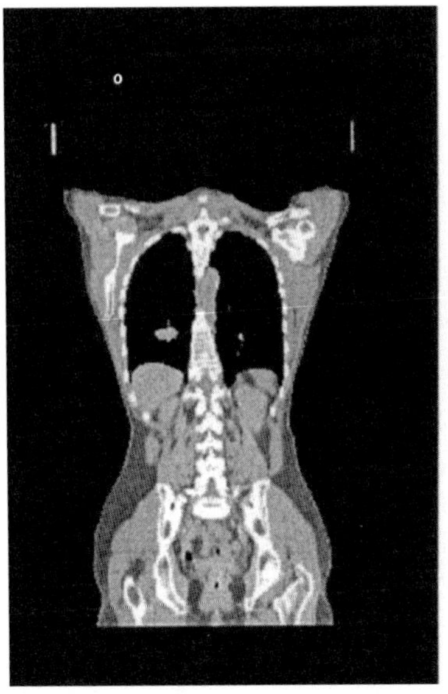

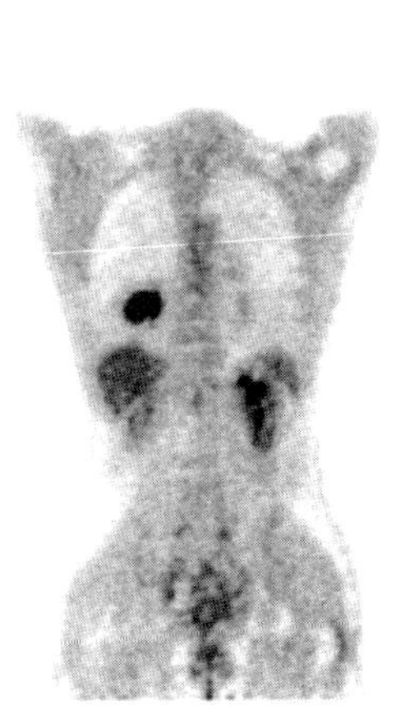

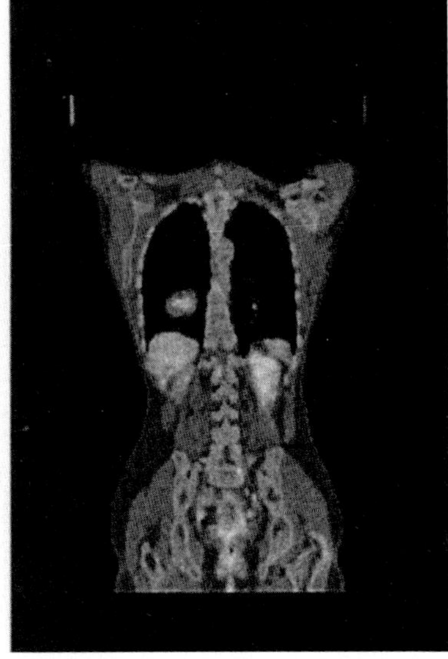

FIGURE 3.9. PET/CT images acquired on the Discovery ST PET/CT scanner of a 63-year-old woman (53 kg) with squamous cell lung cancer. (Courtesy of the M.D. Anderson Cancer Center.)

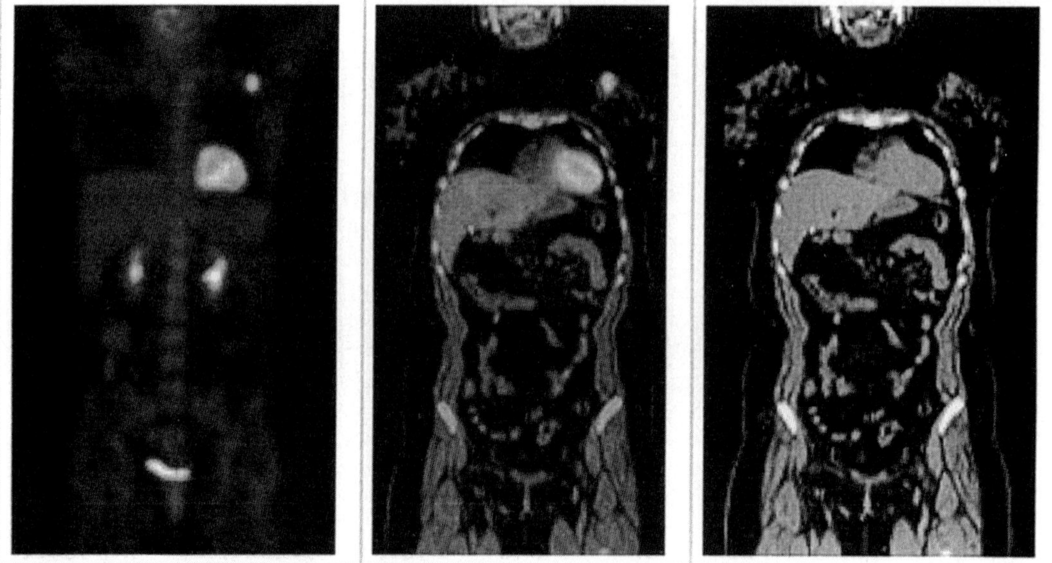

FIGURE 3.10. PET/CT images acquired on the Biograph Sensation 16 of a 54-year-old woman (85 kg) with recently diagnosed breast cancer. (Courtesy of the University of Tennessee.)

transmission scan using a 137-Cs source that acquires single data as well as by using the CT scan. (6) The PET and CT scanners are air-cooled. (7) The patient port size changes from 70 cm at the CT side to 63 cm at the PET side. (8) The separation between the CT and PET scanners is user selectable with a maximum range of 100 cm, thus allowing 195 cm of dual-modality examination range. The minimum separation between the two scanners is 30 cm. (9) The patient couch was completely redesigned to minimize floor space while maximizing scanning length. (10) The weight of the Gemini including the couch is 3700 kg. Its dimensions are 215 cm (W), 160 cm (D), and 206 cm (H). The detector size is 4 mm inplane and 6 mm axial, thereby providing a detector voxel of 0.096 mL. The performance characteristics of the Allegro scanner can be found elsewhere.[50]

Images from the GE Discovery ST and the Biograph LSO/Reveal RT are shown in Figures 3.9 and 3.10, respectively.

References

1. Phelps ME, Huang SC, Hoffman EJ, et al. Tomographic measurement of local cerebral glucose rate in humans with (F-18)2-fluoro-2-deoxy-D-glucose: validation of method. Ann Neurol 1979;6(5):371–388.
2. Huang SC, Phelps ME, Hoffman EJ, et al. Noninvasive determination of local cerebral metabolic rate of glucose in man. Am J Physiol 1980;238(1): E69–82.
3. Smith TA. FDG uptake, tumor characteristics and response to therapy: a review. Nucl Med Commun 1988;19(2):97–105.
4. Delbeke D. Oncological applications of FDG-PET imaging: brain tumors, colorectal cancer, lymphoma and melanoma. J Nucl Med 1999;40(4):591–603.

5. Gambhir SS, Czernin J, Schwimmer J, et al. A tabulated summary of the FDG-PET literature. J Nucl Med 2001;42 (5):1S-93S.
6. Bailey DL. Transmission scanning in emission tomography. Eur J Nucl Med 1998;25:774–787.
7. Zaidi H, Hasegawa B. Determination of the attenuation map in emission tomography. J Nucl Med 2003;44(2) 291–315.
8. Meikle SR, Dahlbom M, Cherry SR. Attenuation correction using count-limited transmission data in positron emission tomography. J Nucl Med 1993;34:143–150.
9. Xu M, Cutler P, Luk W. An adaptive local threshold segmented attenuation correction method for whole-body PET imaging. IEEE Trans Nucl Sci 1996;43:331–336.
10. Bettinardi V, Pagani E, Gilardi M. An automatic classification technique for attenuation correction in positron emission tomography. Eur J Nucl Med 1999;26:447–458.
11. Bengel FM, Ziegler SI, Avril N, et al. Whole-body positron emission tomography in clinical oncology: comparison between attenuation corrected and uncorrected images. Eur J Nucl Med 1997;24:1091–1098.
12. Wahl RL. To AC or not to AC: that is the question. J Nucl Med 1999;40: 2025–2028.
13. Diederichs CG. Prospective comparison of FDG-PET of pancreatic tumors with high end spiral CT and MRI. J Nucl Med 1998;39(5):81.
14. Eubank WB, Mankoff DA, Schmeidl UP. Imaging of oncologic patients: benefit of combined CT and FDG-PET in the diagnosis of malignancy. Am J Radiol 1998;171:1103–1110.
15. Wahl RL, Quint LE, Greenough RL, et al. Staging of mediastinal non-small cell lung cancer with FDG-PET, CT and fusion images: preliminary prospective evaluation. Radiology 1994;191(2):371–377.
16. Wahl RL, Quint LE, Cieslak RD, et al. "Anatometabolic" tumor imaging: fusion of FDG-PET with CT or MRI to localize foci of increased activity. J Nucl Med 1993;34(7):1190–1197.
17. Vanteenkiste JF, Stroobants SG, Dupont PJ, et al. FDG-PET scan in potentially operable non-small cell lung cancer: Do anatometabolic PET-CT fusion images improve the localization of regional lymph node metastases? The Leuven Lung Cancer Group. Eur J Nucl Med 1998;25(11):1495–1501.
18. Woods RP, Cherry SR, Mazziotta J C. Rapid automated algorithm for aligning and reslicing PET images. J Comput Assist Tomogr 1992;16(4):620–633.
19. Kinahan PE, Townsend DW, Beyer T, et al. Attenution correction for a combined 3D PET/CT scanner. Med Phys 1998;25:2046–2053.
20. Hany TF, Steinert HC, Goerres GW, et al. PET diagnostic accuracy: improvement with in-line PET-CT system: initial results. Radiology 2002; 225(2):575–581.
21. Israel O, Mor M, Gaitini D, et al. Combined functional and structural evaluation of cancer patients with a hybrid camera-based PET/CT system using F-18-FDG. J Nucl Med 2002;43(9):1129–1136.
22. Cohade C, Osman M, Leal J, et al. Direct comparison of FDG-PET and PET-CT imaging in colorectal cancer. J Nucl Med 2002;43(suppl 5):78.
23. Freudenberg LS, Antoch G, Mueller SP, et al. Preliminary results of whole-body FDG-PET/CT in lymphoma. J Nucl Med 2002;43(suppl 5):106.
24. Yeung HW, Schoder H, Larson SM. Utility of PET/CT for assessing equivocal PET lesions in oncology—initial experience. J Nucl Med 2002;43(suppl 5):115.
25. Bar-Shalom R, Keidar Z, Guralnik L, et al. Added value of fused PET/CT imaging with FDG in diagnostic imaging and management of cancer patients. J Nucl Med 2002;43(suppl 5):117.

26. Mah K, Caldwell CB, Ung YE, et al. The impact of 18F-FDG-PET on target and critical organs in CT-based tratment planning of patients with poorly defined non-small-cell lung carcinoma: a prospective study. Int J Radiat Oncol Biol Phys 2002;52(2):339–350.
27. Erdi YE, Rosenzweig K, Erdi AK, et al. Radiotherapy treatment planning for patients with non-small-cell lung cancer using positron emission tomography (PET). Radiother Oncol 2002;62:51–60.
28. Mutic S, Grigsby PW, Low DA, et al. PET-guided three-dimensional treatment planning of intracavitary gynecologic implants. Int J Radiat Oncol Biol Phys 2002;52(4):1104–1110.
29. Dizendorf E, Ciernik IF, Baumert B, et al. Impact of integrated PET CT scanning on external beam radiation treatment planning. J Nucl Med 2002; 43(suppl 5):118.
30. Goerres GW, Hany TF, Kamel E, et al. Head and neck imaging with PET and PET/CT: artefacts from dental metallic implants. Eur J Nucl Med Molec Imag 2002;29(3):367–370.
31. Goerres GW, Ziegler SI, Burger C, et al. Artifacts at PET and PET/CT caused by metallic hip prosthetic material. Radiology 2003;226(2):577–584.
32. Antoch G, Freudenberg LS, Egelhof T, et al. Focal tracer uptake: a potential artifact in contrast-enhanced dual-modality PET/CT scans. J Nucl Med 2002;(10):1339–1342.
33. Dizendorf EV, Treyer V, von Schulthess GK, et al. Application of oral contrast media in coregistered positron emission tomography-CT. AJR 2002; 179(2):477–481.
34. Cohade C, Osman M, Nakamoto Y, et al. Initial experience with oral contrast in PET/CT: phantom and clinical studies. J Nucl Med 2003;44(3): 412–416.
35. Antoch G, Freudenberg LS, Stattaus J, et al. A whole-body positron emission tomography-CT: optimized CT using oral and IV contrast materials. AJR 2002;179(6):1555–1560.
36. Mawlawi O, Macapinlac H, Erasmus J, et al. Transformation of CT numbers to PET attenuation factors in the presence of iodinated IV contrast. Eur J Nucl Med Molec Imag 2002;29:S108.
37. Goerres GW, Burger C, Kamel E, et al. Respiration-induced attenuation artifact at PET/CT: technical considerations. Radiology 2003;226(3):906–910.
38. Goerres GW, Kamel E, Heidelberg TNH, et al. PET-CT image co-registration in the thorax: influence of respiration. Eur J Nucl Med Molec Imag 2002;29(3):351–360.
39. Blodgett T, Beyer T, Antoch G, et al. The effect of respiratory motion on PET/CT image quality. J Nucl Med 2002;43(suppl 5):209.
40. Chin BB, Nakamoto Y, Kraitchman DL, et al. Quantitative differences in F-18 FDG uptake due to respiratory motion in PET CT: attenuation correction using CT in end inspiration and end expiration versus Ge-68 correction. J Nucl Med 2002;43(suppl 5):210.
41. Goerres GW, Kamel E, Seifert B, et al. Accuracy of image coregistration of pulmonary lesions in patients with non-small cell lung cancer using an integrated PET/CT system. J Nucl Med 2002;43(11):1469–1475.
42. Carney J, Townsend DW, Kinahan PE, et al. CT-based attenuation correction: the effects of imaging with the arms in the field of view. J Nucl Med 2001;42(suppl 5):211.
43. Cody D, Mawlawi O, Forster K. Preliminary study of CT transmission truncation and beam hardening artifacts on quantitative PET activity. Semin Nucl Med (accepted abstract). J Nucl Med 2003;44(suppl 5):273.
44. Beyer T, Townsend DW, Brun T, et al. A combined PET/CT scanner for clinical oncology. J Nucl Med 2000;41(8):1369–1379.

45. DeGrado TR, Turkington TG, Williams JJ, et al. Performance characteristics of a whole-body PET scanner. J Nucl Med 1994;35(8):1398–1406.
46. Lewellen TK, Kohlmyer SG, Miyaoka RS, et al. Investigation of the performance of the General Electric ADVANCE Positron Emission Tomograph in 3D mode. IEEE Trans Nucl Sci 1996;43(4):2199–2206.
47. Mawlawi O, Kohlmyer S, Williams JJ, et al. Performance characteristics of the GE Discovery ST PET/CT scanner using the NEMA standard. J Nucl Med 2003;44(5):111 p.
48. Brix G, Zaers J, Adam LE, et al. Performance evaluation of a whole-body PET scanner using the NEMA protocol. J Nucl Med 1997;38(10):1614–1623.
49. Reveal RT technical data specification sheet, 2003.
50. Gemini technical specification data sheet, 2003.

4

Radiopharmaceuticals

David J. Yang, Tomio Inoue, and E. Edmund Kim

Radiolabeled Ligands

Several imaging modalities including computed tomography (CT), magnetic resonance imaging (MRI), ultrasound, optical imaging, and gamma scintigraphy have been used to diagnose cancer. Although CT and MRI provide considerable anatomic information about the location and the extent of tumors, they do not adequately differentiate residual or recurrent tumors from edema, radiation necrosis, or gliosis. Ultrasound images provide information about local and regional morphology with blood flow. Though optical imaging showed promising results, its ability to detect deep tissue penetration was not well demonstrated. Radionuclide imaging modalities [positron emission tomography (PET), single photon emission computed tomography (SPECT)] are diagnostic cross-sectional imaging techniques that map the location and concentration of radionuclide-labeled compounds.[1–3] Beyond showing precisely where a tumor is and its size, shape, and viability, PET and SPECT are making it possible to "see" the molecular makeup of the tumor and its metabolic activity. Whereas PET and SPECT can provide a very accurate picture of metabolically active areas, their ability to show anatomic features is limited. As a result, new imaging modalities have begun to combine PET and SPECT images with CT scans for treatment planning. PET-CT and SPECT-CT scanners combine anatomic and functional images taken during a single procedure, without having to reposition the patient between scans. To improve the diagnosis, prognosis, planning, and monitoring of the cancer treatment, characterization of tumor tissue is extensively determined by development of more tumor-specific pharmaceuticals. Radiolabeled ligands as well as radiolabeled antibodies have opened a new era in scintigraphic detection of tumors and have undergone extensive preclinical development and evaluation.

Glucose Transport

^{18}F-fluorodeoxyglucose (FDG)-PET has been used to diagnose and stage tumors,[4–14] myocardial infarction,[15] and neurologic disease.[16,17] 2-Deoxy-2-[^{18}F]fluoro-D-glucose was developed in 1976 for the specific purpose of mapping brain glucose metabolism in living humans. After the first synthesis of ^{18}F-FDG via an electrophilic fluorination with ^{18}F gas, small-volume enriched water targets were developed that made it possible to produce large quantities of [^{18}F]fluoride ion via the high yield ^{18}O(p,n)^{18}F reaction. This was followed by a major milestone, the development of a nucleophilic fluorination method that produced [^{18}F]-FDG in very high yields. These advances and the remarkable properties of ^{18}F-FDG have largely overcome the limitations of the 110-minute half-life of ^{18}F. Although tumor metabolic imaging using [^{18}F]-FDG has been studied in the past two decades, its clinical application is still hampered by its limitations, such as differentiation of infection and tumor recurrence, and differentiation of low-grade and high-grade tumors.[18] To improve the diagnosis, prognosis, planning, monitoring, and predicting results of the cancer treatment, several other PET imaging agents are employed to characterize tumor targets.

Amino Acid Transport

^{11}C-methionine is useful for metabolic imaging of tumors by PET[19]; however, it has too many metabolic pathways that make it difficult to obtain a rate constant.[20,21] Because of its short half-life, it is also difficult to image tumors with slow uptake. To overcome these drawbacks, L-α-methyltyrosine (L-AmT) has been investigated in nuclear medicine, not only because of its biologic importance in the synthesis of protein or thyroid hormone, but also because of its involvement in dopamine or tyramine neurotransmitters.[22] Its analog, ^{123}I-α-methyltyrosine, has also been used for SPECT studies on brain and pancreatic tumors.[23–25] High accumulation of ^{123}I-α-methyltyrosine (I-LAmT) in tumors were reported. PET examination with ^{124}I-labeled α-methyltyrosine has been carried out in patients with brain tumors.[25] L-^{18}F-α-methyltyrosine (L-^{18}FAmT) was also developed. L-^{18}FAmT was synthesized by reacting L-AmT with $CH_3COO^{18}F$. Similar technique has been used to synthesize ^{18}F-labeled meta-tyrosine.[26] An electrophilic reactant $CH_3COO^{18}F$ reacts with L-AmT to give a meta-oriented position on the benzene ring. L-^{18}FAmT is quite stable in vivo compared to 2-^{18}F-fluorotyrosine[27,28] or ^{11}C-tyrosine, which produce too many metabolites, thus making it difficult to obtain quantitative analysis.[29,30] Though the radiochemical yield of L-^{18}FAmT was 20.3 $\pm$ 5.1% ($n = 5$) based on the radioactivity trapped in the reaction vessel, the radiochemistry purification using preparative high-performance liquid chromatography (HPLC) is time-consuming. For instance, ^{19}F-nuclear magnetic resonance (NMR) analysis gave two isomer spectra of L-^{19}FAmT with chemical shifts of -57.5 and -61.0 using trifluoroacetic acid as an internal standard.[31] These two isomer product ratios are 1 to 5.6, which corresponds to 2-L-^{19}FAmT and 3-L-^{19}FAmT, respectively. These assignments were based on the isomer of ^{19}F-meta-tyrosine spectra reported by Dejesus et al.[31] Recently, a rapid synthesis with high yield of O-2-^{18}F-fluoroethyltyrosine was developed.[32–34] Because introducing a methyl group in the α position could slow down the protein incorporation process, ^{18}F-fluoropropyl-AmT (L-^{18}FPAmT) was developed using a similar technique. The synthetic scheme is shown in Figure 4.1. Both L-^{18}FamT and L-^{18}FPAmT are discussed in this chapter.

Markers of Estrogen Receptor Tissue

The presence of sex hormone receptors in both primary and secondary breast tumors is an important indicator for both prognosis and choice of therapy for the disease.[35] Currently, receptors are determined by in vitro analysis of biopsy specimens and the use of antiestrogens. Tamoxifen is the therapy of choice for estrogen receptor–positive (ER+) tumors. The detection and measurement of ER+ tumors by the use of a radiolabeled ligand should provide a useful tool for the detection of primary and secondary tumors, as it may assist in selecting and following the most favorable therapy, as well as predicting its outcome. To this end a number of variations of substituted estradiols have been prepared containing the radioisotope fluorine in the 16 position.[36–38] These compounds have been relatively successful in detecting ER-rich tissue in vivo, but their ability to provide quantitative information on receptor concentration in either animal models or humans has been less clearly demonstrated.

Tamoxifen therapy results are positive in 30% of unselected patients with breast cancer. A response rate of 50% to 60% was obtained in patients with ER+ tumors.[39] Patients with metastatic cancer who do respond to the treatment have a response duration of 10 to 18 months and prolonged survival.[40] A radiolabeled tamoxifen ligand would be useful in diagnosing diseases that produce high levels of ERs, such as ovarian cancer, endometriosis, uterine carcinoma, and meningioma. Our rationale is that if the binding of the ligands with tumors can be

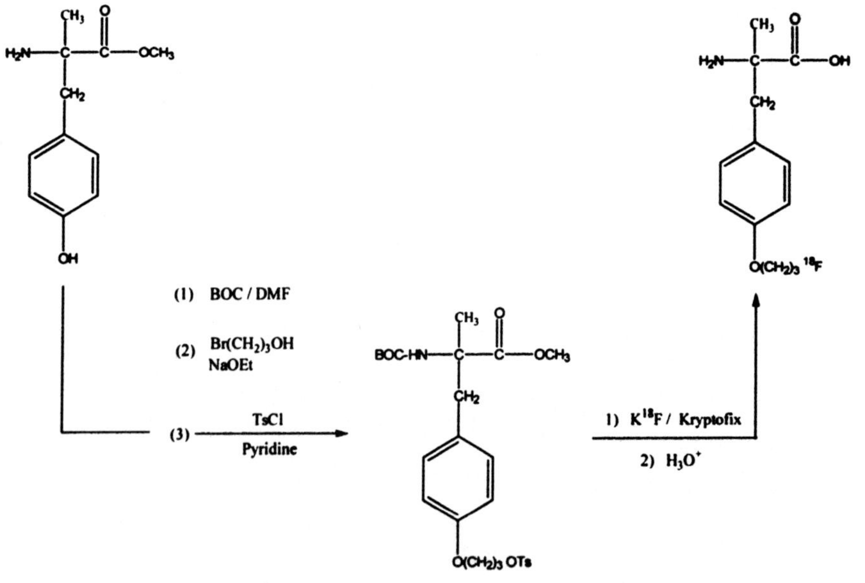

FIGURE 4.1. Synthesis of ^{18}F-fluoropropyl-α-methyltyrosine.

detected with PET or SPECT, then such ligands may predict the response to anticancer agents' therapy for cancer. Radiolabeled tamoxifen would also be useful in investigating tamoxifen's mechanisms of action, since it would provide more accurate information about the effectiveness of antiestrogen (tamoxifen) therapy.

Markers of Tumor Hypoxia

Misonidazole (MISO) is a hypoxic cell sensitizer, and labeling MISO with different halogenated radioisotopes (e.g., fluorine-18 or iodine-131) could be useful for differentiating a hypoxic but metabolically active tumor from a well-oxygenated active tumor by PET or planar scintigraphy.[41–46] [^{18}F]Fluoromisonidazole (FMISO) has been used to assess the hypoxic component in brain ischemia, myocardial infarction, and various tumors.[47–52] Moreover, the assessment of tumor hypoxia with labeled MISO prior to radiation therapy would provide a rational means of selecting patients for treatment with radiosensitizing or bioreductive drugs (e.g., mitomycin C). Such selection of patients would permit more accurate evaluation because the use of these modalities could be limited to patients with hypoxic tumors. It is also possible to select proper modalities of radiotherapy (neutron vs. photon) by correlating labeled MISO results with tumor response.

It has been reported that MISO produced peripheral sensory neuropathy at the dose level required for radiosensitization.[53,54] Thus, we have developed new MISO analogs by adding one hydroxymethyl group to MISO. This new ligand (halogenated erythronitroimidazoles; ETNIM) is more hydrophilic than FMISO. In this report, we used autoradiograms and radionuclide imaging techniques to demonstrate the potential application of FMISO and fluoro-ETNIM (FETNIM) to diagnose tumor hypoxia.

Markers of Lipid Metabolism

An elevated level of phosphatidylcholine has been found in tumors. It is the most abundant phospholipid in the cell membranes of all eukaryotic cells and provides a potential target for tumor imaging. This elevation is thought to be the result of increased uptake of choline, a precursor of the biosynthesis of phosphatidylcholine. Malignant tumors show a high proliferation and increased metabolism of cell membrane components that will lead to an increased uptake of choline.[55] Thus, [^{11}C]choline can be used as a PET marker for imaging cell membrane proliferation in prostate cancer,[56] brain tumors,[57] and many other types of tumors[58] that lack the urinary radioactivity seen with ^{18}F-FDG.[56,59] [^{18}F]Fluorocholine and fluorine-18–labeled choline analogs also have been developed as new and promising oncologic PET tracers for prostate cancer and breast cancer.[60–62]

Markers of Tumor Cell Proliferation

Noninvasive imaging assessment of tumor cell proliferation could be helpful in the evaluation of tumor growth potential and the degree of malignancy, and in the early assessment of treatment response prior to changes in tumor size. Radiolabeled nucleoside/nucleotide analogs should provide proliferative imaging information of primary and secondary tumors.[28–32] They may also assist in selecting and following the most favorable choice of nucleoside/nucleotide therapy and in following its outcome. Our rationale is that if the binding of nucleoside/nucleotide to tumor cell DNA/RNA can be detected with PET, then such a nucleoside/nucleotide analog may be useful to evaluate the response of nucleoside/nucleotide (e.g., 5-fluorouracil, 5-fluorodeoxyuridine, 5-bromodeoxyuridine, cytidine, cytarabine) therapy for tumors. Thus, for DNA/RNA markers, ^{18}F-fluoroadenosine, ^{18}F-fluorothymidine, and fluoro-^{11}C-methyl-arabinofuranosyluracil were developed. These ligands are intended to improve the understanding of the biologic behavior of malignant tumors, which should lead to better prognostic evaluation, treatment follow-up, and patient management.

Gene Expression Markers

Radiolabeled pyrimidine and purine probes for imaging herpes simplex virus type 1 thymidine kinase (HSV-1-*tk*) expression and other reporter genes by PET have been developed. For example, pyrimidine nucleoside (e.g., FIAU, 2′-fluoro-2′-deoxy-5-iodo-1-β-D-ribo-furanosyl-uracil [FIRU], 2′-fluoro-2′-5-methyl-1-β-D-arabinofuranosyl-uracil [FMAU], 2′-fluoro-2′-deoxy-5-iodovinyl-1-β-D-ribofuranosyl-uracil [IVFRU]) and acycloguanosine [9-[(2-hydroxy-1-(hydroxymethyl)ethoxy)methyl]-guanine (GCV) and 9-[4-hydroxy-3-(hydroxymethyl)butyl]guanine (PCV)[63–68]] and other ^{18}F-labeled acycloguanosine analogs, such as 8-fluoro-9-[(2-hydroxy-1-(hydroxymethyl)ethoxy)methyl]guanine (FGCV),[65,66] 8-fluoro-9-[4-hydroxy-3-(hydroxymethyl)butyl]guanine (FPCV),[67,68] 9-[3-fluoro-1-hydroxy-2-propoxymethyl]guanine (FHPG),[69,70] and 9-[4-fluoro-3-(hydroxymethyl)butyl]guanine (FHBG),[71] have been developed as reporter substrates for imaging wild-type and mutant[67] HSV-1-*tk* expression. Recently, imaging, pharmacokinetics, and dosimetry of ^{18}F-FHBG were reported in healthy volunteers as a first step to imaging HSV-1-*tk* reporter expression in clinical gene therapy trials.[72] The difficulty with these probes is that HSV-1-*tk* enzyme expression depends on HSV-1-*tk* gene transduction with adenoviral vectors. The level of HSV-1-*tk* enzyme expression is likely to be different in the different transduced cells and tissues; thus, the application of the HSV-1-*tk* probe is limited. Understanding of tumor proliferative activity could aid in the selection of optimal therapy by estimating patient prognosis and selecting the proper management.

Synthetic Materials and Methods for PET Agents

Glucose Transport

A major advance in the synthesis of ^{18}F-FDG from [^{18}F]fluoride was made using kryptofix to increase the reactivity of [^{18}F]fluoride. Kryptofix masks the potassium ions, which are the counter-ions of the

[^{18}F]fluoride. The reaction of [^{18}F]fluoride with 1,3,4,6-tetra-O-acetyl-2-O-trifluoromethanesulfonyl-B-D-mannopyranase to give 1,3,4,6-tetra-O-acetyl-2-[^{18}F]fluoro-B-D-glycopyranase results in a 95% incorporation of ^{18}F, and the overall synthesis, including purification, proceeds to give about a 60% yield. The synthesis involves two steps: displacement with [^{18}F]fluoride and deprotection with HCl.

Amino Acid Transport

A nucleophilic reactant K^{18}F reacts with L-tosylpropyl-AmT to yield ^{18}F-fluoropropyl-AmT (FPAMT, 40–50%). The synthetic scheme is shown in Figure 4.1.

Markers of Estrogen Receptor Tissue

Using clomiphene, a three-step process to hydroxytamoxifen, tosyl tamoxifen, and halogenated tamoxifen was developed.[73,74] Eight *cis* and *trans* isomers of halogenated tamoxifen analogs were then prepared. In testing these two conformational isomers, we compared their killing power on human breast tumor cells as well as their binding power. Under our approved investigation of new drugs (IND number 40,589) from the Food and Drug Administration (FDA), we have assessed ER+ breast tumors in 10 patients using ^{18}F-FTX (2–12 mCi IV). In a typical study, a patient is positioned supine in the scanner so that the detector rings span the entire breast. A 20-minute attenuation scan is performed with a 4-mCi ^{68}Ge-ring source prior to administering ^{18}F-FTX. After each patient receives ^{18}F-FTX, six consecutive 20-minute scans are taken. Serial transaxial images are performed using the scanner (Posicam 6.5, Positron Corp., Houston, TX), which has a field of view of 42 cm on the transverse and 12 cm on the coronal plane. The axial resolution in the reconstructed plane is 1.2 cm. Twenty-one transaxial slices separated by 5.2 mm are reconstructed. Visual inspection as well as semiquantitative evaluation using standard uptake value (SUV, the activity in tumor/injected dose × body weight) was used. Before PET scanning, the position of breast tumors is determined by contrast-enhanced CT (High Speed Advantages, General Electric Co., Milwaukee, WI) or MRI using the 1.5-T scanner (GE Medical System, Milwaukee, WI). Eight of 10 patients received tamoxifen therapy after the PET study. The response to tamoxifen therapy was evaluated after 6 months.

Markers of Tumor Hypoxia

Synthesis of [^{18}F]FMISO and [^{18}F]FETNIM

Aliquots containing 500 to 800 mCi of ^{18}F activity after 1-hour beam time (18 μA current) were collected. The irradiated water was combined with kryptofix-2,2,2 (26 mg) and anhydrous potassium carbonate (4.6 mg), heated under reduced pressure to remove ^{18}O water, and dried by azeotropic distillation with acetonitrile (3 × 1.5 mL). The tosyl analog of 2-nitroimidazole (20 mg) was dissolved in acetonitrile (1.5 mL), added to the kryptofix-fluoride complex, and then warmed at 95°C for 7 minutes.[42,52] After cooling, the reaction mixture was passed through a silica gel Sep-Pak column (Whatman Inc., Clifton, NJ) and eluted with ether (2 × 2.5 mL). The solvent was evaporated and the resulting mixture hydrolyzed with 2 N HCl (1 mL) at 105°C for 7 minutes. The mixture was cooled under N_2 and neutralized with 2 N NaOH (0.8 mL) and 1 N $NaHCO_3$ (1 mL). The mixture was passed through a short alumina column, a C-18 Sep-Pak column, and a 0.22-μm millipore filter, followed by eluting 6 mL of 10% ethanol/saline. A yield of 80 to 100 mCi of pure product was isolated (25–40% yield, decay corrected) with the end of bombardment (EOB) at 60 minutes. HPLC was done on a C-18 ODS-120T column, 4.6 × 25 mm, with water/acetonitrile, (80/20), using a flow rate of 1 mL/minute. The no-carrier-added product corresponded to the retention time (6.12 minutes) of the unlabeled FMISO under similar conditions. The radiochemical purity was greater than 99%. Under the ultraviolet (UV) ray detector (310 nm), there were no other impurities. A radio-TLC scanner (Bioscan, Washington, DC) showed a retardation factor of 0.6 for FMISO using a 5 × 20 cm silica gel plate (Whatman, Inc., Clifton, NJ), eluted with chloroform/methanol (7:3), which corresponds to the unlabeled FMISO. In addition, kryptofix-2,2,2 was not visualized (developed in the iodine chamber) on the silica-gel–coated plate using 0.1% (v/v) triethylamine in methanol as an eluent. The specific activity of [^{18}F]FMISO and [^{18}F]FETNIM determined were 1 Ci/μmol based on UV and radioactivity detection of a sample of known mass and radioactivity.

PET Imaging of Head and Neck Tumor Hypoxia Using [^{18}F]FMISO

Under our approved IND number 43,997 from the FDA, we have completed three studies using [^{18}F]FMISO. In a typical study, a patient is positioned supine in the scanner so that the detector rings span the entire head and neck. A 20-minute attenuation scan is performed with a 4 mCi ^{68}Ge-ring source prior to administering [^{18}F]FMISO. After each patient receives 10 mCi of [^{18}F]FMISO, six consecutive 20-minute scans are taken. Serial transaxial images are performed using the scanner (Posicam 6.5, Positron Corp., Houston, TX), which has a field of view of 42 cm on the transverse and 12 cm on the coronal plane. The axial resolution in the reconstructed plane is 1.2 cm. Twenty-one transaxial slices separated by 5.2 mm are reconstructed and displayed in SUV, which measures the ratio of tissue [^{18}F]FMISO uptake to that of whole-body uptake (normalized for body weight and injected dose) for each scan. Before PET scanning, the position of head and neck tumors is also determined by contrast-enhanced CT (High Speed Advantages, GE Medical System, Milwaukee, WI).

Autoradiographic Studies of Misonidazole Analogs in Tumor-Bearing Rats

Female Fischer 344 breast tumor–bearing rats and Lewis lung tumor–bearing mice (3/ligand) after receiving [^{18}F]FMISO (1–1.5 mCi IV) were euthanized at 1 hour. The rodent body was fixed in a carboxymethyl cellulose (4%) block. The frozen body in the block was mounted to a cryostat microtome (LKB, Ijamsville, MD), and 100-μm coronal sections were made. The section was freeze-dried and then placed on x-ray film (X-Omat AR, Kodak, Rochester, NY) for 24 hours.

Polar Graphic Oxygen Needle Probe Measurements

To confirm hypoxic tumors detected by imaging, intratumoral pO_2 measurements were performed using the Eppendorf computed histographic system. Twenty to 25 pO_2 measurements along each of two to three linear tracks were performed at 0.4-mm intervals on each tumor (40–75 measurements total). Tumor pO_2 measurements were made on three tumor-bearing rats and three rabbits. Using an on-line computer system, the pO_2 measurements of each track were expressed as absolute values relative to the location of the measuring point along the track, and as the relative frequencies within a pO_2 histogram between 0 and 100 mm Hg with a class width of 2.5 mm.

Markers of Lipid Metabolism

After ^{11}C-carbon dioxide production in a cyclotron and the subsequent ^{11}C-methyl-iodide synthesis, methyl-^{11}C-choline was synthesized by the reaction of ^{11}C-methyl-iodide with "neat" dimethylaminoethanol at 120°C for 5 minutes. Purification was achieved by evaporation of the reactants followed by passage of the aqueous solution of the product through a cation-exchange resin cartridge. The time required for overall chemical processing, excluding the cyclotron operation, was 15 minutes. Radiochemical yield was >98%. Radiochemical purity was >98%. Chemical purity was >90% (dimethylaminoethanol was the only possible impurity). Specific radioactivity of the product was >133 GBq/μmol. PET was performed on cancer patients from the level of the pelvis to the lower abdomen. After transmission scanning, 370 MBq ^{11}C-choline was injected intravenously. The emission scan was performed 5 to 15 minutes postinjection. Finally, PET images were displayed so that each pixel was painted by a specified color representing the degree of SUV. The ^{11}C-choline image was compared with the ^{18}F-FDG image obtained from the same patient.

No-carrier-added [^{18}F]fluoroethyl choline [^{18}F]FECh was synthesized by two-step reactions: first, tetrabutylammonium (TBA) ^{18}F-fluoride was reacted with 1,2-bis(tosyloxy)ethane to yield 2-^{18}F-fluoroethyl tosylate; second, 2-^{18}F-fluoroethyl tosylate was reacted with *N,N*-dimethylethanolamine to yield ^{18}F-FECh, which was then purified by chromatography. An automated apparatus was constructed for preparation of the ^{18}F-FECh injection solution. In vitro experiments were performed to examine the uptake of ^{18}F-FECh in Ehrlich ascites tumor cells, and the metabolites were analyzed by solvent extraction followed by various kinds of chromatography. Clinical studies of ^{18}F-FECh PET were performed on patients with untreated primary prostate cancer, and the data were compared with those of ^{11}C-choline PET on the same patients.

Markers of Tumor Cell Proliferation

Synthesis of ^{18}F-Fluoro-2′-Deoxyadenosine [9-(2′-Deoxy-2′-Fluoro-b-D-Arabinofuranosyl)Adenine](FAD)

2′-O-p-toluenesulfonyladenosine (100 mg, 0.238 mmol) was derivatized along with N^6, O-3′, and O-5′ acetylated analogs by dissolving in tetrahydrofuran (5 mL) and acetic anhydride (2 mL), along with pyridine (2 mL).[76,76] The reaction was stirred overnight. The solvent, excess of pyridine, and unreacted acetic anhydride were removed by evaporation, and the residue was chromatographed on silica gel (with ethyl acetate as eluent). Aliquots containing 20 to 40 mCi of [^{18}F]fluoride were combined with kryptofix-2,2,2 and anhydrous potassium carbonate and heated to remove [^{18}O]H_2O. The triacetylated tosyl analog of adenosine was dissolved in acetonitrile, added to the kryptofix-fluoride (fluorine-18) complex, and then heated at 95°C for 10 minutes. After cooling, the reaction mixture was passed through a silica-gel–packed column (SPE 500 mg) and eluted with acetonitrile (ACN, 2 mL). After solvent evaporation, the acetyl groups were deprotected with 2 N HCl (1 mL) at 105°C for 10 minutes. The product was neutralized with 2 N NaOH (0.8 mL) and 1 N $NaHCO_3$ (1 mL). The product was then eluted through a reverse phase C-18 column (Sep-Pak Cartridge, Waters, Milford, MD) and a 0.22-mm filter, followed by saline (3 mL).

Markers of Gene Expression

Using a known procedure, di-tritylated tosylbutylguanine (TsHBG) was synthesized. Mass spectrum and NMR spectrum were determined. Under similar conditions for the synthesis of ^{18}F-fluorinated adenosine, ^{18}F-FHBG was synthesized. A C-18 reverse-phase Sep-Pak was used to purify the compound.

Results of Synthesis for PET Agents

The overall synthesis of ^{18}F-FDG including purification proceeds to result in about a 60% yield after displacement with [^{18}F]fluoride and deprotection with HCl. The simplest method to remove kryptofix is the incorporation of a short cation exchange resin in the synthesis system so that the hydrolysate (HCl) passes through the cartridge before final purification; 2-deoxy-2-chloro-D-glucose (ClDG) was identified as an impurity with less than 100 μg during chromatographic determination of the specific activity of ^{18}F-FDG preparations from the nucleophilic route.

Amino Acid Transport

Proton NMR spectrum of L-tosylpropylAmT is shown in Figure 4.2. Figures 4.3 and 4.4 show HPLC and radio-TLC analysis of [^{18}F]FPAMT. There was a similarity in cellular uptake both in vitro (Fig. 4.5) and in vivo (Fig. 4.6) between [^{18}F]FPAMT and [^{18}F]FDG. Due to a zwitterion, there was much less uptake in brain compared to [^{18}F]FDG. Clinical images indicated that low-grade brain tumor could be imaged with [^{18}F]FPAMT (Figs. 4.7 and 4.8).

Markers of Estrogen Receptor Tissues

Using MCF-7 cells incubated for 72 hours, we observed that the eight new compounds were superior in killing power compared to tamox-

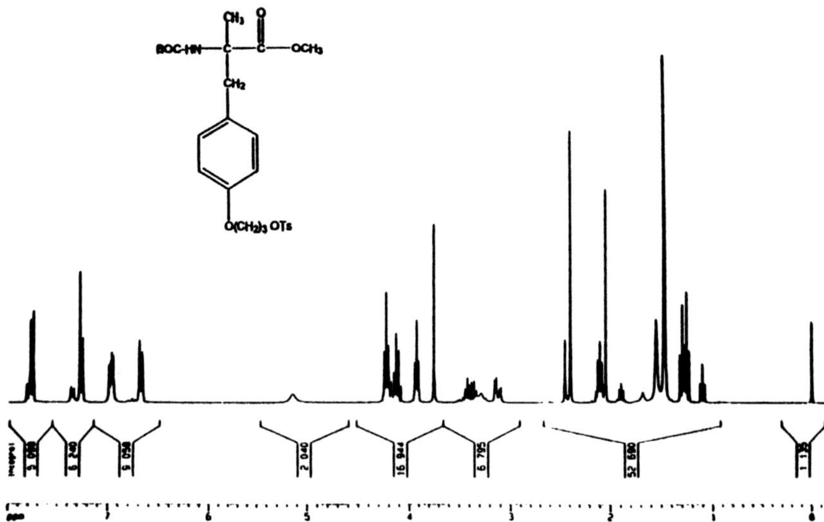

FIGURE 4.2. ^{1}H-NMR of N-BOC-tosylpropyl-α-methyltyrosine methyl ester.

ifen; for example, the bromo had almost 25 times the killing power of tamoxifen.[77,78] By using pig uterine cytosol, we noted that halogenated tamoxifen had a better binding affinity than tamoxifen itself. Bromotamoxifen was 150 times better than tamoxifen, and fluorotamoxifen had a binding power 30 times that of tamoxifen.

Of these eight different agents, we pursued fluorotamoxifen for its killing and binding power and were interested in using this technol-

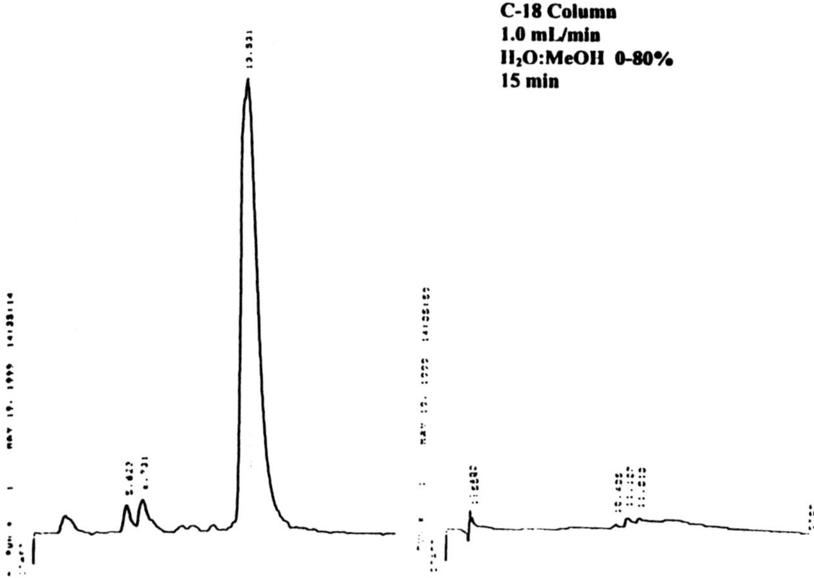

FIGURE 4.3. High-performance liquid chromatography (HPLC) analysis of ^{18}F-FPAMT (left: radioactive, right: UV).

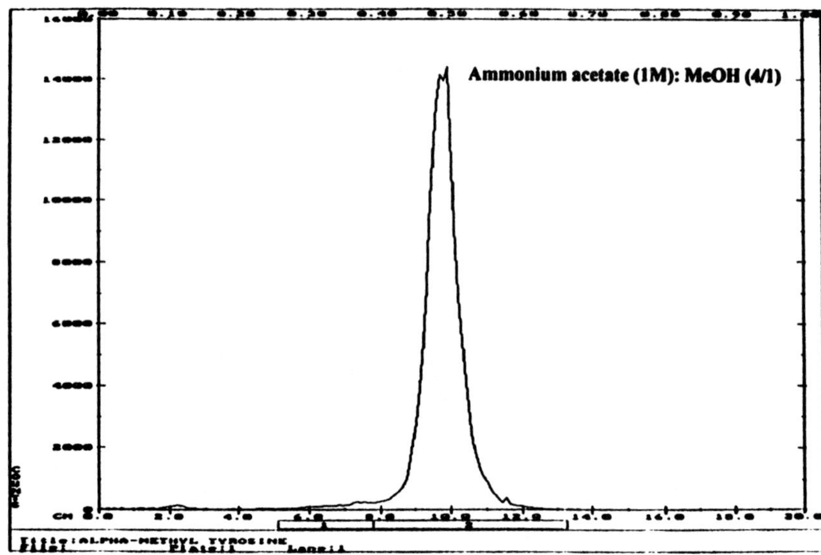

FIGURE 4.4. Radio-TLC analysis of ^{18}F-FPAMT.

ogy as a PET imaging agent. Using the PET camera, the uterus of a pig was defined. We then administered the fluorotamoxifen and noted a configuration that was much like what we saw in the anatomic specimen, with the uterus and the fallopian-tube–ovarian complex (Fig. 4.9). From the cross-sectional configuration it appears that fluorotamoxifen can be used as an imaging agent as well (Fig. 4.10). By administering tamoxifen, or diethylstilbestrol (DES), the uptake in the target organ

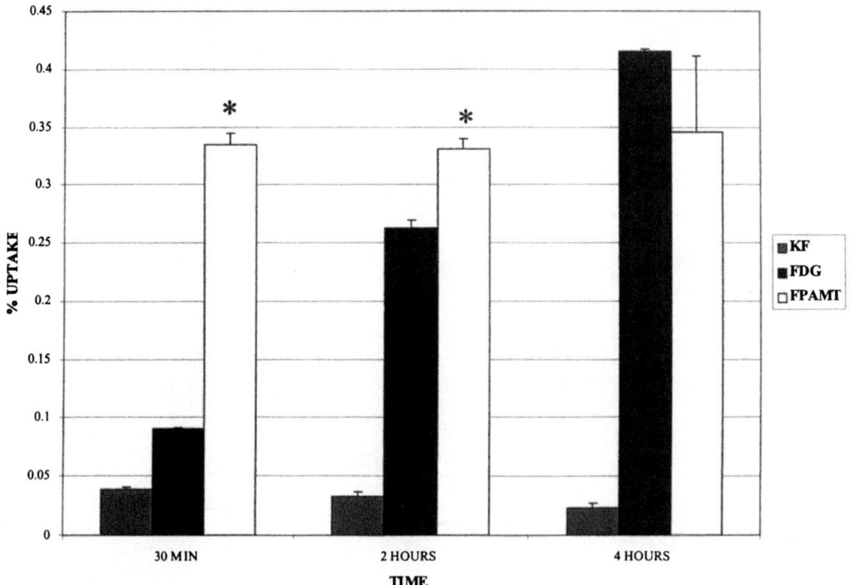

FIGURE 4.5. Cellular uptake of ^{18}F-FDG and ^{18}F-FPAMT in breast cancer cell line.

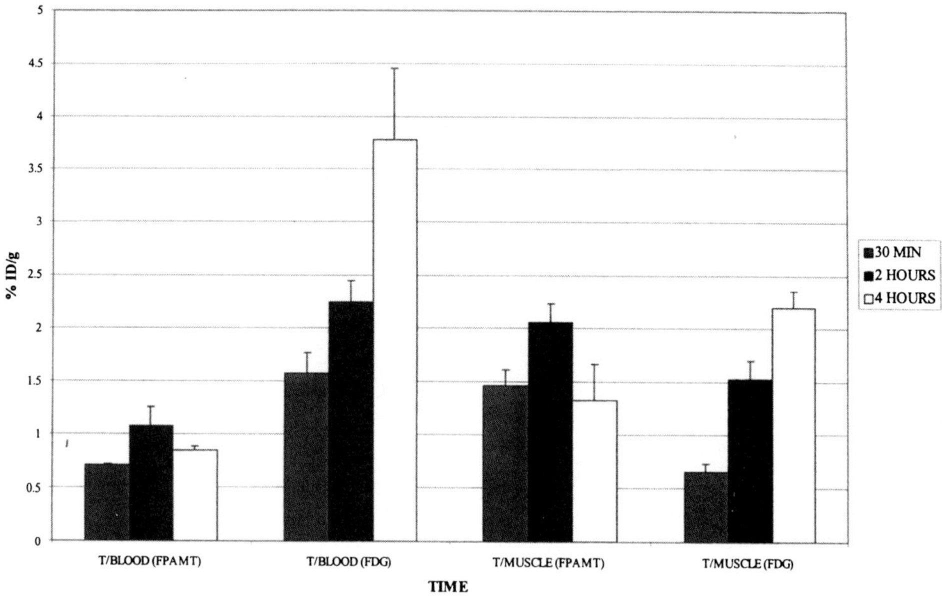

FIGURE 4.6. Tumor-to-tissues count density ratios of ^{18}F-FDG and ^{18}F-FPAMT in breast tumor–bearing rats.

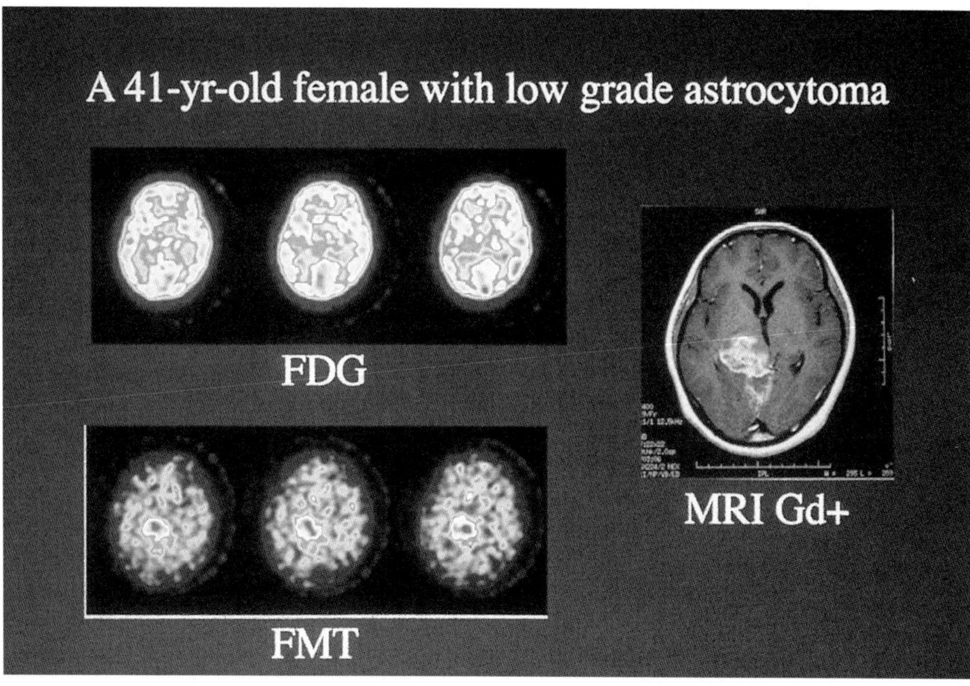

FIGURE 4.7. Imaging comparison between FDG and FPAMT indicated that low-grade brain tumor could be imaged with FPAMT.

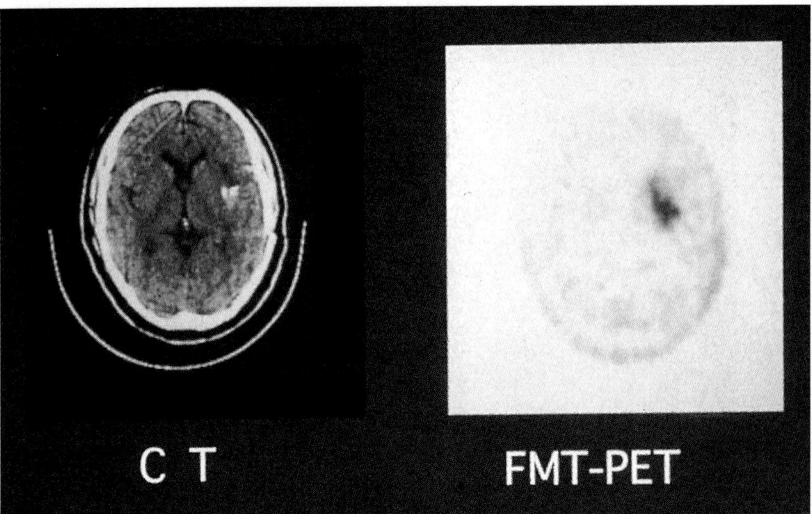

FIGURE 4.8. A select PET image indicated that recurrent glioma could be imaged with ^{18}F-FAmT.

could be blocked (Fig. 4.11).[79] As a breast tumor model, we used a rat with deposition of ER+ tumor cells (NF 13762 cell line) in the flank. In utilizing fluorotamoxifen, we observed uptake within the uterus as well as in the tumor in the flank, which suggests we have a fluorinated tamoxifen that can readily visualize ER sites, even in the implanted neoplasm. In studying the distribution, we noted fairly good uptake in the tumor, brain, and liver. We found fairly good biodistribution in the uterus/blood count ratio. The count ratio was 13.5, and the uterine uptake could be blocked somewhat by any of the estrogens or by tamoxifen itself. Fluorotamoxifen can be prepared as an analog of tamoxifen itself with high specific activity, and it can image ER+ sites in the animal models and in humans.[80,81] In addition, such ligands might help in determining the causes of occasional failure of tamoxifen therapy when biopsy indicators are ER+.

To date we have used an ^{18}F-labeled tamoxifen ligand (2–12 mCi IV) to image 10 patients with ER+ breast tumors (IND number 40,589) by PET. We found it is possible to visualize both primary and metastatic breast tumors by their uptake of the radiolabeled tamoxifen ligand (Fig. 4.12). Of the 10 patients, three had tumors that showed good uptake of the radiolabeled ligand and positive responses to tamoxifen therapy.[82,83] However, we observed high uptake in the liver and lung, which affected the imaging and created difficulty in interpretation of tumors near those organs. Others have also reported that liver and lung tamoxifen uptake levels can remain high between 3 and 14 days of therapy.

Markers of Tumor Hypoxia

Autoradiographs of ^{18}F-FMISO showed that tumor necrotic region could be differentiated (Figs. 4.13 and 4.14). Clinical PET studies

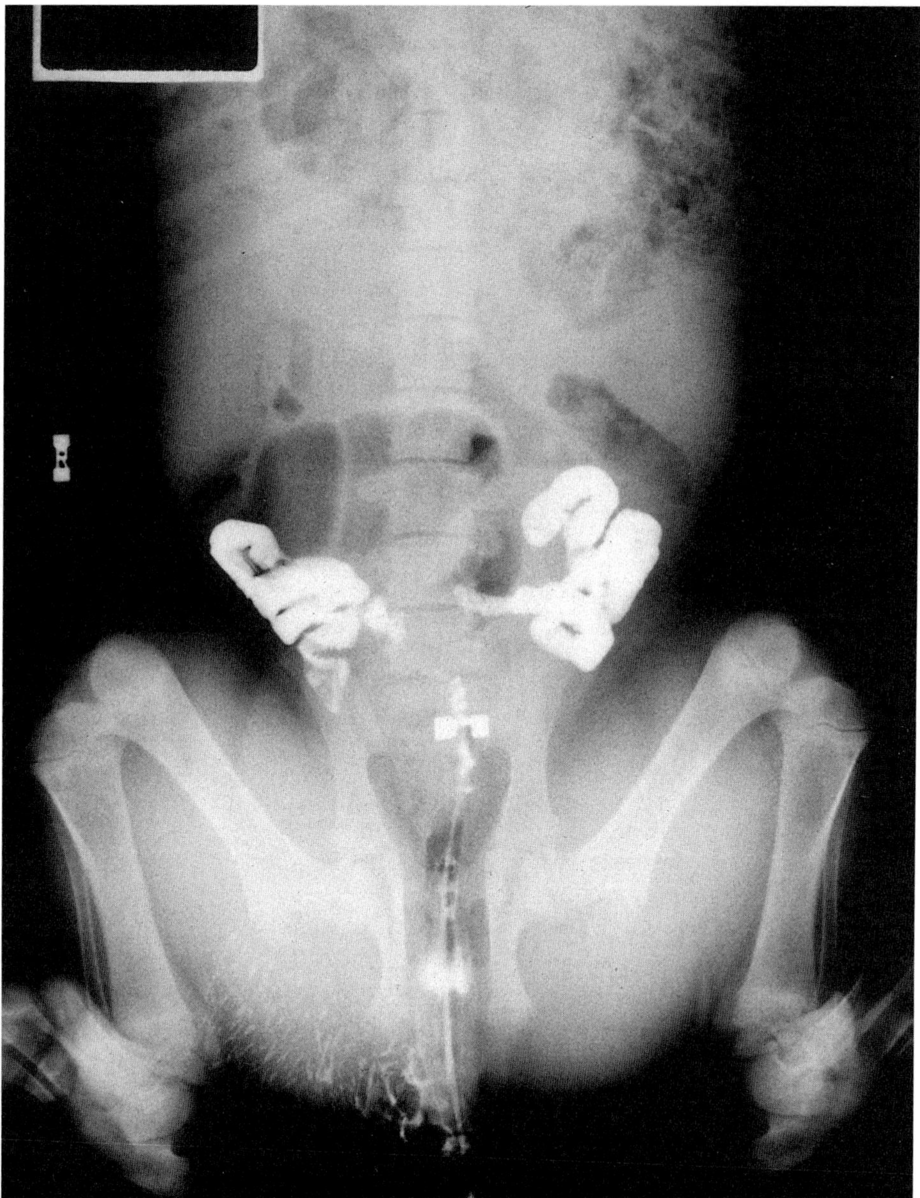

FIGURE 4.9. Salpingogram showed the localization of a pig uterine tissue.

showed that the tumors could be well visualized on ^{18}F-FMISO and ^{18}F-FETNIM tests (Figs. 4.15 to 4.17). The tumor oxygen tension was 3 to 6 mm Hg as compared to the normal, 30 to 40 mm Hg.

Marker of Lipid Metabolism

Imaging of prostate cancer and its local metastasis was difficult when ^{18}F-FDG was used because, within the pelvis, the areas of high uptake

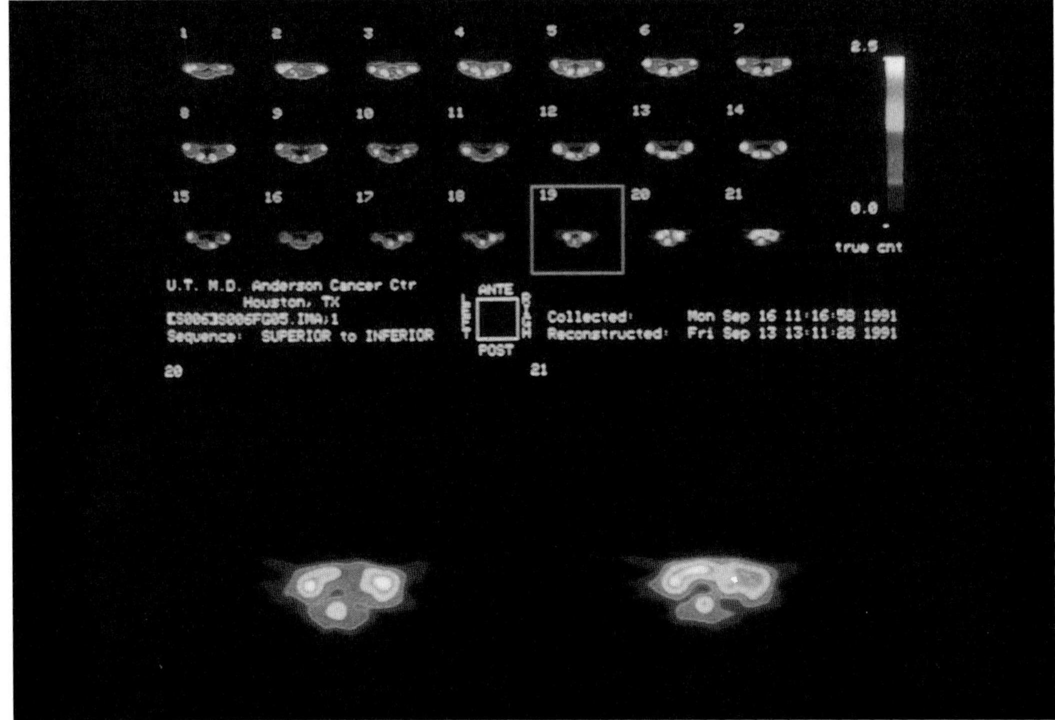

FIGURE 4.10. PET-fluorotamoxifen images showed that the uterine tissue of a pig could be imaged.

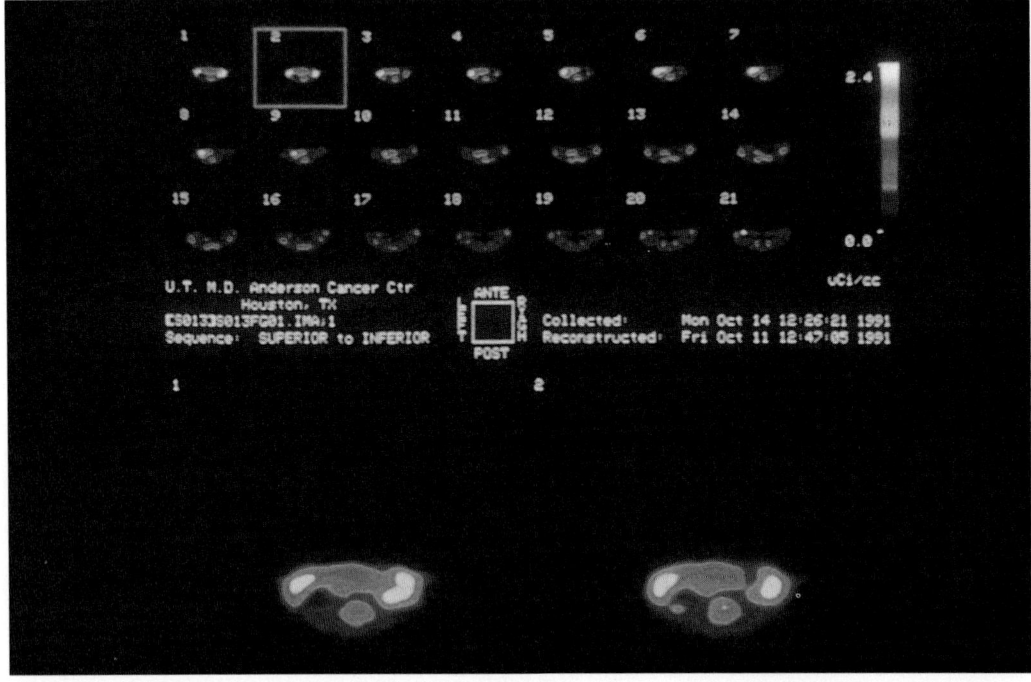

FIGURE 4.11. Pretreatment of a pig with diethylstilbestrol could decrease uptake of ^{18}F-fluorotamoxifen.

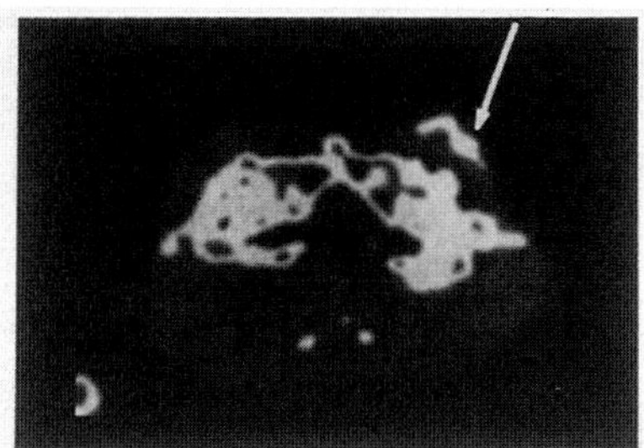

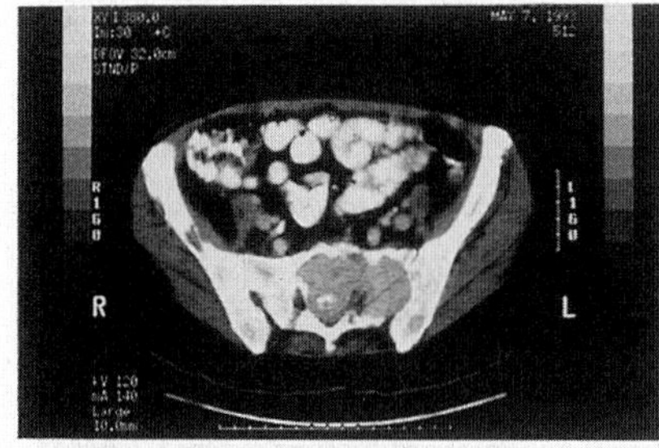

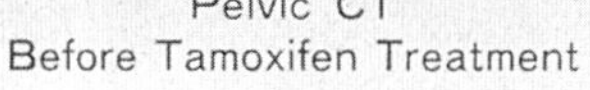

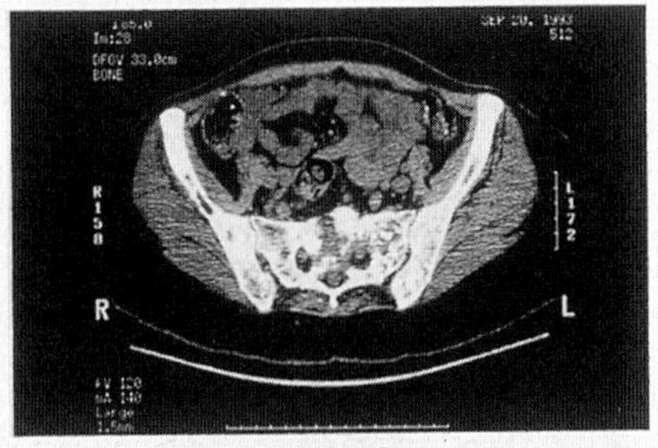

FIGURE 4.12. PET-18F-fluorotamoxifen showed that an estrogen receptor positive (ER+) tumor could be imaged. The patient showed positive response to hormonal therapy.

were concealed by the overwhelmingly abundant radioactivity in urine (in ureters and bladder). By contrast, it was easy when ^{11}C-choline was used because the urinary activity was negligible and tumor uptake was marked. The radioactivity concentration of ^{11}C-choline in prostate cancer and metastatic sites was at an SUV of more than three in most cases. The SUV of ^{18}F-FDG was considerably lower than that of ^{11}C-choline (Fig. 4.18). The sensitivity and specificity of ^{18}F-FDG and ^{11}C-choline are shown in Table 4.1. ^{18}F-FECh was prepared in high yield and purity. The in vitro experiment revealed that ^{18}F-FECh was incorporated into tumor cells by active transport, then phosphorylated (yielding phosphoryl^{18}F-FECh) in the cells, and finally integrated into phospholipids. The clinical PET studies showed marked uptake of ^{18}F-FECh in prostate cancer.[60,61] A dynamic PET study on one patient revealed that the blood level of ^{18}F-FECh decreased rapidly (in 1 minute), the prostate cancer level became almost maximal in a short period (1.5 minutes) and it remained constant for a long time (60 minutes), and the urinary radioactivity became prominent after a short time lag (5 minutes). Static PET studies conducted under bladder irrigation showed no difference between ^{18}F-FECh uptake and ^{11}C-choline uptake in prostate cancer. However, ^{18}F-FECh gave a slightly higher spatial resolution of the image, which was attributed to the shorter positron range of ^{18}F. The synthesis of ^{18}F-FECh was easy and reliable. ^{18}F-FECh PET was very effective in detecting prostate cancer in patients.

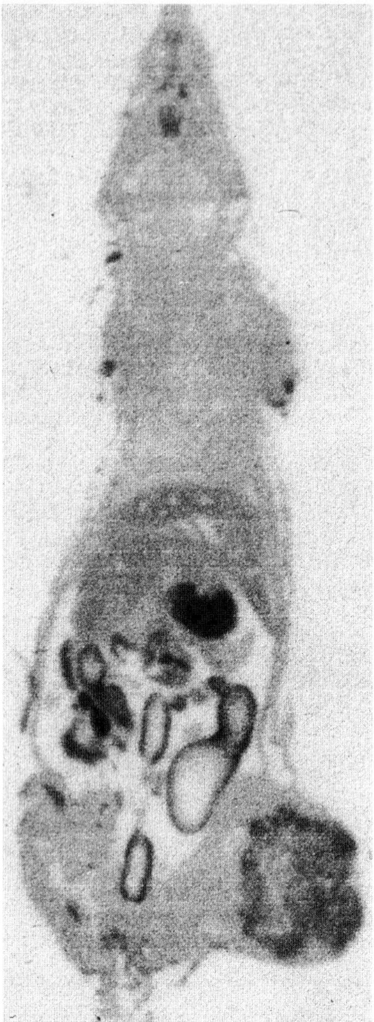

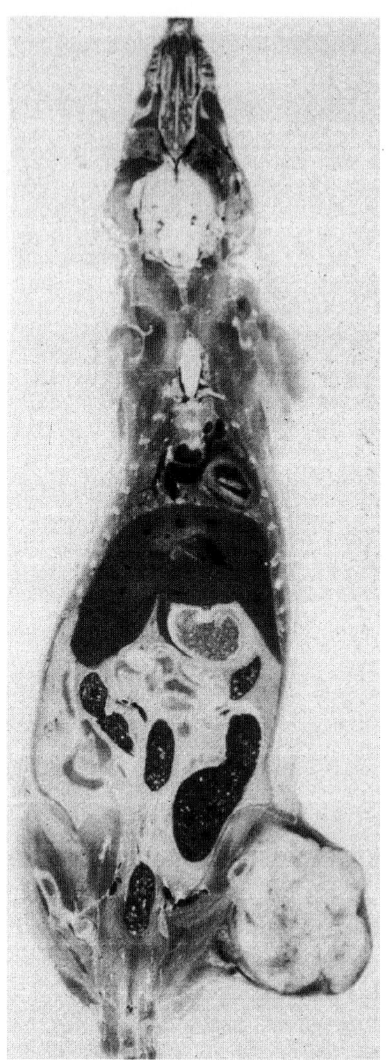

FIGURE 4.13. Autoradiogram of ^{18}F-FMISO indicated that tumor necrotic region could be assessed.

Markers of Tumor Cell Proliferation

The radioactivity of the final product (structure shown in Fig. 4.19 was 7 to 15 mCi, 50% to 60%, decay corrected) with the end of bombardment at 70 minutes. Under similar condition, ^{18}F-fluorinated uracil (structure shown in Fig. 4.20) was synthesized. Autoradiogram showed that the tumor could be visualized with ^{18}F-fluorinated uracil (Fig. 4.21).

Markers of Gene Expression

Using a known procedure, di-tritylated tosylpenclovir (TsHBG) was synthesized. Mass spectrum and NMR spectrum are shown in Figures 4.22 and 4.23. Under similar condition for the synthesis of ^{18}F-fluorinated adenosine, ^{18}F-FHBG was synthesized. A C-18 reverse phase Sep-Pak was used to purify the compound. The radiochemical yield of ^{18}F-

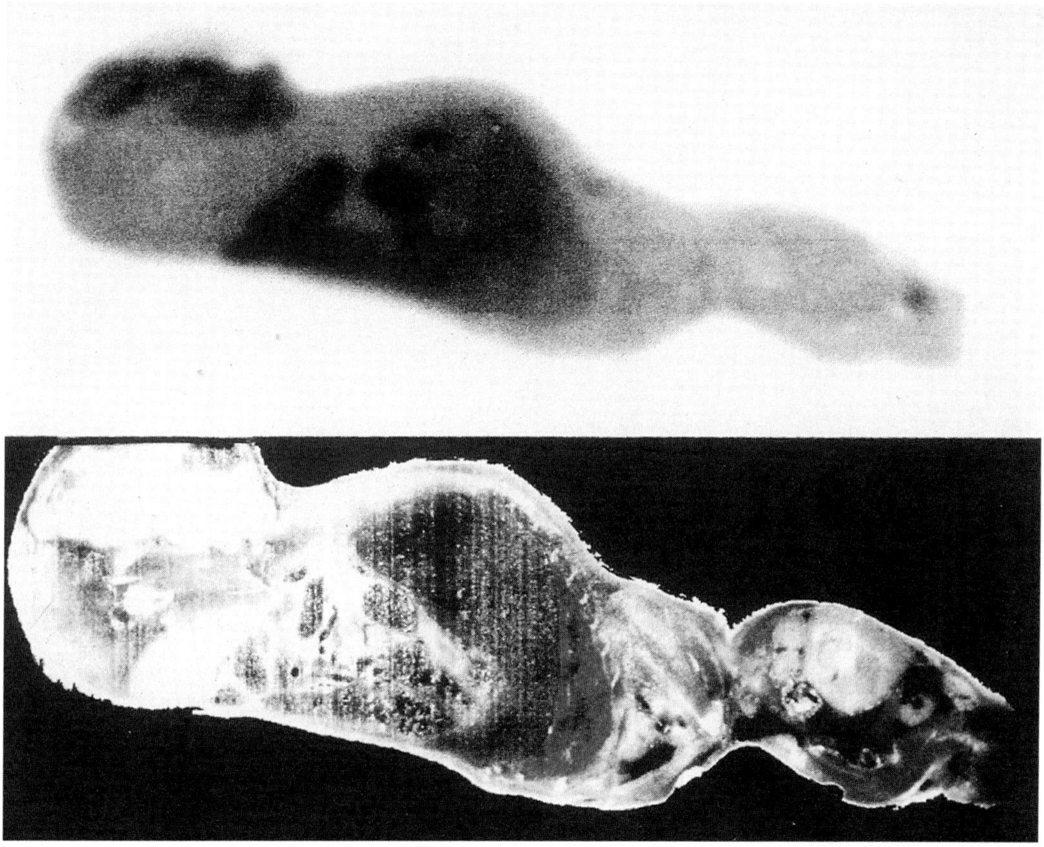

FIGURE 4.14. Autoradiogram of ^{18}F-FMISO showed that lung tumor could be imaged.

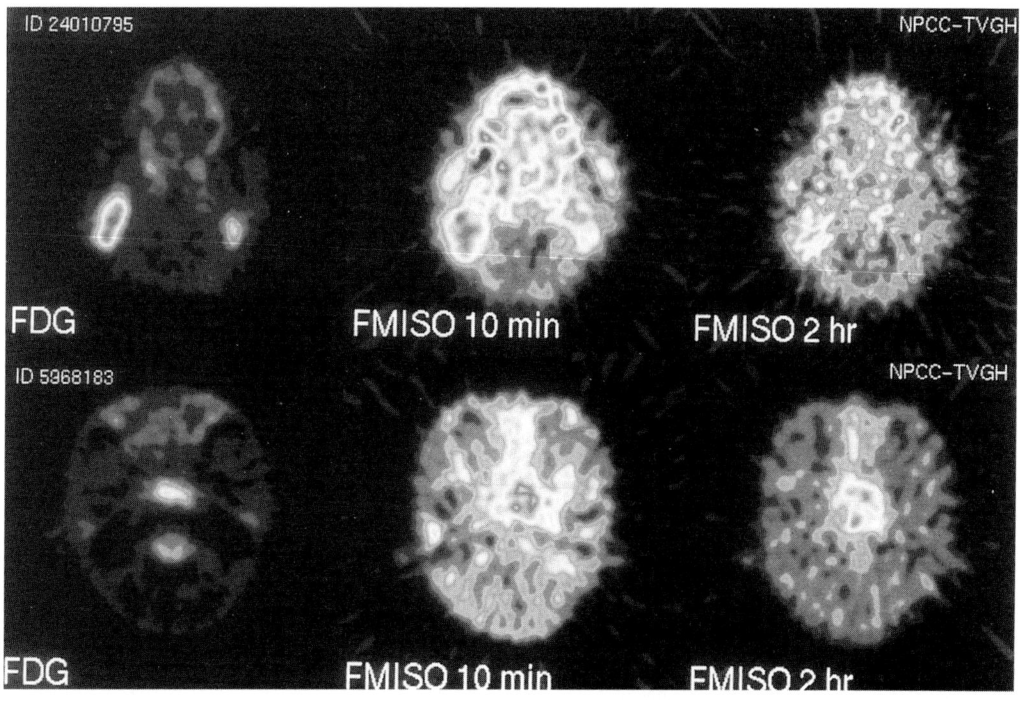

FIGURE 4.15. PET ^{18}F-FMISO showed that tumor hypoxia could be assessed.

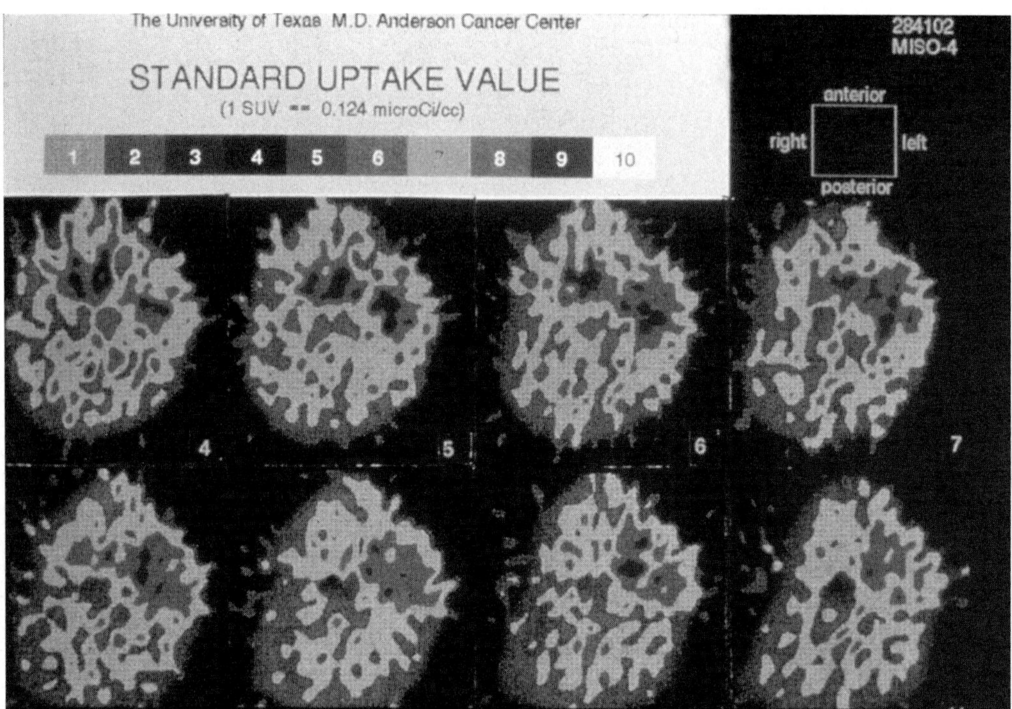

FIGURE 4.16. PET ^{18}F-FMISO showed that tumor hypoxia could be imaged.

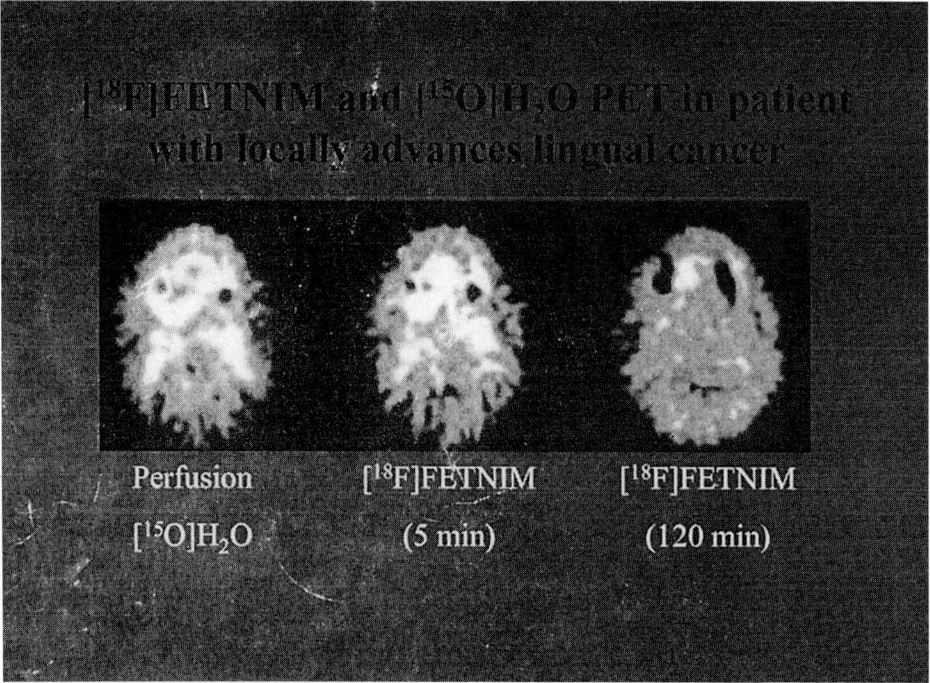

FIGURE 4.17. In the early phase, [^{18}F]FETNIM uptake is associate with blood flow, and later there is differential uptake between well- and poorly oxygenated tissues.

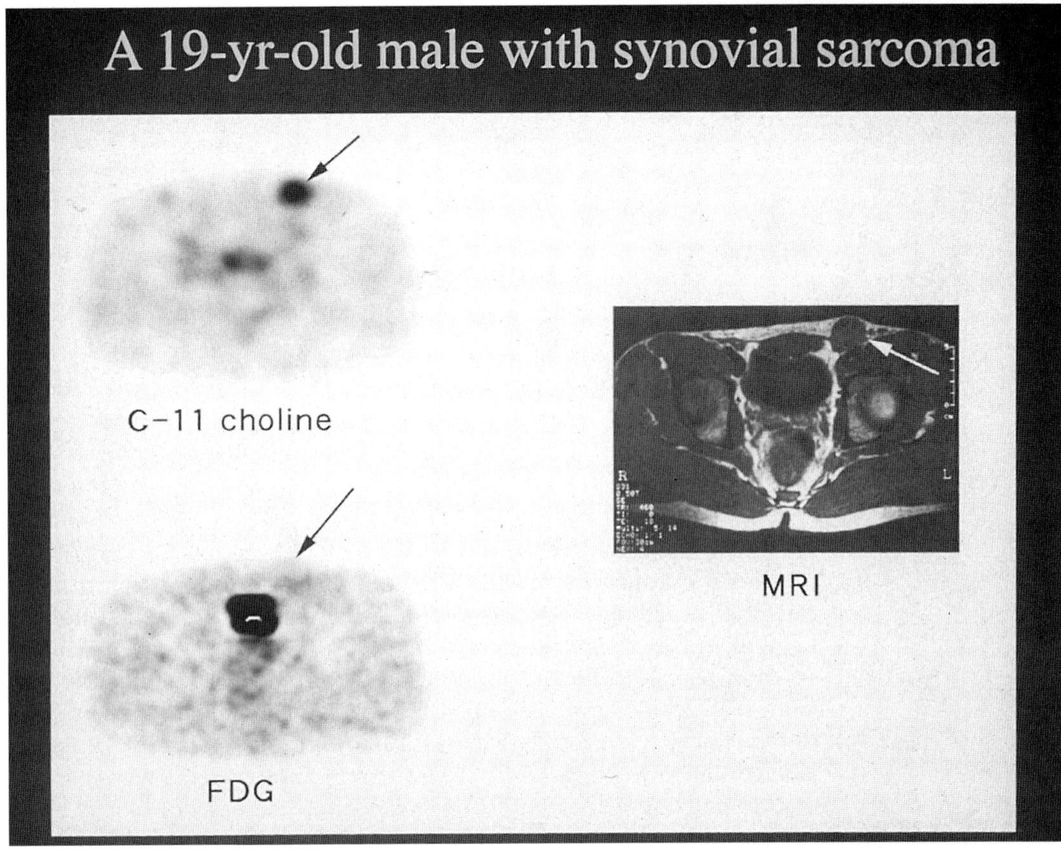

FIGURE 4.18. PET ^{11}C-choline showed that tumor could be imaged due to less bladder uptake.

FHBG was 10% to 15% (decay corrected), with the end of bombardment at 90 minutes. Radio-TLC is shown in Figure 4.24.

Discussion

Placing an iodine atom or a fluorine atom on the aromatic ring of tamoxifen has been previously reported.[84,85] These analogs produced either low affinities for estrogen receptors or low specific activities, neither suitable for imaging estrogen responsive tissues. When ^{11}C-labeled tamoxifen was synthesized, the specific activity was also low.[86] Placing a chlorine atom on the aliphatic side chain of tamoxifen produced a higher affinity than that of tamoxifen.[87] However, this compound is

TABLE 4.1. PET results of diagnostic accuracy

	Sensitivity	Specificity
C-11 choline	67% (18/27 lesions)	95% (53/56 lesions)
FDG	48% (13/27 lesions)	100% (56/56 lesions)

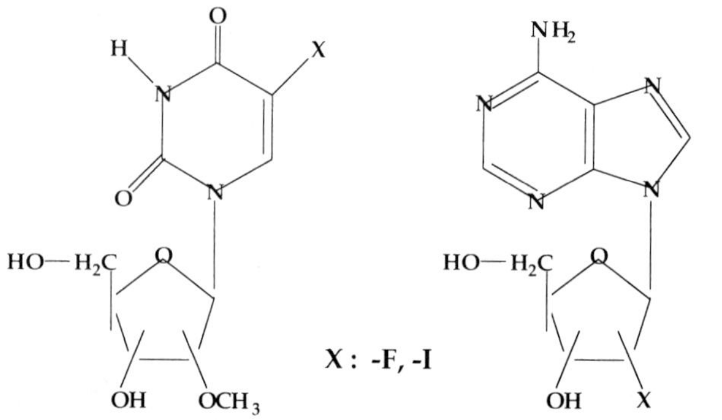

2'-O-Methyluridine 2'-Deoxyadenosine

X : -F, -I

FIGURE 4.19. Structure of ^{18}F-fluorinated adenosine.

not suitable for imaging purposes since there is no existing cyclotron-produced isotope for chlorine. Previous studies from our group indicate that replacing a chlorine with a halomethyl group develops a higher binding affinity for tamoxifen.

At present, 10 patients with ER+ breast tumors (IND number 40,589) using ^{18}F-labeled tamoxifen ligand (2–12 mCi IV) were imaged by PET. Both primary and metastatic breast tumors could be diagnosed by ^{18}F-labeled tamoxifen ligands. Three lesions in three patients were considered to be truly negative for breast cancer on the basis of biopsy specimens and/or clinical course. Five (71.4%) of seven patients and 16 (80%) of 20 lesions were interpreted to be truly positive for breast cancer. The mean SUV of the radiotracer in tumor was 2.8 on delayed images. There was no significant correlation between the SUV of [^{18}F]fluorotamoxifen in the lesion and the ER concentration in primary or metastatic lesions. Eight of 10 patients received tamoxifen therapy after the PET study. Three patients who had a good response to tamoxifen therapy showed an SUV of [^{18}F]fluorotamoxifen of more than 2.4 in the tumor, whereas four of five patients who had a poor response to tamoxifen therapy showed an SUV of [^{18}F]fluorotamoxifen of less than 2.0 in the lesion. PET imaging using [^{18}F]fluorotamoxifen as the radiotracer provides useful information in predicting the effect of tamoxifen therapy in patients with recurrent or metastatic ER+ breast cancer. Results from the present study also indicate that radioiodinated and indium-labeled tamoxifen analogs are feasible to diagnose ER+ lesions.

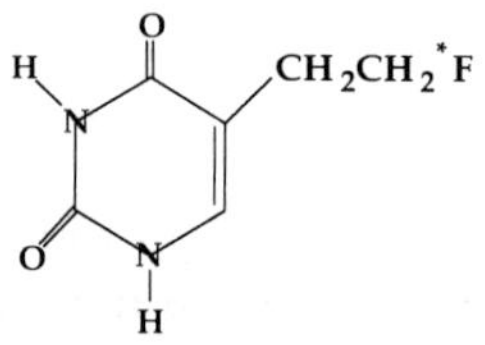

FIGURE 4.20. Structure of ^{18}F-fluorinated fluoroethyl uracil.

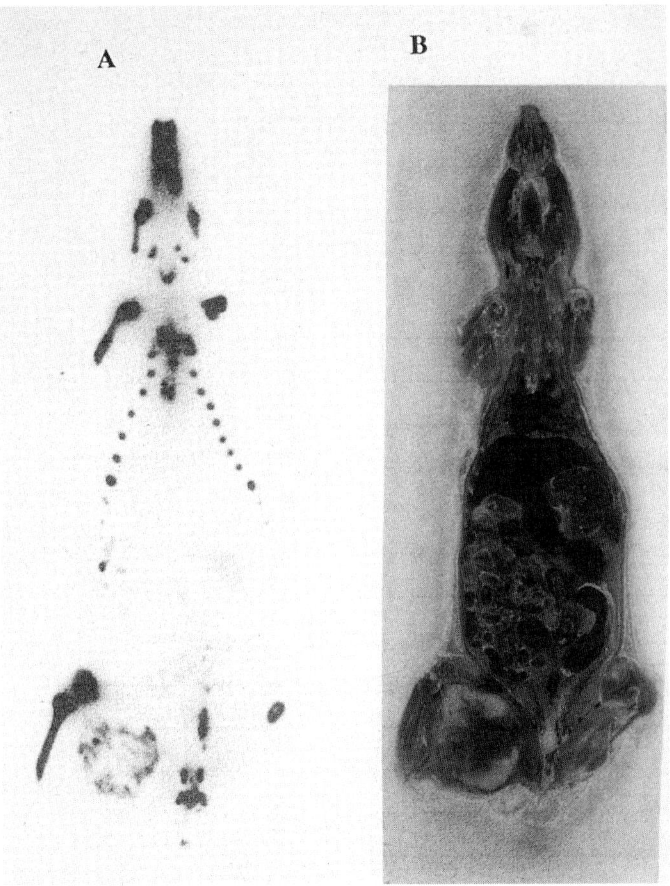

FIGURE 4.21. Autoradiogram of ^{18}F-fluorinated uracil showed that the tumor could be imaged.

The key to the development of ^{18}F-FMISO is to prepare (2′-nitro-1′-imidazolyl)-2-O-acetyl-3-O-tosylpropanol precursor. This intermediate could be prepared easily by treatment of 2-acetyl-1,3-ditosyl glycerol and 2-nitroimidazole as described previously. Both labeled compounds produced sufficient radioactivity and high radiochemical purity. Others have used ^{18}F-epifluorohydrin with 2-nitroimidazole or 1,3-ditosyl-O-tetrahydropyran to react with 2-nitroimidazole, followed by ^{18}F-displacement. These reactions take longer synthetic steps, have a longer reaction time, or provide lower radiochemical yield. Numerous in vitro and in vivo experiments have shown that cells irradiated under low oxygen tensions are more resistant to the lethal effects of low linear energy transfer (LET) ionized radiation compared to cells irradiated under "normal" oxygen tensions. Our clinical trial with PET demonstrated that ^{18}F-FMISO is capable of providing functional images of tumor hypoxia. Autoradiographs of all four analogs showed that tumor hypoxia could be easily demonstrated in rodents. Tumor oxygen tension was determined to be 3.2 to 6.0 mm Hg, whereas normal muscle tissue had 30 to 40 mm Hg.

Mass Spec

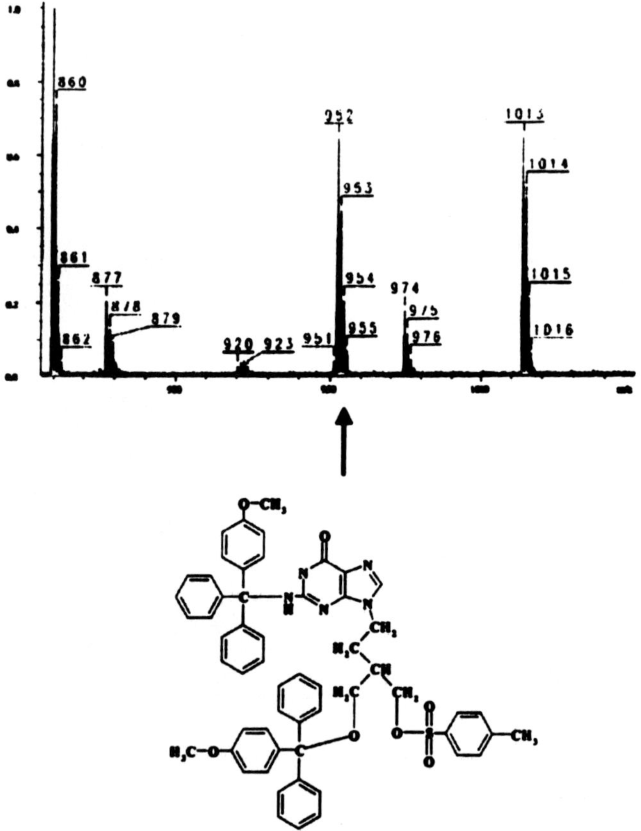

FIGURE 4.22. Mass spectrometry of di-tritylated tosylpenciclovir.

Because tumor uptake of ^{11}C-choline is higher than that of ^{18}F-FDG (i.e., synovial sarcoma), and shorter imaging time is required for ^{11}C-choline, ^{11}C-choline appeared to be a promising PET tracer. There was no effect on tumor uptake in patients with diabetes mellitus. ^{11}C-choline is feasible for detecting intrapelvic lesions due to low urinary excretion. ^{18}F-fluorinated choline revealed in vitro phosphorylation was similar to that of choline. The PET images of a patient with recurrent prostate cancer showed uptake of ^{18}F-fluorinated choline in the prostatic bed and in metastases to lymph nodes. ^{18}F-fluorinated choline PET showed uptake in malignancies in a patient with metastatic breast cancer. PET revealed ^{18}F-fluorinated choline uptake in biopsy-proven recurrent brain tumor with little confounding uptake by normal brain tissues. The ^{18}F-fluorinated choline may serve as a probe of choline uptake and phosphorylation in cancer cells. Preliminary PET studies on patients with prostate cancer, breast cancer, or brain tumor support further studies to evaluate the usefulness of fluorocholin (FCH) as an oncologic probe.

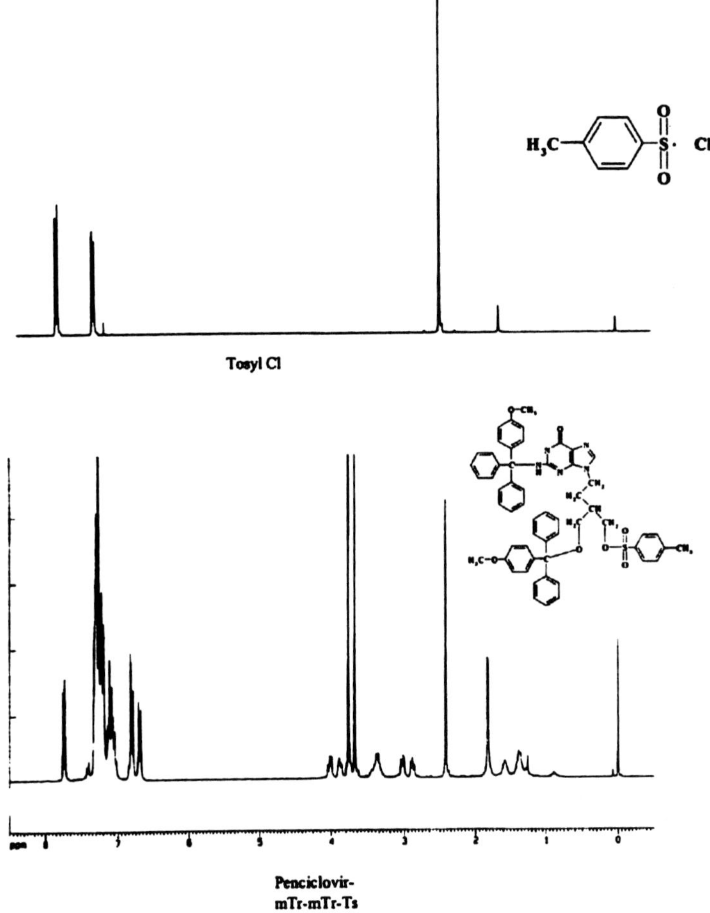

FIGURE 4.23. NMR of tosyl chloride and di-tritylated tosylpenciclovir.

To enhance the biologic activity and increase chemical or metabolic stability, fluorine substitution at the C2′ position of the sugar moiety (arabino configuration) has been widely investigated in drug research.[88–90] [^{18}F]FAD is structurally closer to 2′-deoxyadenosine due to the similarity in the Van der Waals radii between the C-H bond and C-halogen bond. Deep-seated tumors in blood-rich organs may require significantly higher ratios for assessment of proliferation. Tumor-to-muscle ratios of [^{18}F]FAD at 2 and 4 hours postinjection were 5.2 and 14.3, respectively. Tumor-to-blood ratio at the same time intervals were 2.8 and 5.3, respectively. These data were considered to be acceptable as a tumor imaging agent. Although many other radiopharmaceuticals could be used for assessment of tumor proliferation or metabolic activity, the choice should be determined not only by the biologic behavior of radiopharmaceuticals but also by their ease of preparation, as well as by the logistics of imaging.

Although we have synthesized FHBG, we have not conducted preclinical studies. Results from other studies showed that FHBG is a

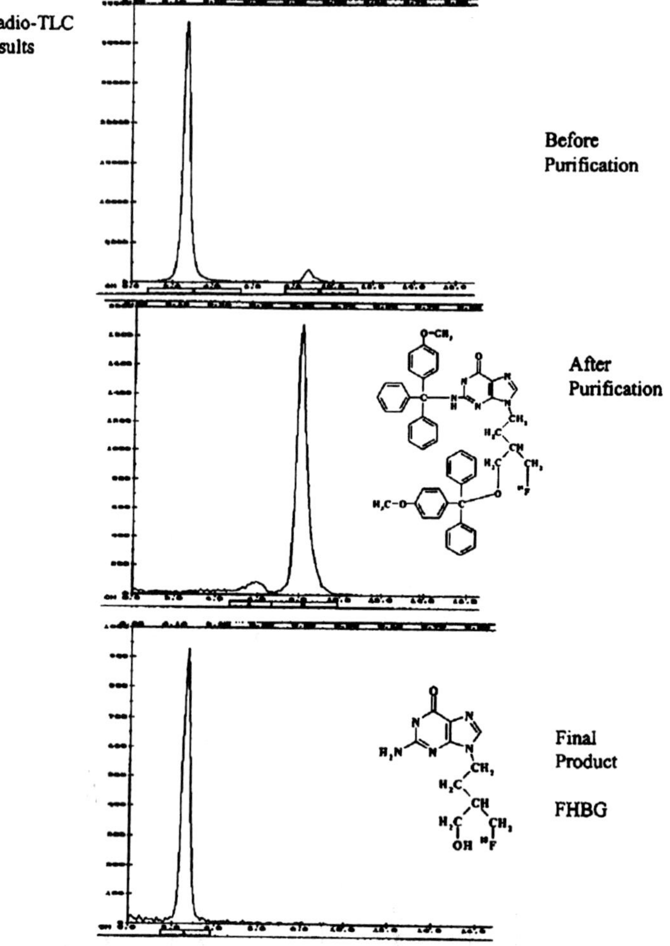

FIGURE 4.24. Radiosynthesis of ^{18}F-FHBG.

promising PET gene expression probe. For instance, Inubushi et al[91] showed that HSV-1-*sr39tk* reporter gene expression can be monitored with ^{18}F-FHBG and micro-PET in rat myocardium quantitatively and serially with high detection sensitivity. Cardiac PET reporter gene imaging offers the potential of monitoring the expression of therapeutic genes in cardiac gene therapy. Tjuvajev et al[92] also concluded that the in vitro and in vivo results (including the PET images) show that FIAU is a substantially more efficient probe than FHBG or FHPG for imaging HSV1-*tk* expression, with greater sensitivity and contrast as well as lower levels of abdominal background radioactivity at 2 and 24 hours. Alauddin et al[71] concluded that ^{18}F-FHBG may yield high-contrast PET images of HSV-*tk* expression in tumors. Thus, it is a very promising radiotracer for monitoring of gene therapy of cancer with PET.

Acknowledgment. The animal research reported here is supported by a Cancer Center Core grant, NIH-NCI CA-16672.

References

1. Bar-Shalom R, Valdivia AY, Blaufox MD. PET imaging in oncology. Semin Nucl Med 2000;30:150–185.
2. Plowman PN, Saunders CA, Maisey M. On the usefulness of brain PET scanning to the paediatric neuro-oncologist. Br J Neurosurg 1997;11:525–532.
3. Weber WA, Avril N, Schwaiger M. Relevance of positron emission tomography (PET) in oncology. Strahlenther Onkl 1999;175:356.
4. Lau CL, Harpole DH, Patz E. Staging techniques for lung cancer. Chest Surg Clin North Am 2000;10(4):781–801.
5. Schulte M, Brecht-Krauss D, Heymer B, et al. Grading of tumors and tumor like lesions of bone: evaluation by FDG PET. J Nucl Med. 2000;41(10): 1695–1701.
6. Yutani K, Shiba E, Kusuoka H, et al. Comparison of FDG-PET with MIBI-SPECT in the detection of breast cancer and axillary lymph node metastasis. J Comput Assist Tomogr 2000;24(2):274–280.
7. Franzius C, Sciuk J, Daldrup-Link HE, et al. FDG-PET for detection of osseous metastases from malignant primary bone tumors: comparison with bone scintigraphy. Eur J Nucl Med 2000;27(9):1305–1311.
8. Folpe AL, Lyles RH, Sprouse JT, et al. (F-18) fluorodeoxyglucose positron emission tomography as a predictor of pathologic grade and other prognostic variables in bone and soft tissue sarcoma. Clin Cancer Res 2000; 6(4):1279–1287.
9. Meyer PT, Spetzger U, Mueller HD, et al. High F-18 FDG uptake in a low-grade supratentorial ganglioma: a positron emission tomography case report. Clin Nucl Med 2000;25(9):694–697.
10. Franzius C, Sciuk J, Brinkschmidt C, et al. Evaluation of chemotherapy response in primary bone tumors with F-18 FDG positron emission tomography compared with histologically assessed tumor necrosis. Clin Nucl Med 2000;25(11):874–881.
11. Carretta A, Landoni C, Melloni G, et al. 18-FDG positron emission tomography in the evaluation of malignant pleural diseases—a pilot study. Eur J Cardiothorac Surg 2000;17(4):377–383.
12. Torre W, Garcia-Velloso MJ, Galbis J, et al. FDG-PET detection of primary lung cancer in a patient with an isolated cerebral metastasis. J Cardiovasc Surg 2000;41(3):503–505.
13. Brunelle F. Noninvasive diagnosis of brain tumors in children. Childs Nerv Syst 2000;16(10–11):731–734.
14. Mankoff DA, Dehdashti F, Shields AF. Characterizing tumors using metabolic imaging: PET imaging of cellular proliferation and steroid receptors. Neoplasia 2000;2:71.
15. Fitzgerald J, Parker JA, Danias PG. F-18 fluorodeoxyglucose SPECT for assessment of myocardial viability. J Nucl Cardiol 2000;7(4):382–387.
16. Schwarz A, Kuwert T. Nuclear medicine diagnosis in diseases of the central nervous system. Radiology 2000;40(10):858–862.
17. Roelcke U, Leenders KL. PET in neuro-oncology. J Cancer Res Clin Oncol 2001;127(1):2–8.
18. Brock CS, Meikle SR, Price P. Does ^{18}F-fluorodeoxyglucose metabolic imaging of tumors benefit oncology? Eur J Nucl Med 1997;24:691–705.
19. Syrota A, Comar D, Cerf M, et al. [^{11}]C-methionine pancreatic scanning with positron emission computed tomography. J Nucl Med 1979; 20:778–781.
20. Syrota A, Duquesnoy N, Dasaf A, et al. The role of positron emission tomography in the detection of pancreatic disease. Radiology 1982;143:249–253.

21. Kubota K, Yamada K, Fukuda H, et al. Tumor detection with carbon-11 labeled amino acid. Eur J Nucl Med 1984;9:136–140.
22. Hagenfeldt L, Venizelos N, Bjerkenstedt L, et al. Decreased tyrosine transport in fibroblasts from schizophrenic patients. Life Sci 1987;41:2749–2757.
23. Tisljar U, Kloster G, Stocklin G. Accumulation of radioiodinated L-alpha-methyltyrosine in pancreas of mice: concise communication. J Nucl Med 1979;20:973–976.
24. Kloss G, Leven M. Accumulation of radioiodinated tyrosine derivatives in the adrenal medulla and in melanomas. Eur J Nucl Med 1979;4:179–186.
25. Langen KJ, Coenen HH, Roosen N, et al. SPECT studies of brain tumors with L-3-[^{123}I]-Iodo-alpha-methyl tyrosine: comparison with PET, ^{124}IMT and first clinical results. J Nucl Med 1990;31:281–286.
26. Tomiyoshi K, Hirano T, Inoue T, et al. Positron emission tomography for evaluation of dopaminergic function using a neurotransmitter analog L-^{18}F-m-tyrosine in monkey brain. Bioimages 1996;4(1):1–7.
27. Wienhard K, Herholz K, Coenen HH, et al. Increased amino acid transport into brain tumors measured by PET of L-(2-^{18}F)fluorotyrosine. J Nucl Med 1991;32:1338–1346.
28. Coenen HH, Kling P, Stocklin G, et al. Metabolism of L2-^{18}F-fluorotyrosine, new PET tracer for protein synthesis. J Nucl Med 1989;301:367–1372.
29. Ishiwata K, Valvurg W, Elsigna PH, et al. Metabolic studies with L-^{11}C-tyrosine for the investigation of a kinetic model of measuring protein synthesis rate with PET. J Nucl Med 1988;29:524–529.
30. Bolster JM, Valburg W, Paans AMJ, et al. Carbon-11 labeled tyrosine to study tumor metabolism by positron emission tomography (PET). Eur J Nucl Med 1986;12:321–324.
31. Dejesus OT, Sunderland JJ, Nicles R, et al. Synthesis of radiofluorinated analogs of m-tyrosine as potential L-dopa tracers via direct reaction with acetylhypofluorite. Appl Radiat Isot 1990;41(5):433–437.
32. Tang G, Wang M, Tang X, et al. Pharmacokinetics and radiation dosimetry estimation of O-(2-[18F]fluoroethyl)-L-tyrosine as oncologic PET tracer. Appl Radiat Isot 2003;58(2):219–225.
33. Hamacher K, Coenen HH. Efficient routine production of the 18F-labelled amino acid O-2-18F fluoroethyl-L-tyrosine. Appl Radiat Isot 2002;57(6):853–856.
34. Rau FC, Weber WA, Wester HJ, et al. O-(2-[(18)F]Fluoroethyl)-L-tyrosine (FET): a tracer for differentiation of tumour from inflammation in murine lymph nodes. Eur J Nucl Med Mol Imag 2002;29(8):1039–1046.
35. Fernandez MD, Burn JI, Sauven PD, et al. Activated estrogen receptors in breast cancer and response to endocrine therapy. Eur J Cancer Clin Oncol 1984;20:41–46.
36. McGuire AH, Dehdashti F, Siegel BA, et al. Positron tomographic assessment of 16-alpha-[^{18}F]fluoro-17-beta-estradiol uptake in metastatic breast carcinoma. J Nucl Med 1991;32:1526–1531.
37. McManaway ME, Jagoda EM, Kasid A, et al. [^{125}I]17-beta-iodovinyl-11-beta-methoxyestradiol: interaction in vivo with ERS in hormone independent MCF-7 human breast cancer transfected with V-ras H oncogene. Cancer Res 1987;47:2945–2948.
38. Jagoda EM, Gibson RE, Goodgold H, et al. [^{125}I]17-Iodovinyl-11-beta-methoxyestradiol: in vivo and in vitro properties of a high affinity estrogen-receptor radiopharmaceutical. J Nucl Med 1984;25:472–477.
39. Hamm JT, Allegra JC. Hormonal therapy for cancer. In: Witts RE, ed. Manual of Oncologic Therapeutics. New York: Lippincott, 1991:122–126.

40. Wittliff JL. Steroid-hormone receptor in breast cancer. Cancer Res 1984; 53:630–643.
41. Rasey JS, Nelson NJ, Chin L, et al. Characterization of the binding of labeled fluoromisonidazole in cells in vitro. Radiat Res 1990;122:301–308.
42. Cherif A, Yang DJ, Tansey W, et al. Synthesis of [^{18}F]fluoromisonidazole. Pharm Res 1994;11:466–469.
43. Hwang DR, Dence CS, Bonasera TA, et al. No-carrier-added synthesis of 3-[^{18}F]fluoro-1-(2-nitro-1-imidazolyl)-2-propanol. A potential PET agent for detecting hypoxic but viable tissues. Int J Radiat Appl Instrum A 1989; 40:117–126.
44. Jerabeck PA, Patrick TB, Kilbourn D, et al. Synthesis and biodistribution of ^{18}F-labeled fluoronitroimidazoles: potential in vivo markers of hypoxic tissue. Appl Radiat Isot 1986;37:599–605.
45. Parliament MB, Chapman JD, Urtasun RC, et al. Noninvasive assessment of tumor hypoxia with ^{123}I-iodoazomycin arabinoside: preliminary report of a clinical study. Br J Cancer 1992;65:90–95.
46. Valk PET, Mathis CA, Prados MD, et al. Hypoxia in human gliomas: demonstration by PET with [^{18}F]fluoromisonidazole. J Nucl Med 1992;33: 2133–2137.
47. Martin GV, Caldwell JH, Rasey JS, et al. Enhanced binding of the hypoxic cell marker [^{18}F]fluoromisonidazole in ischemic myocardium. J Nucl Med 1989;30:194–201.
48. Martin GV, Cardwell JH, Graham MM, et al. Nonivasive detection of hypoxic myocardium using [^{18}F]fluoromisonidazole and PET. J Nucl Med 1992;33:2202–2208.
49. Yeh SH, Liu RS, Hu HH, et al. Ischemic penumbra in acute stroke: demonstration by PET with fluorine-18 fluoromisonidazole. J Nucl Med 1994;35: 5:205 (abst).
50. Yeh SH, Liu RS, Wu LC, et al. Fluorine-18 fluoromisonidazole tumour to muscle retention ratio for the detection of hypoxia in nasopharyngeal carcinoma. Eur J Nucl Med 1996;23(10):1378–1383.
51. Liu RS, Yeh SH, Chang CP, et al. Detection of odontogenic infections by [F-18]fluoromisonidazole. J Nucl Med 1994;35:5:113 (abst).
52. Yang DJ, Wallace S, Cherif A, et al. Development of F-18-labeled fluoroerythronitroimidazole as a PET agent for imaging tumor hypoxia. Radiology 1995;194:795–800.
53. Cherif A, Wallace S, Yang DJ, et al. Development of new markers for hypoxic cells: [^{131}I]iodomisonidazole and [^{131}I]iodoerythronitroimidazole. J Drug Targeting 1996;4(1):31–39.
54. Inoue T, Yang DJ, Wallace S, et al. Evaluation of [131I]iodoerythronitroimidazole as a predictor for the radiosensitizing effect. Anticancer Drugs 1996;7(8):858–865.
55. Podo F. Tumor phospholipid metabolism. NMR Biomed 1999;12:413–439.
56. Hara T, Kosaka N, Kishi H. PET imaging of prostate cancer using carbon-11-choline. J Nucl Med 1998;39:990–995.
57. Hara T, Kosaka N, Shinoura N, et al. PET imaging of brain tumor with [methyl-^{11}C]choline. J Nucl Med 1997;38:842–847.
58. Hara T, Kosaka N, Kishi H, et al. Imaging of brain tumor, lung cancer, esophagus cancer, colon cancer, prostate cancer, and bladder cancer with [C-11]choline. J Nucl Med 1997;38:250P.
59. Kotzerke J, Prang J, Neumaier B, et al. Experience with carbon-11 choline positron emission tomography in prostate carcinoma. Eur J Nucl Med 2000;27:1415–1419.
60. DeGrado TR, Baldwin SW, Wang S, et al. Synthesis and evaluation of (18)F-

labeled choline analogs as oncologic PET tracers. J Nucl Med 2001;42(12): 1805–1814.
61. Price DT, Coleman RE, Liao RP, et al. Comparison of [18F]fluorocholine and [18F]fluorodeoxyglucose for positron emission tomography of androgen dependent and androgen independent prostate cancer. J Urol 2002; 168(1):273–280.
62. DeGrado TR, Reiman RE, Price DT, et al. Pharmacokinetics and radiation dosimetry of 18F-fluorocholine. J Nucl Med 2002;43(1):92–96.
63. Haberkorn U, Khazaie K, Morr I, et al. Ganciclovir uptake in human mammary carcinoma cells expressing herpes simplex virus thymidine kinase. Nucl Med Biol 1998;25:367–373.
64. Gambhir SS, Barrio JR, Wu L, et al. Imaging of adenoviral-directed herpes simplex virus type 1 thymidine kinase reporter gene expression in mice with radiolabeled ganciclovir. J Nucl Med 1998;39:2003–2011.
65. Gambhir SS, Barrio JR, Phelps ME, et al. Imaging adenoviral-directed reporter gene expression in living animals with positron emission tomography. Proc Natl Acad Sci USA 1999;96:2333–2338.
66. Namavari M, Barrio JR, Toyokuni T, et al. Synthesis of 8-[^{18}F]fluoroguanine derivatives: in vivo probes for imaging gene expression with positron emission tomography. Nucl Med Biol 2000;27:157–162.
67. Gambhir SS, Bauer E, Black ME, et al. A mutant herpes simplex virus type 1 thymidine kinase reporter gene shows improved sensitivity for imaging reporter gene expression with positron emission tomography. Proc Natl Acad Sci USA 2000;97:2785–2790.
68. Iyer M, Barrio JR, Namavari M, et al. 8-[^{18}F]Fluoropenciclovir: an improved reporter probe for imaging HSV1-tk reporter gene expression in vivo using PET. J Nucl Med 2001;42:96–105.
69. Alauddin MM, Conti PS, Mazza SM, et al. 9-[(3-[^{18}F]-Fluoro-1-hydroxy-2-propoxy)methyl]guanine ([^{18}F]-FHPG): a potential imaging agent of viral infection and gene therapy using PET. Nucl Med Biol 1996;23:787–792.
70. Alauddin MM, Shahinian A, Kundu RK, et al. Evaluation of 9-[(3-^{18}F-fluoro-1-hydroxy-2-propoxy)methyl]guanine ([^{18}F]-FHPG) in vitro and in vivo as a probe for PET imaging of gene incorporation and expression in tumors. Nucl Med Biol 1999;26:371–376.
71. Alauddin MM, Conti PS. Synthesis and preliminary evaluation of 9-(4-[^{18}F]-fluoro-3-hydroxymethylbutyl)guanine ([^{18}F]FHBG): a new potential imaging agent for viral infection and gene therapy using PET. Nucl Med Biol 1998;25:175–180.
72. Yaghoubi S, Barrio JR, Dahlbom M, et al. Human pharmacokinetic and dosimetry studies of [^{18}F]FHBG: a reporter probe for imaging herpes simplex virus type-1 thymidine kinase reporter gene expression. J Nucl Med 2001;42:1225–1234.
73. Yang DJ, Cherif A, Tansey W, et al. N,N-diethylfluoromethyltamoxifen: synthesis assignment of ^{1}H and ^{13}C spectra and receptor assay. Eur J Med Chem 1992;27:919–924.
74. Yang D, Tewson T, Tansey W, et al. Halogenated analogs of tamoxifen: synthesis, receptor assay and inhibition of MCF7 cells. J Pharm Sci 1992;81: 622–625.
75. Kim CG, Yang DJ, Kim EE, et al. Assessment of tumor cell proliferation using [^{18}F]fluorodeoxyadenosine and [^{18}F]fluoroethyluracil. J Pharm Sci 1996;85(3):339–344.
76. Cherif A, Yang DJ, Tansey W, et al. Radiosynthesis and biodistribution studies of [F-18]fluoroadenosine and [I-131]-5-iodo-2′-O-methyl-uridine for the assessment of tumor proliferation rate. Pharm Res 1995;12(9):128.

77. Yang D, Wallace S. High affinity tamoxifen derivatives and uses thereof. U.S. Patent number 5,192,525, 1993.
78. Yang D, Wallace S, Wright KC, et al. Imaging of estrogen receptors with PET using ^{18}F-fluoro analogue of tamoxifen. Radiology 1992;182:185–186.
79. Yang DJ, Kuang L-R, Cherif A, et al. Synthesis of ^{18}F-alanine and ^{18}F-tamoxifen for breast tumor imaging. J Drug Targeting 1993;1:259–267.
80. Yang DJ, Li C, Kuang L-R, et al. Imaging, biodistribution and therapy potential of halogenated tamoxifen analogues. Life Sci 1994;55:(1)53–67.
81. Yang DJ, Wallace S. High affinity halogenated tamoxifen derivatives and uses thereof. U.S. Patent number 5,219,548, 1993.
82. Inoue T, Kim EE, Wallace S, et al. Positron emission tomography using [18F]fluorotamoxifen to evaluate therapeutic responses in patients with breast cancer: preliminary study. Cancer Biother Radiopharm 1996;11(4): 235–245.
83. Inoue T, Kim EE, Wallace S, et al. Preliminary study of cardiac accumulation of F-18 fluorotamoxifen in patients with breast cancer. Clin Imaging 1997;21(5):332–336.
84. Hanson RN, Seitz DE. Tissue distribution of the radiolabeled antiestrogen [^{125}I]iodotamoxifen. Int J Nucl Med Biol 1982;9:105–107.
85. Ram S, Spicer LD. Radioiodination of tamoxifen. J Labelled Compd Radiopharm 1989;27:661–668.
86. Kangas L, Nieminen A-L, Blanco G, et al. A new triphenylethylene, FC-1157a, antitumor effects. Cancer Chemother Pharmacol 1986;17:109–113.
87. Kallio S, Kangas L, Blanco G, et al. A new triphenylethylene, FC-1157a, hormonal effects. Cancer Chemother Pharmacol 1986;17:103–108.
88. Kawai G, Yamamoto Y, Kamimura T, et al. Conformational rigidity of specific pyrimidine residues in tRNA arises from posttranscriptional modifications that enhance steric interaction between the base and the 2′-hydroxyl group. Biochemistry 1992;31:1040–1045.
89. Uesugi S, Kaneyasu T, Ikehara M. Synthesis and properties of ApU analogues containing 2′-halo-2′-deoxyadenosine. Effect of 2′ substituents on oligonucleotide conformation. Biochem 1982;21:5870–5877.
90. Ikehara M, Miki H. Studies of nucleosides and nucleotides. Cyclonucleosides. Synthesis and properties of 2′-halogeno-2′-deoxyadenosines. Chem Pharm Bull 1978;26:2449–2453.
91. Inubushi M, Wu JC, Gambhir SS, et al. Positron-emission tomography reporter gene expression imaging in rat myocardium. Circulation 2003; 107(2):326–332.
92. Tjuvajev JG, Doubrovin M, Akhurst T, et al. Comparison of radiolabeled nucleoside probes (FIAU, FHBG, and FHPG) for PET imaging of HSV1-tk gene expression. J Nucl Med 2002;43(8):1072–1083.

5

Automated Synthesis of Radiopharmaceuticals

David J. Yang, Ali Azhdarinia, and E. Edmund Kim

Positron emission tomography (PET) and single photon emission computed tomography (SPECT) are in vivo imaging methods that use gamma radiotracers to track biochemical processes in humans and animals. Positron-emitting isotopes are produced by a cyclotron facility. The four major positron emitters used to label compounds are ^{11}C ($t\frac{1}{2}$ = 20.4 minutes); ^{18}F ($t\frac{1}{2}$ = 110 minutes); ^{13}N ($t\frac{1}{2}$ = 10 minutes) and ^{15}O ($t\frac{1}{2}$ = 2.0 minutes). The commonly used SPECT radioisotopes are ^{131}I ($t\frac{1}{2}$ = 7 days), ^{123}I ($t\frac{1}{2}$ = 13 hours), ^{111}In ($t\frac{1}{2}$ = 67 hours) and ^{99m}Tc (technetium 99m) ($t\frac{1}{2}$ = 6 hours). Among these isotopes, ^{18}F and ^{123}I are the most suitable for the preparation of a more complex chemistry and for a longer observation period in biologic experiments.

Radiosynthesis of PET and SPECT must be rapid because of the higher risk of radiation exposure during radiosynthesis. An automated apparatus is needed to assure production efficiency and minimize the radiation exposure by PET and SPECT isotopes. ^{18}F-fluorodeoxyglucose (^{18}F-FDG) has been widely used in various PET centers. In cancer patients, ^{18}F-FDG uptake in tumors is increased due to the faster glycolysis of tumor cells. At present, commercially available black boxes are suitable only for production of ^{18}F-FDG but not for the preparation of other compounds or research purposes.[1] We have developed an automated radiotracer production apparatus (ARPA) that is able to synthesize various radiotracers (water soluble and oil soluble) using valve components that are modular, accessible, and easy to maintain. To demonstrate the ability of this box to make different tracers, five agents were tested: (1) ^{18}F-FDG, (2) [^{123}I]tamoxifen ([^{123}I]ITX), (3) [^{18}F]tamoxifen ([^{18}F]FTX), (4) [^{18}F]fluoropropyl-α-methyltyrosine ([^{18}F]FPAMT), and (5) [^{18}F]nitroimidazole ([^{18}F]FETNIM).

The rationale for selecting tamoxifen, an antiestrogen, was its effectiveness in 30% of all patients with breast tumors. Patients with estrogen receptor–positive tumors have a response rate of 50% to 60% to tamoxifen. Radiolabeled tamoxifen would be useful to image functioning estrogen receptors by PET and SPECT.[2–9] Such a ligand may be useful in predicting tumor response to tamoxifen therapy. The other three agents were tissue hypoxia markers ([^{18}F]FMISO and [^{18}F]FET-NIM)[10–16] and fluorinated amino acid ([^{18}F]FPAMT). This ARPA device provides rapid synthesis of radiopharmaceuticals and can recover [^{18}O]-enriched water, which makes it cost-effective.

Existing Automated Devices

Commercially available boxes are built by General Electric (GE), Siemens, Sumitomo, Bioscan, and EBCO. Presently, commercially available black boxes are suitable only for production of ^{18}F-FDG, [^{18}F]DOPA, [^{18}F]fluorothymidine, [^{18}F]α-methyltyrosine, [^{11}C]choline, [^{13}N]NH_3, and [^{15}O]H_2O, but not for the preparation of other compounds or for research purposes. Each box's function is described below.

TRACERlab M_XFDG—Kit-Based Synthesizer (Fig. 5.1): High-Performance FDG Synthesizer by GE Medical Systems[17]

Selected by major radiopharmaceutical companies for its high and reliable output, ease of use, and compliance with pharmaceutical practices, the GE TRACERlab M_X produces FDG ready for quality control with high yield and high purity. The easy-to-use, disposable sterilized cassettes allow for multiple, back-to-back production runs, with easy setup and high FDG yield in a disposable, fluid pathway design.

Features

- High and reproducible yields
- Fast and easy setup of disposable cartridge, allowing multiple back-to-back productions
- Sterilized disposable cartridge meets pharmaceutical standards and prevents cross-contamination
- Low maintenance: no cumulative damage on disposable fluid pathway

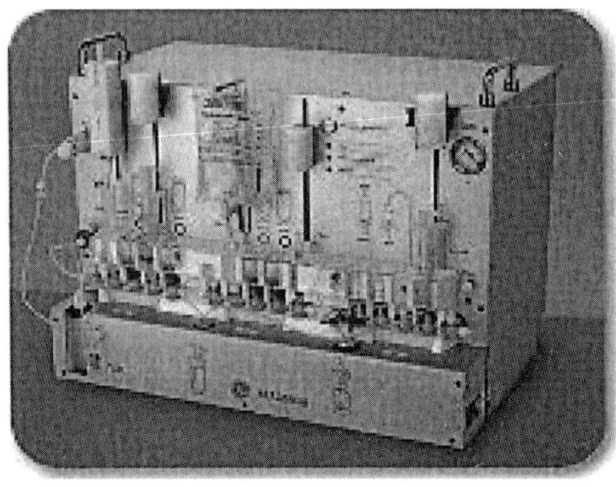

FIGURE 5.1. TRACERlab M_XFDG—kit-based synthesizer.

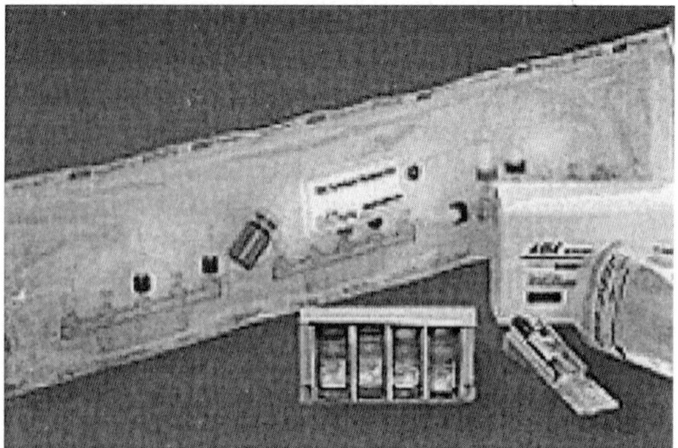

FIGURE 5.2. Sterilized cassette and reagent set.

- User-friendly graphical interface with automated record keeping
- Unsurpassed service and warranty programs to optimize the investment
- Synthesis preparation time: <5 minutes
- Synthesis time: 25 minutes
- Production yield (not corrected for decay): typically 60%
- Radiochemical yield (corrected for decay): typically 70%
- Residual activity at end of synthesis (EOS) <0.5%; sterilized cassette and reagent set (Fig. 5.2)

TRACERlab F_XFDG (Fig. 5.3): The Load-Once, Run-Twice FDG Synthesizer by GE Medical Systems[17]

Designed for those PET Tracer distribution centers that may need twice-a-day production runs, the TRACERlab F_X Synthesizer allows for two consecutive FDG runs without reloading and without opening the hot cell. TRACERlab F_X is designed as two independent synthesis units within a single housing. The GE TRACERlab F_X Synthesizer does the

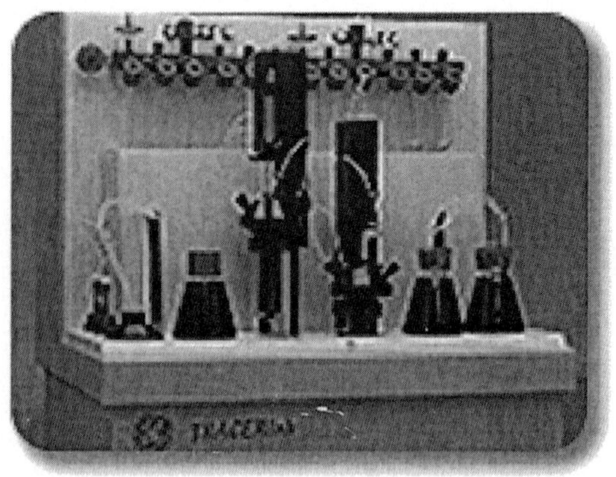

FIGURE 5.3. TRACERlab F_XFDG.

work of two separate units, but not at twice the price or with a double space requirement.

Features

- High output due to high yield and load-once, run-twice concept
- High reliability due to well-established technology
- Low operational cost
- Unsurpassed service and warranty programs to optimize the investment
- Synthesis preparation time: <15 minutes dual setup
- Synthesis time: <30 minutes
- Production yield (not corrected for decay): typically 60%
- Radiochemical conversion yield (corrected for decay): typically 70%

TRACERlab F_XDOPA (Fig. 5.4): Fully Automated [^{18}F] FDOPA Production from [^{18}F] F_2 by GE Medical Systems[17]

TRACERlab F_XDOPA is an automated, dedicated synthesizer for easy and efficient production of F-DOPA via electrophilic substitution with [^{18}F]fluorine in the form of F_2. Purification is achieved by an integrated preparative high-performance liquid chromatography (HPLC) system. TRACERlab F_XDOPA is easy to operate and compatible with the GE PET trace F_2 target system, making the training of staff in doing this usually difficult synthesis fast and economical.

Features

- Easy to operate
- Fully automated [^{18}F] F-DOPA production
- Built-in preparative HPLC for complete preparation of injectable solution
- Closed system allowing clean synthesis operation in any hot cell environment

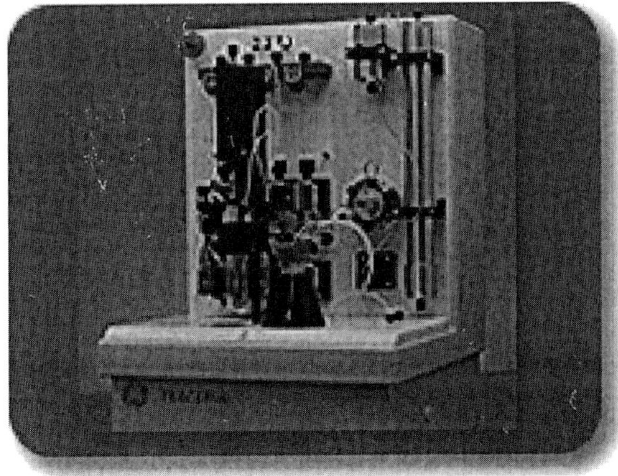

FIGURE 5.4. TRACERlab F_XDOPA.

- Automated cleaning procedure for easy, fast preparation
- Unsurpassed service and warranty programs to optimize the investment
- Synthesis preparation time: <15 minutes
- Synthesis time: <40 minutes
- Production yield (not corrected for decay): typically 20%
- Radiochemical conversion yield (corrected for decay): typically 25%
- Enantiomeric purity: ≥99%

TRACERlab F_XF-N (Fig. 5.5): Fully Automated Nucleophilic Fluorination with [^{18}F] Fluoride by GE Medical Systems[17]

TRACERlab F_XF-N is an automated versatile synthesizer for easy and efficient production of [^{18}F] tracers via nucleophilic substitution with [^{18}F]fluoride trapped from [^{18}O] water. Purification is achieved by an integrated, preparative HPLC system. Through application software, all process steps are easily programmed to produce the required tracers.

Features

- Easy to operate
- Flexible concept for easy setup of numerous PET radiopharmaceuticals
- Built-in preparative radiofrequency/ultraviolet (UV)-HPLC for complete preparation of injectable solution
- Closed system allowing clean synthesis operation in any hot cell environment
- Automated cleaning procedure for easy, fast preparation
- Unsurpassed service and warranty programs to optimize the investment

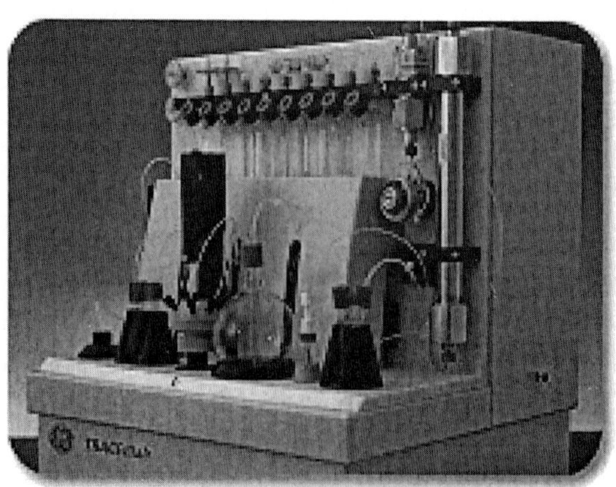

FIGURE 5.5. TRACERlab F_XF-N.

Examples of [^{18}F] Tracers

- [^{18}F] labeled long chain fatty acids—[^{18}F]fluoro-6-thia-heptadecanoic acid (FTHA): for anaerobic metabolism and cardiac ischemia
- [^{18}F]fluoromisonidazole: for poorly perfused tumors
- [^{18}F]methylbenperidol: dopaminergic D2 receptor: for schizophrenia and drug addiction
- [^{18}F]methylspiperone: dopaminergic D2 receptor for schizophrenia and drug addiction
- [^{18}F]fluoroestradiol: for steroid metabolism and estrogen-dependent breast cancer
- [^{18}F]altanserine: (serotonergic S2 receptor) for depression
- [^{18}F]FLT (fluoro-L-thymidine): for DNA synthesis in tumor proliferation
- ^{18}F-FDG: for glucose metabolism in cancers, myocardial viability, and Alzheimer's disease

TRACERlab F_XF-E (Fig. 5.6): Fully Automated Electrophilic Fluorination by Use of [^{18}F] F_2 by GE Medical Systems[17]

TRACERlab F_XF-E is an automated, versatile synthesizer for easy and efficient production of general ^{18}F tracers via electrophilic substitution with [^{18}F]fluorine in the form of F_2. Purification is achieved by an integrated, preparative HPLC system. Through application software, all process steps are easily programmed to efficiently produce the required tracers.

Features

- Easy to operate
- Flexible concept for easy setup of numerous PET radiopharmaceuticals
- Built-in preparative radiofrequency/UV-HPLC for complete preparation of injectable solution

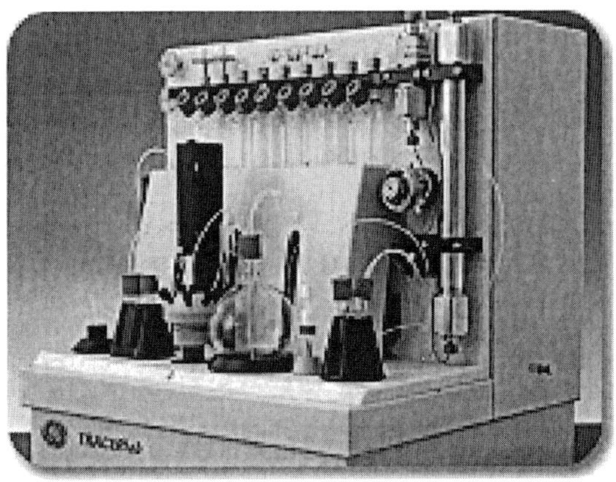

FIGURE 5.6. TRACERlab F_XF-E.

- Closed system allowing clean synthesis operation in any hot cell environment
- Automated cleaning procedure for easy, fast preparation
- Unsurpassed service and warranty programs to optimize the investment

Examples of [^{18}F] Tracers

- [^{18}F]F-DOPA: dopamine synthesis for Parkinson's disease
- [^{18}F]fluoro-L-m-tyrosine: dopamine synthesis for Parkinson's disease
- [^{18}F]fluoro-L-tyrosine: protein synthesis, amino acid transport for lung cancer
- [^{18}F]fluorouracil: RNA component for oncology therapy planning in colon cancer

TRACERlab F_XC (Fig. 5.7): Fully Automated Methylation with Integrated Gas Phase Methyliodide Production by GE Medical Systems[17]

TRACERlab F_XC is an automated versatile synthesizer for easy and efficient production of ^{11}C-labeled tracers, mainly through methylation reactions with [^{11}C]methyliodide. Purification is achieved by an integrated preparative HPLC system. Through the application software, all process steps are easily programmed to produce the required tracers.

Features

- Easy to operate
- Allows methylation starting from [^{11}C]CO_2 or [^{11}C]CH_4
- Flexible concept for easy setup of numerous PET radiopharmaceuticals
- Built-in preparative radiofrequency/UV-HPLC for complete preparation of injectable solution

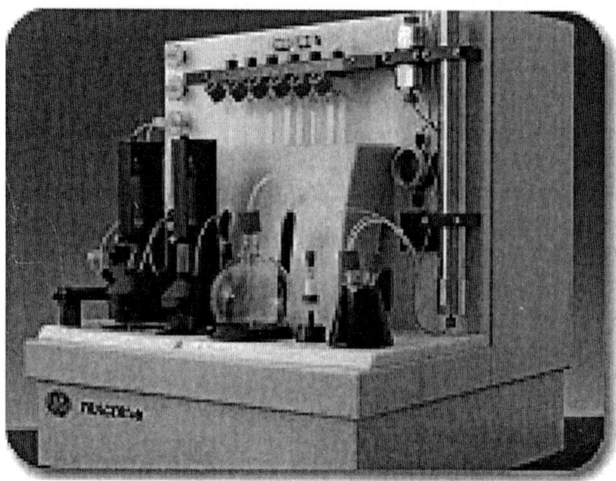

FIGURE 5.7. TRACERlab F_XC.

- Closed system allowing clean synthesis operation in any hot cell environment
- Unsurpassed service and warranty programs to optimize the investment

Examples of [^{11}C] Compounds

- [^{11}C]raclopride: for dopamine postsynaptic receptors in schizophrenia and drug addiction
- [^{11}C]metahydroxyephedrine: for adrenergic neurotransmission in heart failure
- [^{11}C]methylspiperone: for dopamine postsynaptic receptors in schizophrenia and drug addiction
- [^{11}C]methionone: for protein synthesis in fast-growing tumors
- [^{11}C]acetate: for cell metabolism/cardiac metabolism
- [^{11}C]palmitate: for fatty acid metabolism cardiac ischemia

^{18}F-FDG Synthesizer (Figs. 5.8 and 5.9): PET Tracer Production System by Sumitomo[18]

Sumitomo installed the first in-house cyclotron for PET diagnosis in 1979. Since then Sumitomo has developed cyclotron technologies for PET, and a large number of references have accumulated, some of which are listed in the reference list. Sumitomo has the majority of the market in Japan. The remarkable technology for which Sumitomo is highly reputed is not only in cyclotrons, but also in radiochemistry production systems, such as FDG synthesis modules, MeI modules, etc., which are used for experimental study of PET.

Sumitomo deals with cyclotrons, target chemistry, and the method of the production of commonly used radio-compounds labeled with the positron emitters such as ^{11}C, ^{13}N, ^{15}O, and ^{18}F, which must be manufactured by in-house cyclotrons because of their short half-life.

Description

Featuring disposable kits that fit easily onto the unit's front panel, the Coincidence unit reduces preparation time and cleaning requirements

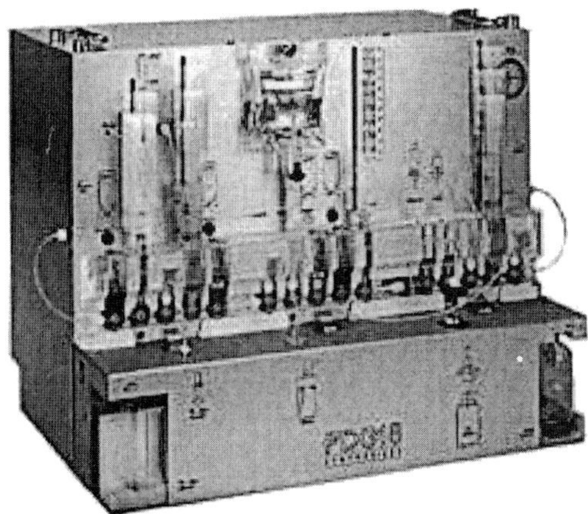

FIGURE 5.8. FDG synthesizer.

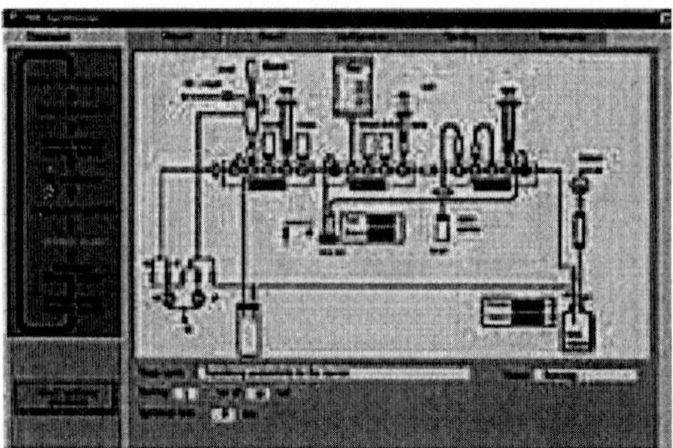

FIGURE 5.9. FDG synthesis software.

to a minimum. The kit and reagent set contain everything for one production run, and low residual activity allows the user to replace the kit and begin a new synthesis immediately. Operator intervention is minimized, as a self-diagnostic routine is performed automatically and all cartridges are conditioned during the synthesis.

The synthesis unit is controlled by a dedicated industrial programmable logic controller (PLC) interfaced to a graphical menu-driven program on a PC. All relevant parameters are displayed and recorded. The operator is informed when the FDG synthesis is complete. The final product can be delivered to a remote location. The Coincidence synthesizer allows the recovery of [^{15}O] water, the most expensive raw material in the process, and has built-in radiation detectors.

FDG Synthesis

Mannose triflate is labeled with [^{18}F] by nucleophilic substitution. The resulting tetraacetyl-[^{18}F]glucose is trapped on a reverse-phase cartridge and any impurities are eluted. The acetyl groups are hydrolyzed on the cartridge in less than 2 minutes using sodium hydroxide, and the FDG is eluted with water and then buffered, purified, and filtered.

Features

- Time of synthesis: 23–26 minutes
- Decay corrected yields of 64–80%
- Radiochemical yield: routinely 60–65% (EOS)
- Radiochemical purity: >98%
- Residual acetonitrile: <1 mg/batch
- Residual kryptofix: <150 μg/batch
- Residual kit activity: <4% of end of bombardment (EOB) activity
- Footprint: 22 × 15 inches
- Residual box activity: zero (allows back-to-back production runs)
- Target water recovered
- Easy setup with preassembled kits

Radiochemistry System for PET

The in-house cyclotron produces mainly four radionuclides: ^{15}O, ^{13}N, ^{11}C, and ^{18}F. Sumitomo can provide research laboratories with the most radiochemistry modules, as requested, such as the ^{15}O gas system.

[^{15}O] Gas System by Sumitomo (Fig. 5.10)[18]

Features

- Target material: O_2
- Process: [^{15}O] is produced in target and transferred to the gas synthesis unit with nitrogen. After the purification, the gas is transferred to the PET room and introduced to the patient via the inhalation module. The radioactive waste gas is stored at the reservoir [medical device No. (03B) No.1381].

[^{18}O] Water Purifier by Sumitomo (Fig. 5.11)[18]

This unit is used to purify the used [^{18}O] water for a production of ^{18}F. [^{18}O] water is purified by the combination of UV irradiation and evaporation. This unit is manufactured by Sumitomo under the license of KFA, Germany.

Features

- 16 g is generated in one operation.
- Over 98% of water can be recovered after the purification.
- Organic compounds, metals, and gases can be eliminated efficiently.

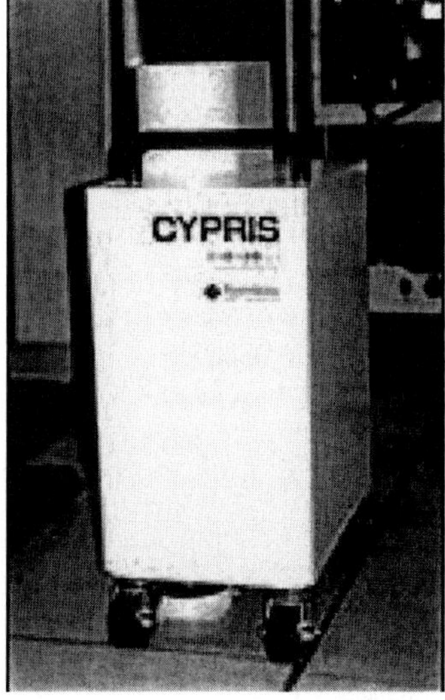

FIGURE 5.10. [^{15}O] gas system.

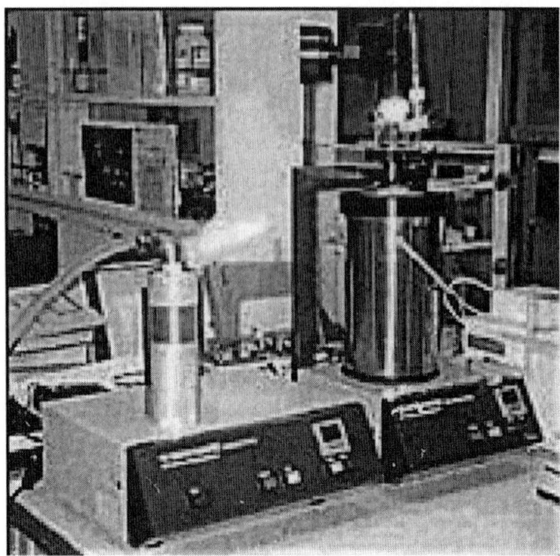

FIGURE 5.11. [^{18}O] water purifier.

Lead-Shielded Box for Automated Modules by Sumitomo (Fig. 5.12)[18]

Features

- Hot cell for module (right two units): This box is used for RI modules. Four modules are stored in both sides. The door is opened electrically, and the lead windows and the small access door are equipped in each side.
- Hot cell for research and development (left one unit): The shield door can be fully opened, and the box in the inner space can be arranged to suit one's purpose.

FDG Module by EBCO (Figs. 5.13 and 5.14)[19]

The module design is less complicated, more reliable, easier to operate, and less expensive than other FDG modules available in the marketplace.

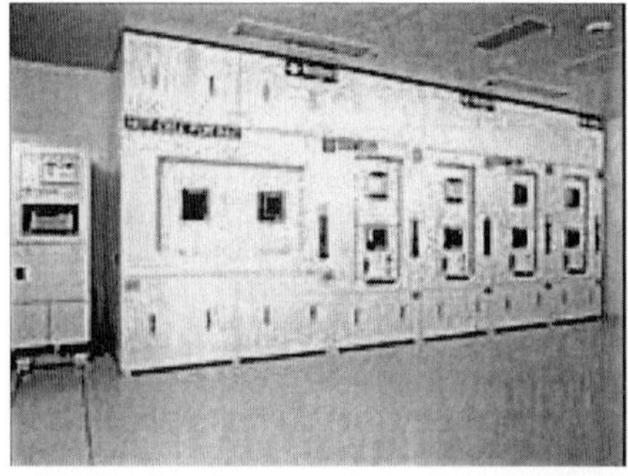

FIGURE 5.12. Lead-shielded box for automated modules.

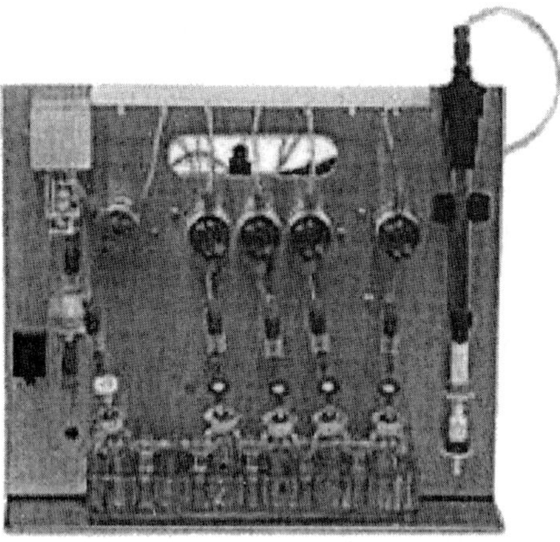

FIGURE 5.13. Reliable and easy to operate FDG module.

Features

- Automated mode of operation
- Decay corrected yields >65%
- Radiochemical purity >98%
- 95% reliability and >90% reproducibility from run to run
- Capable of producing multiple curies of FDG
- Uses the Hamacher method, the no-carrier-added nucleophilic fluorination of mannose triflate
- Can be used for other nucleophilic fluorination labeling reactions
- Either tetrabutylammonium bromide (TBAB) or kryptofix-2,2,2, can be used as a phase transfer catalyst
- Each reagent follows its own flow path through its separate tubing
- Controlled flow of helium or nitrogen gas is used to transfer the reactants

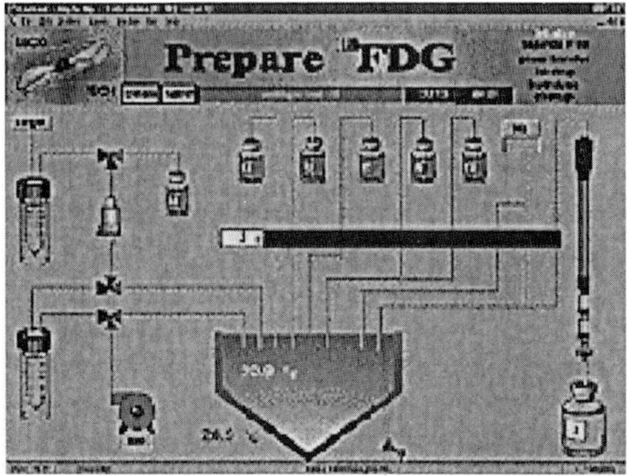

FIGURE 5.14. FDG module software.

- Two-step rinse of the reaction vessel and columns to maximize yield
- Sealed-septum dispensing vial and sealed reactant vials
- Simplified design
- Simplified control system and user-friendly, graphic user interface
- Automatic pre-run aseptic cleaning, and pressure and vacuum testing
- Thermocouple temperature sensor on reaction vessel
- An improved reaction vessel allows both heating and cooling real-time control of synthesis process
- Real-time data logging
- Compact size requiring less shielding
- Low maintenance requirements
- Ability to recover [^{18}O] water through distillation (with appropriate equipment)
- Radiation detectors at key points in process (optional)
- Automated bolus transfer to and from target system (optional)

Automated Modules for Production of [^{11}C], [^{13}N], [^{15}O], and [^{18}F] Radiochemicals by EBCO (Figs. 5.15 and 5.16)[19]

Features

- Reliable and easy to operate radiochemistry modules
- Automated mode of operation
- High decay-corrected yields
- High radiochemical purity
- 95% reliability and >90% reproducibility from run to run

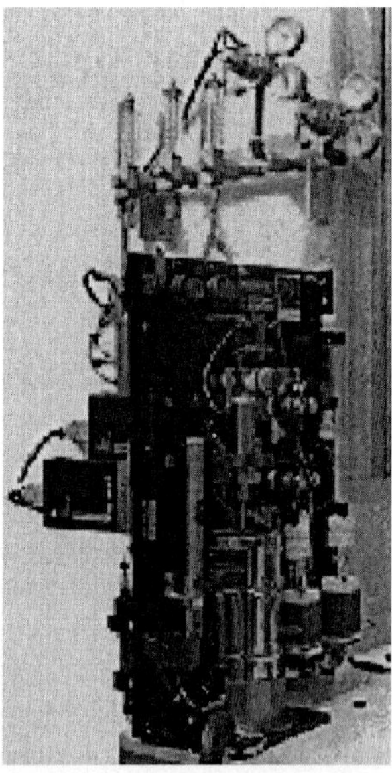

FIGURE 5.15. Automated module for the radiochemical production.

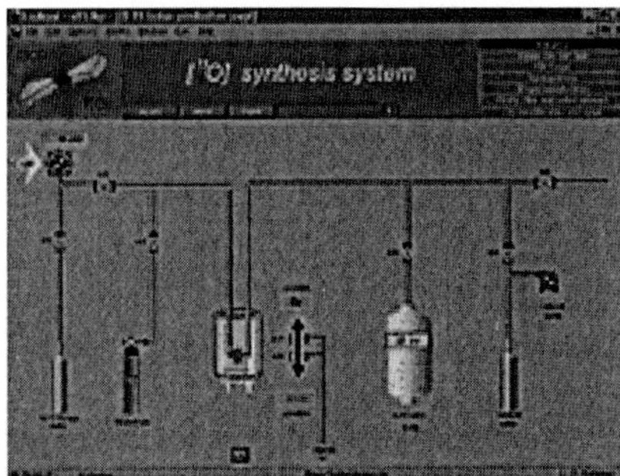

FIGURE 5.16. Automated module software.

- Can be used for a variety of labeling reactions
- Controlled flow of helium or nitrogen gas is used to transfer the reactants
- Sealed-septum dispensing vial and sealed reactant vessels
- Simplified design
- Simplified control system and user-friendly, graphic user interface
- Automatic pre-run aseptic cleaning and pressure and vacuum testing
- Thermocouple temperature sensors
- Real-time control of synthesis process
- Real-time data logging
- Compact size requiring less shielding
- Low maintenance requirements
- Radiation detectors at key points in process (optional)
- Automated bolus transfer to and from target system (optional)

Automated Radiotracer Production Apparatus (ARPA) (Fig. 5.17)

Our box system consists of an apparatus and a computer unit. This system uses 32 valves as well as other fittings and is housed in the lead-shielded hot cell. In addition to the main unit, a vacuum pump is used to generate sufficient vacuum for waste collection and venting; a +24V DC power supply is used to supply electrical current to drive the valves. The same power supply is used to drive the carousel motor. A personal computer (Pentium) hosting two 24-channel parallel I/O cards is used to operate the relays by software. The software is a simple Microsoft Windows graphical user-interface (GUI) that allows the operator to turn individual solenoid valves on and off by clicking graphical buttons.

The electrical system is located above the fluid system to prevent a potential electrical hazard due to fluid leakage. Three modules on each side, each corresponding to a product stage, are mounted on cards that can easily slide in and out of the chassis for servicing and replacement. A printed circuit board (PCB) backplane used to connect the solenoid

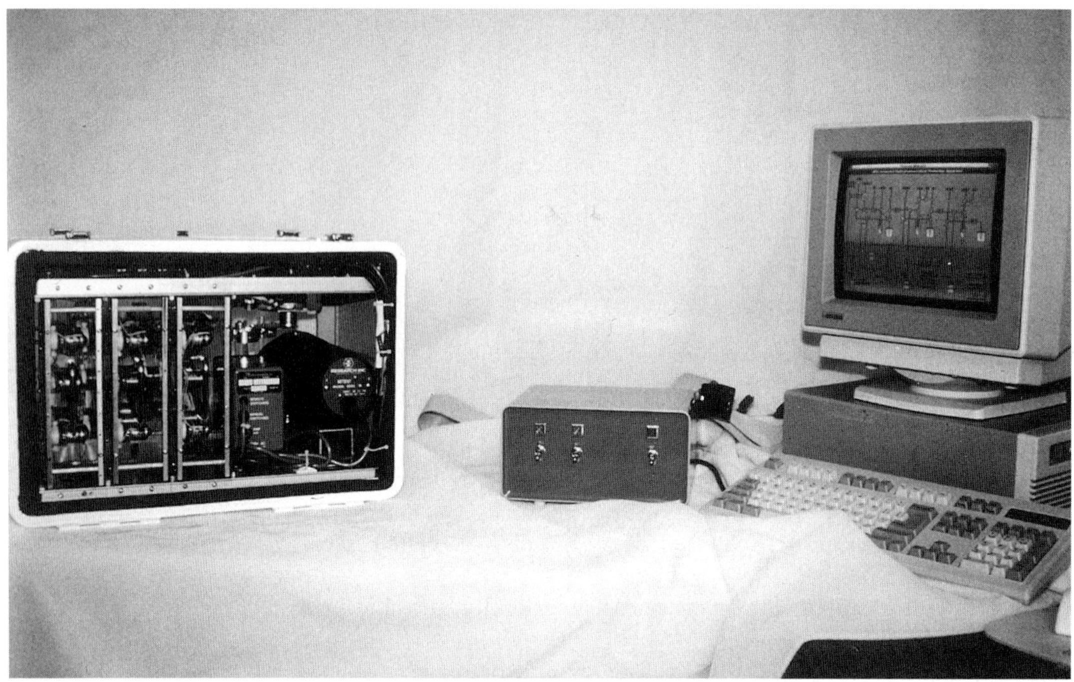

FIGURE 5.17. Automated radiotracer production apparatus (ARPA).

valves on each module to the relay circuits reduces the amount of point-to-point wiring, and therefore reduces the overall bulk. The motorized test tube carousel is used to eliminate the need to manually insert individual test tubes into the heater for heating. An infrared spot heater is used for rapid, focused heating via a side opening. The front and back covers are removed to expose the apparatus for visibility, and the use of high-density valve packaging permits the unit to be portable.

Production of ^{18}F-FDG (a Water-Soluble Compound) (Fig. 5.18)

Preparation of Columns

Two ^{18}C silica Sep-Pak columns and one alumina Sep-Pak column are washed first with 10 mL of 95% ethanol and then with 20 mL of water. The ^{18}C silica column between the vessels (tube 1 to tube 2) is left wet. The remaining two columns are purged with air until dry. Then 10 mg of ion exchange resin AG1-X8 in the $^{-}$OH form is added to the column connected to the ^{18}F target system.

Synthesis

[^{18}F]fluorine, in 1 mL of 95% [^{18}O]-enriched water, is transferred from the cyclotron target to an anion exchange column (in the $^{-}$OH form) where the ^{18}F is trapped, and the [^{18}O] water passes through and is collected in a bottle. The ^{18}F is washed from the column with 1.5 mL of 0.01 mol/L potassium carbonate into a reaction vessel containing 26 mg of kryptofix-2,2,2. The resulting potassium fluoride/kryptofix com-

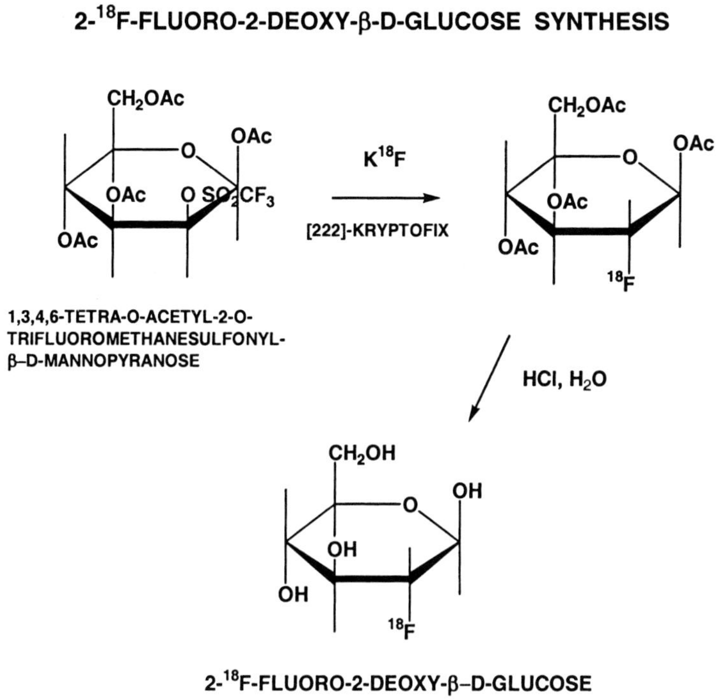

2-^{18}F-FLUORO-2-DEOXY-β-D-GLUCOSE SYNTHESIS

CH_2OAc OAc O OAc O SO_2CF_3 OAc

1,3,4,6-TETRA-O-ACETYL-2-O-TRIFLUOROMETHANESULFONYL-β-D-MANNOPYRANOSE

$K^{18}F$

[222]-KRYPTOFIX

CH_2OAc O OAc OAc OAc ^{18}F

HCl, H_2O

CH_2OH O OH OH OH ^{18}F

2-^{18}F-FLUORO-2-DEOXY-β-D-GLUCOSE

FIGURE 5.18. Production of ^{18}F-FDG.

plex is subsequently dried, first by distillation under vacuum and then by azeotropic distillation of the remaining water with the addition of three 1.5-mL portions of acetonitrile. The ^{18}F complex is allowed to exchange with the trifluoromethylsulfonyl group on 20 mg of 1,3,4,6-tetra-O-acetyl-2-O-trifluoromethanesulfonyl-β-D-mannopyranose (triflate), which is dissolved in 2 mL of dry acetonitrile and added to the reaction vessel. This exchange takes 5 minutes, and then the solvent is removed by distillation under vacuum.

The product ([^{18}F]triflate) is redissolved in 0.25 mL of acetonitrile and 6 mL of water and is passed onto an ^{18}C silica Sep-Pak. The ^{18}C silica Sep-Pak is subsequently washed with 4 mL of water, and 4 mL of 0.1 normal hydrochloric acid to remove the kryptofix from the mixture. The product is then washed off the ^{18}C silica Sep-Pak to the second reaction vessel by washing twice with 2-ml portions of tetrahydrofuran.

The tetrahydrofuran is removed by distillation under vacuum, 2 mL of 2.0 normal hydrochloric acid is added, and the reaction is then allowed to reflux for 8 minutes in order to hydrolyze the acetyl protecting groups. The vessel is removed from the heat source and is partially neutralized by the addition of 1.8 mL of 2.0 normal sodium hydroxide. Neutralization and buffering are then accomplished by the addition of 4 mL of a saturated sodium bicarbonate solution (1.2 mol/L). The resulting solution is passed through a neutral alumina Sep-Pak to remove unreacted fluoride, an ^{18}C silica Sep-Pak to remove organic impurities, and then passed through a 0.22 μm filter for sterilization. The final product is analyzed for sterility and by HPLC for radiochemical purity. Synthesis takes 40 to 45 minutes. Production yield (not corrected for decay) is typically 50% to 60%.

Synthesis of 3-[^{18}F]Fluoropropyl-α-Methyltyrosine ([^{18}F]FPAMT) (Fig. 5.19)

Fluorine-18/Kryptofix Preparation (Routine Procedure)

[^{18}F]fluorine, in 1.0 mL of 95% [^{18}O]-enriched water, is transferred from the cyclotron target to an anion exchange column (in the OH form) where the ^{18}F is trapped, and the [^{18}O]water passes through and is collected in a bottle. The ^{18}F is washed from the column with 1.5 mL of 0.01 mol/L potassium carbonate into a reaction vessel containing 26 mg of kryptofix-2,2,2. The resulting potassium fluoride/kryptofix complex is subsequently dried, first by distillation under vacuum and then by azeotropic distillation of the remaining water with the addition of three 1.5-mL portions of acetonitrile.

Displacement and Hydrolysis Reactions

The ^{18}F complex is allowed to exchange with the tosyl group on 4 mg of N-t-butoxycarbonyl-O-[3-tosylpropyl]-α-methyltyrosine methylester

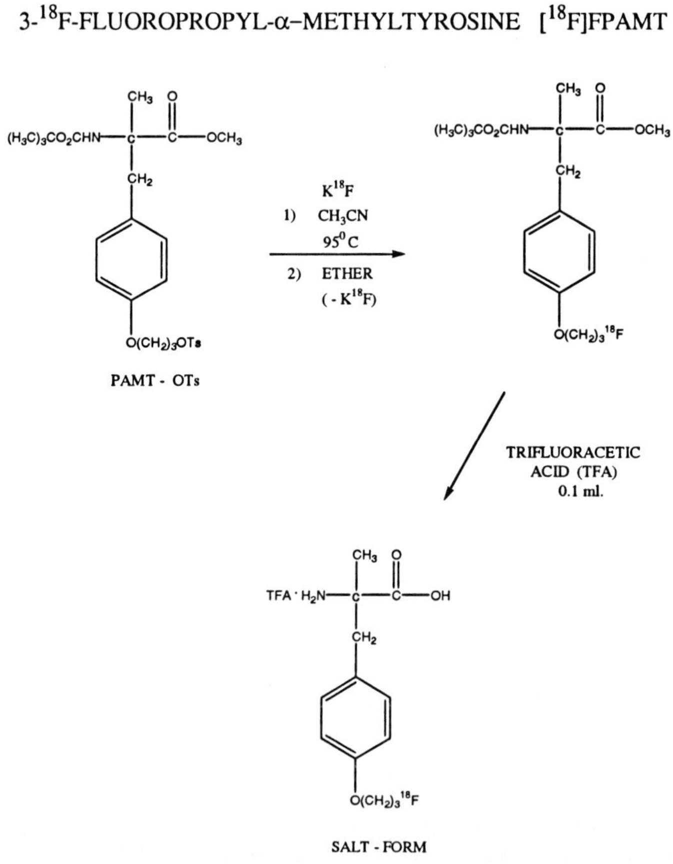

3-^{18}F-FLUOROPROPYL-α–METHYLTYROSINE [^{18}F]FPAMT

PAMT - OTs

1) $K^{18}F$, CH_3CN, 95^0C

2) ETHER ($-K^{18}F$)

TRIFLUORACETIC ACID (TFA) 0.1 ml.

SALT - FORM

FIGURE 5.19. Synthesis of 3-[^{18}F]Fluoropropyl-α-methyltyrosine ([^{18}F]FPAMT).

(tosyl precursor; PAMT-OTs), which is dissolved in 0.5 mL of acetonitrile (tube 1). The reaction is heated for 15 minutes at 95°C. The cooled acetonitrile solution is passed onto a dry normal 500-mg silica column. This material is eluted (washed from the column) with 3 mL of diethyl ether into tube 2, where the solvents (ether/acetonitrile) are evaporated to about 1 mL. To remove the protecting group, 0.1 mL of trifluoroacetic acid is added. The reaction sits for 20 minutes at room temperature. The solution is evaporated to dryness and 2 mL of HCl (2 N) is added and heated at 100°C for 10 minutes. After cooling, sodium hydroxide (1.8 mL, 2 N) and $NaHCO_3$ (1 mL, 1 N) are added. Water (2 mL) is added to tube 2. After warming (40°C), the water solution is passed through a 0.22-μm filter for sterilization.

Production of [^{123}I]ITX (an Oil-Soluble Compound)

Synthesis
The tosyl precursor of tamoxifen is placed in vessel 1. After ^{123}I-displacement, the product is purified by a column (F1, silica) and hydrolyzed in a second vessel. The product is extracted and purified by a column (F2A, F2B, silica). The solvent is evaporated. The product is formulated in citrate, filtered through a 0.22-μm filter, and placed in the final bottle.

Production of [^{18}F]FTX (an Oil-Soluble Compound)

Synthesis
The tosyl precursor of tamoxifen (2,3) is placed in vessel 1. After ^{18}F-displacement, the product is purified by a column (F1, silica) and hydrolyzed in a second vessel. The product is extracted and purified by a column (F2A, F2B, silica). The solvent is evaporated. The product is formulated in citrate, filtered through a 0.22-μm filter, and placed in the final bottle.

Production of n-(4-[^{18}F]-fluoro-2,3-Dihydroxybutyl-2-Nitroimidazole) [^{18}F]FETNIM (Fig. 5.20)

Synthesis
[^{18}F]fluorine, in 1.0 mL of 95% [^{18}O]-enriched water, is transferred from the cyclotron target to an anion exchange column (in the OH form) where the ^{18}F is trapped, and the [^{18}O] water passes through and is collected in a bottle. The ^{18}F is washed from the column with 1.5 mL of 0.01 mol/L potassium carbonate into a reaction vessel containing 26 mg of kryptofix-2,2,2. The resulting potassium fluoride/kryptofix complex is subsequently dried, first by distillation under vacuum and then by azeotropic distillation of the remaining water with the addition of three 1.5-mL portions of acetonitrile. The ^{18}F complex is allowed to exchange with the tosyl group on 10 mg of *N*-(4-tosyl-2,3-isopropylidene-butyl)-2-nitroimidazole (tosyl precursor), which is dissolved in 1.5 mL of acetonitrile and added to tube 1. This exchange takes 7 minutes at 97°C. The cooled acetonitrile solution is passed onto a dry normal 500-mg silica column. This material is eluted (washed from the column) with 5 mL of diethyl ether into tube 2 where the solvents (ether/ace-

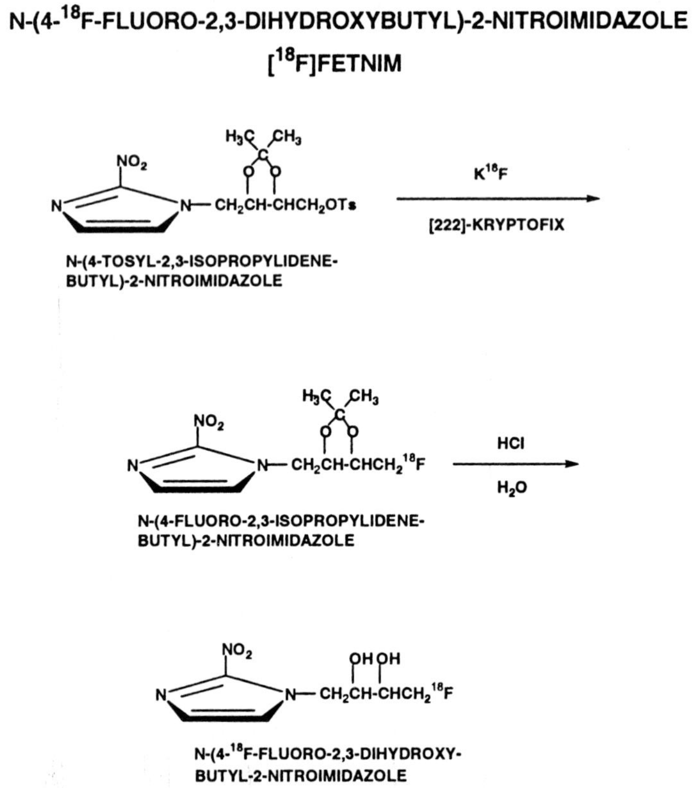

N-(4-^{18}F-FLUORO-2,3-DIHYDROXYBUTYL)-2-NITROIMIDAZOLE
[^{18}F]FETNIM

N-(4-TOSYL-2,3-ISOPROPYLIDENE-BUTYL)-2-NITROIMIDAZOLE

$K^{18}F$ / [222]-KRYPTOFIX

N-(4-FLUORO-2,3-ISOPROPYLIDENE-BUTYL)-2-NITROIMIDAZOLE

HCl / H_2O

N-(4-^{18}F-FLUORO-2,3-DIHYDROXY-BUTYL-2-NITROIMIDAZOLE

FIGURE 5.20. Production of n-(4-[^{18}F]-fluoro-2,3-dihydroxybutyl-2-nitroimidazole) [^{18}F]FETNIM.

tonitrile) are evaporated. Addition of 1.0 mL of 2 N hydrochloric acid for 7 minutes at 100°C removes the ether protecting group. Once cooled, the solution is neutralized with 0.8 mL of 2 N sodium hydroxide and then buffered with 1.0 mL of sodium bicarbonate.

The resulting solution is passed through a neutral alumina Sep-Pak to remove unreacted fluoride, and then through a ^{18}C Sep-Pak to remove organic impurities, and finally eluted from the column with 5.0 mL of 10% ethanol, and then passed through a 0.22-μm filter for sterilization. The final product is analyzed for sterility and by HPLC for radiochemical purity.

References

1. Brock CS, Meikle SR, Price P. Does [^{18}F]fluorodeoxyglucose metabolic imaging of tumors benefit oncology? Eur J Nucl Med 1997;24:691–705.
2. Yang DJ, Cherif A, Tansey W, et al. N,N-diethylfluoromethyltamoxifen: synthesis assignment of ^{1}H and ^{13}C spectra and receptor assay. Eur J Med Chem 1992;27:919–924.
3. Yang D, Tewson T, Tansey W, et al. Halogenated analogs of tamoxifen: synthesis, receptor assay and inhibition of MCF7 cells. J Pharm Sci 1992;81: 622–625.
4. Yang D, Wallace S, Wright KC, et al. Imaging of estrogen receptors with PET using [^{18}F]fluoro analogue of tamoxifen. Radiology 1992;182:185–186.

5. Yang DJ, Kuang L-R, Cherif A, et al. Synthesis of [^{18}F]fluoroalanine and [^{18}F]fluorotamoxifen for breast tumor imaging. J Drug Targeting 1993;1: 259–267.
6. Yang DJ, Li C, Kuang L-R, et al. Imaging, biodistribution and therapy potential of halogenated tamoxifen analogues. Life Sci 1994;55(1):53–67.
7. Inoue T, Kim EE, Wallace S, et al. Positron emission tomography using [^{18}F]fluorotamoxifen to evaluate therapeutic responses in patients with breast cancer: preliminary study. Cancer Biother Radiopharm 1996;11(4): 235–245.
8. Inoue T, Kim EE, Wallace S, et al. Preliminary study of cardiac accumulation of [^{18}F]fluorotamoxifen in patients with breast cancer. Clin Imaging 1997;21(5):332–336.
9. Hanson RN, Seitz DE. Tissue distribution of the radiolabeled antiestrogen [^{125}I]iodotamoxifen. Int J Nucl Med Biol 1982;9:105–107.
10. Yeh SH, Liu RS, Hu HH, et al. Ischemic penumbra in acute stroke: demonstration by PET with [^{18}F]fluoromisonidazole. J Nucl Med 1994;35:5:205 (abst).
11. Yeh SH, Liu RS, Wu LC, et al. [^{18}F]fluoromisonidazole tumour to muscle retention ratio for the detection of hypoxia in nasopharyngeal carcinoma. Eur J Nucl Med 1996;23(10):1378–1383.
12. Liu RS, Yeh SH, Chang CP, et al. Detection of odontogenic infections by [^{18}F]fluoromisonidazole. J Nucl Med 1994;35:5:113(abst).
13. Yang DJ, Wallace S, Cherif A, et al. Development of [^{18}F]fluoroerythronitroimidazole as a PET agent for imaging tumor hypoxia. Radiology 1995; 194:795–800.
14. Valk PET, Mathis CA, Prados MD, et al. Hypoxia in human gliomas: demonstration by PET with [^{18}F]fluoromisonidazole. J Nucl Med 1992;33: 2133–2137.
15. Martin GV, Caldwell JH, Rasey JS, et al. Enhanced binding of the hypoxic cell marker [^{18}F]fluoromisonidazole in ischemic myocardium. J Nucl Med 1989;30:194–201.
16. Martin GV, Cardwell JH, Graham MM, et al. Noninvasive detection of hypoxic myocardium using [^{18}F]fluoromisonidazole and PET. J Nucl Med 1992;33:2202–2208.
17. http://www.gemedicalsystems.com/rad/nm_pet/products/cyclotron/index.html.
18. http://www.shi.co.jp/quantum/eng/product/product_index.html.
19. http://www.ebcotech.com/mainframes.html.

6

Economics of Clinical Operation

E. Edmund Kim and Franklin C.L. Wong

Positron emission tomography (PET) has been used for almost 30 years to quantify normal physiology and metabolism, to characterize disease, and to evaluate the changes resulting from disease processes. The data that have been developed from these research applications have led to the clinical applications. Clinical PET is one of the many uses of PET, including clinical care, and it is reimbursed by insurance companies. Clinical PET became a reality only after widespread reimbursement became available for the procedure. Rapid growth in the utilization of PET is directly related to changes in radiopharmaceutical regulation and reimbursement. In the Food and Drug Administration (FDA) Modernization and Accountability Act passed by Congress in 1997, it was stated that PET radiopharmaceuticals have the equivalence of FDA approval until a new process for regulating PET radiopharmaceuticals is developed. In 1998, the Health Care Financing Administration (HCFA) began covering fluorodeoxyglucose (FDG)-PET for the evaluation of solitary pulmonary nodules (G code 0125), initial staging of lung cancer (G0126), detection of recurrent colorectal cancer with rising carcinoembryonic antigens (G0163), staging of lymphoma (G0164), and detection of recurrent malignant melanoma (G0165). The HCFA-approved indications were paid using G codes, and hospital outpatients have been reimbursed using the Ambulatory Payment Classification (APC). The PET imaging devices, both dedicated and hybrid systems, have been also covered.[1] The growing recognition of the cost-effectiveness of FDG-PET in cancer management has made oncology the focus for most clinical PET studies.[2]

The coverage for breast cancer and Alzheimer's disease as well as myocardial viability has been recently approved. The revenue generated by PET is now a substantial portion of the total nuclear medicine department income. With the expanded coverage of PET in oncology and cardiology by Medicare, the trend of clinical PET applications seems to be toward continued growth.[3] However, the survival of PET centers may be affected by the potential decrement in reimbursement and by competition for patients from nearby PET centers. The shortage of human resources may be another challenge in the future, and the reimbursement for tracers other than ^{18}F and ^{82}Rb may be necessary for further growth in clinical PET.

PET Facility

To ensure a financially successful PET center, whether hospital-based or in a private practice, several steps should be followed in the initial planning and developing of the facility. A mission statement should be created to define the type of facility and its goals, which can be clinically based or research oriented, or a combination of both. The decision-making process for purchasing a PET scanner is very complicated, entailing choice of equipment, potential clinical use in the service area, physician knowledge, and FDG availability. The equipment options are dedicated PET scanners with or without a cyclotron, a coincidence camera-based PET, and a mobile PET service. There are multiple camera options with varied capabilities and differences in purchasing and operating costs. The least costly venture with the lowest financial risk is either a mobile PET service or a dual-head coincidence camera for both FDG and general nuclear imagings. The most costly and financially risky venture is a dedicated PET scanner with a cyclotron, which costs as much as $5 million. The operating cost of the cyclotron increases the operating cost of the facility by as much as a half-million dollars per year (Table 6.1). The physical location of the facility should meet federal, state, and city requirements.

The purchase of the equipment should include having the vendor as a continuous resource, as the vendor's support is critical for a new technology. The following programs also should be included: initial and ongoing technician training, preceptorship and over-read programs for physicians, assistance of reimbursement, and marketing program (speakers, materials, and a resource library). Minimum space planning should include estimations for the cyclotron room (500 sq. ft.), the heat exchanger room (150 sq. ft.), the hot/cold pharmacy laboratory (800 sq. ft.), the clinical laboratory (450 sq. ft.), the imaging suite (400 sq. ft.), the equipment control areas (100 sq. ft.), the patient preparation rooms (125 sq. ft.), and specialized support areas.[4] The cyclotron room must be capable of supporting at least 120,000 lbs for cyclotron and ancillary shielding. Adequate bench space, atmospheric exhaust hoods to hold up to 1500 lbs, and laminar exhaust hoods should be included in the design of the pharmacy facility. Hot cells cost around $70,000 each, and remote manipulators usually cost $25,000 per arm. Computer-assisted robotic systems for radiochemical synthesis cost approximately $100,000, and the automated synthesis modules for ^{18}F products cost around $55,000 each. Specific equipment includes high-pressure liquid chromatography ($75,000), gas chromatography ($25,000), radionuclide dose calibrators, flammable safety storage cabinets, incubation ovens, and glassware. In the clinical laboratory, a glucose analyzer, a blood gas analyzer, microfuges, and a sampling device are needed for assaying blood samples. Patient preparation rooms should be config-

TABLE 6.1. Expenses of cyclotron operation

1. Salaries	$400,000	
a. Staff physicists		$150,000
b. Accelerator operation or software engineer		$100,000
c. Electronic technicians (4)		$150,000
2. Maintenance and operation		
a. Expendables	$ 31,150	
Extractor foils (47/yr)		$ 1500
Pullers (12/yr)		$ 9600
Cathodes (50/yr)		$ 2500
Anodes (12/yr)		$ 4800
Foil holders (2/yr)		$ 1600
Insulator rods (20/yr)		$ 200
Hydrogen gas (3/yr)		$ 90
Oils (8 gal/yr)		$ 7660
Batteries		$ 200
Office supplies		$ 3000
b. Contract maintenance	$ 6900	
De-ionizers		$ 800
Hydraulic systems		$ 3900
Computers		$ 2200
c. Spare parts	$ 27,000	
Power supplies		$ 5000
Radiofrequency system		$ 7000
Vacuum system		$ 5000
Water cooling system		$ 2000
Radiation monitors		$ 3000
Profile scanners		$ 1000
Electricals and electronics		$ 4000
d. Utilities	$126,500	
Electrical		$ 96,000
Chilled water		$ 30,500
3. Replacement equipment for maintenance test	$ 8800	
a. Lead detector (5 yrs)		$ 4000
b. Mass spectroscopy (5 yrs)		$ 2000
c. Oscilloscopes (5 yrs)		$ 2800
4. Travel (2 trips/yr)	$ 2000	
5. Consultation	$ 10,000	
6. Total direct cost	$612,350	

ured conveniently with the imaging suite, and should be of adequate size with a nurse call system as well as a sound- and light-controlled environment.

Feasibility Study

To prepare a feasibility study of the PET operation, information should be gathered about the number of prospective referring physicians, the physicians' clinical awareness of PET, the reimbursement by third-party carriers, the competition in the service area, and the commercial availability of FDG. The list of physicians to be interviewed include medical, surgical, and radiation oncologists; neurologists and neurosurgeons; and cardiologists and radiologists. Patient demographics are important if non-reimbursed procedures will constitute a significant portion of the work. Before interviewing the physicians, a matrix should be prepared that lists the local and national insurance carriers and their PET policy by covered clinical indications. After the interviews are completed, the potential number of requested scans can be estimated, and the potential financial success of the project may be computed. Total revenue (numbers of scan × $2,000 per scan) minus bad debt (25% of revenue) yields the net revenue. Expenses include costs of equipment leasing, facility (utilities and insurance, maintenance, radiopharmaceuticals, and supplies), and staffing (technicians, a secretary, and their benefits). There are three options for purchasing equipment: direct purchase, direct financed lease/bank debt, and operating lease. Most manufacturers have capital finance companies that can assist in the financing of the equipment. To review the ability to collect fees for the studies completed, a review must be undertaken of existing practices by the payers (Medicare and private insurers), to gather information related to covered indications, preauthorization, precertification, and payment for services.

Financial Decision and Marketing

The most common business structure is for the hospital or private practice to purchase the equipment. In a fee-for-service contract, the hospital enters into an agreement with a company, usually a mobile provider. The hospital is responsible for the purchase of the radiopharmaceuticals and related supplies. The joint venture structure has been very effective in the PET market for both scanners and cyclotrons. The FDG vendors develop a distribution network to provide other sites with FDG by either ground or air transport. The price of FDG is approximately $800 per 10 mCi and is often negotiable. Projected financial stability both on a cash and accrual basis should be maintained. There should be enough funds to carry the PET center during the start-up phase and during difficult periods for collecting accounts receivable. The marketing plan is as critical as the financial analysis. Education is the key to developing a successful marketing program. A series of grand rounds or lectures for a broad overview of PET and its clinical uses should be set up. A general brochure and scientific articles on PET as well as information for the patients also should be sent to the physicians.

Computed tomography (CT) and PET are clinically useful in the staging of non–small cell lung cancer because it reduces unnecessary surgeries.[5] It also has been shown to be economical, with the saving of $1,154 per patient.[5] It saves significantly more by not pursuing biopsy in patients with positive CT and PET results. Significant additional savings would result if PET was used to rule out surgical candidates based on the detection of distant metastases. Compared with optimized Ga 67 single photon emission computed tomography (SPECT), FDG-PET achieves a higher detection rate and more accurate staging in patients with high-risk melanoma and can also detect synchronous or metachronous primary malignancies more sensitively.[6] This incremental information can alter management in around 10% of patients at only marginally higher cost, providing a cost-effective alternative. The entire community, including the general population, insurance providers, and the administration of the hospital, in addition to physicians, needs to be educated on all aspects of PET. The newest and fastest-growing source for consumers is the Internet. A public relations company places articles about PET, such as features and patient stories, in newspapers, magazines, and on television and radio.

References

1. Coleman RE, Tesar R, Phelps M. HCFA and expanded coverage of PET. J Nucl Med 1999;42:11–12N.
2. Coleman RE. PET in lung cancer. J Nucl Med 1999;40:814–820.
3. Wong CO, Hill J. A review of trends and demands for PET imaging; one community hospital's experience. J Nucl Med 2001;42:21–24N.
4. Chilton HM. Planning and financing a PET center. J Nucl Med 1991;32:35–38N.
5. Gambhir SS, Hoh CK, Phelps ME, et al. Decision tree sensitivity analysis for cost-effectiveness of FDG-PET in the staging and management of non-small cell lung carcinoma. J Nucl Med 1996;37:1428–1436.
6. Kalff V, Hicks RJ, Ware RE, et al. Evaluation of high-risk melanoma: comparison of F-18 FDG PET and high dose Ga-67 SPECT. Eur J Nucl Med 2002;29:506–515.

7

Technical Considerations

E. Edmund Kim and Franklin C.L. Wong

The role of positron emission tomography (PET) in clinical practice is increasing. Clinical decisions based on PET studies are changing patient management by adding functional information to that obtained from conventinal morphologic modalities. Focal areas of abnormally increased fluorodeoxyglucose (FDG) uptake are considered suspicious for malignant disease, as metabolic changes often precede the anatomic changes associated with disease. Disease management depends on the tumor type, the extent and aggressiveness of the lesion, and on local and distant metastases. Whole-body FDG-PET is becoming a standard procedure for imaging cancer, and FDG-PET can play a significant role in establishing therapeutic response.

There is difficulty in interpreting FDG-PET scans, particularly in the neck and abdomen, due to the absence of identifiable anatomic structures. The low contrast and resolution in the PET scan is insufficient for precise anatomic structures and anatomic localization of abnormal uptake. A combined PET/CT scanner successfully acquires co-registered anatomic and functional images in a single scanning session. Technical factors must be considered when evaluating organ function because they may introduce artifacts and findings that are, in reality, normal variants. These include the time between injection and scanning, the dose administered, filtering and processing steps, test–retest variability, and the type of scanner. Patient preparation, with good instructions and a questionnaire, is vitally important for optional PET scanning.

Radiopharmaceutical, Dosimetry, and Instrument

^{18}F-FDG (2-F-18-fluoro-2-deoxy-d-glucose), 5 to 20 mCi, is administered IV through an intracatheter (23–25 gauge) or butterfly needle and flushed with 10 to 20 cc of normal saline. The IV system should then be removed and a residual should be taken. If whole-body imaging will be acquired in addition to the brain study then 15 to 20 mCi of ^{18}F-FDG should be given. If 3D imaging is necessary, a lower dose of ^{18}F-FDG should be given so that the ratio between trues and randoms remains in an ideal range.

The bladder wall is the critical organ and receives 3.15 rad per 5 mCi ^{18}F-FDG. Radiation dose estimates for the bladder, heart, and brain are 1.10, 2.20, and 1.20 rads per 5 mCi ^{18}F-FDG, respectively.

The Siemens/CTI ECAT HR+ dedicated full-ring PET scanner and the discovery LS GE Medical Systems PET/CT system are commonly utilized instruments.

General Procedure

1. Patient checks in at the reception area.
2. Nurse confirms the chart and required paperwork.
3. Nurse reviews and answers any of the patient's questions regarding the procedure, and ensures that all of the required preparation before the exam has been followed.
4. Patient can change into a hospital gown or simply remove all metal objects, prostheses, etc.
5. Nurse should alert the technologist or physician if there is reason to believe the patient cannot tolerate the procedure.
6. Patient's height and weight should be measured.
7. Patient's blood sugar levels should be measured and recorded with a glucometer. If the patient's blood sugar level exceeds 200 mg/dL, the nurse should notify the technologist/physician.
8. Patients should answer questionnaire, and females should sign the consent form.
9. Nurses will then begin a 20- to 23-gauge intracatheter or butterfly.
10. The dose should be checked out from the radiopharmacy.
11. Give the dose of 5 to 20 mCi of ^{18}F-FDG and flush with 10 to 20 cc of normal saline. The syringe should be checked to determine the residual, which should be noted in the documentation.
12. Patient waits comfortably in the holding area for 30 to 45 minutes postinjection.
13. Position the patient in the scanner supine with the head toward the gantry. The head should be secured to limit patient movement.
14. Set up the protocol (energy window centered at 511 keV with lower limit (LLD) of 350 and upper limit (ULD) of 650, and assure that the correct time of injection, dose administered, and patient height and weight are entered for the procedure.
15. Scan the patient, taking care to ensure correct positioning.
16. If no transmission scan is needed because emission and norm data will be used to calculate attenuation, the study may be stopped after completion of the emission scan.
17. Upon completion of the scan, patients may change back into their clothes and wait for the images to be reviewed before leaving. The gown or scrubs used should be placed in the linen bags to ensure there is no radiation contamination from urine.

Protocol for Whole-Body PET Using ^{18}F-FDG

Procedure

1. Set up the protocol. Ensure that the patient's height is represented in Database Utilities. Also assure that the correct time of injection, dose administered minus residual, and patient weight are entered for the procedure.
    - Use 2D, seven planes of overlap, or 3D, 15 planes of overlap whole-body imaging.
    - Check the number of bed positions based on the height of the patient.
2. Position the patient from the orbits to 2 cm below the pubic symphysis. The first bed position should be over the pelvis to avoid artifacts in the retrovesical region from later accumulation of radioactive urine in the bladder.
3. Data acquisition of PET/CT. A combined PET/CT system (Discovery LS, GE Medical Systems, Waukesha, WI) is able to acquire CT images and PET data of the same patient in one session (Fig. 7.1). A GE Advance Nxi PET scanner and a multidetector-row helical CT (LightSpeed plus) are integrated in this dedicated system. The table excursion permits scanning of six continuous PET sections covering 867 mm. This gives adequate coverage from head to pelvic floor in all patients. The PET and CT data sets are acquired on two independent computer consoles, which are connected by an interface to transfer CT data to the PET scanner. For viewing of the images, the PET and CT data sets are transferred to an independent, PC-based computer workstation by DICOM transfer. All viewing of co-registered images is performed with dedicated software (eNTEGRA, ELGEMS, Haifa, Israel). While PET images are acquired during free breathing and each image is acquired over multiple respiratory cycles, CT scans are acquired during shallow breathing.

    The patients are fasted for at least 4 hours prior to the intravenous administration of 10 mCi (370 MBq) of FDG. Forty-five minutes postinjection, the combined examination starts. The CT data are acquired first. The patient is positioned on the table in a head-first, supine position. The arms of the patient are placed in an elevated position above the head to reduce beam-hardening artifacts. However, in patients unable to maintain this position, arms are positioned in front of the abdomen. For the CT data acquisition, the following parameters are used: tube-rotation time 0.5 sec/evolution, 140 kV, 80 mA, 22.5 mm/rotation, slice pitch 6 (high-speed mode), reconstructed slice-thickness 5 mm, scan length 867 mm, acquisition-time 22.5 seconds per CT scan. No intravenous or oral contrast agents are used.

    After the CT data acquisition is completed, the table top is automatically advanced into the PET gantry, and acquisition of PET emission data is started at the level of the pelvic floor. Six incremental table positions are acquired with minimal overlap, thereby covering

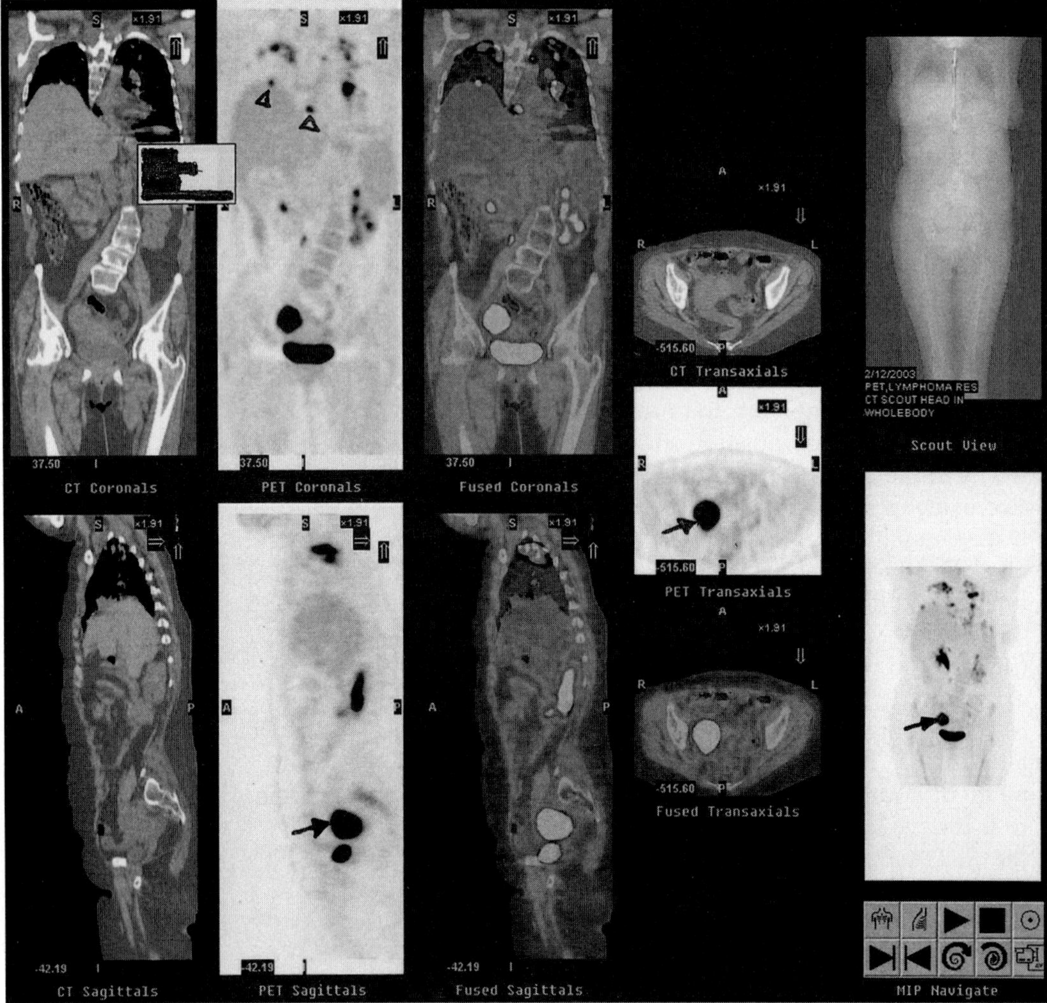

FIGURE 7.1. Selected coronal and sagittal images of the axial body as well as an axial image of the lower pelvis are shown by CT, ^{18}F-FDG-PET, and PET/CT co-registered images with lymphoma lesions in the right external iliac (*arrows*), and bilateral perihilar and diaphragmatic (*arrowheads*) nodes.

867 mm of table travel. For each position, 35 2D non–attenuation-corrected scans are obtained simultaneously over a 5-minute period. No transmission scans are obtained since CT data are used for transmission correction. Transaxial, attenuation-corrected slices are reconstructed using iterative reconstruction. Image reconstruction matrix is 128 × 128 with a transaxial field of view (FOV) of 49.7 × 49.7 cm.

4. Image analysis of PET/CT: Clinical preimaging data are available for reviewers. This information includes location of primary tumor, suspicion of local recurrence, and/or metastases. Image interpretation is performed without any objective measurements concerning FDG uptake. However, the images are consistently windowed so that brain FDG activity is in the overrange and the lower window level is close to zero. On a grading scale from 0 to 4, activity com-

parable to brain was 4, between brain and liver 3, liver 2, and below liver 1. Lesions are called positive only if they had FDG uptake of at least level 3 in PET, while in PET/CT small lesions noted on CT such as multiple intrapulmonary lesions are called positive even in the face of negative PET.

For lesion-based image analysis, the following three categories are evaluated if applicable: recurrence of primary, metastases, and second primary tumor. Since localization of the lesion is crucial for staging, all lesions are assigned to an anatomic region. Therefore, the full evaluation of a data set includes status as well as location of recurrence, number and location of regional and distant metastases, and possible number and location of second primary tumors.

Billing

Table 7.1 lists the service codes for billing purposes.

Table 7.1. Billing with service code numbers in the United States

Service code	Description	Comments
2320927	PET, tumor imaging—miscellaneous indications	This code should be utilized when a private payer covers the patient.
2320922 G0213 G0214 G0215	Recurrence of colorectal CA, PET of whole body (WB) (diagnosis, staging, and restaging)	This code should be utilized when Medicare covers the patient.
2320923 G0220 G0221 G0222	Staging of Lymphoma, PET WB (initial staging and restaging of Hodgkin's and non-Hodgkin's lymphomas)	This code should be utilized when Medicare covers the patient.
2320924 G0216 G0217 G0218	Recurrence of melanoma, PET WB (diagnosis, initial staging, and restaging, NOT including evaluation of regional nodes)	This code should be utilized when Medicare covers the patient.
2320925 G0125	Characterization of single pulmonary nodule (SPN) PET WB	This code should be utilized when Medicare covers the patient.
2320926 G0210 G0211 G0212	Initial staging of non–small cell lung cancer (NSCLC), PET WB (diagnosis, initial staging, and restaging of NSCLC)	This code should be utilized when Medicare covers the patient.
July 2001 G0226 G0227 G0228	Diagnosis, initial staging, and restaging of esophageal CA, PET WB	This code should be utilized when Medicare covers the patient.
July 2001 G0223 G0224 G0225	Head and Neck CA, PET WB (CNS and thyroid CA is NOT covered)	This code should be utilized when Medicare covers the patient.
July 2001 G0229	PET for pre-surgical evaluation for patients with refractory seizures	This code should be utilized when Medicare covers the patient.
PETNC	^{18}F-FDG (fluorodeoxyglucose)	This code should be utilized to show that the radiopharmaceutical has been given.

Protocol for PET Using ^{15}O Water or Gases and ^{11}C Methionine

1. ^{15}O water is used to measure blood flow. PET data can be acquired in 3D mode with a model-based correction applying to account for 35% of 3D scatter fraction. Images are reconstructed with a Hanning filter (cutoff Nyquist). For each ^{15}O water study, 15 to 20 mCi are injected in 5 mL saline as a rapid bolus using an automated injector with simultaneous sampling of arterial blood and 4-minute gynamic PET scan (23 frames; 10 × 3 seconds, 3 × 10 s, 4 × 15 s, and 6 × 20 s). The arterial blood data (input function) are collected over 4 minutes. Blood is withdrawn at a 6-mL/min rate and radioactive events are detected. Eight sequential PET scans are obtained at 20-minute. intervals. The data are analyzed using the tissue compartment model.
2. ^{15}O gases are used to measure blood flow and volume as well as oxygen extraction and metabolism. ^{15}O gases, O_2, CO_2, and CO, are administered sequentially in one session to provide three separate data sets.

   The ^{15}O O_2 and ^{15}O CO_2 gases are delivered continuously during the study period at flows of 10 mCi/min at 80 mL/min, and 5 mCi/min at 60 mL/min, respectively. Labeled gases are mixed with 200 mL/min of medical air, and are supplied to the patient through a plastic face mask. Once inhalation of the labeled gas is initiated, equilibrium will be established over a 12-minute period, followed by scans with 1.5 to 2.5 million for each ^{15}O O_2 image and 2 to 4 million ^{15}O for each CO_2 image. ^{15}O CO is administered at 80 mCi at 100 mL/min for 4 minutes. The ^{15}O CO supply is then discontinued, and after a 1-minute equilibrium period, images can be obtained with 300,000 to 500,000 true coincidences. Blood samples are obtained from an arterial line for the measurement of blood gases throughout these studies.

   The oxygen analysis program generates maps for the functional parameters for each anatomic plane as a composite data set. The oxygen extraction fraction and metabolic rate are corrected for blood volume.
3. ^{11}C-Methionine PET

   ^{11}C-methionine is another tracer for PET that can be used to assess metabolic demand for amino acids in cancer cells. Methionine PET has been useful in differential diagnosis of benign and malignant lesions in the brain and lung. Patients fast at least 6 hours before the PET scan. Transmission scan is acquired for 20 minutes using a rotating ^{68}Ge source, and the total counts per slice is more than 7 million. Emission scans are obtained over a 15-minute scanning period, 20 to 30 minutes after intravenous injection of 10 mCi ^{11}C-methionine, with more than 3 million counts per slice. Image reconstruction in a 128 × 128 matrix using measured attenuation correction is performed using a Shepp and Logan filter.

Common Questions and Answers Asked by Patients

What Is PET?

PET is a technology that combines the fields of medicine, computer science, chemistry, physics, and physiology to study the function of organs such as the heart, brain, and bone. It is different from conventional imaging equipment, such as x-ray, CT, ultrasound, and MRI, in that PET images contain information about how tissue functions. The other imaging modalities show what the tissues look like.

What Does a PET Scanner Look Like?

The PET scanner is similar in shape to a CT or MRI scanner; however, a PET scanner makes no noise. The bed on the scanner moves during the exam so that each area of the body can be imaged.

What Can I Expect?

- You will be asked questions about your illness.
- Your blood glucose (sugar) levels will be checked.
- A small IV tube will be placed in your arm to administer a very small quantity of a radioactive material. This allows for the PET scanner to "see" where sugar metabolizes in your body.
- Because the injection you will receive is radioactive and because it is important that you are relaxed and quiet after the injection, family members are not allowed in the area while you are in the PET suite.
- Depending on the type of PET scan that you are receiving, you may be given a medicine called Lasix through the same IV line that the radioactive sugar was injected. Lasix is a diuretic that will stimulate you to urinate.
- Again, depending on the type of PET scan, you might need to have a tube, also known as a Foley catheter, placed in your bladder. This is done so that the scanner can "see" the area surrounding your bladder.
- After the injection, you will need to rest quietly until it is time for your scan. Again, the amount of quiet time depends on the study, but be prepared to wait for between 45 and 90 minutes.
- During the scan, you will lie on your back on a table.
- The amount of time the scan takes depends on how tall you are and why you are having the test.
- When the exam is over, the data will be processed and the results will be reported to your physician the next day.

Can I Eat?

No. We cannot emphasize this enough. If you eat within 6 hours of your test, there is an exceptionally high chance that your exam will be canceled. The reason for this is that the scan relies on how your body absorbs sugar, and if you have eaten, your body is saturated with sugar and the medication we give will not distribute properly.

If your PET scan is scheduled in the morning, you must only drink water. No caffeine or sugar products may be consumed. If your scan is later in the afternoon, do not eat for at least 6 hours before your test. You may take all of your medications. If the medication needs to be taken with food, we will contact your physician and give you further instructions.

How Long Does the Test Take?

Overall, you should allow about 3 hours for your test. The preparation for the scan takes about 45 minutes. The scan typically takes a little over an hour. However, the physician might want to perform additional images.

Is PET Safe?

PET is a noninvasive technique that provides maximum information to your physicians with minimal radiation exposure. The radiotracers remain in the body for only short periods of time and have no known side effects.

Questionnaire for Patients

Table 7.2 is an example of a questionnaire given to patients.

TABLE 7.2. Questionnaire

Patient Name ________________	Patient ID ________		
Weight ______lb ________ kg	Height ____________cm		
Blood sugar level mg/dL: (1)______(2)______(3)______			
1. Have you been fasting?	Yes	No	Comment:__________
2. Are you hydrated?	Yes	No	
3. Surgical history ________________			
4. Where are your incision sites?________________			
5. Have you had any biopsies recently?	Yes	No	If yes, where? ________
6. Have you had chemotherapy?	Yes	No	If yes, when?________
7. Have you had radiation therapy?	Yes	No	If yes, when?________
8. Do you have an ostomy site?	Yes	No	If yes, where? ________
9. Do you have a catheter (CVC or porta-cath) placed? Yes No			
If yes, where? ____________ when?____________			
10. Do you have any metal objects or prostheses on?		Yes	No
11. Do you have a pacemaker?	Yes	No	
12. Have you had any of the following:			
Inflammation	Yes	No	If yes, when?________
Recent injury	Yes	No	If yes, when?________
Infection (sinus, throat, bladder, etc.)	Yes	No	If yes, when?________
13. Are you positive for any of the following inflammatory diseases?			
Tuberculosis	Yes	No	
Rheumatoid arthritis	Yes	No	
Toxoplasmosis	Yes	No	
14. Were you instructed not to eat 6 hours prior to the study?		Yes	No
15. Were you instructed to drink six to eight glasses of water?		Yes	No
16. Are you aware that the study takes approximately 3 hours to complete?		Yes	No
17. Were you told that family members are not allowed into the PET suite?	Yes	No	

TABLE 7.2. Questionnaire (*continued*)

18. Do you have any questions or issues?
    If so, what were they?____
    Scheduled__________________________ Time
    Scheduled __________________________ AM/PM
    Patient information completed by:________________________________

Worksheet for PET

Table 7.3 is an example of a worksheet for staff.

TABLE 7.3. Worksheet

1. General Information
   Patient Name____
   Medical Record Number (MRN)_______________ Height_____________
   Outpatient [ ] Inpatient [ ] (room #________) DOB________________
   Weight__________
   Male [ ] Female [ ] (Pregnant? Yes [ ] No [ ])
   Translation services required? No [ ] Yes [ ] language:_______________
   Contact numbers:
   Home_________________________ Work_______________
   (Local/cell)______________________
   Requesting physician_______________________________________
2. Patient instructions
   a. Is the patient a diabetic? Yes [ ] No [ ]
      If yes, what was the last reading? __________ <200? Yes [ ] No [ ]
      Note: If the pt.'s glucose level is 200 or higher, contact the nuclear medicine special procedures physician
   b. Is the patient able to lie on his/her back for over an hour? Yes [ ] No [ ]
      Note: If the patient is unable to lie on his/her back for this time, he/she may wish to contact his/her physician for a dose of pain medication.
   c. Is the patient claustrophobic? Yes [ ] No [ ]
      Has the patient ever had a problem having an MRI or CT? Yes [ ] No [ ]
      Note: If the patient answers yes to either of these questions, refer this case to a PET nurse to evaluate for conscious sedation.
   d. Has the patient had radiation therapy? Yes [ ] No [ ]
      (If yes, is the patient currently undergoing treatment, or when was the radiation therapy completed?______________)
   e. Is the patient receiving chemotherapy? Yes [ ] No [ ]
      (If yes, include list of medications in the next question.)
   f. Has the patient had a previous PET/gallium scan? Yes [ ] No [ ]
      If answer is yes, date:_____________
   g. List medications (name, dosage, and frequency) that the patient is taking.
      ____
   h. Was the patient instructed not to eat 6 hours prior to the study? Yes [ ] No [ ]
   i. Was the patient instructed to drink six to eight glasses of water? Yes [ ] No [ ]
   j. Is the patient aware the study takes approximately 3 hours to complete? Yes [ ] No [ ]
   k. Was the patient told that family members are not allowed into the PET suite? Yes [ ] No [ ]
   l. Did the patient have any questions or issues? Yes [ ] No [ ]
      If so, what were they?
      ____
      Scheduled__________________________________Time
      Scheduled__________________________________AM/PM
      Patient information completed by : ______________________________

Checklist for Female Patients

Table 7.4 is an example of a checklist for female patients.

TABLE 7.4. Checklist for female patients

Question		
1. Have you passed menopause: If your answer is yes, go to question 6. If your answer is no, please answer all of the following questions.	Yes	No
2. Are you pregnant or do you believe you might be pregnant?	Yes	No
3. How many days has it been since the beginning of your last menstrual cycle? _____		
4. Are you practicing any form of birth control?	Yes	No
5. Are you nursing a baby?	Yes	No
6. Are you currently taking any hormones?	Yes	No
7. Do you have young children at home?	Yes	No
8. Have you had surgery on your breasts? Implants, reconstruction?	Yes	No
9. Do you understand the above questions?	Yes	No
10. Do you have any questions about using radioactive substances or about the questions above that you would like to discuss with a physician?	Yes	No

8

Normal and Variable Patterns

Ho-Young Lee, Myung-Chul Lee, and E. Edmund Kim

The clinical applications and investigations of positron emission tomography (PET) have been recently increasing. The majority of the clinical PET studies and the use of ^{18}F-fluoro-2-deoxyglucose (FDG) are related to oncology, but the uptake of this radiopharmaceutical is not specific to malignant tissue. There are several physiologic uptakes and artifacts, which make it difficult to evaluate or detect malignant tissue. It is important to be aware of normal variants and benign diseases that may mimic more serious pathology. Uptake of FDG in a number of sites may be variable and may be seen normally in the skeletal muscle after exercise or under tension, in the myocardium, in parts of the gastrointestinal tract, especially the stomach and cecum, and in the urinary tract. Some causes of increased physiologic uptake are avoidable, and measures can be taken to minimize accumulation.[1]

In certain clinical situations, the lack of specificity of ^{18}F-FDG uptake has led to the applications of L-[methyl-^{11}C]-methionine. Due to the short half-life of ^{11}C, use of this radiopharmaceutical is limited to those PET scanners that are not far from a cyclotron. However, ^{11}C-methionine has now become one of the most commonly used radiopharmaceuticals in clinical PET.[2]

PET Imaging with ^{18}F-FDG

Uptake Mechanism

^{18}F-FDG is an analog of glucose that is an energy substrate of metabolism.[3] Although tumors show increased glycolysis compared to normal tissues, the uptake of ^{18}F-FDG is not specific to malignant tissue. ^{18}F-FDG is transported into tumor cells by glucose transporter membrane proteins (Glut-1 to Glut-5). In particular, the expression of Glut-1 is increased in many tumors. After transported into the cell, ^{18}F-FDG is converted to ^{18}F-FDG-6-phosphate by hexokinase. After that it does not enter further enzymatic metabolic process. Due to its negative charge, it remains trapped in tissue. Glucose-6-phosphatase mediates dephosphorylation of the ^{18}F-FDG-6-phosphate. It occurs slowly in myocardium and brain. Many tumors have low concentrations of this enzyme, and hence the accumulation of ^{18}F-FDG-6-phosphate is proportional to the rate of glycolysis. Conversely, tissues such as liver, kidney, intestine, and resting skeletal muscle with high glucose-6-phosphatase activity may show lower activity.

Tumor uptake of ^{18}F-FDG is poor in acute hyperglycemia due to competition between ^{18}F-FDG and glucose. To optimize the accumulation in tumors, patients are usually fasted for 4 to 6 hours prior to scanning. Fortunately, it appears that chronic hyperglycemia, as seen in diabetic patients, only minimally reduces tumor uptake, but that insulin-induced hypoglycemia may actually impair tumor identification by reducing tumor uptake and increasing background muscle activity.

It has also been noted that the hypoxia in tumors may increase the accumulation of ^{18}F-FDG, and this also probably occurs through the activation of the anaerobic glycolytic pathway.

Normal Physiologic Distribution of ^{18}F-FDG

In the abdomen, low-grade accumulation of FDG is usually seen in the liver and the spleen. Small and large bowel activity may be variable, and unlike glucose, ^{18}F-FDG is excreted in the urine, leading to variable appearance in the urinary tract.

Skeletal muscle at rest usually shows low-grade uptake of ^{18}F-FDG (Fig. 8.1), but active skeletal muscle, after exercise, shows increased ac-

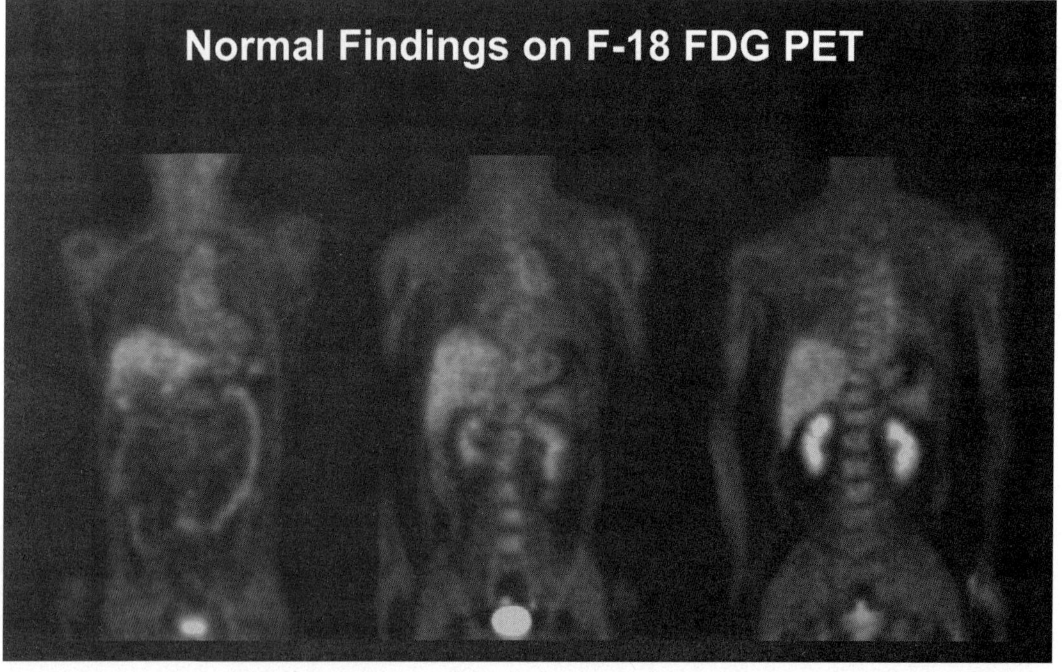

FIGURE 8.1. Coronal PET images of the axial body (*anterior to posterior on left to right*) using ^{18}F-FDG show normal distribution of FDG after fasting. Note significant activity in urinary and gastrointestinal tracts as well as liver and bone marrow. Note also mild diffuse and symmetrical activities in the muscles.

cumulation. Low-grade FDG uptake in muscles is part of the normal biodistribution pattern.[4] When this uptake is symmetric and corresponds to the location of a specific group of muscles, it is easily recognized.

Myocardial uptake of ^{18}F-FDG (Figs. 8.2, 8.3, and 8.4) is also very variable.[4,5] Normal myocardial metabolism depends on free fatty acids and glucose. Optimal uptake of ^{18}F-FDG in myocardial metabolic studies can be encouraged by the administration of oral glucose to increase glucose metabolism with or without insulin to enhance the myocardial uptake of glucose and hence ^{18}F-FDG.

The hyperinsulinemic euglycemic clamping technique may further improve myocardial ^{18}F-FDG uptake but is technically more difficult. This technique allows maximal insulin administration without rendering the patient hypoglycemic. An alternative method to encourage glu-

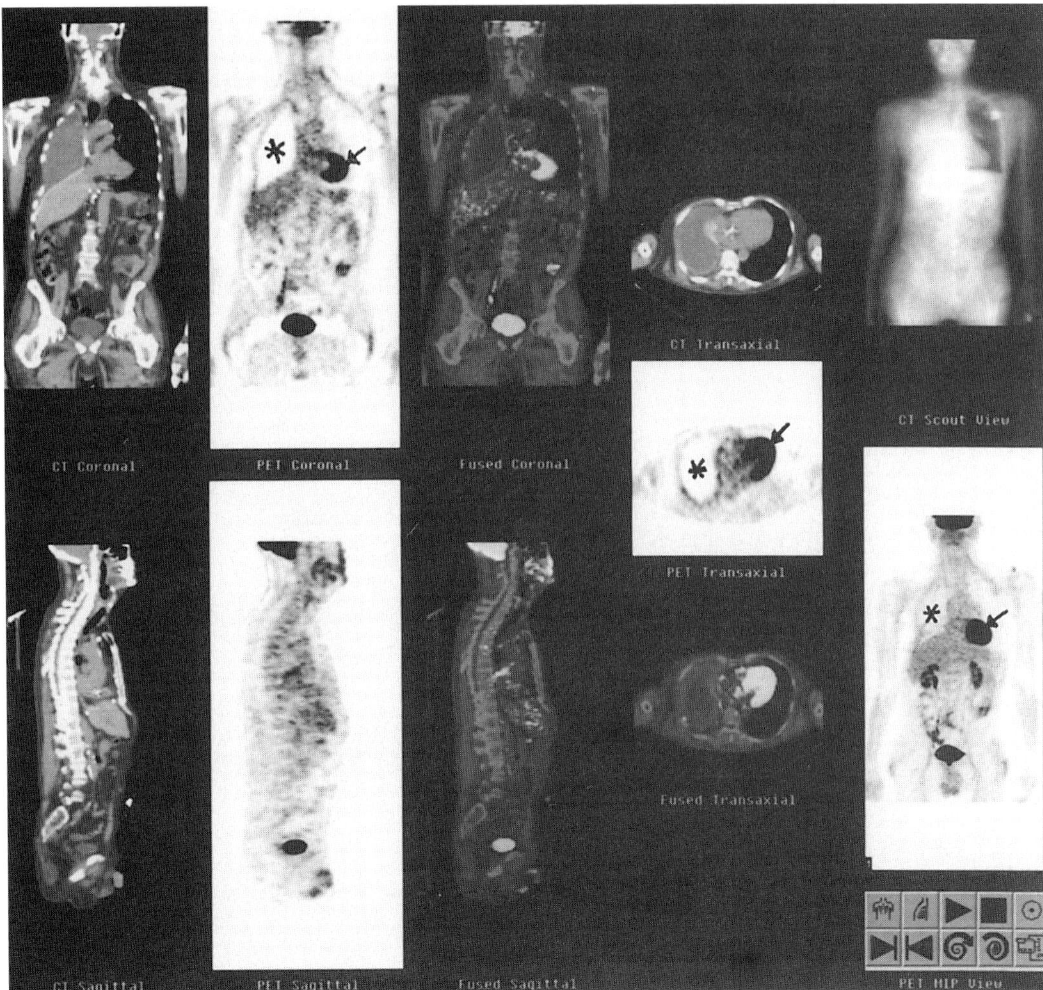

FIGURE 8.2. Selected coronal and sagittal PET/CT images of the axial body and an axial image of the lower chest show markedly increased uptake of ^{18}F-FDG in the left ventricular myocardium (*arrows*) and no activity in the right lung with fluid collection (*) after pneumonectomy.

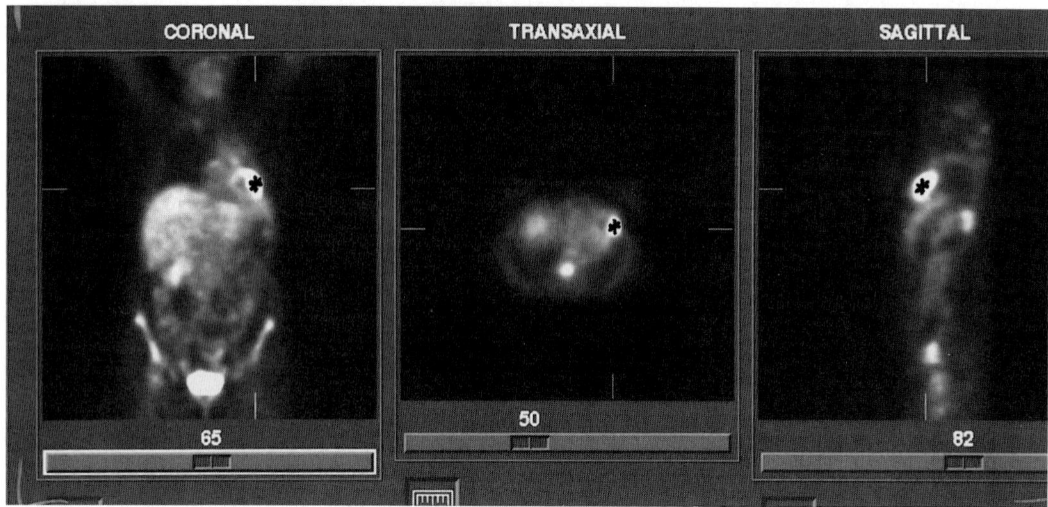

FIGURE 8.3. Selected coronal and sagittal PET images of the axial body and an axial image of the lower chest show markedly increased uptake of ^{18}F-FDG in thick left ventricular myocardium (*). No significant cardiac disease was found. Note heterogeneous hepatic activity.

cose metabolism in the myocardium is to reduce circulating free fatty acids pharmacologically. Improved cardiac uptake after administration of oral nicotinic acid derivatives has been reported. This is a simple and safe intervention that may also be effective in diabetic patients.

The brain typically shows high uptake of ^{18}F-FDG (Fig. 8.5) in the cortex, basal ganglia, and thalamus, but a generalized reduction in cor-

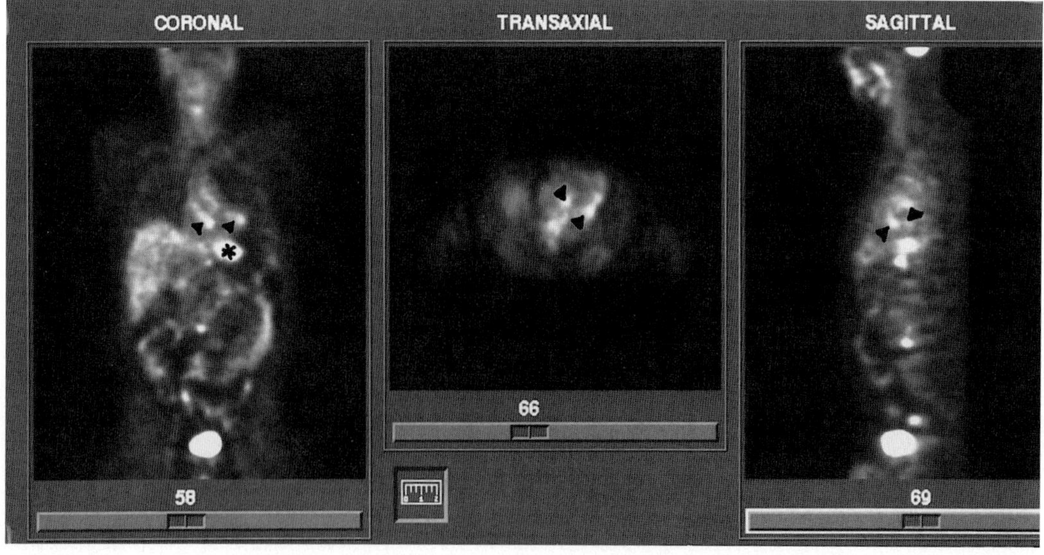

FIGURE 8.4. Selected coronal and sagittal PET images of the axial body and an axial image of the lower chest with ^{18}F-FDG show curvilinear increased activity in the upper left ventricular myocardium and possibly left atrium (*arrowheads*). No significant cardiac disease was found. Note markedly increased activity in the gastric fundus (*).

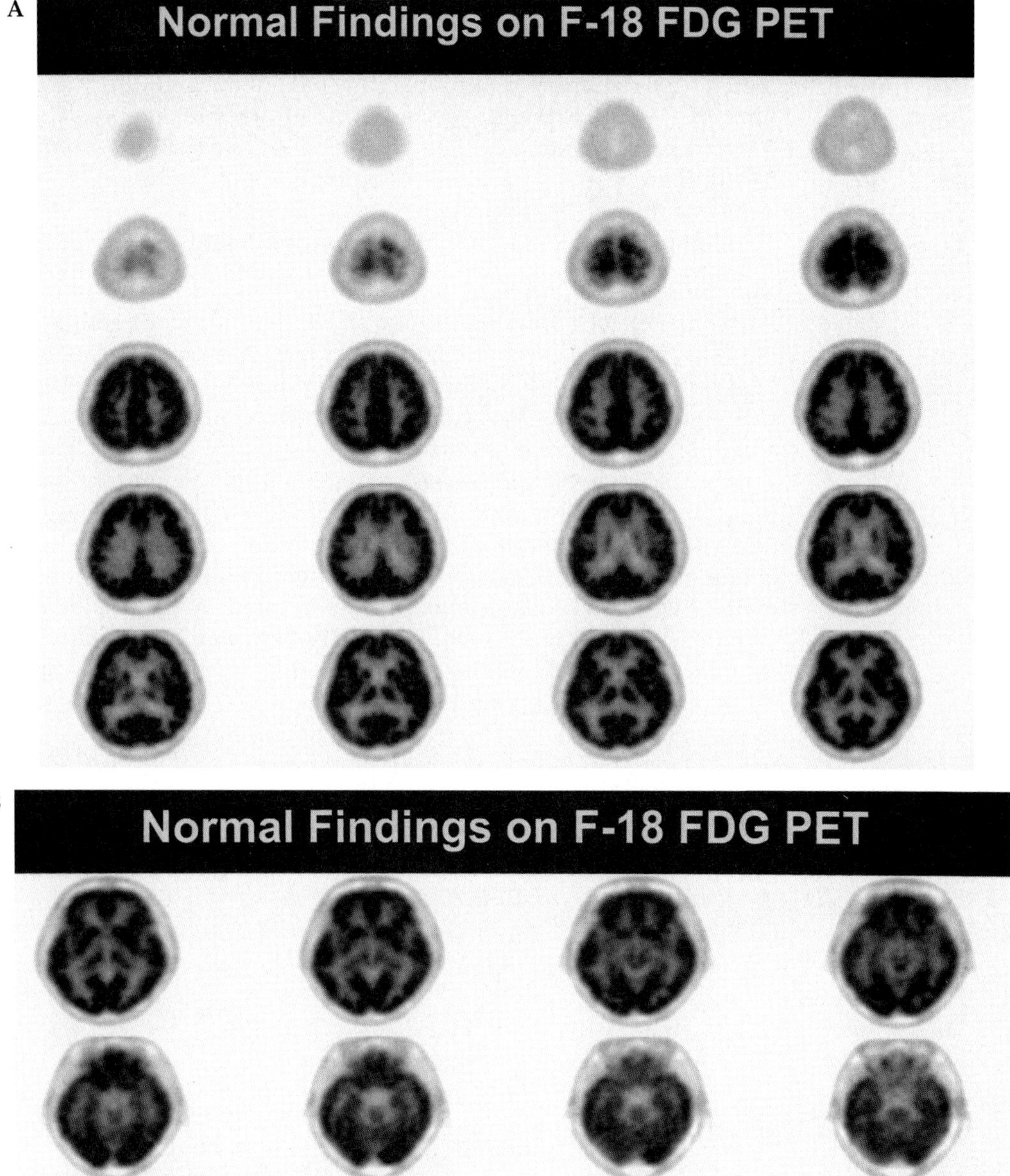

FIGURE 8.5. **A.** Transaxial PET images of the upper head with ^{18}F-FDG show symmetrical significant activity in the cerebral gray matter, basal ganglia, and thalamus. **B.** Transaxial image of the lower head using ^{18}F-FDG show symmetric activity in temporal and cerebellar gray matter.

tical activity may be seen with sedative and general anesthetic drugs that may be required for uncooperative patients and children. This may limit PET's sensitivity for the detection of areas of hypometabolism. Also, there is a general decline in metabolic activity in the frontal and somatosensory areas with normal aging.[6]

Physiological Variants That May Mimic Pathology

Skeletal Muscle

At rest, skeletal muscle does not show significant accumulation of ^{18}F-FDG, but after exercise or if contraction takes place during the uptake period after ^{18}F-FDG injection, there is an increased uptake in active skeletal muscle (Figs. 8.6 to 8.9), which relates to increased aerobic glycolysis of active muscle tissue.

Increased aerobic glycolysis of active skeletal muscle such as paraspinal, posterior cervical, or trapezius muscle may lead to increased accumulation of ^{18}F-FDG after exercise or due to tension, and is one of the most common causes of interpretation problems. Symmetric FDG uptake in the shoulders, neck, and thoracic spine region (Figs. 8.10 and 8.11) is possibly related to activated brown fatty tissue in underweight patients during increased sympathetic nerve activity due to cold stress.[7] Laryngeal muscle activity (Fig. 8.12) may be related to speech, and swallowing may cause hyoid and tongue base activities. Hyperventilation may create a diaphragmatic uptake. Exercise should be prohibited on the day of scanning to minimize muscle up-

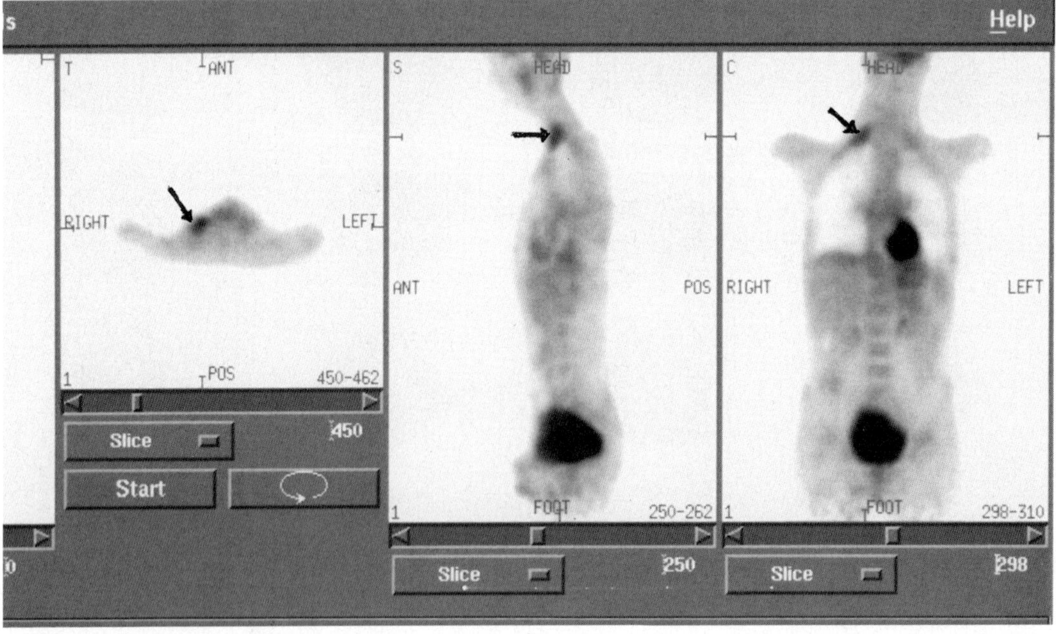

FIGURE 8.6. Selected axial PET image of the neck (*left*) and sagittal (*middle*) view, as well as coronal (*right*) PET images of the axial body with ^{18}F-FDG show a stressed sternocleidomastoid muscle (*arrows*).

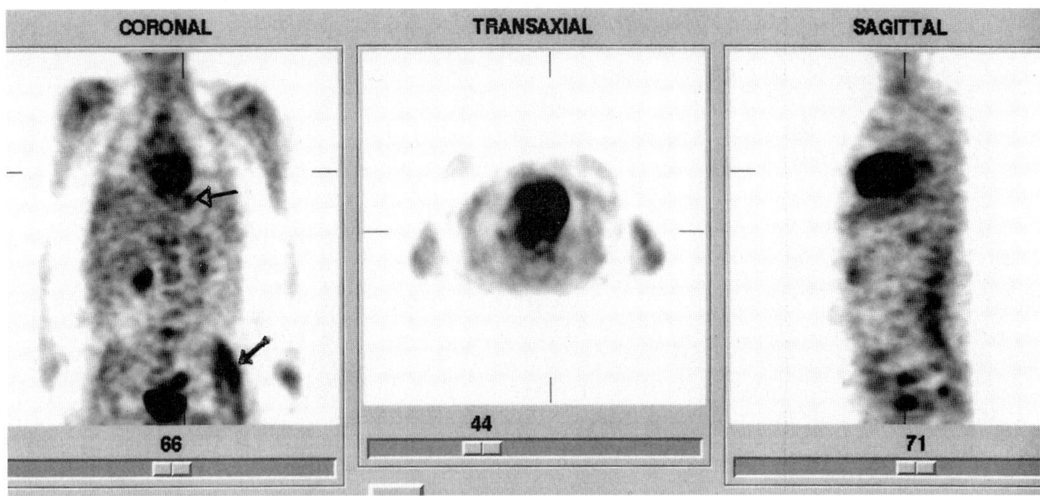

FIGURE 8.7. Selected coronal (*left*) and sagittal (*right*) PET images of the axial body with ^{18}F-FDG show diffusely increased activity in the stressed left gluteus muscles (*closed arrow*) and also focal increased activity in the gastric fundus (*open arrow*). Note also nonuniform activities due to obesity.

take, and benzodiazepines may be used to abolish the characteristic paraspinal and posterior cervical muscle uptake often seen in tense patients. Even with these precautions, skeletal muscle activity may still be seen. Anxiety-related increased muscular tension may cause symmetric or asymmetric uptake in neck and paravertebral muscles.

Problems may also result from involuntary muscle spasm such as that seen with torticollis, which may lead to asymmetric, unilateral uptake in the sternocleidomastoid muscle, and that may either mimic or obscure the pathology in the neck. Accurate interpretation of asymmetric muscle activity in the neck, shoulder, or arm is at times diffi-

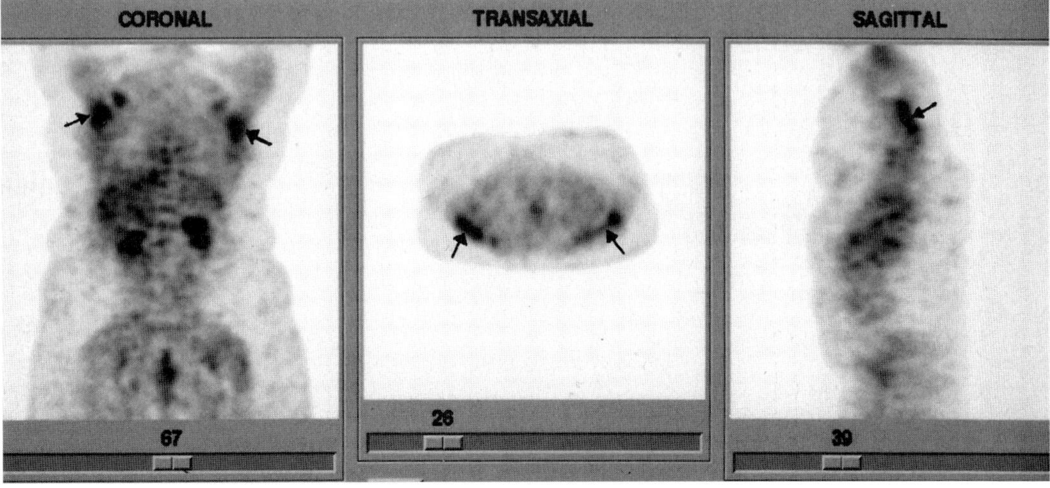

FIGURE 8.8. Selected coronal and sagittal PET images of the axial body and an axial image of the upper chest show symmetrically increased uptake of ^{18}F-FDG in bilateral infraspinatus muscles (*arrows*).

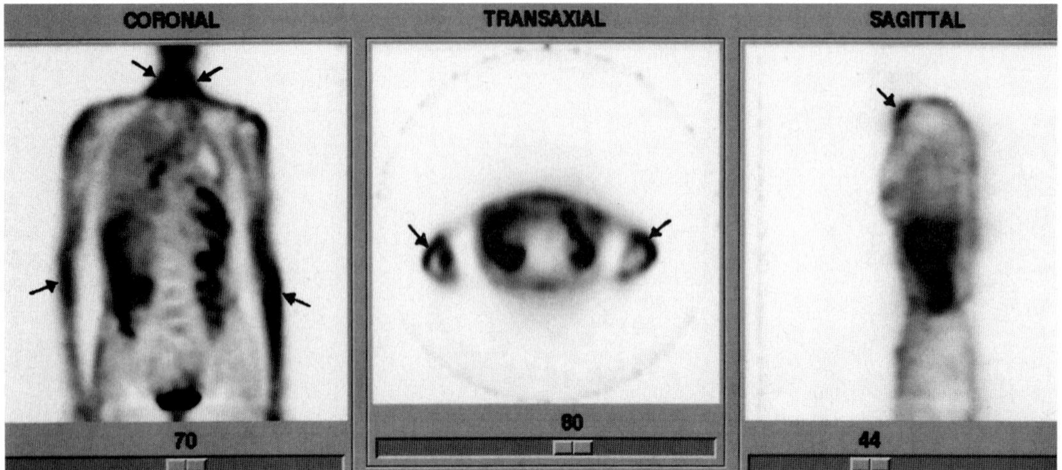

FIGURE 8.9. Selected coronal and sagittal PET images of the axial body and an axial image of the upper abdomen with ^{18}F-FDG show diffusely increased activity in the neck and arm muscles (*arrows*).

cult.[8] Trauma and inflammation may also cause enhanced skeletal muscle activity.

Gastrointestinal System

A number of regions in the gastrointestinal system may show uptake of ^{18}F-FDG. This uptake may be partly due to smooth muscle activity, although it has been shown that gastrointestinal uptake of ^{18}F-FDG in rats may be reduced either by bowel lavage or by use of antimicrobials, suggesting an alternative mechanism such as smooth muscle peristalsis.[9] In humans, ^{18}F-FDG activity is most noticeable in the large

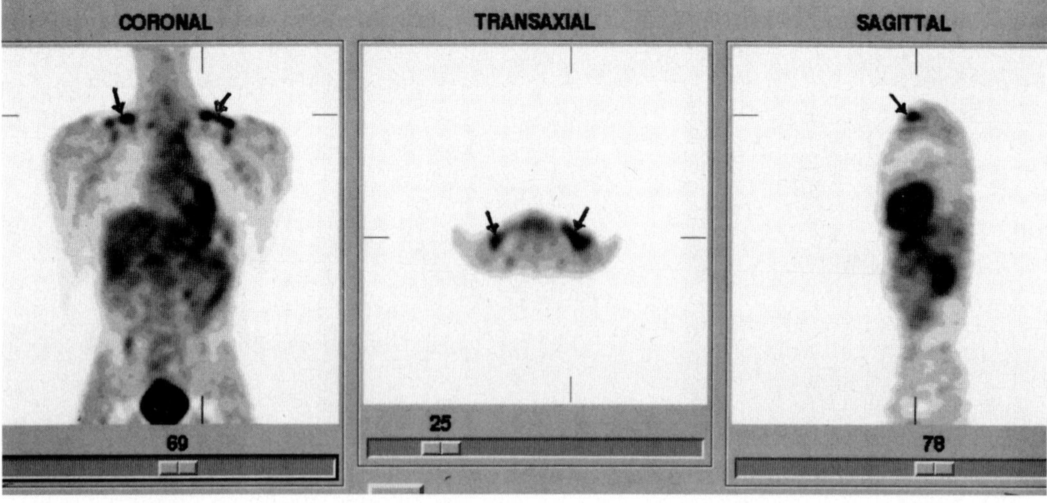

FIGURE 8.10. Selected coronal and sagittal PET images of the axial body and an axial image of the upper chest show symmetrically increased uptake of ^{18}F-FDG in the anterior neck muscles or brown fatty tissues (*arrows*).

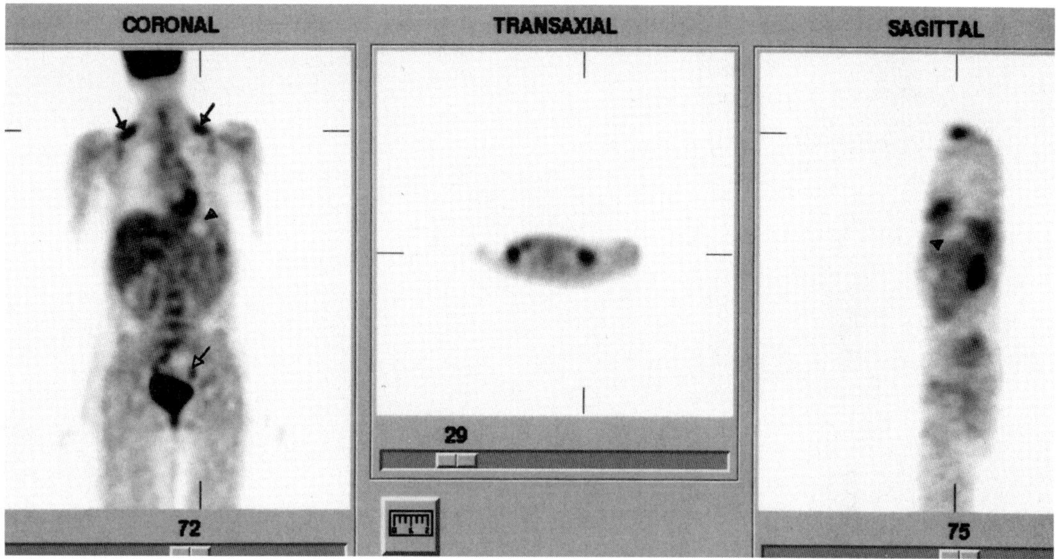

FIGURE 8.11. Selected coronal and sagittal PET images of the axial body and an axial image of the upper chest with ^{18}F-FDG show symmetrically increased activity in the anterior neck muscles or brown fatty tissues (*closed arrows*). Note gastric fundus with fluid (*arrowhead*) and focal increased activity in the left distal ureter (*open arrow*).

bowel and to a lesser extent in the stomach and small intestine. Low-to-moderate stomach wall activity, particularly fundal activity, is commonly noted and may be mistaken for a tumor mass (Figs. 8.4 and 8.13). Sagittal slices may be helpful in defining the oblique position of the stomach as it passes caudally. Marked activity on occasion may be

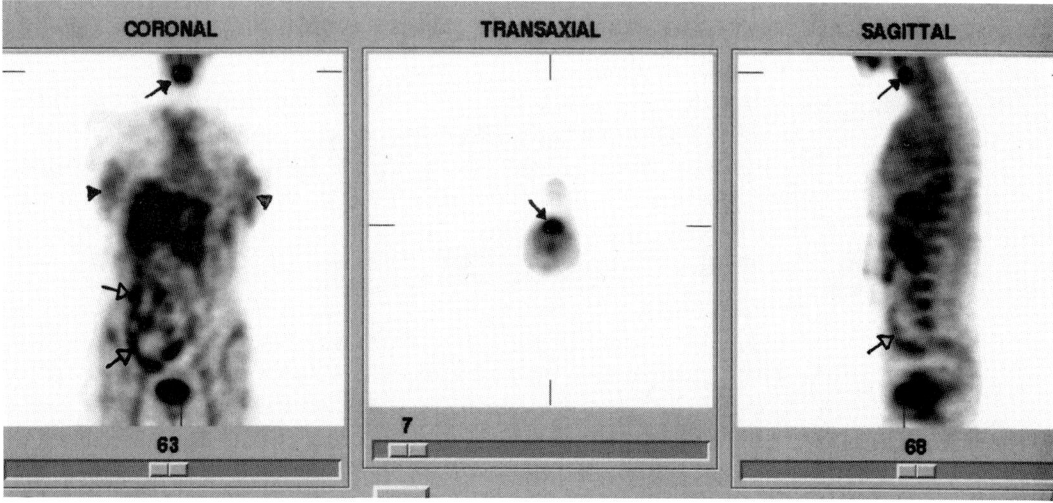

FIGURE 8.12. Selected coronal PET image (*left*) of the axial body with ^{18}F-FDG shows markedly increased activity in the laryngeal muscle (*closed arrows*). Note curvilinear intestinal (*open arrows*) and also breast (*arrowheads*) activity.

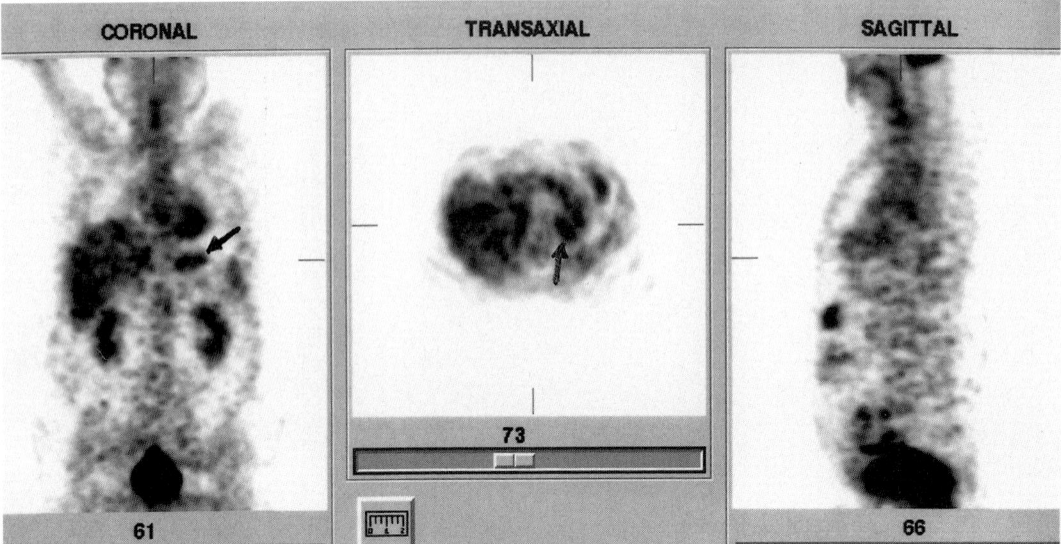

FIGURE 8.13. Selected coronal (*left*) and sagittal (*right*) PET images of the axial body as well as an axial (*middle*) image of the upper abdomen with ^{18}F-FDG show focal increased activity in the gastric fundus (*arrows*). Note nonuniform activity in the body due to obesity.

seen in the cecum and sigmoid/rectum, leading to difficulties in interpretation when assessing local recurrence of large bowel tumors (Fig. 8.12).

Lymphoid tissues may also demonstrate the significant uptake of ^{18}F-FDG, and the normal appearance of the tonsils and adenoids (Fig. 8.14) (which may be particularly marked in children) would be recognized.[5] After radiotherapy or surgery, pharyngeal lymphoid activity may become asymmetric, making it more difficult to differentiate from physiologic activity. It is also possible that cecal activity, which is often seen as the normal variant, may be due to lymphoid tissue present in this region.[1]

Apart from excreted ^{18}F-FDG through the urinary system, which could be seen anywhere within the urinary tract, prior knowledge of any urinary diversion procedure may be helpful in avoiding errors in interpretation. An ileal conduit or other urinary intestinal diversions may produce unusual images unless the alteration in anatomy is appreciated.

Urinary Tract

Unlike glucose, FDG is not totally reabsorbed in the renal tubules.[1] Significant and variable urinary activity is seen in all patients. Renal collecting system activity is easily recognized but may limit the use of FDG in the investigation of tumors in the urinary tract (Fig. 8.15). If there is a significant holdup in the renal collecting system of an obstructed kidney, reconstruction artifacts may interfere with visualization of the upper abdomen. Imaging may be improved in a nonobstructed but dilated system by keeping the patients well hydrated, and by administering diuretics.

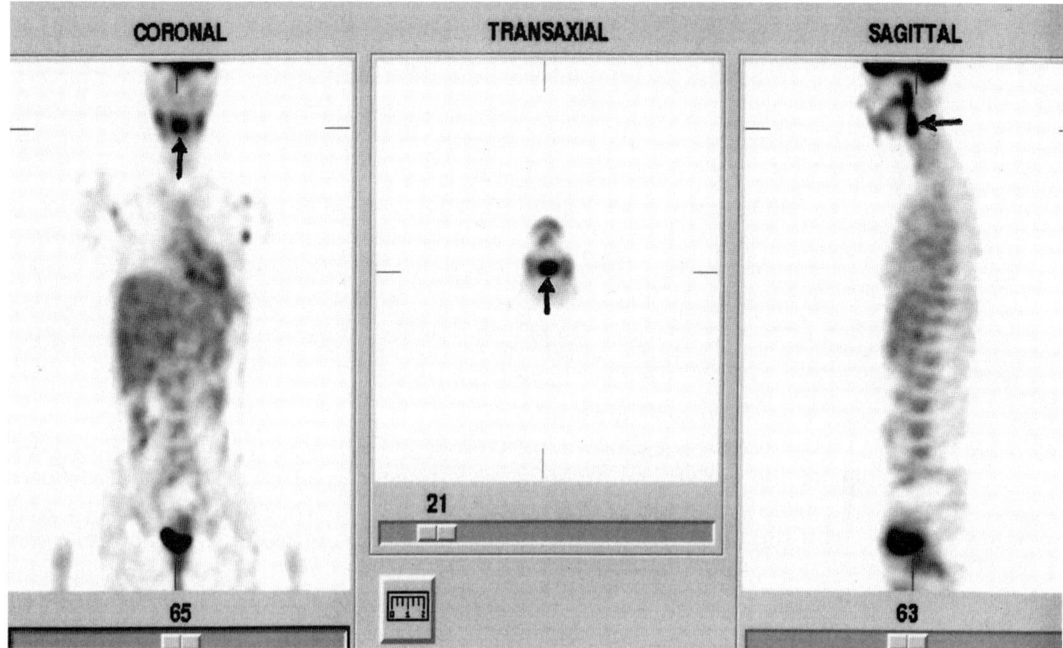

FIGURE 8.14. Selected coronal (*left*) and sagittal (*right*) PET images of the axial body as well as an axial (*middle*) image of the upper neck show markedly increased activity in the lingual tonsil (*closed arrows*) and slightly increased activity in bilateral axillary nodes, possibly due to viral infection.

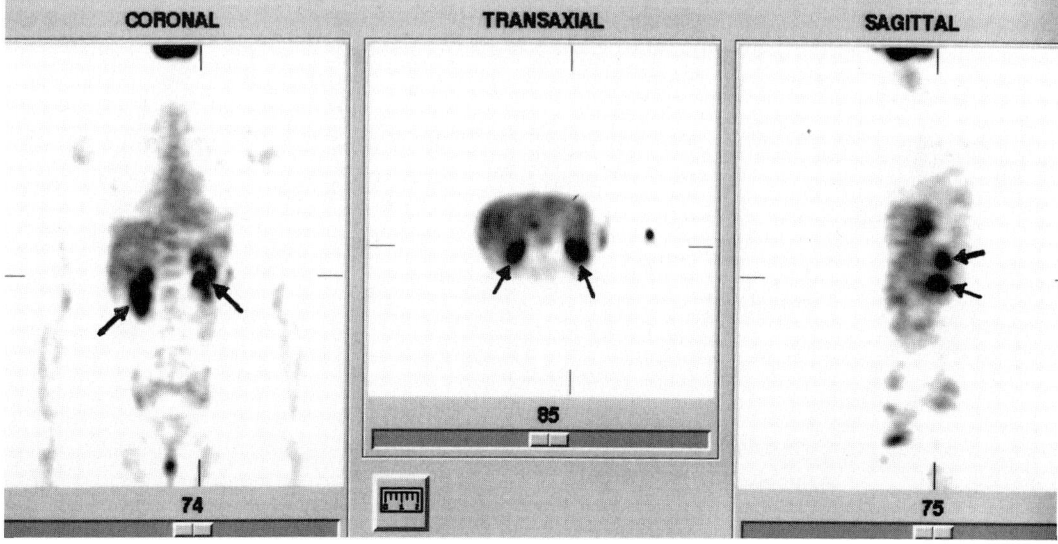

FIGURE 8.15. Selected coronal (*left*) and sagittal (*right*) PET images of the axial body as well as an axial (*middle*) image of the upper abdomen with ^{18}F-FDG show intense activity (*arrows*) accumulated in bilateral kidneys without hydronephrosis.

Reticuloendothelial System

Hepatic and splenic activities on an attenuation-corrected image (Fig. 8.4) are slightly nonuniform, and thus small metastatic lesions are very difficult to be identified. Hepatic activity on uncorrected images is similar to lung uptakes with slightly increased activity in the periphery. There is no gallbladder activity (Fig. 8.1).

Bone marrow and thymus harbor many white cells, which are known to take up ^{18}F-FDG. When these cells are activated by the growth factors or cytokine therapy, the activities in the bone marrow and spleen are markedly increased (Figs. 8.16 and 8.17). Increased marrow activity is also seen in patients with acute infection due to increased production of white cells.[10]

Miscellaneous Variants

On occasion, skin contamination from urinary activity may be limited at the superficial areas, which is usually easily recognized as such. Breast uptake may be variable, and focal increased uptake may be seen at the nipple. Asymmetric uptake may be noted in a woman who fed her baby on one side. Thymic activity (Fig. 8.18 and 8.19) may be seen in children or late teens with an inverted V shape.[1]

Other Variants

Glandular breast tissue often demonstrates moderate uptake of ^{18}F-FDG in premenopausal women. After menopause there is little breast activity, but women on estrogen for hormone replacement therapy (HRT) may also show enhanced uptake. The symmetric nature would suggest taking HRT, but there is the potential for lesions to be obscured by this physiologic activity.

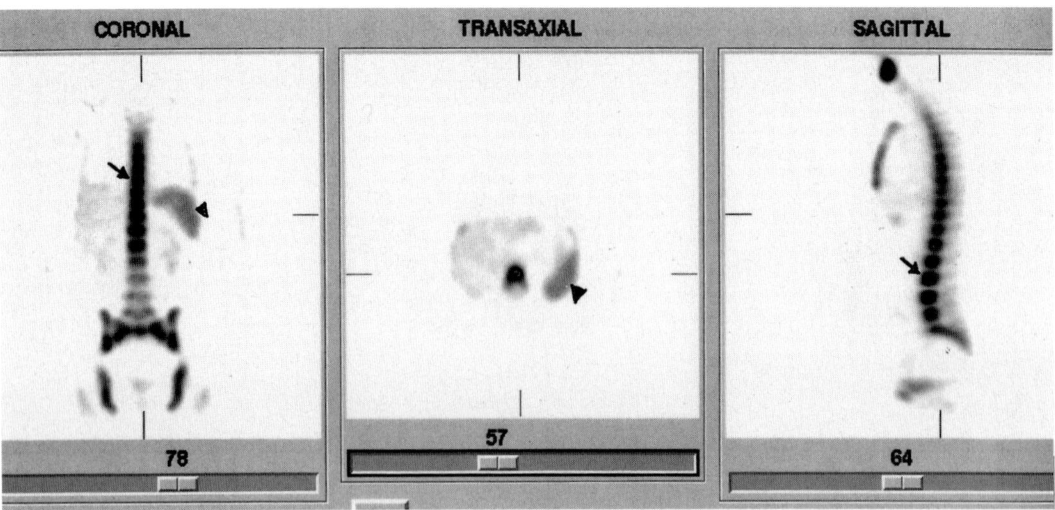

FIGURE 8.16. Selected coronal (*left*) and sagittal (*right*) PET images of axial body and an axial image (*middle*) of the upper abdomen with ^{18}F-FDG show diffusely increased activity in the bone marrow (*arrows*) and spleen (*arrowheads*) due to granulocyte-macrophage colony-stimulating factor (GM-CSF) therapy.

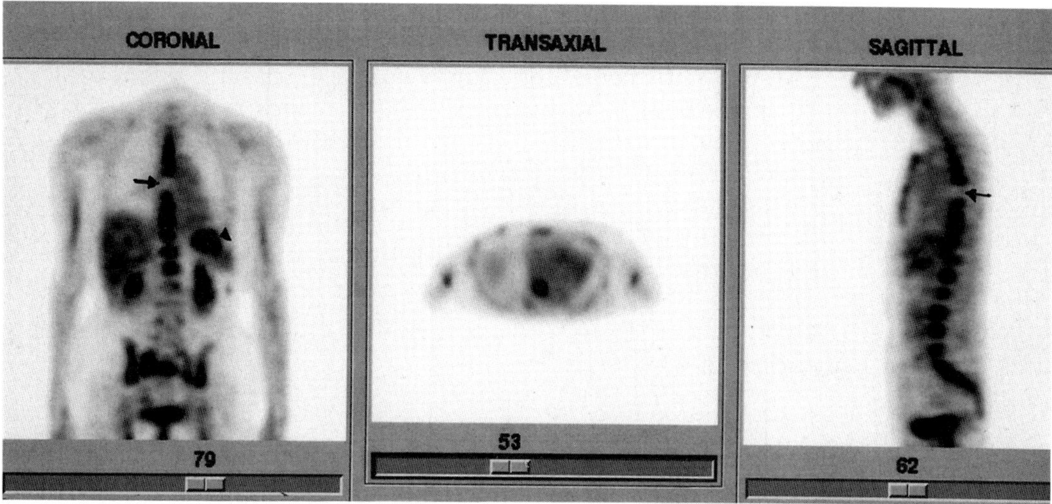

FIGURE 8.17. Selected coronal and sagittal PET images of the axial body as well as an axial image of the lower chest with ^{18}F-FDG in a patient with cytokine (interferon) therapy show diffusely increased activity in the spleen (*arrowhead*) and bone marrow except for T6 (*arrows*). No significant abnormality was noted on the MRI of the thoracic spine.

Artifacts

If attenuation correction is not performed on whole-body PET imaging, there may be higher apparent activity in superficial structures such as the skin, which may obscure lesions, e.g., cutaneous melanoma metastases (Fig. 8.20). A common artifact resulting from this phenomenon is caused by the axillary skinfold, where a double layer of skin

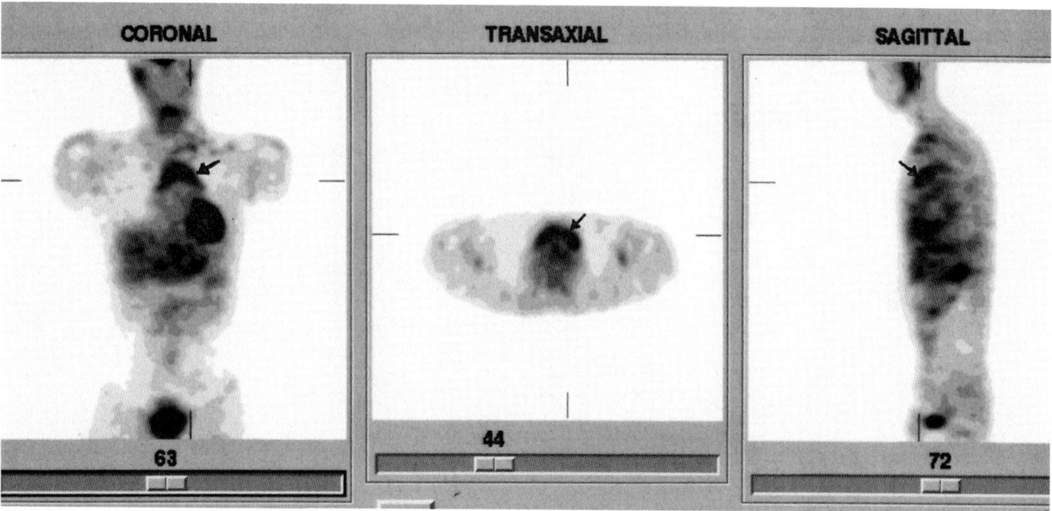

FIGURE 8.18. Selected coronal (*left*) PET image of the axial body, and transaxial (*middle*) and sagittal (*right*) images of the left thigh show a markedly increased uptake of ^{18}F-FDG in triangular thymus (*arrows*).

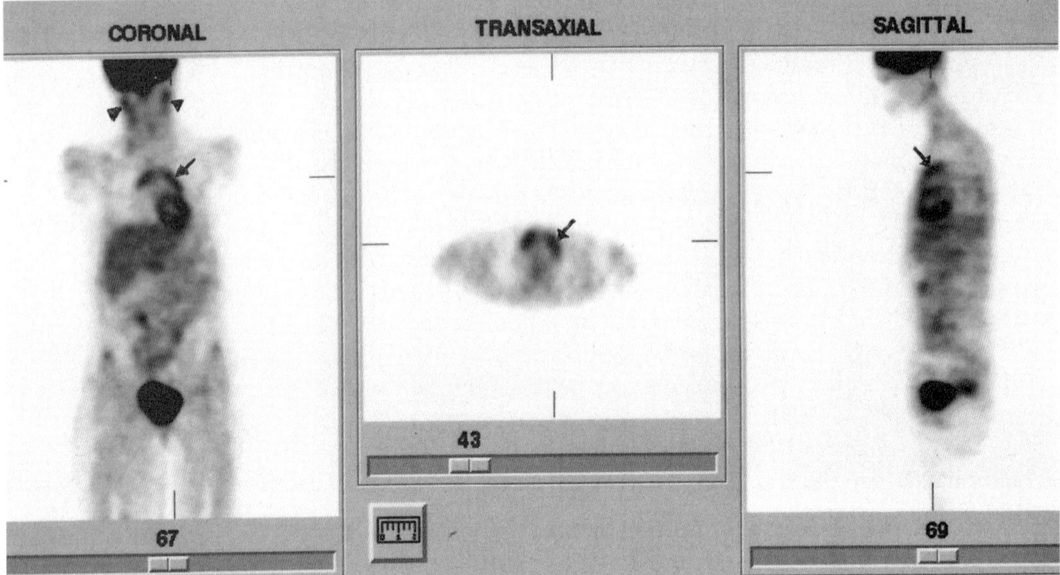

FIGURE 8.19. Selected coronal and sagittal PET images of the axial body and an axial image of the upper chest show moderately increased uptake of ^{18}F-FDG in butterfly-shaped thymus (*arrows*) and stressed neck muscles (*arrowheads*).

may mimic focal lymphadenopathy on coronal sections. The linear distribution of activity on axial or sagittal planes would help to prevent a misinterpretation.

Artifacts caused by prostheses are usually readily recognizable. Photon-deficient areas may result from metallic hip prostheses, breast prostheses and implants, medallions, coins and keys in pockets, etc. Ring

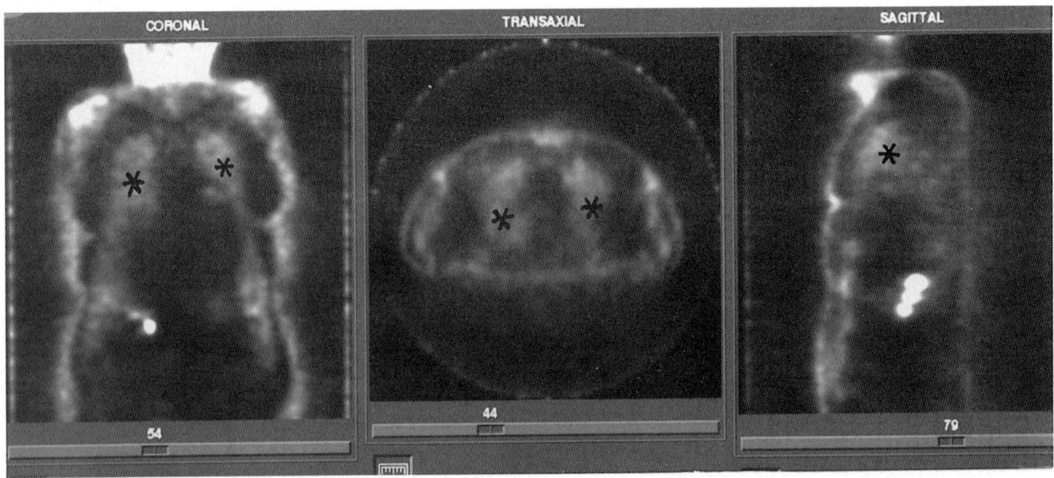

FIGURE 8.20. Selected coronal and sagittal PET images of the axial body as well as an axial image of the upper chest without attenuation correction show slightly increased uptake of ^{18}F-FDG diffusely in the lungs (*). Note also exaggerated increased activity in degenerative shoulder joints bilaterally.

artifacts may occur if there is a misregistration between transmission and emission data, e.g., due to slight patient movement, and are especially apparent at borders where there are sudden large changes in activity, e.g., at a metal prosthesis.

Patient's movement may compromise image quality. In brain imaging, splitting the study into a number of time frames may be helpful, so that if movement occurs in one frame this can be discarded before summation of the data. Whole-body imaging can lead to unusual appearances if the patient moves between bed scan positions with, for example, the upper part of an arm being visible in the higher scanning positions but being absent or "amputated" lower down when moved out of the field of view of the scanning positions.

Problems with injections may interfere with image interpretation. A partly infiltrated injection not only may cause reconstruction artifacts across the trunk, but also may result in a low count study and inaccuracies in the standard uptake value (SUV) measurement. Local axillary lymph node uptake may occur following subcutaneous extravasation, and thus radiopharmaceuticals should be administered on the opposite side to a known or questioned pathologic lesion, if possible. Although rare, an inadvertent intraarterial injection may be easily recognized.

PET Imaging with ^{11}C-Methionine

Uptake Mechanism

^{11}C-L-methionine represents the amino acid with which there is a sufficient clinical experience in PET imaging. Increased transport and utilization of amino acids are common in cancers. The use of L-methionine in cancer imaging is based on this observation and the increased activity of the transmethylation in some cancers. There is normally substantial uptake of ^{11}C-methionine in the pancreas, salivary glands, liver, and kidneys. As a natural amino acid, there is some metabolism of L-methionine in the bloodstream. This tracer is mostly used in imaging of brain tumors, head and neck cancers, lymphoma, and lung cancers as well as several other clinical settings. Early clinical studies demonstrated the stereospecificity of tumor uptake. L-methionine uptake is much greater in brain tumors than the uptake of D-methionine when an intact brain–blood barrier was present.[2]

Physiologic Distribution of ^{11}C-Methionine

By far the greatest experience with ^{11}C-methionine lies in brain tumor imaging. Uptake of ^{18}F-FDG into brain tumors is closely related to the grade of malignancy. As there is high uptake of ^{18}F-FDG into the normal brain cortex and basal ganglia, it may be difficult to identify a low- or intermediate-grade tumor with similar or less activity. The relatively high uptake of ^{18}F-FDG in a normal structure, however, may allow better anatomic localization of those tumors that are visible, or similarly, may give a number of anatomic landmarks to aid image registration with magnetic resonance imaging (MRI) or computed tomography (CT). In constrast to ^{18}F-FDG, ^{11}C-methionine typically shows low-grade uptake in the normal cortex (Fig. 8.21) and is better suited for detection of low- and intermediate-grade tumors. However, while tumor margins and extent may be more easily identified with ^{11}C-methionine, the correlation between tumor grade and uptake appears less strong than that with ^{18}F-FDG.

One of the most difficult problems in the management of primary brain tumors is in the assessment of tumor recurrence versus post-treatment scar and gliosis, which often remains problematic with anatomic imaging such as MRI and CT, and where functional imaging with PET has a role. Soon after radiation therapy, accumulation of ^{18}F-FDG may occur in macrophages surrounding necrotic areas in addition to any viable tumor cells. By contrast, methionine has low uptake by macrophages and other cellular components but accumulates in viable cancer cells. Uptake of ^{11}C-methionine therefore correlates better with tumor extent when compared with surgical and biopsy findings. Unlike ^{18}F-FDG, there is no significantly increased uptake of ^{11}C-methionine in stressed muscles (Fig. 8.22).

Tumor imaging in the pelvis may be problematic since normal excreted activity in the urine may interfere with tumor identification. Because there is very little urinary ^{11}C-methionine activity in the majority of patients, the use of this tracer has been evaluated in a number of urinary and gynecologic cancers. Besides the response of invasive

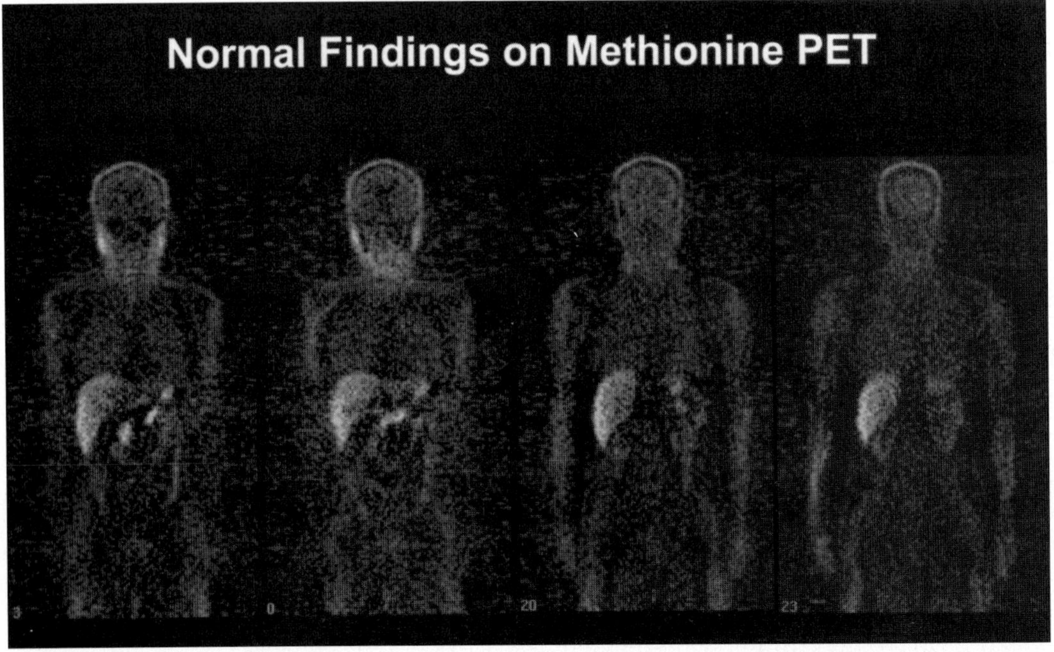

FIGURE 8.21. Coronal PET images of the axial body with ^{11}C-methionine (*anterior to posterior on left to right*) show no significantly increased activity in the brain, thyroid, heart, or urinary bladder. Note the curvilinear increased activity in the pancreas (*upper mid-abdomen on second image*).

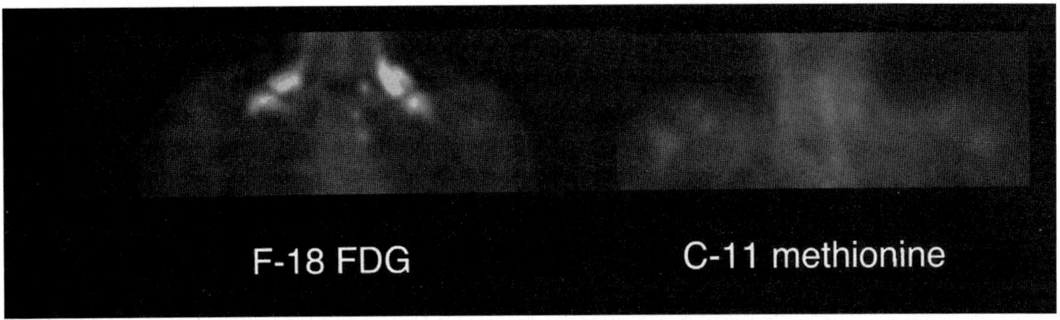

FIGURE 8.22. Selected coronal PET images of the neck show markedly increased activity in the stressed sternocleidomastoid muscles bilaterally with ^{18}F-FDG but no significantly increased activity with ^{11}C-methionine.

bladder tumor to chemotherapy, ovarian and uterine cancers have been assessed with this radiopharmaceutical.

Physiologic Variants

As with all imaging techniques, thorough knowledge of normal distribution and anatomic, physiologic, and pathologic variants is required to avoid misinterpretaion. As the clinical use of ^{11}C-methionine PET develops, more and more potential pitfalls will be recognized. Here we summarize the status from our own and others' experience.

During brain tumor imaging there are a number of structures in the head that normally show accumulation of ^{11}C-methionine. The lacrimal glands may show moderately intense uptake, but may be easily recognized by virtue of the symmetric distribution and the anterior position below the frontal lobes. Normal bone marrow uptake within the sphenoid and clivus may cause confusion at the skull base, however. Pathologic variants that we have experienced include uptakes within a recent biopsy tract, into an incidental benign meningioma, and within the pons following radiotherapy to the surrounding area.

In the neck, bone marrow activity that may appear quite focal at the medial tips of the clavicles may cause false-positive interpretations when investigating hyperparathyroidism or focal metastatic lymph node. The majority of patients show no thyroid ^{11}C-methionine activity (Fig. 8.22); however, a small percentage show low-grade activity that is lower than the activity seen in abnormal parathyroid glands. This actually may be helpful in identifying anatomic landmarks for the surgeon. Unfortunately, as with other nuclear medicine procedures for investigating hyperparathyroidism, the uptake within the thyroid may on occasion interfere with diagnosis. We have noted diffusely increased uptake in patients with coincidental Hashimoto's thyroiditis and thyrotoxicosis due to Graves' disease. Uptake also may be seen in benign thyroid nodules, and thus correlative imaging may be required with this technique in specific cases.

High salivary gland activity is demonstrated by ^{11}C-methionine PET (Fig. 8.23). This is unlikely to cause confusion, but asymmetric activity

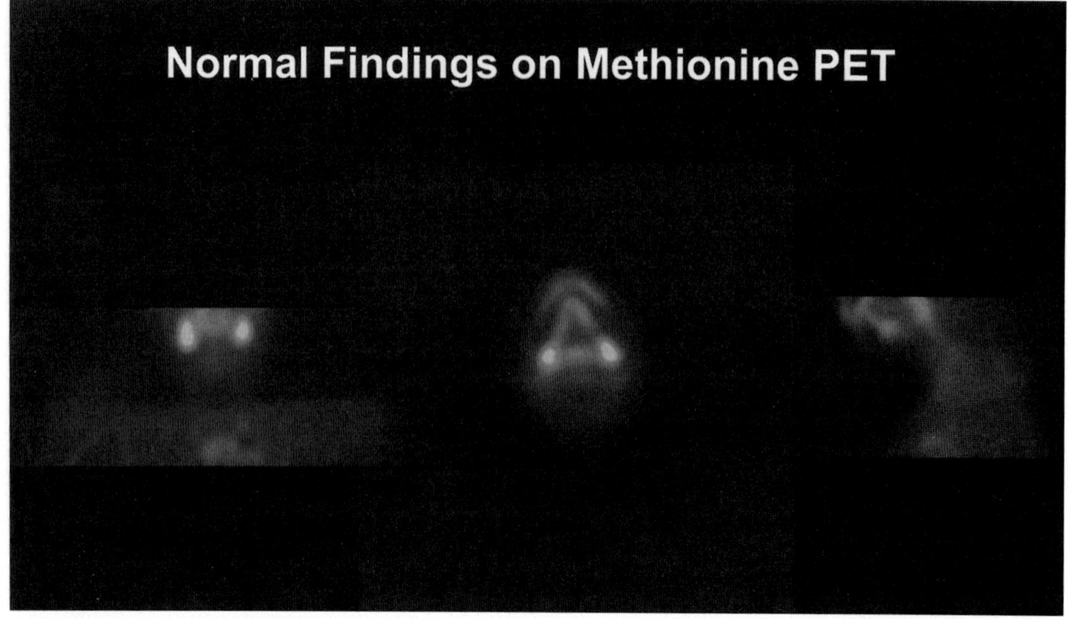

FIGURE 8.23. Selected coronal, axial and sagittal images of the neck show markedly increased uptake of ^{11}C-methionine in the parotid glands symmetrically.

following unilateral radiotherapy or extensive surgery for head and neck cancers may be problematic.

In the abdomen, physiologic accumulation within the bowel may cause difficulties and limit the use of this tracer in the investigation of bowel cancer and pelvic tumors. High pancreatic uptake in the upper mid-abdomen is normally identified (Fig. 8.21), although it may obscure the uptake within pancreatic tumors. We have found that anatomic information obtained from a ^{11}C-methionine scan complements an ^{18}F-FDG scan where no significant pancreatic accumulation normally occurs.

The presence of urinary ^{11}C-methonine activity is variable but occurs in the minority of patients. It may nevertheless lead to interpretative problems in the pelvis. In our experience there is low-grade renal cortical activity, which would not be expected to interfere with renal tumor evaluation.

References

1. Cook GJR, Fogelman I, Maisey MN. Normal physiological and benign pathological variants of F-18 deoxyglucose PET scanning: potential for error in interpretation. Semin Nucl Med 1996;26:308–314.
2. O'Tuama LA, Phillips PC, Smith IR, et al. L-methionine uptake by human cerebral cortex. Maturation from infancy to old age. J Nucl Med 1991;32: 16–20.
3. Newberg A, Alvi A, Reivich M. Determination of regional cerebral function with FDG-PET imaging in neuropsychiatric disorders. Semin Nucl Med 2002;32:13–34.

4. Tashiro M, Fujimoto T, Itoh M, et al. ^{18}F-FDG PET imaging of muscle activity in runners. J Nucl Med 1999;40:70–76.
5. Shreve PD, Anzai Y, Wahl R. Pitfalls in oncologic diagnosis with FDG PET imaging: physiologic and benign variants. Radiographics 19(1):61–77; Quiz 150-1.
6. Loessner A, Alvi A, Lewandrowski KU, et al. Regional cerebral function determined by FDG-PET in healthy volunteers: normal patterns and changes with age. J Nucl Med 1995;36:1141–1149.
7. Hany TF, Gharehpapagh E, Kamel EM, et al. Brown adipose tissue: a factor to consider in symmetrical tracer uptake in the neck and upper chest region. Eur J Nucl Med 2002;29:1393–1398.
8. Yasuda S, Fuji H, Takahashi W, et al. Elevated ^{18}F-FDG uptake in the psoas muscle. Clin Nucl Med 1998;23:716–717.
9. Kim S-K, Chung J-K, Kim B-T, et al. Relationship between gastrointestinal ^{18}F-FDG accumulation and gastrointestinal symptoms in whole-body PET. Clin Pos Imag 1999;2:273–280.
10. Sugawara Y, Fisher SJ, Zasadny KR, et al. Preclinical and clinical studies of bone marrow uptake of ^{18}F-FDG with or without granulocyte colony stimulating factor during chemotherapy. J Clin Oncol 1998;16:173–180.

9

Artifacts in FDG-PET

Tomio Inoue, Noboru Oriuchi, and E. Edmund Kim

As the number of clinical positron emission tomography (PET) units is increasing, interpretation of PET images requires a knowledge of the possible pitfalls that may occur due to artifacts and mimic pathology. These artifacts may be caused by various factors such as injection, attenuation material, image reconstruction, contamination, patient movement, and pathologic variants (Table 9.1).[1]

Injection-related artifacts (Figs. 9.1 to 9.4) may interfere with image interpretation. A partly infiltrated injection causes a reconstruction artifact across the trunk. It also results in inaccuracy of the standard uptake value (SUV). If the injection leak on fluorodeoxyglucose (FDG)-PET images is demonstrated, the SUV derived from these images should be carefully evaluated. Following the subcutaneous extravasations of FDG solution, the tracer may flow into the lymphatic channel (Fig. 9.5) and may be trapped in local lymph nodes.[2] It mimics an abnormal FDG uptake in the lymph node metastases. The tracer should be administered on the opposite site to the known lesion.

Increased levels of insulin in the peri-injection period cause extracardiac uptake in diabetic patients or patients who did not fast (Fig. 9.6).[3] Attenuation materials such as coins and keys in a pocket, prostheses, pacemakers, and silicon in breast implants may cause photo deficient areas on FDG-PET images. The use of attenuation correction can result in the generation of artifacts of apparently increased FDG uptake around hip prostheses.[4,5] Such artifacts are visible with all types of scanners because of the inherent problem of partial-volume mapping at the borders of metal and adjacent tissues. The shape of the prosthesis, the absorption properties of the surrounding tissues, and the method of transmission scanning influence the appearance of such artifacts. Since patient movement worsens these artifacts, it is important to verify attenuation-corrected images against non–attenuation-corrected images to avoid false-positive results.

Regarding the image reconstruction, attenuation correction is essentially needed to obtain the quantitative image data such as the SUV. However, if emission data and transmission data for a whole-body FDG-PET are obtained separately, patients have to keep the same position on the diagnostic bed for more than 90 minutes after the injec-

TABLE 9.1. Artifacts in FDG-PET

Factors of artifact	Artifact
Injection	Reconstruction artifact from extremely high counts Lymph node uptake after infiltrated injection Diffuse uptake in periphery area from injection site by intraarterial injection Inaccuracy in SUV measurement
Attenuation material	Coins and keys in pocket, prostheses, pacemakers, silicon in breast implants, etc.
Image reconstruction	Apparent superficial increase in activity on the image without attenuation correction Attenuation-correction–induced artifact at the joint space between the metallic prosthetic surfaces Non–attenuation-correction–induced artifact of high activity structure such as urinary bladder Streak artifact induced by inappropriate ML-EM algorithm Ring artifact induced by misregistration between transmission and emission data
Contamination	Urinary contamination
Patient movement	Reduced image quality Apparent "amputation" of body part Underestimation of SUV and obscured the lesion or lesions by respiratory movement

tion. In many PET centers, whole-body images without attenuation correction are employed. If attenuation correction is not performed in whole-body FDG-PET imaging, higher apparent activity in superficial structures such as the skin may obscure cutaneous melanoma metastases (Fig. 9.7).[5] A common artifact resulting from higher apparent activity in superficial structures on non–attenuation-corrected images is caused by the skinfold, where a double layer of skin may mimic focal lymphadenopathy on coronal images. If the linear distribution of activity on axial or sagittal images is observed, an artifact of the image reconstruction without attenuation correction should be suspected with the axillary uptake on the coronal image. The artifacts observed on pelvic FDG images without attenuation correction can be positive and negative around the increased activity in the urinary bladder. Positive artifacts are observed in anteroposterior projection, and negative artifacts are observed around high activity in the urinary bladder. Positive artifacts are observed in the anteroposterior projection and negative artifacts are shown in the lateral projection. They are caused by the inequality of detected activity in low-attenuation anteroposterior projections and high-attenuation lateral projections of the body (Fig. 9.8). Attenuation correction is effective in eliminating artifacts.

However, image processing of attenuation correction may produce artifacts if there are inappropriate conditions, such as the existence of attenuation material, or misregistration of emission and transmission data. Attenuation-correction–induced artifacts on FDG-PET imaging

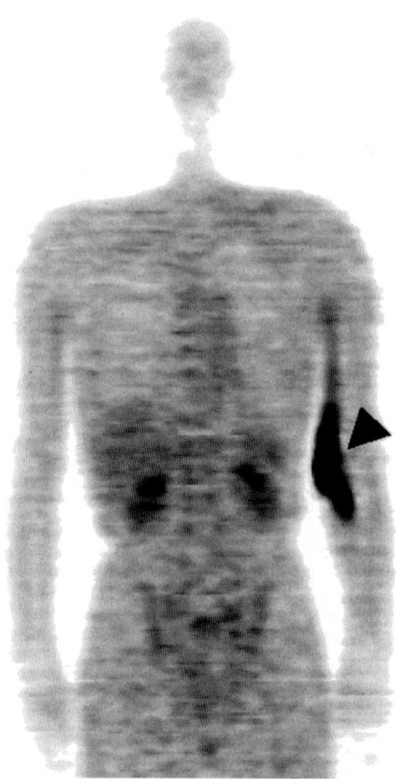

FIGURE 9.1. Selected coronal whole-body PET images show a subcutaneous extravasation of FDG solution (*arrowhead*). The tracer may flow into subcutaneous lymphatic channel.

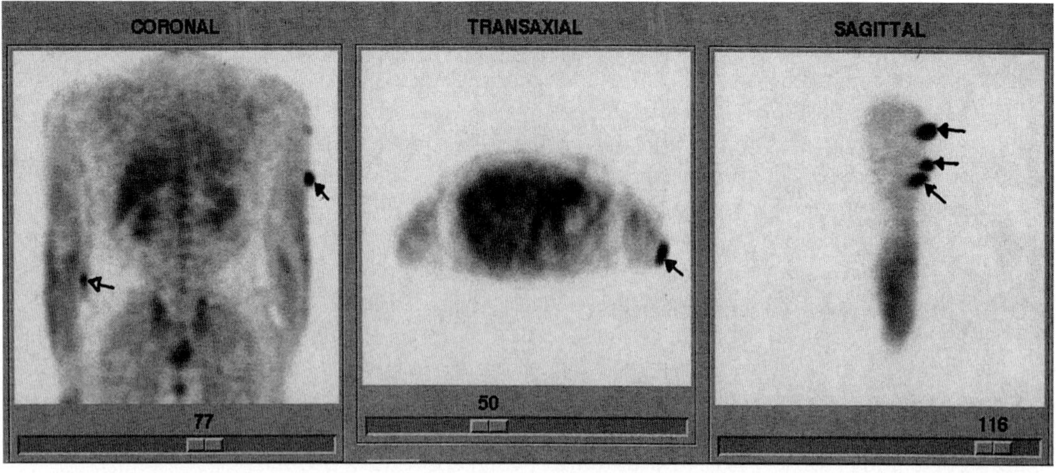

FIGURE 9.2. Selected coronal and sagittal PET images of the axial body as well as an axial image of the upper abdomen with ^{18}F-FDG show multiple focal areas of markedly increased activity at the site of injection (*open arrow*) and biopsy (*closed arrows*).

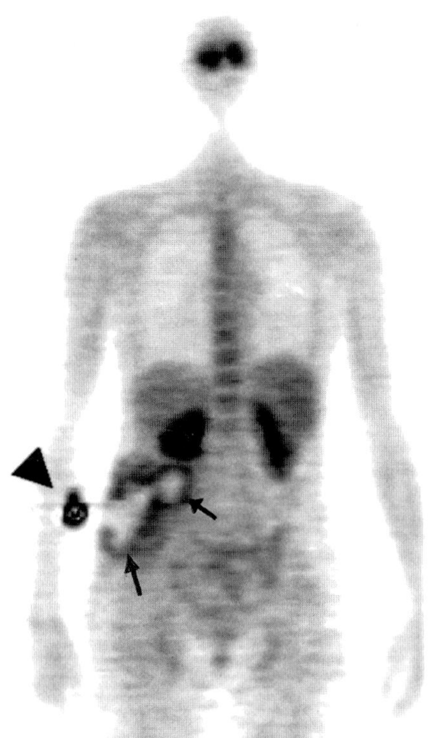

FIGURE 9.3. Selected coronal PET image of the axial body shows a focal area of markedly increased activity (*arrowhead*) in the right forearm, producing an irregular photopenic area with increased activity in the rim overlying the right abdomen (*arrows*), probably representing reconstruction artifacts.

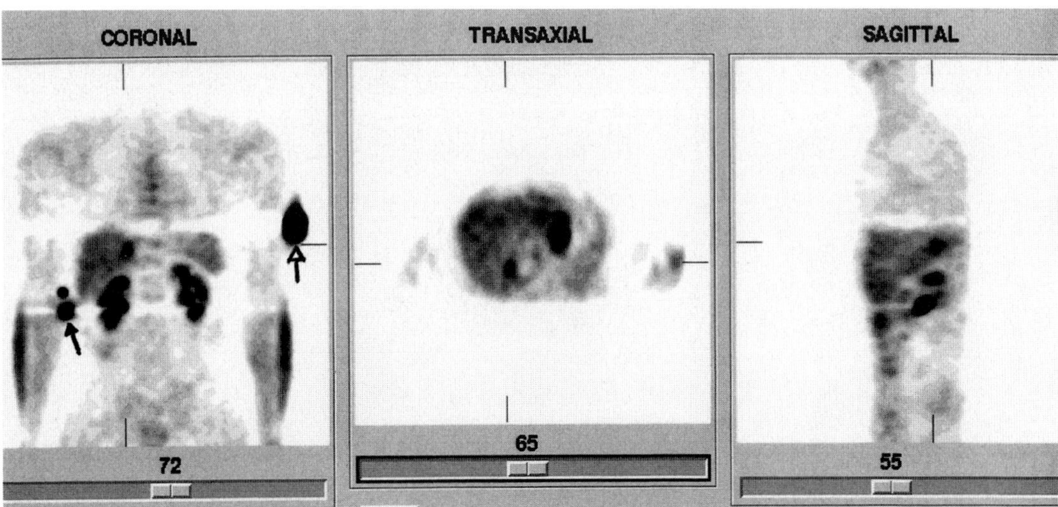

FIGURE 9.4. Selected coronal and sagittal PET images of the axial body with ^{18}F-FDG show focal increased activity infiltrated into right elbow (*closed arrow*) as well as left upper arm (*open arrow*) from the intravenous injection. Note horizontal linear photon deficiency along the extravasated activities, probably representing reconstruction artifacts.

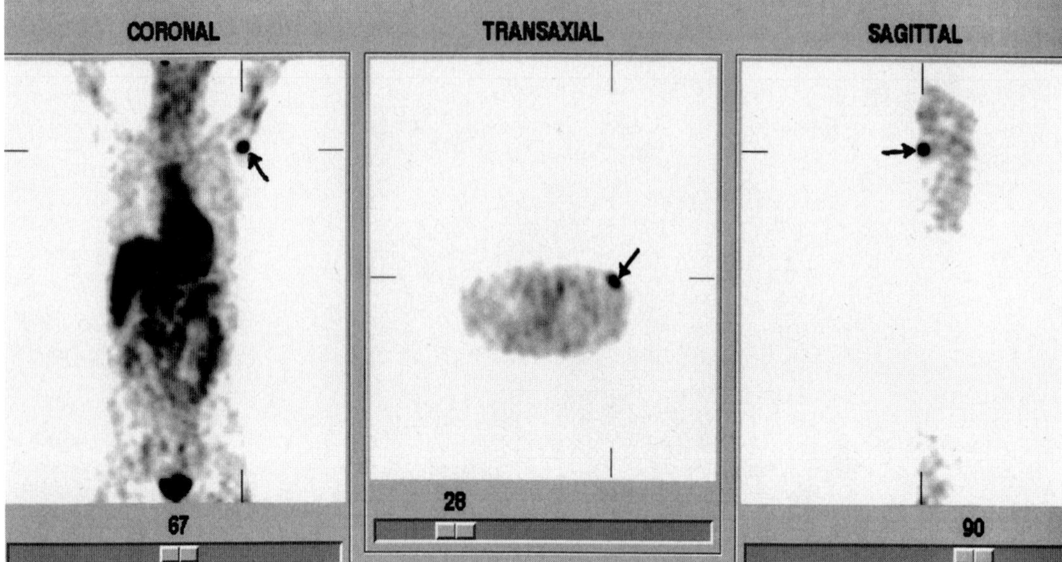

FIGURE 9.5. Selected coronal (*left*) and sagittal (*right*) PET images of the axial body as well as an axial (*middle*) image of the upper chest with ^{18}F-FDG show a focal area of markedly increased activity in the left axillary lymph node (*arrows*) after extravasation of the activity injected into left elbow.

following total knee or hip replacement.[6] Heiba et al[7] presented two false-positive cases of FDG-PET obtained by a dual-head coincidence camera. On attenuation-corrected images, they demonstrated unusual intense activity at the joint space between the metallic prosthetic surfaces at the level of knee joint, which was not shown on the images without attenuation correction. Ring artifacts may occur if there is a

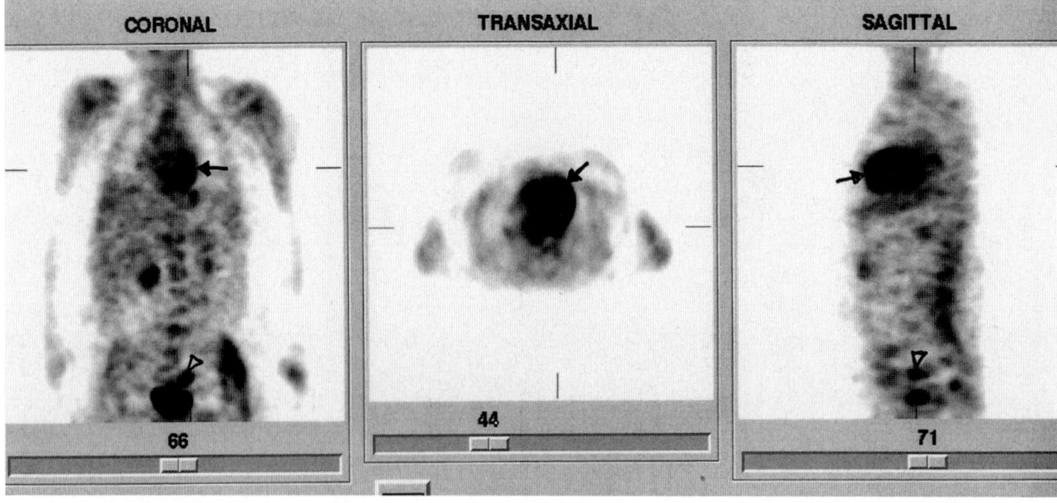

FIGURE 9.6. Selected coronal and sagittal PET images of the axial body as well as an axial image of the lower chest show markedly increased uptake of ^{18}F-FDG in the left ventricular myocardium (*arrows*) in a patient with no significant fasting.

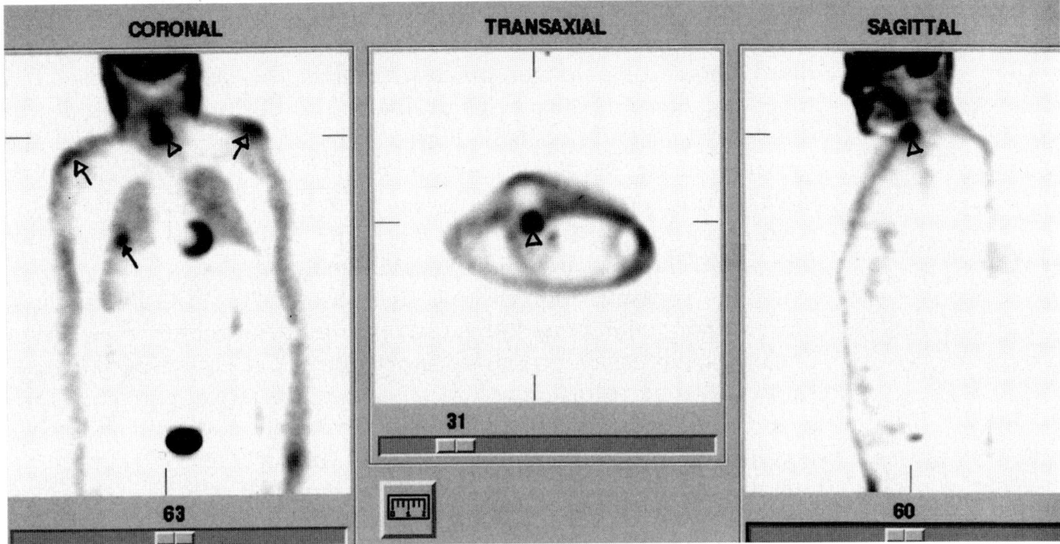

FIGURE 9.7. Selected coronal and sagittal PET images of the axial body as well as an axial image of the neck without attenuation correction show diffusely increased uptake of ^{18}F-FDG in the lungs with carcinoma (*closed arrow*) and also along the body surface. Note also exaggerated increased activity in the vocal muscles (*open arrowhead*) and arthritic shoulders (*open arrows*).

misregistration between transmission and emission data due to slight patient movement, and are especially apparent at borders (e.g., at a metal prosthesis) where there are sudden large changes in activity.

The two major classes of reconstruction method in PET imaging are the filtered back-projection (FBP) method and statistical model based

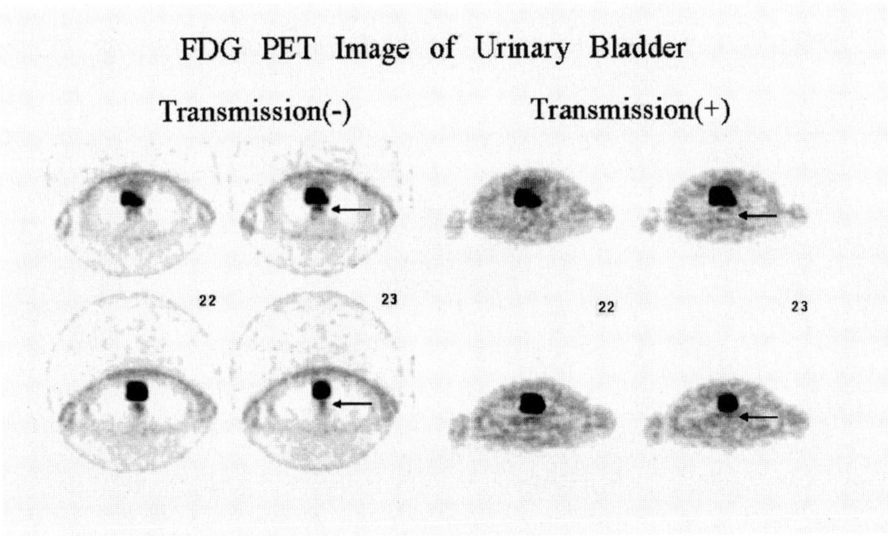

FIGURE 9.8. Positive artifact is observed just behind the bladder (*arrows*) on axial PET images of the lower pelvis in the anteroposterior projection, and negative artifact is noted around the bladder without attenuation correction (*left*). Attenuation correction is effective in eliminating artifacts (*right*).

on iterative algorithms such as the maximum likelihood expectation maximization (ML-EM) method. Although the ML-EM method has the disadvantage of a longer processing time, the ordered subset EM (OSEM) method resolved this problem. The FBP method could produce streak artifacts near the high-activity area (Fig. 9.9) such as the urinary bladder and myocardium on FDG-PET images. However, streak artifacts on a PET image can be induced by an inappropriate condition for using the ML-EM algorithm.[8] The ML-EM algorithm requires that the data are Poisson distributed.

Urinary contamination is sometimes observed on FDG-PET images. Since urinary contamination is usually superficial activity on the skin or clothes, it is easily recognized as artifact. FDG-PET is especially useful in detecting recurrent colorectal cancer in surgical patients. However, the interpretation of FDG-PET images of the abdomen and pelvis is complicated by urinary (Fig. 9.10) and colonic (Fig. 9.11) concentration of FDG. Elimination of artificial accumulation of FDG in the colon and urinary system is essential if primary colorectal cancer, regional lymphadenopathy, or subtle recurrences are to be evaluated in the FDG-PET imaging of the abdomen and pelvis.[9] Elimination of artificial accumulation of FDG requires good patient preparation, which begins with scanning. Patients also need sufficient hydration after the injection of FDG. After administration of furosemide, a Foley catheter with a drainage bag is placed. Normal saline can be delivered retrogradely into the urinary bladder just prior to imaging over the pelvis. After the first PET scan patients void, and repeated PET images of the pelvis may be taken.[9]

Patient movements degrade the image quality of FDG-PET (Fig. 9.12). Whole-body FDG-PET imaging can lead to an unusual appear-

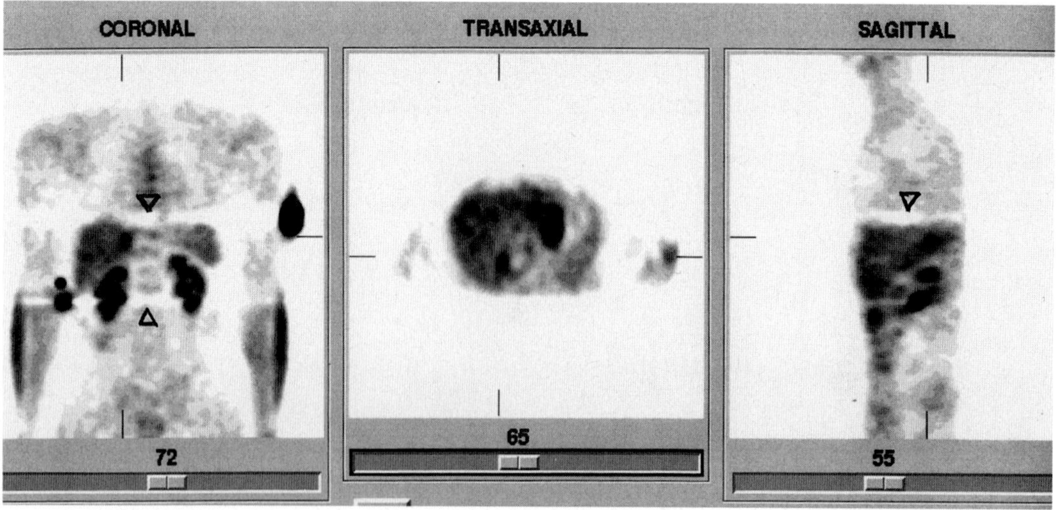

FIGURE 9.9. Selected coronal and sagittal PET images of the axial body with ^{18}F-FDG injected into the right elbow as well as the left upper arm show streak negative artifacts (*arrows*) due to the reconstruction problem.

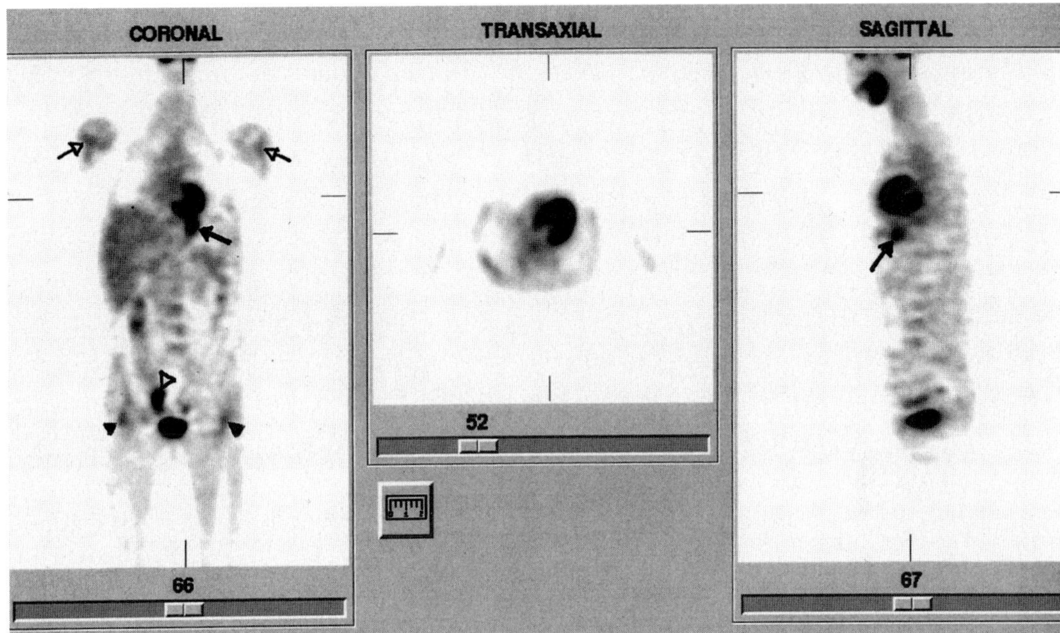

FIGURE 9.10. Selected coronal and sagittal PET images of the axial body with ^{18}F-FDG show focal areas of markedly increased activity in the slightly dilated right distal ureter (*open arrowhead*) and gastric fundus (*closed arrow*). Note also symmetrically increased activities in the arthritic shoulders (*open arrows*) and hips (*closed arrowheads*).

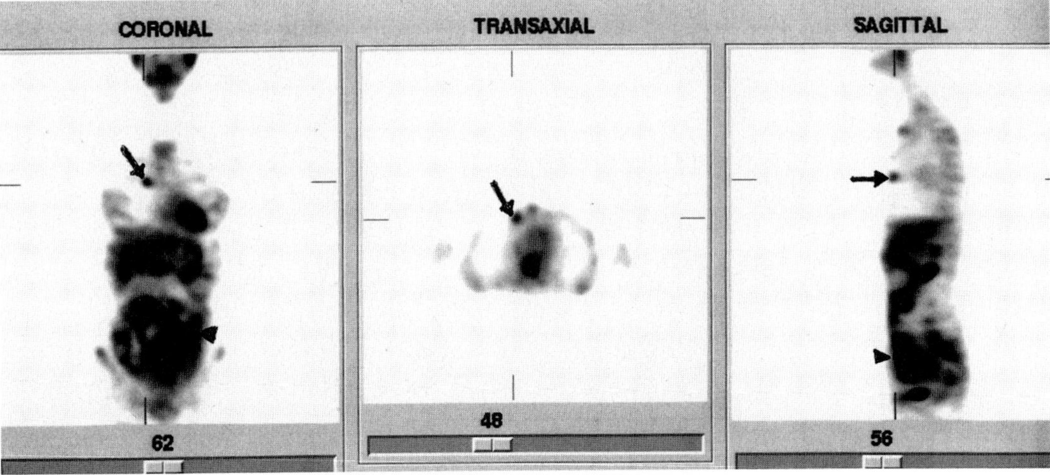

FIGURE 9.11. Selected coronal and sagittal PET images of the axial body as well as an axial image of the upper chest with ^{18}F-FDG show a small focal area of moderately increased activity (*arrows*). Biopsy revealed an inflammatory granuloma. Note markedly increased activity in the bowel loops (*arrowhead*).

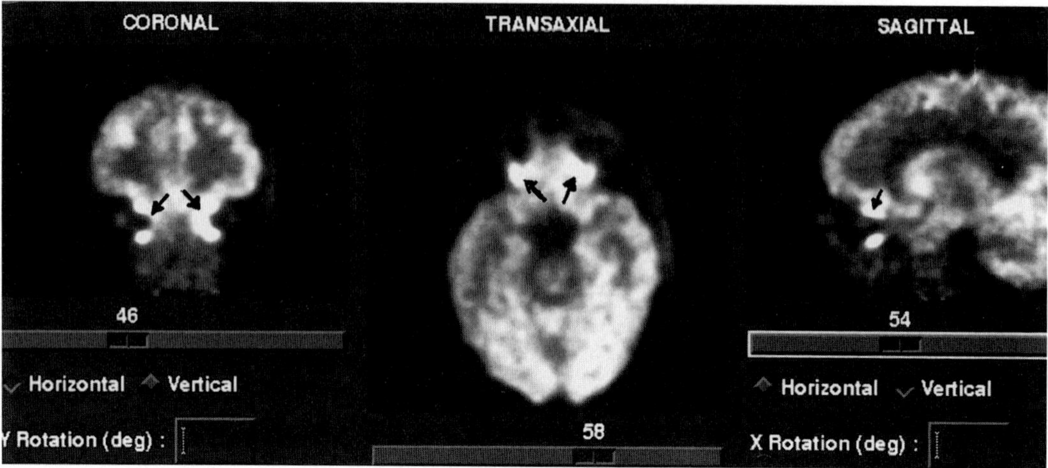

FIGURE 9.12. Selected coronal, axial, and sagittal PET images of the brain with ^{18}F-FDG show markedly increased activity in the bilateral ocular muscles (*arrows*) due to excessive eye movement.

ance if the patient moves between the bed scan positions, with the upper part of an arm, for example, being visible in the higher scanning positions but absent or "amputated" lower down when moved out of the field of view for lower scanning positions (Fig. 9.13). Respiratory movement also may degrade the image quality and quantification of a FDG-PET scan.[10] It affects not only lung lesions but also lesions in the upper abdomen near the diaphragm. Motion artifacts lead to two major effects: First, it affects the accuracy of quantification, producing

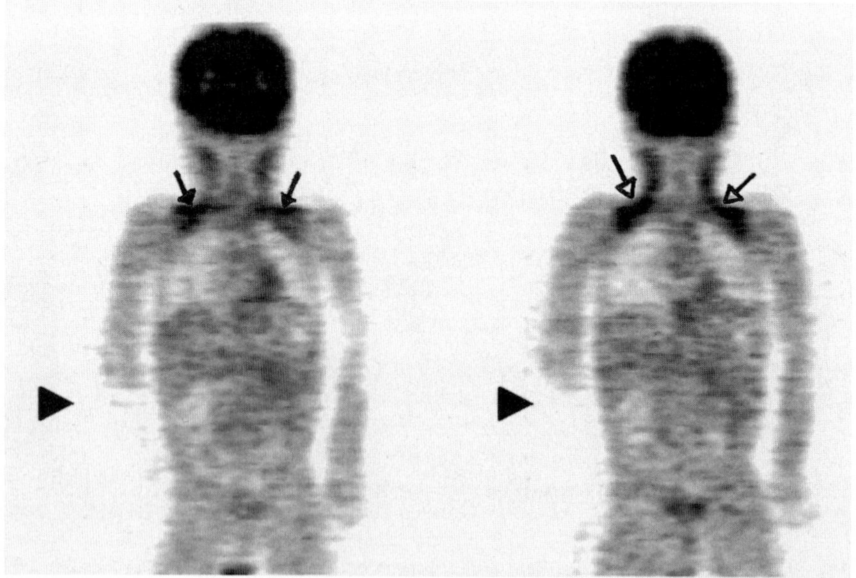

FIGURE 9.13. Selected coronal whole-body FDG-PET images show an unusual appearance with absent activity in the right forearm (*arrowhead*) due to patient's movements between bed scan positions.

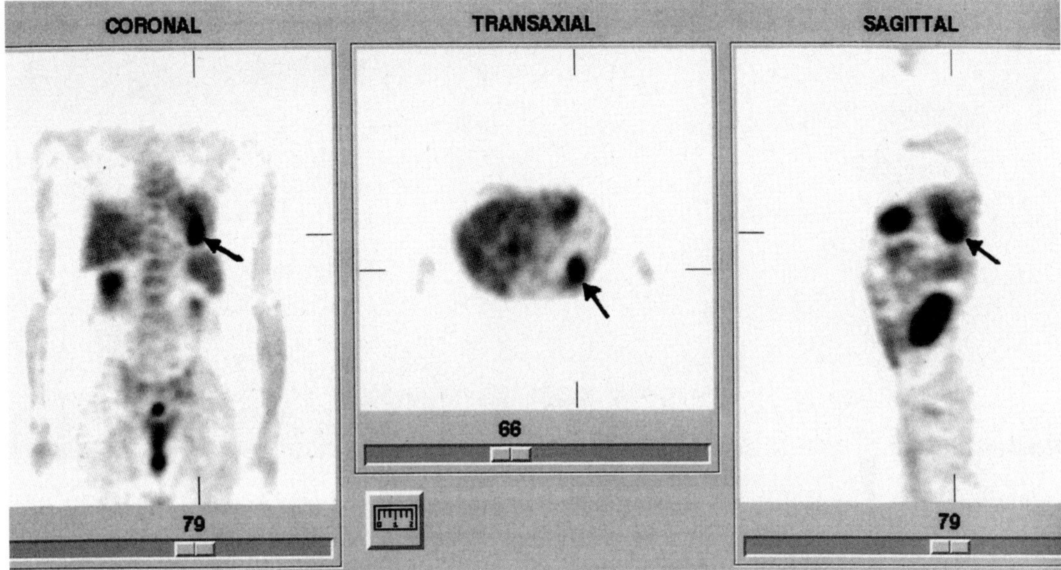

FIGURE 9.14. Selected coronal and sagittal PET images of the axial body as well as an axial image of the lower chest with ^{18}F-FDG show a herniated stomach (*arrows*) in the left lower chest posteriorly (Bochdalek hernia) with markedly increased activity.

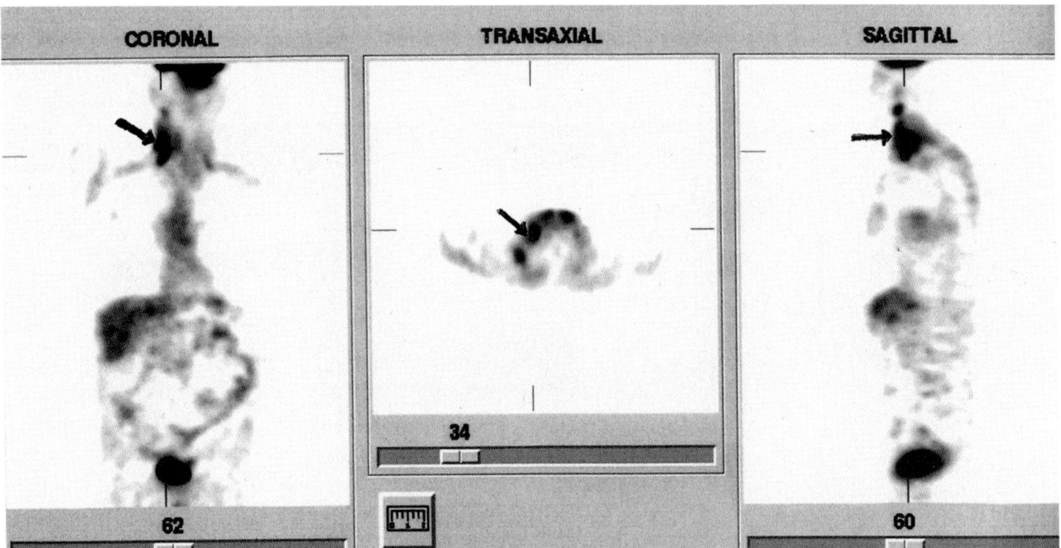

FIGURE 9.15. Selected coronal (*left*) and sagittal (*right*) PET images of the axial body as well as an axial (*middle*) image of the neck with ^{18}F-FDG show irregular markedly increased activity (*arrows*) in the right lower neck due to inflammatory reaction related to radiation therapy for the metastatic lung cancer. PET scan was obtained 1 month after radiation. Biopsy revealed inflammatory findings with residual microscopic tumor cells.

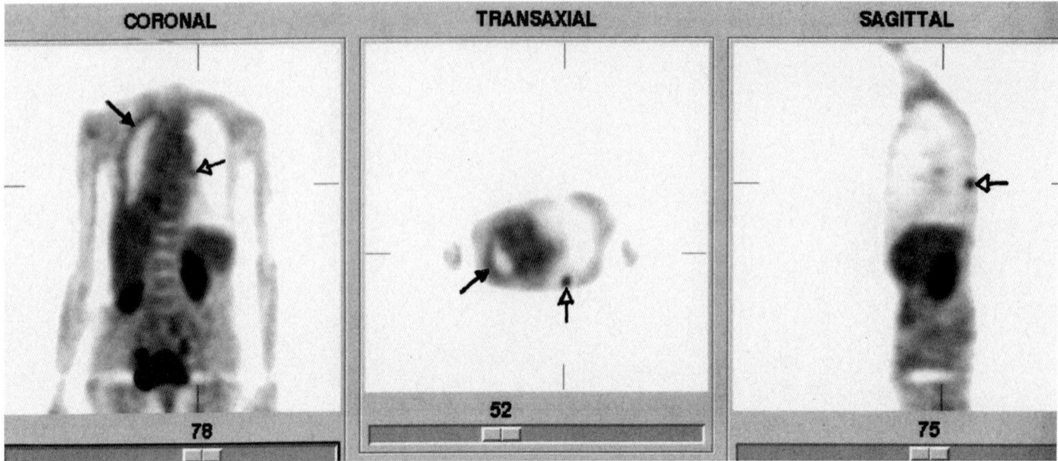

FIGURE 9.16. Select coronal (*left*) and sagittal (*right*) PET image of the axial body as well as an axial (*middle*) image of the mid-chest with ^{18}F-FDG show a curvilinear increased activity in the right chest wall (*closed arrows*) following pneumonectomy. Note small focal increased activity in the medial posterior aspect of left lung due to metastasis (*open arrows*).

a reduction of the measured SUV. Second, the apparent lesion volume is overestimated. Respiratory gating by applying a multiple-frame capture technique, with which PET data are acquired in synchronization with the respiratory motion, compensates for these effects.

A number of benign diseases (Fig. 9.14) may cause significant uptake of FDG that may simulate malignant lesion. In the chest, active tuberculosis, sarcoidosis, and histoplasmosis have been reported as showing increased FDG uptake (Fig. 9.11).[11] These disorders may lead

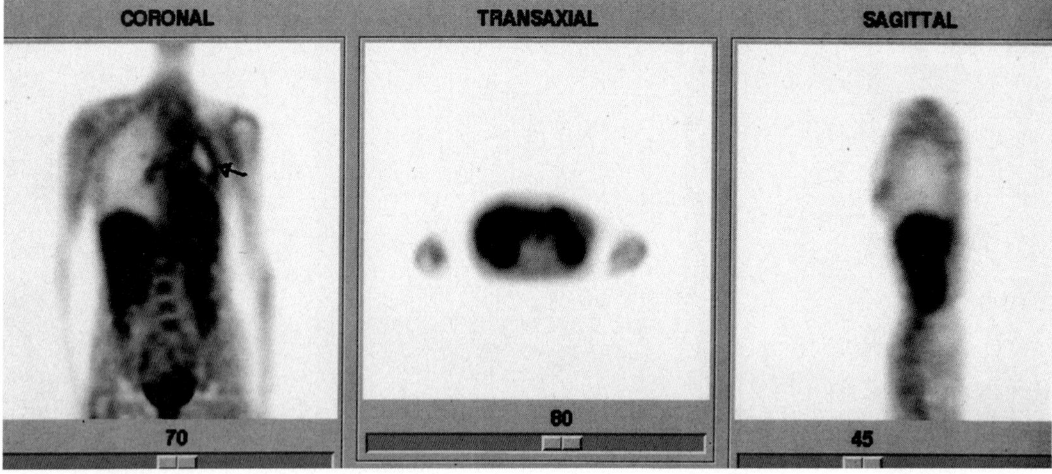

FIGURE 9.17. Selected coronal PET image of the axial body with ^{18}F-FDG shows a curvilinear increased activity (*arrow*) along the left chest with mediastinal shift to the left side following left pneumonectomy.

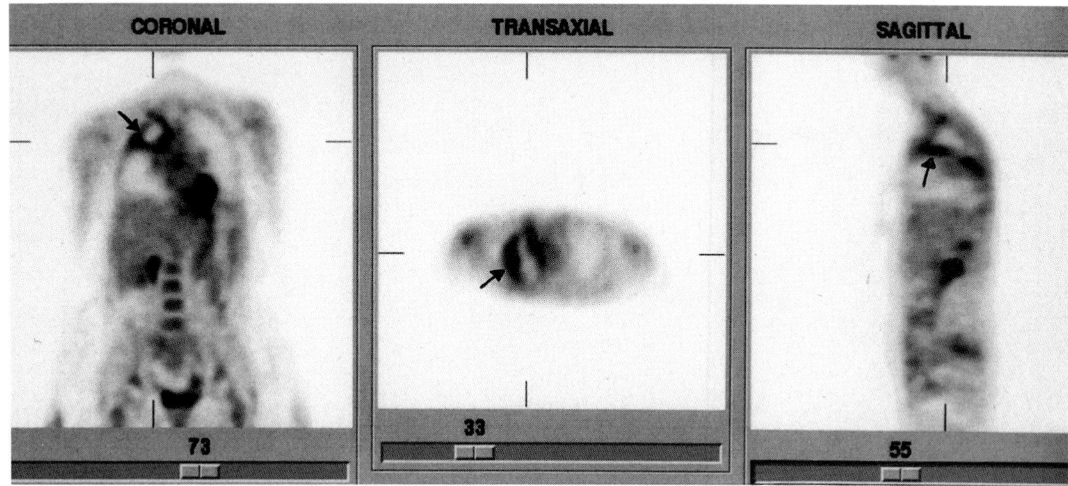

FIGURE 9.18. Selected coronal and sagittal PET images of the axial body as well as an axial image of the upper chest with ^{18}F-FDG show curvilinear increased activity (*arrows*) in the right upper chest after right upper lobectomy.

to FDG uptake (SUV) in the borderline or low-malignant range. Inflammation in any tissue may cause increased FDG uptake (Fig. 9.15). Common sites of inflammatory activity are operative areas (Figs. 9.16 to 9.18) where tumors have been removed, and amputation stumps. These activities may last for several weeks after surgery. Increased uptake of FDG has been noted in the area of treated brain tumors (Fig. 9.19).[12] This may be related to increased macrophage activity in the healing phase after radiotherapy (Figs. 9.20 to 9.22).[11] Active degenerative changes in the joints usually demonstrate curvilinear

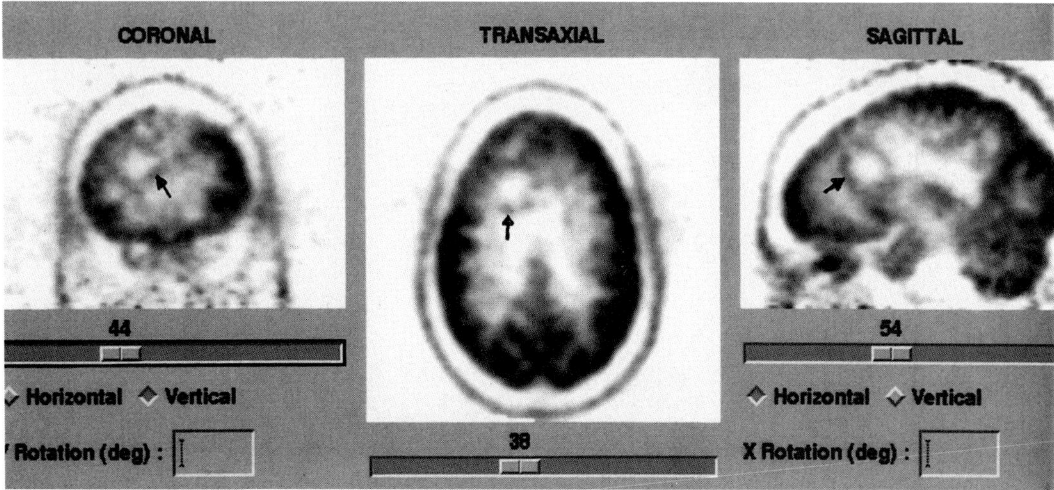

FIGURE 9.19. Selected coronal, axial, and sagittal PET images of the brain with ^{18}F-FDG show slightly increased activity outlining surgical cavity (*arrows*).

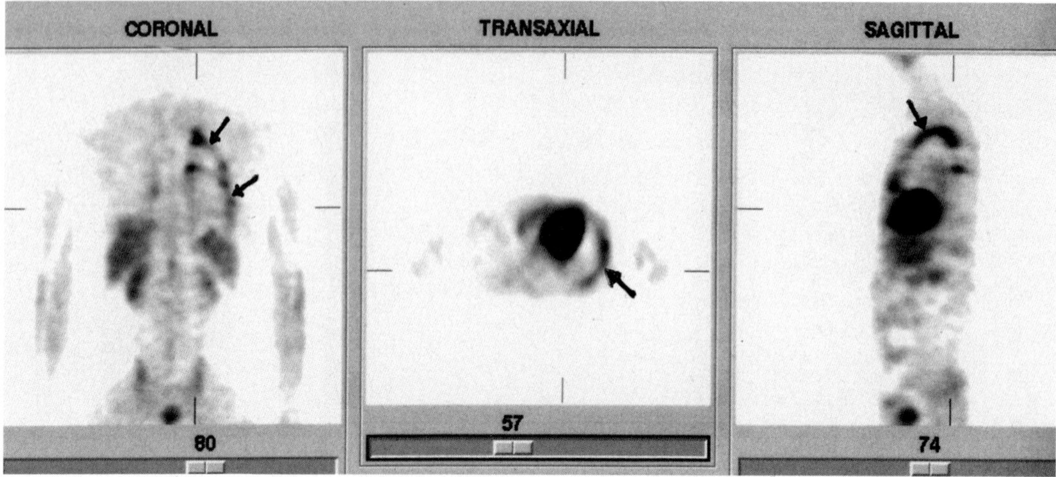

FIGURE 9.20. Selected coronal (*left*) and sagittal (*right*) PET images of the axial body as well as an axial (*middle*) image of the lower chest with ^{18}F-FDG show curvilinear increased activity along the chest wall (*arrows*) due to inflammatory pleural reaction following radiation therapy.

increased uptakes of ^{18}F-FDG around the joint capsule (Figs. 9.10 and 9.23).

Disease may cause intense diffuse uptake of FDG in the thyroid (Figs. 9.24 and 9.25). A follicular ovarian cyst in the pelvis may show high FDG uptake in the periphery of an active but benign cyst. PET/CT fusion may help avoid misinterpretation in this instance.

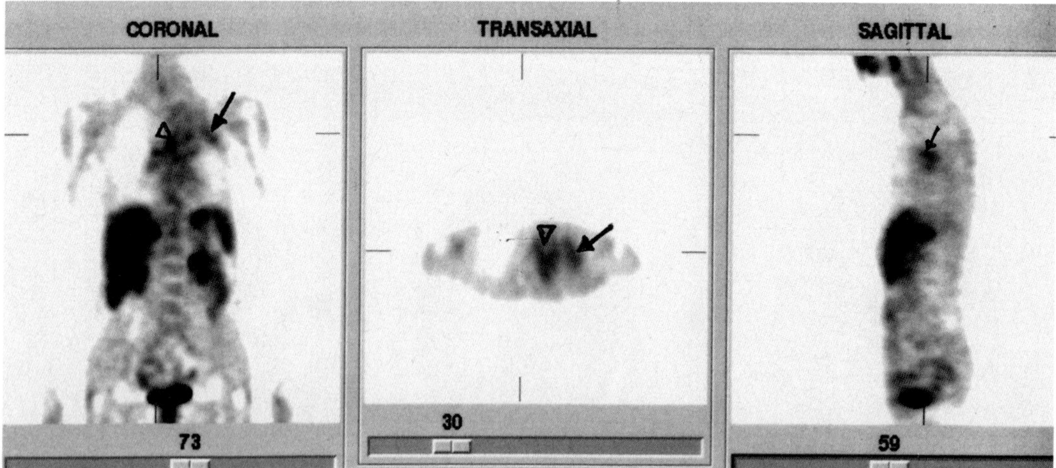

FIGURE 9.21. Selected coronal and sagittal PET image of the axial body as well as an axial image of the upper chest with ^{18}F-FDG shows curvilinear increased activity in the left upper lung (*arrows*) and also irregular increased activity in the superior mediastinum (*arrowheads*) due to inflammatory reaction following the radiation therapy.

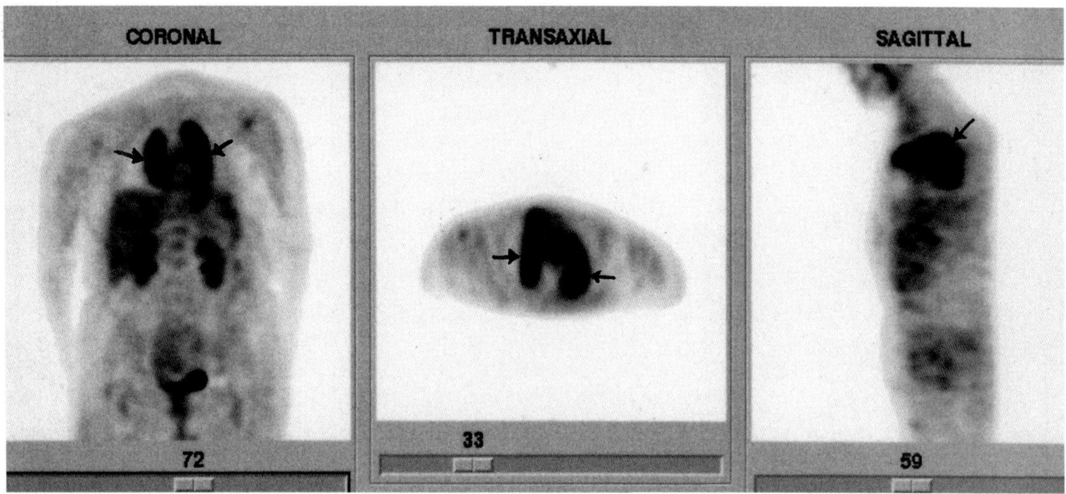

FIGURE 9.22. Selected coronal and sagittal PET images of the axial body as well as an axial image of the upper chest with ^{18}F-FDG show markedly increased activity along the bilateral paramediastinal linings (*arrows*) following the radiation therapy.

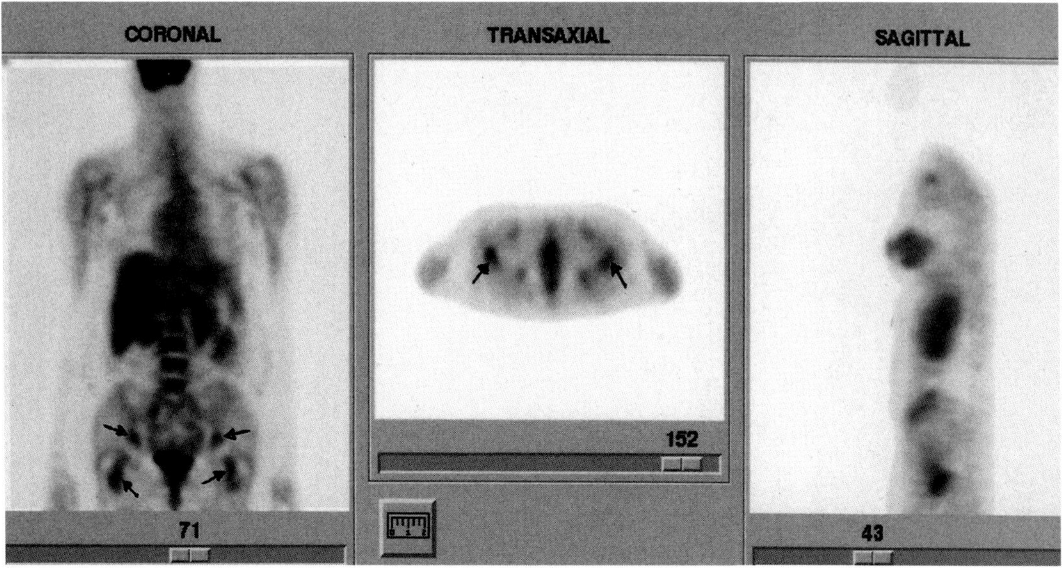

FIGURE 9.23. Selected coronal PET image of the axial body and an axial image of the lower pelvis with ^{18}F-FDG show curvilinear increased activity around the joint capsules (*arrows*) of degenerative hips bilaterally.

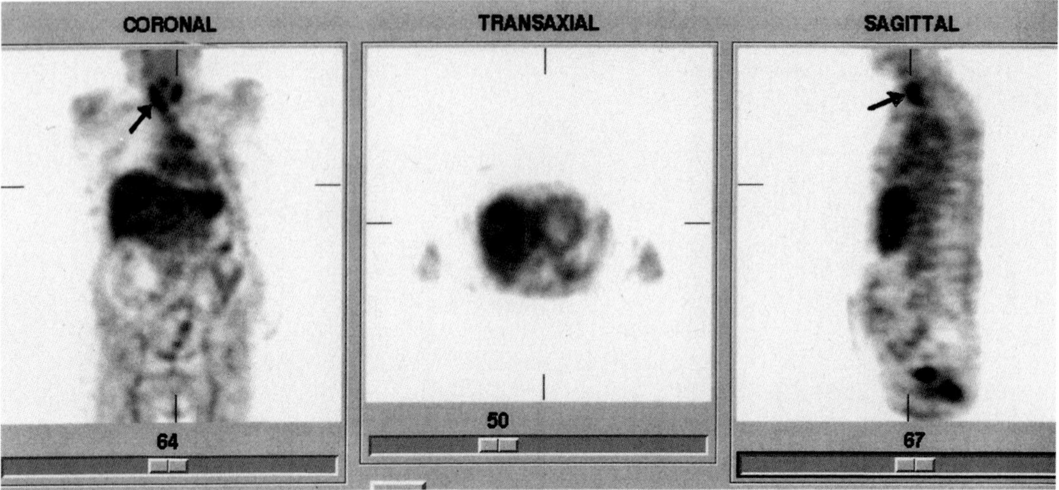

FIGURE 9.24. Selected coronal (*left*) and sagittal (*right*) PET images of the axial body with ^{18}F-FDG show markedly increased activity (*arrows*) on the thyroid gland due to thyroiditis.

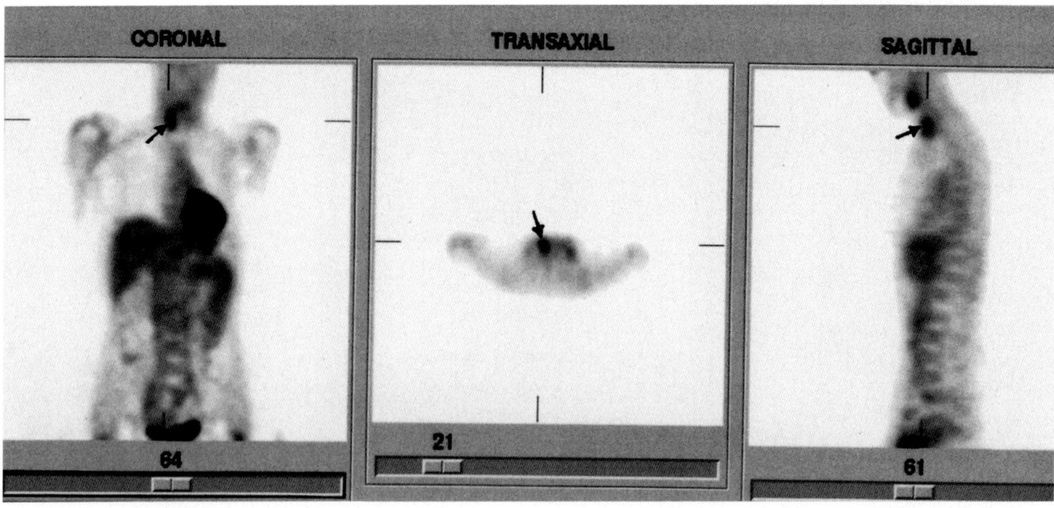

FIGURE 9.25. Selected coronal and sagittal PET images of the axial body as well as an axial image of the neck show an incrased uptake of ^{18}F-FDG in the right thyroid lobe (*arrows*) with Graves' disease. Left thyroid lobe has been removed.

References

1. Cook GJR, Maisey MN, Fogelman I. Normal variants, artifacts and interpretable pitfalls in PET imaging with 18-fluoro-2-deoxyglucose and carbon-11 methionine. Eur J Nucl Med 1999;26:1363–1378.
2. Alibazoglu H, Megremis D, Ali A, et al. Injection artifact on FDG-PET imaging. Clin Nucl Med 1998;23:264–265.
3. Minn H, Nuutila P, Lindholm P, et al. In vivo effects of insulin on tumor and skeletal muscle glucose metabolism in patients with lymphoma. Cancer 1994;73:1490–1498.
4. Goerres GW, Ziegler SI, Burger C, et al. Artifacts at PET and PET/CT caused by metallic hip prosthetic material. Radiology 2003;226:577–584.
5. Zhuang H, Chacko TK, Hickeson M, et al. Persistent non-specific FDG uptake on PET imaging following hip arthroplasty. Eur J Nucl Med 2002;29: 1328–1333.
6. Engel H, Steinert H, Buck A, et al. Whole-body PET: physiological and artifactual fluorodeoxyglucose accumulations. J Nucl Med 1996;37:441–446.
7. Heiba SI, Luo J, Sadek S, et al. Attenuation-correction induced artifact in F-18 FDG-PET imaging following total knee replacement. Clin Positron Imaging 2000;3:237–239.
8. Nuyts J, Michel C, Dupont P. Maximum likelihood expectation: maximization reconstruction of sinograms with arbitrary noise distribution using NEC-transformation. IEEE Trans Med Imaging 2001;20:365–375.
9. Miradli F, Vessell H, Faulharber P, et al. Elimination of artifactual FDG in PET imaging of colorectal cancer. Clin Nucl Med 1998;23:3–7.
10. Nehmeh SA, Erdi YE, Ling CC, et al. Effect of respiratory gating on reducing lung motion artifact in PET imaging of lung cancer. Med Phys 2000;29:366–371.
11. Cook GJR, Fogelman I, Maisey MN. Normal physiological and benign pathological variants of F-18 deoxyglucose PET: potential for error in interpretation. Semin Nucl Med 1996;26:308–324.
12. Kubota R, Kubota K, Yamada S, et al. Methionine uptake by tumor tissue: a microautoradiographic comparison with FDG. J Nucl Med 1995;36:484–492.

PART II

Clinical Applications

10

Epilepsy

Dong-Soo Lee and Myung-Chul Lee

It is well established today that the success rate of operations for epilepsy reaches almost 85%.[1–3] To localize epileptogenic zones, preoperative evaluation of surgical candidates by ^{18}F-fluorodeoxyglucose (^{18}F-FDG) positron emission tomography (PET) has become a routine practice. The diagnostic performance of ^{18}F-FDG-PET was recently improved by new image processing methods based on technologic advancements in neuroscience fields.

A 1995 review of the literature regarding the diagnostic performance of various imaging methods in finding epileptogenic zones showed the variable sensitivity of the several methods used in medial temporal lobe and neocortical epilepsies.[4] The diagnostic performance for medial temporal lobe epilepsy is different from that for extratemporal neocortical epilepsy.[4–7] Lateral temporal lobe epilepsy falls into the group of neocortical epilepsy.[2] Until 1995, the sensitivity of FDG-PET was not particularly high, especially in the case of extratemporal epilepsy; however, recent progress has increased the sensitivity.[4]

The sensitivity of FDG-PET was compared in a head-to-head fashion with that of magnetic resonance imaging (MRI) or ictal single photon emission computed tomography (SPECT) using technetium (Tc-99m) hexamethyl propylene amine oxime (HMPAO) or cysteinate dimer (ECD)[8] (Table 10.1). Among 118 patients who were operated for medial temporal and neocortical epilepsies and followed up for more than a year, the sensitivity of FDG-PET was 85%.

Diagnostic Performance of ^{18}F-FDG-PET in Medial Temporal Lobe Epilepsy

Medial temporal lobe epilepsy is well known for its pathologic diagnostic criteria of hippocampal sclerosis and atrophy. These hippocampal changes are easily found by the recent generation of MRI machines. Both quantitative and qualitative MRI interpretation give similar diagnostic effectiveness for temporal lobe epilepsy with the recent generation of MRI machines. FDG-PET reveals equally well the epileptogenic zones in medial temporal lobe epilepsy (Fig. 10.1A). Cases without any abnormal findings on MRI exist but are rare.[9]

TABLE 10.1. Correct localization of magnetic resonance imaging (MRI) ^{18}F-FDG-PET, and ictal single photon emission computed tomography (SPECT)

	Pathology (%)	Surgical outcome (%)
MRI	72	77
^{18}F-FDG-PET	85	86
Ictal SPECT	73	78

Modified from Won et al.[8]

Thus, FDG-PET is helpful only for three types of cases in medial temporal lobe epilepsy. The first type is ambiguous sclerosis (Fig. 10.1B). In a few patients with medial temporal lobe epilepsy, hippocampal sclerosis is not prominent even on three-dimensional multiplanar (MP)-PAGE MR images. The second type is bilateral sclerosis and atrophy (Fig. 10.1C). A few confusing cases have been filed among 600 fully in-

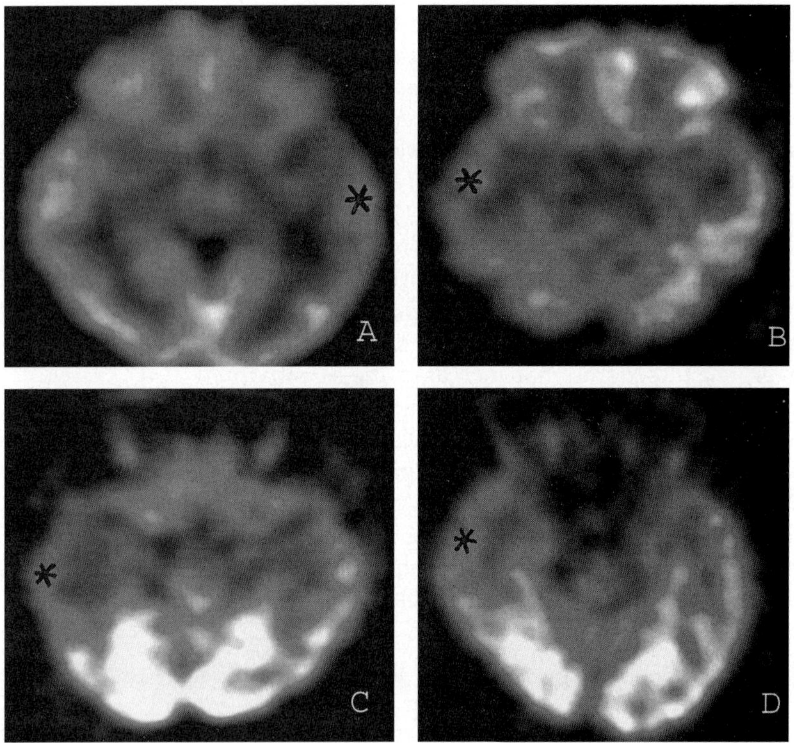

FIGURE 10.1. Selected axial FDG-PET images of the lower brain for medial temporal lobe epilepsy. A: A typical matching case with hippocampal atrophy and hypometabolism with decreased uptake of ^{18}F-FDG (*) in the left temporal lobe. B: A case with ambiguous ictal EEG but with definite hypometabolism with decreased activity (*) in the right temporal lobe. C: An example of bilateral hippocampal atrophy on MRI but unilateral hypometabolism (*) in the right temporal lobe. D: A nonlesional cryptogenic case on MRI but with mild hypometabolism (*) in the right temporal lobe. All four of these patients underwent operations and had surgical outcomes of Engel class 1.

vestigated epilepsy patients at our institution. The third type is nonlesional cases with normal MRI findings (Fig. 10.1D). FDG-PET and ictal SPECT were found to be similarly effective at localizing epileptogenic zones in nonlesional (MRI-negative) medial temporal lobe epilepsy.[9]

Diagnostic Performance of FDG-PET in Neocortical Epilepsy

In contrast to temporal lobe epilepsy, neocortical epilepsy poses several problems in terms of the localization of epileptogenic zones. About one third to one half of intractable patients are usually suspected of having neocortical epilepsy,[10,12] which consists of lateral temporal, frontal, occipital, and parietal lobe epilepsy, in decreasing order of prevalence.[11]

Neocortical epilepsy poses two kinds of problems in localization of epileptogenic zones. First, if the MRI shows multiple-candidate foci of epileptogenic zones, one cannot be sure which is the culprit lesion for the seizure induction. Second, if the MRI does not show any structural lesion, that is to say, the lesion is cryptogenic, it is difficult to determine where to apply subdural grids and strips during subdural EEG studies. FDG-PET is helpful in these cases. It may make it clear that a lesion is epileptogenic or it may localize a lesion in a totally cryptogenic case. In some patients, FDG-PET can at least lateralize cryptogenic lesions, although it cannot localize a lesion.

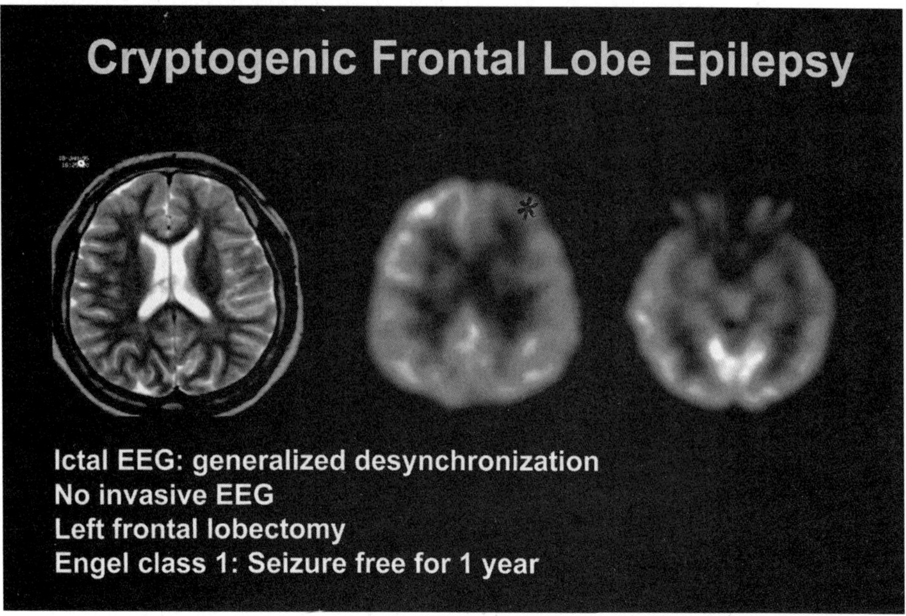

FIGURE 10.2. A case with cryptogenic frontal lobe epilepsy. Selected axial T2-weighted MRI of the brain was normal, and ictal EEG was also nonlocalizing. Selected axial FDG-PET showed images of the head, and definitive hypometabolism with decreased uptake of ^{18}F-FDG (*) in the left frontal lobe. After successful frontal lobectomy, the patient became seizure-free.

According to our previous study,[13] the positive predictive value of FDG-PET in cryptogenic epilepsy is over 70%.[13] Localization rates are different for different epileptogenic lobes. Among the complex partial seizure patients, lateral temporal lobe or frontal lobe epilepsies are relatively easy to diagnose. The sensitivity of FDG-PET was 36% in patients without structureal lesions on MRI and 73% in patients with structural lesions in frontal lobe epilepsy.[14] In nonlesional cryptogenic cases, epileptogenic zones yield decreased metabolism (Fig. 10.2).

In contrast, it is not easy to localize epileptogenic zones in occipital lobe epilepsy.[15] Areas showing the most severe hypometabolism are limited to the occipital lobes in some patients (Fig. 10.3); however, this is not true in all patients. The areas of highest perfusion also were not limited to the occipital lobes. In some patients the hypometabolism was localized to the ipsilateral temporal lobes (Fig. 10.4). Moreover, epilep-

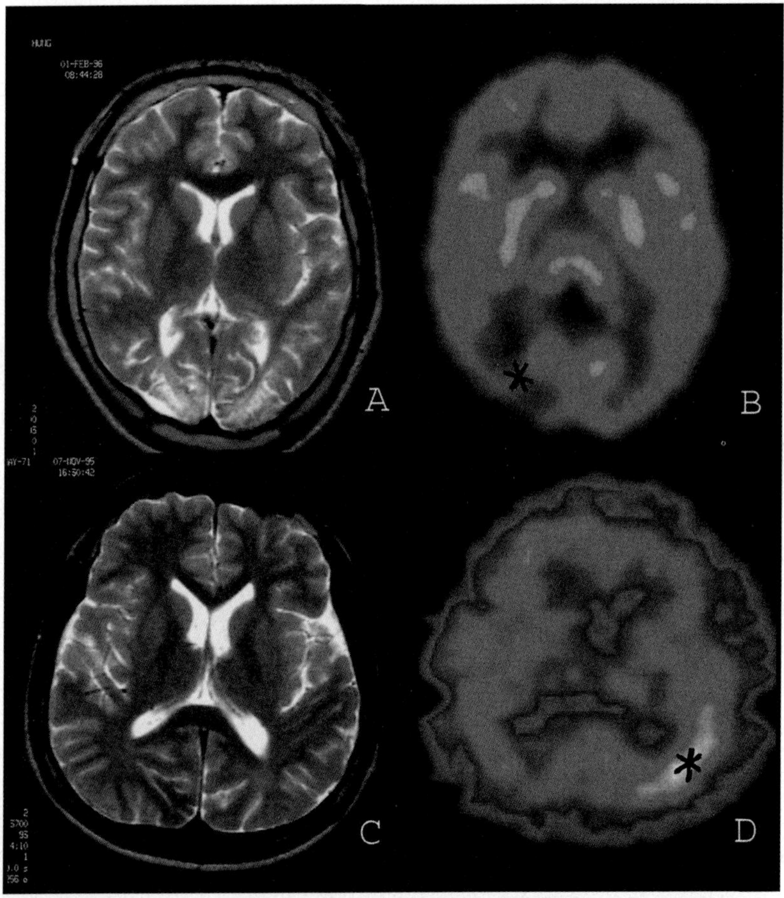

FIGURE 10.3. Cases of occipital lobe epilepsy. Selected T2-weighted axial MRI of the brain (A) was normal, but metabolism with ^{18}F-FDG was decreased in the right occipital lobe epilepsy (*) on the axial image of the head (B). In another case, the MRI (C) was normal, but perfusion with Tc-99m HMPAO was increased in the left occipital lobe (*) on ictal SPECT of the head (D). Both of the patients became seizure-free after neocortical resection.

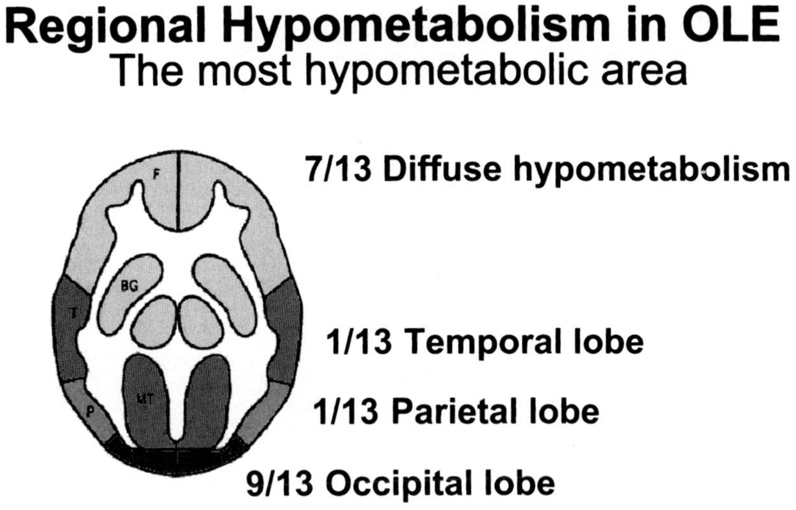

Regional Hypometabolism in OLE
The most hypometabolic area

F
BG
T
MT
P
7/13 Diffuse hypometabolism
1/13 Temporal lobe
1/13 Parietal lobe
9/13 Occipital lobe

FIGURE 10.4. Regional prevalence of interictal hypometabolism on ^{18}F-FDG-PET in occipital lobe epilepsy (OLE). The occipital lobe is the most common site of hypometabolism.

togenic zones could have been misdiagnosed for the temporal lobes. As for occipital lobe epilepsy, the localization rate was found to be 47% by MRI and 60% by PET.[15] In confusing cases of occipital lobe epilepsy, the examination of visual symptoms and visual field is mandatory.[15]

Comparison of Interictal FDG-PET with Interictal Perfusion SPECT

The sensitivity of interictal perfusion SPECT was 44% on average according to a meta-analysis.[5] However, in our cohort study, the sensitivity was lower (34%) in temporal and neocortical epilepsy. When we consider the dogma of metabolism and perfusion coupling in brain, the significance of, or the reason for, this finding is important. The reason why interictal FDG-PET is excellent but interictal SPECT is poor for the localization of epileptogenic zones could be explained as follows. Among more than 300 patients, we identified 14 patients with increased perfusion in the epileptogenic zones as determined by surgical outcome or invasive studies.[16] Four of these were the patients in whom interictal SPECT was performed on the second day after the ictal study. Another four patients who were seemingly hyperperfused were studied on the 3rd to 5th day after the ictal study (Fig. 10.5A,B). This means that interictal SPECT was not really an interictal one. Subclinical seizure activity just before or during interictal studies could have resulted in this increased perfusion at the epileptogenic zones.

On the other hand, delayed postictal perfusion abnormalities even long after the previous ictus could have resulted in the increased perfusion.[17] When we performed delayed postictal SPECT at 6 hours after ictal SPECT, we found remnant hyperperfusion in half of the pa-

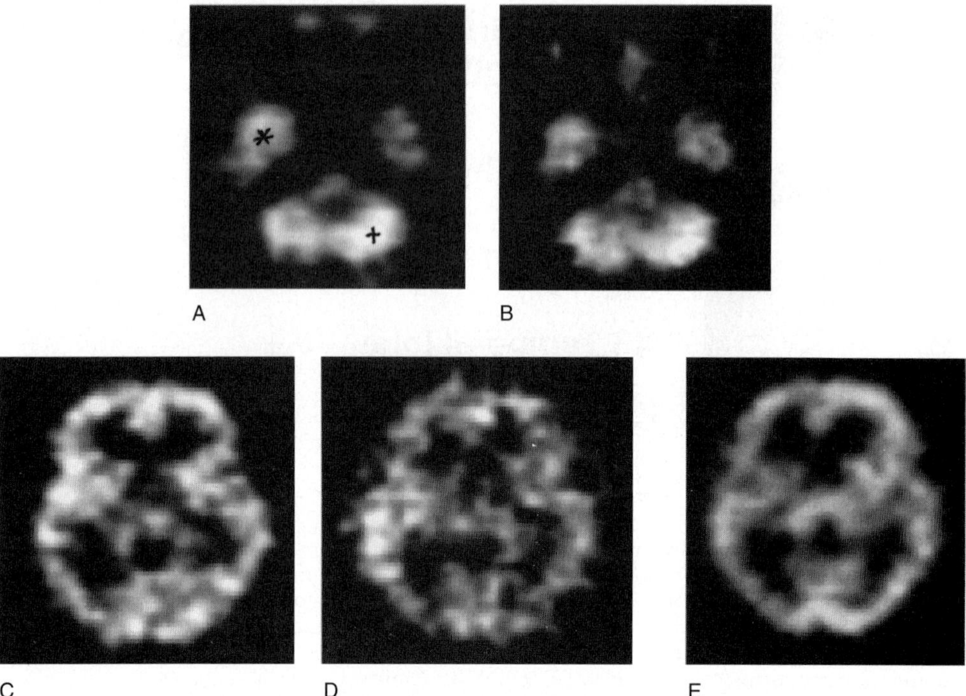

FIGURE 10.5. Hyperperfusion on interictal SPECT using Tc-99m HMPAO and delayed postictal hyperperfusion after ictus. In a patient with surgically confirmed right temporal lobe epilepsy, axial images of the head on interictal SPECT (B) taken on the fourth day after ictal study (A) showed the similar increased perfusion in the right temporal lobe (*) and crossed cerebellar hyperperfusion (+). In the other patient with right temporal lobe epilepsy, perfusion was increased in the right temporal lobe (*) on ictal SPECT (C) and also in 6-hour delayed SPECT (D). On interictal SPECT (E), perfusion was relatively decreased in this temporal lobe (*).

tients (Fig. 10.5C–E). In one patient, severe hypoperfusion was found on delayed postictal SPECT, which recovered on interictal SPECT. Based on this investigation, we suggest that even with the EEG monitoring during interictal SPECT, one cannot be sure that the true interictal SPECT has been obtained.

Voxel-Based Analysis of FDG-PET

Statistical parametric mapping (SPM) is a voxel-based approach for determining the significantly different area from normal controls (Fig. 10.6). After spatially transforming and smoothing the individual PET data, using the general linear model, the voxel count of the individual patient is compared with that of the normal controls. This analysis method is easy to perform and very robust, and has become popular.[14,18,19] The SPM analysis of ^{15}O water PET, ^{18}F-FDG-PET, and Tc-99m HMPAO interictal SPECT revealed that in the same patients the areas of hypoperfusion were concordant with, but smaller than, the areas of hypometabolism[20] (Fig. 10.7). This uncoupling of perfusion and metabolism in epileptogenic zones was another reason why interictal

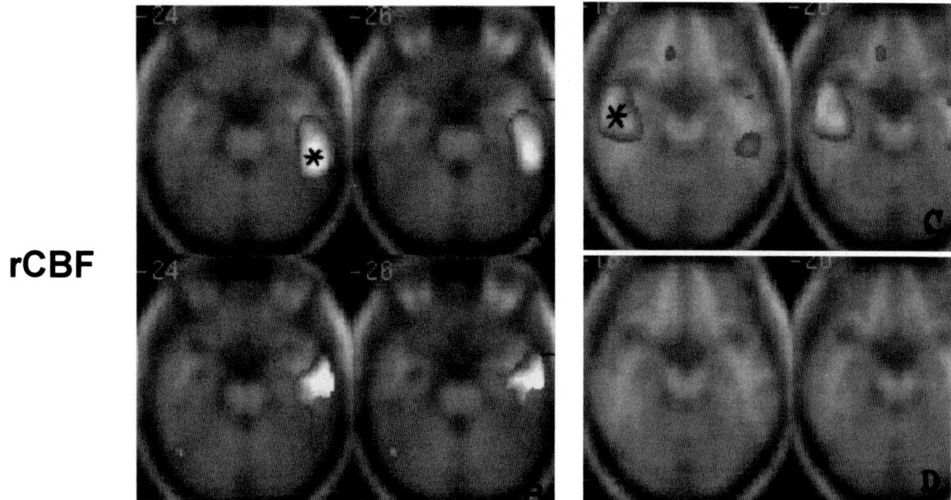

FIGURE 10.6. Statistical parametric mapping (SPM) analysis of the result of ^{18}F-FDG-PET and ^{15}O-water PET superimposed on MRI. Activities are the voxels that differ from the normal controls. In a coupled case (*left*), the left temporal lobe (*) was found to have hypometabolic voxels on axial FDG-PET images (A) and hypoperfused voxels on water PET (B). In an uncoupled case (*right*), the right temporal lobe (*) was found to have hypometabolic voxels on FDG-PET axial images (C); however, there was no area of hypoperfusion on water PET (D). rCBF, regional cerebral blood flow.

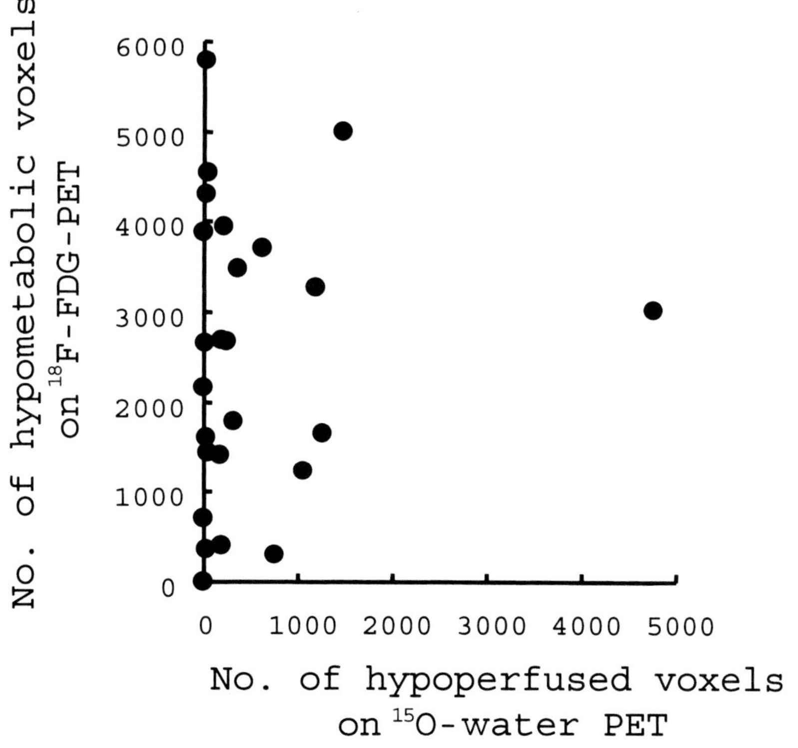

FIGURE 10.7. Number of hypoperfused voxels and hypometabolic voxels on ^{15}O-water PET and ^{18}F-FDG-PET in the epileptogenic temporal lobes. Each data point represents voxel number per epileptogenic whole temporal lobe per patient. Numbers of hypometabolic voxels tended to be much larger than those of hypoperfused voxels.

FDG-PET was superior to interictal perfusion SPECT in localizing epileptogenic zones.

In frontal lobe epilepsy, on SPM analysis, using an uncorrected probability value of .005 as the threshold, the sensitivity of SPM analysis reached that of visual assessment. The sensitivity decreased according to the decrease in probability value (Fig. 10.8).

Quantification Using Automatic Volume of Interest on a Population-Based Atlas

This method uses the population-based standard anatomy, which was developed at the Montreal Neurological Institute and named "statistical probabilistic anatomical map" (SPAM) (Fig. 10.9). SPAM differs from SPM in that SPM is a voxel-based approach, whereas SPAM is an area-based approach. SPAM is an objective and operator-independent method of volume-of-interest (VOI) drawing. We use a population-averaged anatomic definition of gyri and lobes in MRI template format. To construct SPAM, the Montreal group collected, parceled, and segmented normal MR images from 152 young people. Original PET images are transformed to an MRI template and multiplied by the probabilities obtained from the SPAM template. For ex-

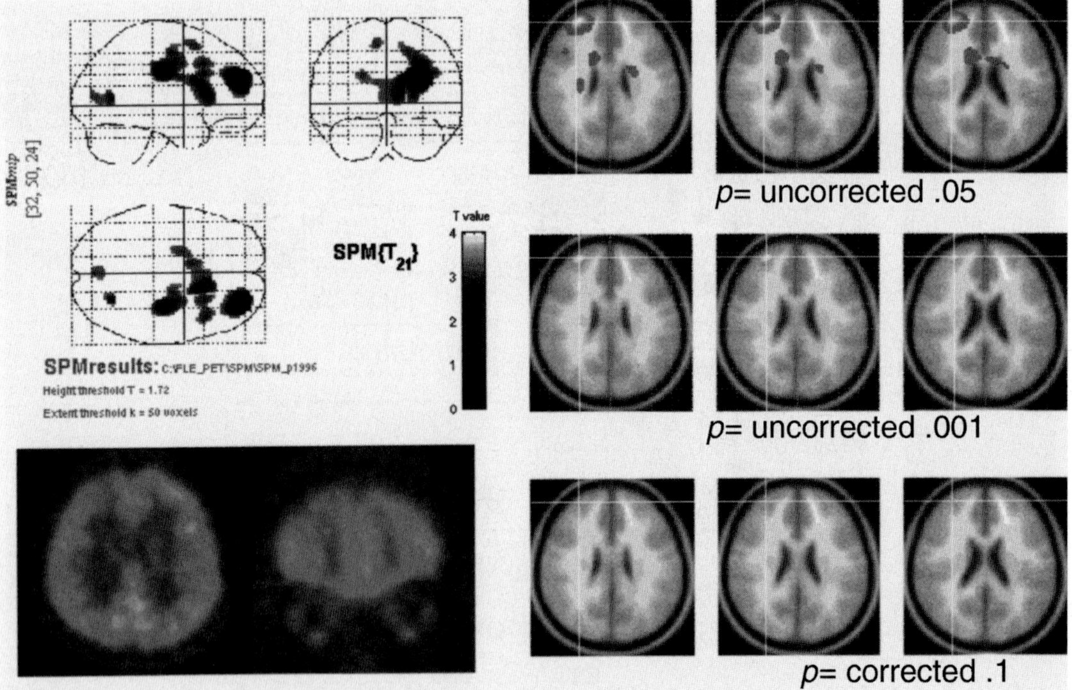

FIGURE 10.8. Example of SPM analysis with varying threshold. According to the cutoff value of voxel height, SPM analysis became less sensitive when a stricter criterion was applied. The sensitivity decreases according to the decrease in the probability value.

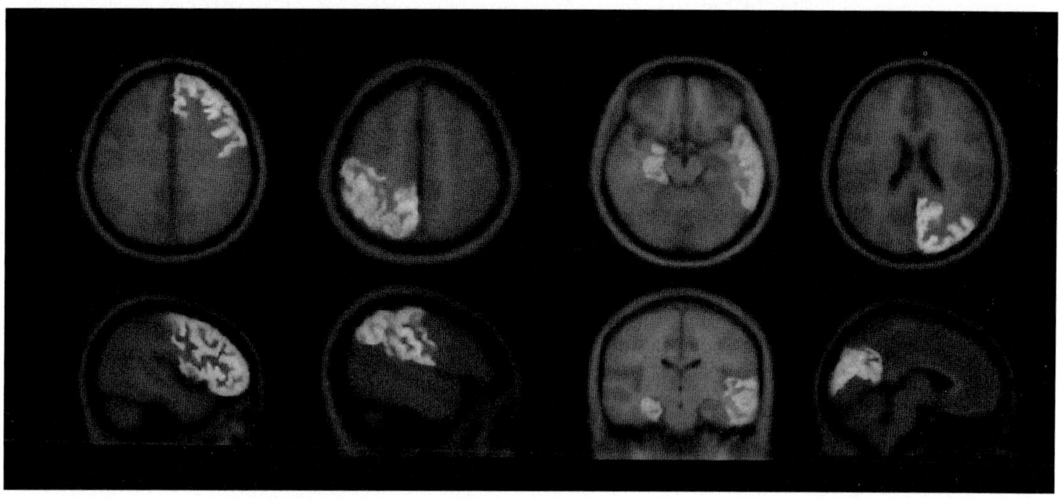

FIGURE 10.9. Statistical probabilistic anatomical map (SPAM) as an objective volume of interest (VOI) in PET image processing. Frontal and parietal (*left*) as well as temporal and occipital (*right*) lobes were displayed on the MRI template. These SPAM masks can be used as a VOI on the MRI template.

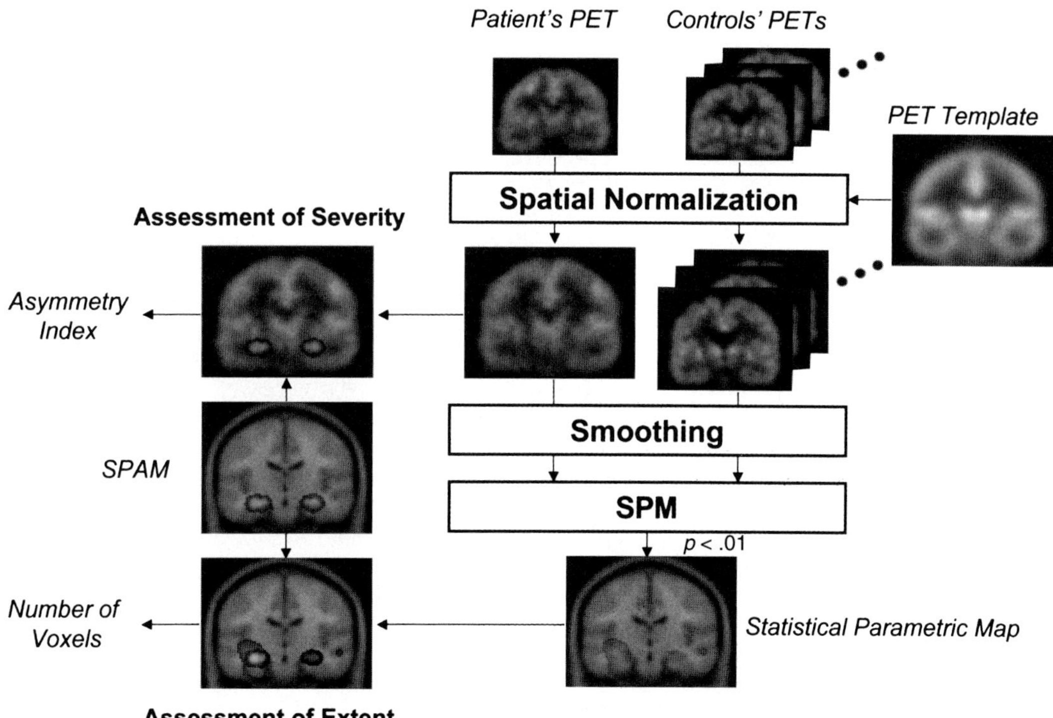

FIGURE 10.10. Assessment of the severity and extent of hypometabolism. Asymmetric indexes were calculated on six pairs of volumes of interest (VOIs) to represent the temporal lobe. Significant regional hypometabolism was estimated by comparing the PET images with those of controls by using SPM. The extent of hypometabolic area for each VOI was determined by counting the number of voxels with significantly decreased hypometabolism in each VOI segmented by SPAM.

ample, if the right hippocampus is chosen, the resulting image shows the counts in the probabilistic area of the right hippocampus. This method was first used to quantify objectively the asymmetric index, and these asymmetric indices could be used to localize the epileptogenic zones on FDG-PET.[21]

Figure 10.10 describes the method of using SPAM to evaluate the extent and severity of hypometabolism on FDG-PET in epileptogenic zones. The relation of hypometabolism to surgical prognosis of medial temporal lobe epilepsy could be evaluated. By the successful application of SPAM of six gyri of temporal lobes, this analysis revealed that focal severity and extent were not related to the surgical outcome in medial temporal lobe epilepsy.[22]

Conclusion

FDG-PET is helpful in localizing the epileptogenic zones, especially in patients with nonlesional epilepsy on MRI. Quantitative methods, such as SPM and SPAM, are believed to be able to enhance the objectivity of the analysis to find the epileptogenic zones by revealing the hypometabolic areas.

References

1. Wiebe S, Blume WT, Girvin JP, et al. A randomized, controlled trial of surgery for temporal-lobe epilepsy. N Engl J Med 2001;345:311–318.
2. Schramm J, Kral T, Grunwald T, et al. Surgical treatment for neocortical temporal lobe epilepsy: clinical and surgical aspects and seizure outcome. J Neurosurg 2001;94:33–42.
3. Foldvary N, Nashold B, Mascha E, et al. Seizure outcome after temporal lobectomy for temporal lobe epilepsy: a Kaplan-Meier survival analysis. Neurology 2000;54:630–634.
4. Spencer SS, Theodore WH, Berkovic SF. Clinical applications: MRI, SPECT, and PET. Magn Reson Imaging 1995;13:1119–1124.
5. Devous MD Sr, Thisted RA, Morgan GF, et al. SPECT brain imaging in epilepsy: a meta-analysis. J Nucl Med 1998;39:285–293.
6. Hwang SI, Kim JH, Park SW, et al. Comparative analysis of MR imaging, positron emission tomography, and ictal single-photon emission CT in patients with neocortical epilepsy. AJNR 2001;22:937–946.
7. Lewis PJ, Siegel A, Siegel AM, et al. Does performing image registration and subtraction in ictal brain SPECT help localize neocortical seizures? J Nucl Med 2000;41:1619–1626.
8. Won HJ, Chang KH, Cheon JE, et al. Comparison of MR imaging with PET and ictal SPECT in 118 patients with intractable epilepsy. AJNR 1999;20:593–599.
9. Son YJ, Chung CK, Lee SK, et al. Comparison of localizing values of various diagnostic tests in non-lesional medial temporal lobe epilepsy. Seizure 1999;8:465–470.
10. Nam H, Lee SK, Chung CK, et al. Incidence and clinical profile of extramedial-temporal epilepsy with hippocampal atrophy. J Korean Med Sci 2001;16:95–102.
11. Kutsy RL. Focal extratemporal epilepsy: clinical features, EEG patterns, and surgical approach. J Neurol Sci 1999;166:1–15.

12. Zentner J, Hufnagel A, Ostertun B, et al. Surgical treatment of extratemporal epilepsy: clinical, radiologic, and histopathologic findings in 60 patients. Epilepsia 1996;37:1072–1080.
13. Lee DS, Lee SK, Chung J-K, et al. Predictive values of ^{18}F-FDG-PET and ictal SPECT to find epileptogenic zones in cryptogenic neocortical epilepsies. J Nucl Med 1997;38:272P(abst).
14. Kim YK, Lee DS, Lee SK, et al. ^{18}F-FDG-PET in localization of frontal lobe epilepsy: comparison of visual and SPM analysis. J Nucl Med 2002;43: 1167–1174.
15. Kim SK, Lee DS, Lee SK, et al. Diagnostic performance of ^{18}F-FDG-PET and ictal [99mTc]-HMPAO SPECT in occipital lobe epilepsy. Epilepsia 2001;42:1531–1540.
16. Lee DS, Kim SK, Lee SK, et al. Frequencies and implications of discordant findings of interictal SPECT and ictal SPECT in patients with intractable epilepsy. Eur J Nucl Med 1997;24:983(abst).
17. Lee DS, Lee SK, Kim SK, et al. Late postictal residual perfusion abnormality in epileptogenic zone found on 6-hour postictal SPECT. Neurology 2000;55:835–841.
18. Signorini M, Paulesu E, Friston K, et al. Rapid assessment of regional cerebral metabolic abnormalities in single subjects with quantitative and nonquantitative ^{18}F-FDG-PET: a clinical validation of statistical parametric mapping. Neuroimage 1999;9:63–80.
19. Van Bogaert P, Massager N, Tugendhaft P, et al. Statistical parametric mapping of regional glucose metabolism in medial temporal lobe epilepsy. Neuroimage 2000;12:129–138.
20. Lee DS, Lee JS, Kang KW, et al. Disparity of perfusion and glucose metabolism of epileptogenic zones in temporal lobe epilepsy demonstrated by SPM/SPAM analysis on ^{15}O-water PET, ^{18}F-FDG-PET, and [99mTc]-HMPAO SPECT. Epilepsia 2001;42:1515–1522.
21. Kang KW, Lee DS, Cho JH, et al. Quantification of ^{18}F-FDG-PET images in temporal lobe epilepsy patients using probabilistic brain atlas. Neuroimage 2001;14:1–6.
22. Lee SK, Lee DS, Yeo JS, et al. FDG-PET images quantified by probabilistic atlas of brain and surgical prognosis of temporal lobe epilepsy. Epilepsia 2002;43:1032–1038.

11

Dementia and Cerebrovascular Disease

Sang-Eun Kim and Myung-Chul Lee

Dementia is a major public health challenge, not only for clinicians, but also for society as a whole. Prevalence rates of dementia are dependent on age, being reported as high as 24% to 48% in those older than 85 years.[1,2] The overall prevalence in North America in those older than 65 years is 8% to 10%, or more than 27 million people.[2] Furthermore, mortality is increased threefold in those with dementia.[1] The proportion of elderly in our population is growing rapidly; with current prevalence rates, the number of individuals with dementia older than 65 years will more than double by 2021.[2] Thus, there is an increasing demand on the health care system and public resources to care for people with dementia.

A wide variety of disorders have been identified as causes of dementia, including primary brain disease and diseases of other organ systems that lead to secondary brain dysfunction. Between 10% and 20% of the dementias may be reversible, and thus distinguishing patients with potentially reversible conditions from those with degenerative dementias is crucial.[3] Some irreversible dementias may have important interventions (e.g., vascular dementia), and accurate diagnosis is necessary in the degenerative disorders to provide prognostic and genetic counseling. Neuroimaging plays a critical role in the diagnostic evaluation of the dementia patient. Vascular dementia, hydrocephalus, neoplasms, subdural hematomas, and some infectious and degenerative processes can be identified with contemporary imaging technology.

The majority of the dementias are insidiously progressive, leading to cognitive failure and premature death.[3] Beyond the age of 65 years, the most common cause of dementia is Alzheimer's disease (AD). Since the original case report of AD in 1907, clinicians have sought to find accurate antemortem tests to aid in the diagnosis of this disorder. Until now, however, no peripheral biochemical or genetic marker for AD has been found. A biopsy or postmortem examination of cerebral tissue is needed if confirmation of the presumptive clinical diagnosis is required, making clinicians rely on clinical diagnostic criteria. Currently, there is clinical ambiguity in diagnosing AD in its early stages, and it is essentially a diagnosis of exclusion. The patients, the family, and the physician are typically faced with a battery of negative test results and an ambiguous clinical impression that leads to periodic repetition of tests, entailing cost, inconvenience, potential morbidity to the patient, and lack of a definitive diagnosis. As the percentage of elderly people grows, and because the incidence of dementia increases with age, the economic, social, and health care consequences of dementing illnesses, and AD in particular, will increase with time. In 1986, the cost of care for patients with dementia was estimated to exceed $25 billion per year in the United States. The ability to diagnose AD early in its course, noninvasively and reliably with positron emission tomography (PET), will have significant impact on these medical and economic realities.

This chapter describes the application of functional neuroimaging in the evaluation of AD and other dementias as well as cerebrovascular diseases.

Alzheimer's Disease

Alzheimer's disease, which affects 5% to 10% of people over 65 years of age and up to 47% of those aged 85 years or older,[4] is the most common cause of primary progressive dementia, followed by cerebrovascular and other neurodegenerative diseases, including diffuse Lewy body disease and frontotemporal dementia. Alzheimer's disease is characterized by a progressive, global, and irreversible deterioration of cognitive function, which usually begins with memory problems, followed by deficits in language, mathematical and visuospatial skills, abstract thinking, and planning, as well as personality and behavioral changes.

Neuropathology

One of the pathologic hallmarks of AD is senile plaques, which accumulate extracellularly in the brain. They are found most characteristically in the gray matter of the neocortex and hippocampus, but also occur in the basal ganglia, thalamus, and cerebellum. A few are found in hemispheric white matter. Neurofibrillary tangles are intracellular characteristics of AD. Generally, tangles are formed by the large neurons of the brain—the pyramidal cells of the hippocampus and neocortex, the large neurons in the olfactory cortex, amygdala, basal forebrain nuclei, and several brainstem nuclei, including the locus ceruleus and the raphe nucleus.

The AD brain also is characterized by neuronal cell loss and change in neuronal morphology. This is reflected by a decreased brain weight and by atrophy of the cortex. Although the pattern and degrees of atrophy vary considerably from individual to individual, it is most prominent in the frontal anterior temporal parietal lobe. Neuronal loss is most notable in the hippocampus, frontal, parietal, and anterior temporal cortices, amygdala, and the olfactory system. Profound loss also occurs in the nucleus basalis, a large cholinergic system at the base of the forebrain. This cell loss also occurs in the locus ceruleus and is likely to account for the reduction in the brain level of norepinephrine noted in some AD. As expected, neuronal loss is generally seen in areas that show plaque or tangle pathology. In the hippocampus the most prominently affected zones are the CA1 region, the subiculum, and the entorhinal cortex. Other areas of the limbic system, including olfactory bulbs, olfactory cortices, amygdala, cingulate gyrus, and hypothalamus, are also affected.

Many individuals (at least 20% to 30%) diagnosed antemortem with AD demonstrate cortical Lewy bodies at autopsy in addition to the neuropathologic findings of AD. Alzheimer's disease with Lewy bodies has been associated with excess cognitive burden, extrapyramidal symptoms, and more frequent psychotic symptoms.[5]

Neurochemistry

Alzheimer's disease is associated with deficits in several neurotransmitter systems, both those that project to the neocortex and those that reside within the cortex. The basal forebrain contains a well-characterized group of magnocellular cholinergic neurons extending from the medial septal region through the nucleus basalis of Meynert, Ch1–Ch4, which provide the majority of cholinergic innervation to the hippocampus and neocortex.[6] In patients with AD, postmortem studies have consistently documented a selective loss of cholinergic neurons in the basal forebrain[7] and a marked reduction in choline acetyltransferase, the enzyme that catalyzes the synthesis of acetylcholine, in the projection areas that correlate with dementia severity.[8] Cholinergic deficits are not the transmitter deficit in AD. There are cortical losses of norepinephrine and serotonin that can be traced to cell loss in the locus ceruleus and raphe nuclei. In addition to deficits in systems that project to the cortex, there are abnormalities in pathways that are intrinsic to the cortex. A large number of peptide transmitters are found in cortical interneurons. These losses of somatostatin, neuropeptide Y, corticotropin-releasing factor, and substance P have been described in AD.

Presumably, the deficits in these various transmitter systems in AD are all a reflection of the degeneration and death of neuronal populations. Another indication of neuronal degeneration in AD is the loss of synapses and presynaptic marker proteins in the neocortex and hippocampus. The loss is likely a result of both deafferentation of cortical and hippocampal neurons and of atrophy of the neurons themselves. Synaptic loss thus provides another neuroanatomic marker for the development and severity of dementia and may be even a better correlate of cognitive impairment than plaques or tangles.[9]

Identification of the loss of cholinergic neurons in the basal forebrain and cholinergic innervation of the cerebral cortex in AD was followed by investigations into the involvement of cholinergic receptors. In contrast to choline acetyltransferase, no major or consistent changes in muscarinic acetylcholine receptors (mAChRs) were observed in the cerebral cortex,[10] although moderate reductions in the cortical M2 receptor subtype have been reported.[11] In contrast, reductions in nicotinic acetylcholine receptors (nAChRs) with high affinity for agonists ranging between 20% and 50% were consistently observed at autopsy in a number of neocortical areas and hippocampi of patients with AD.[12,13] Recent immunochemical analyses indicate that this deficit is predominantly associated with the loss of $\alpha 4$ subunits. A significant reduction in the binding of ^{125}I-α-bungarotoxin, which binds to homomeric $\alpha 7$-containing nAChRs, was also reported in the temporal but not the frontal cortex in AD.[14,15] Changes of nAChRs in AD are distinct from those in normal aging and are likely to contribute to clinical features and possibly neuropathology. The cortical nAChR deficits significantly correlate with cognitive impairment in AD patients.[16]

A reduction in the density of the presynaptic vesicular acetylcholine transporter binding sites measured by H-3 vesamicol was also seen in the AD cortical tissue, but the decrease in H-3 vesamicol binding was less than that in nAChRs. This observation suggests that the vesamicol binding sites may be more preserved in the existing presynaptic terminals of AD cortical tissue, thereby expressing a compensatory capacity to maintain cholinergic activity. The reduction in vesicular acetylcholine transporter radioligand binding was less than that in choline acetyltransferase activity in AD neocortex. Thus, there is a possibility that these two presynaptic cholinergic markers may be differentially regulated or differentially lost in AD. There may be an upregulation of vesicular acetylcholine transporter expression to compensate for cholinergic terminal losses, or alternatively, choline acetyltransferase expression may be reduced within otherwise intact presynaptic nerve terminals.[17]

Prominent reductions in postmortem measures of presynaptic dopamine have been reported in AD with Lewy bodies.[18–20] These reductions, however, are not as severe as those seen in Parkinson disease.[19,20]

Clinical Diagnosis

There is no definitive antemortem diagnostic test for AD, and brain biopsy may miss subsequently proven cases. Clinicians therefore must rely on clinical diagnostic criteria for senile or presenile dementia of the Alzheimer type. When compared against the "gold standard" of pathologic AD, the diagnostic accuracy in dementia of the Alzheimer type varies widely, the average being about 75%, with false-positive rates ranging from more than 50% down to 11% for a maximum sensitivity or detection rate of approximately 90%.[21–23] In the early stages of the disease, the clinical diagnosis is often questionable.[24]

Structural Imaging

In AD, structural imaging such as magnetic resonance imaging (MRI) and computed tomography (CT) shows a progressive cortical atrophy associated with increases in the ventricular and cortical cerebrospinal fluid space. These imaging techniques are excellent in identifying the causes of dementia that have structurally identifiable basis on the microscopic level. Such entities include multiple infarcts, subdural hematomas, brain tumors, and hydrocephalus. These techniques, however, are of little use in differentiating AD from other degenerative dementias, such as dementia with Lewy bodies, frontotemporal dementia,[25] early Huntington's disease,[26–28] and progressive supranuclear palsy.[29,30] MRI and CT in these degenerative diseases demonstrate the presence of cerebral atrophy of variable degree, focal or diffuse to the whole brain, usually unrelated to the neurologic and neuropsychological symptoms presented by the patients.

Functional Imaging

PET assesses and maps a regional brain function. The signal measured in PET is derived from the decay of radioactive positron-emitting nuclides that are introduced into the body via intravenous injection or inhalation. Common nuclides including ^{15}O, ^{11}C, and ^{18}F are used to label compounds such as glucose and oxygen for the purpose of evaluating cerebral metabolism or measuring regional cerebral blood flow (rCBF). Radiolabeled receptor ligands have been developed and are widely used for the assessment of neurotransmitter systems. The short half-life of some of these tracers (minutes) facilitates repeat studies within a single scanning session, while ensuring low radiation exposure for the patient. A circumferential detector placed around the head maps the distribution of the positron-emitting nuclide with a resolution of approximately 5 mm.

Metabolic and Blood Flow Imaging

$^{F}18$-fluoro-2-deoxy-D-glucose (FDG)-PET has the ability to provide objective, accurate, and noninvasive diagnostic information about patients with dementia of various causes. FDG-PET studies have shown a characteristic pattern of metabolic impairment of cortical association areas in AD (Fig. 11.1).[31–33] Impairment of glucose metabolism seen in AD (usually 1 to 2 years after onset of the disease) typically involves the temporoparietal cortex, and often is bilateral. As the disease progresses, the areas of cortical involvement with hypometabolism expand. Later, decreased metabolism is found in the frontal cortex, but the primary visual cortex and primary sensorimotor cortices typically appear to be relatively spared until the late stages of the disease, in accord with pathologic data. Subcortical structures such as basal ganglia and the thalamus and brainstem also remain relatively unaffected. Cerebellar metabolism is relatively preserved in mild to moderate AD. A significant reduction in cerebellar glucose metabolism has been reported in severe AD with no evident cerebellar atrophy.[34] In early stages of the disease, the typical pattern may not yet be complete. In particular, frontal involvement may be missing, and only temporoparietal metabolism may be unilaterally impaired. In spite of these limitations, it has been suggested that FDG-PET may be used for early diagnosis of AD, which would be very valuable for therapeutic trials in early stages of the disease.[32]

In a very early stage of AD, even before clinical diagnosis of probable AD is possible, a decrease of blood flow and glucose metabolism in the posterior cingulate gyrus and precuneus has been reported

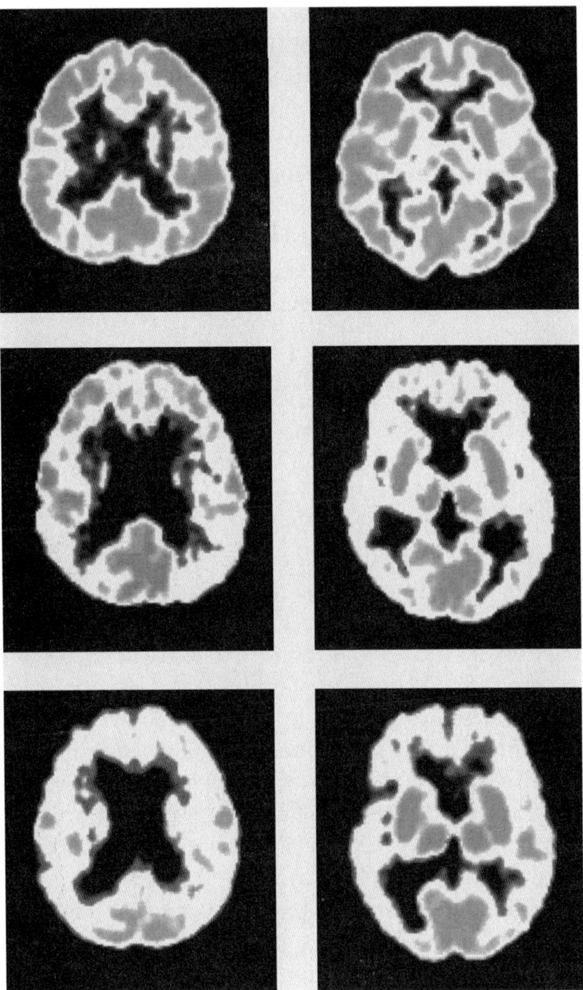

FIGURE 11.1. Selected axial PET images of the brain in control (*top*) and patients with Alzheimer's disease (*middle* with 1.0 CDR and *bottom* with 2.0 CDR), showing a characteristic pattern of metabolic impairment with decreased uptakes of ^{18}F-FDG in the bilateral temporoparietal association cortex, with relative sparing of primary sensorimotor and visual areas, basal ganglia, thalamus, and cerebellum (not shown here). In early stages of the disease, frontal involvement may be missing and temporoparietal metabolism may be only unilaterally impaired.

using PET[33] or single photon emission computed tomography (SPECT).[34,35] These structures are important in memory. The metabolic and flow reduction in these regions may be due to functional deafferentation from the entorhinal cortex, which is among the first regions pathologically affected in AD.[36] As the disease progresses, the medial temporal structures and parietotemporal association cortex show flow and metabolic reductions. Most pathologic and morphologic studies demonstrated that the medial temporal structures, including the amygdala, hippocampal formation, entorhinal cortex, and parahippocampal and fusiform gyri, are the first structures affected in AD with histological changes, including amyloid deposits and neurofibrillary changes. This is in accordance with the finding that the episodic memory loss is the earliest neuropsychological deficit in AD.[37] The reduced rCBF in the medial temporal structures demonstrated by PET and SPECT is consistent with these pathologic findings.[38–40] Following the involvement of the medial temporal structures, the neuropathological changes spread to the basal forebrain and anterior cingulate gyrus before encroaching on the neocortical association areas.[41] It is likely that the anterior cingulate gyrus is functionally involved since attention is the first nonmemory domain affected in AD before deficits in language and visuospatial functions occur.[42] However, few reports have described involvement of the anterior cingulate gyrus.

As described above, PET and SPECT imaging of patients with AD demonstrates progressive reductions of brain glucose metabolism and blood flow in the resting state in relation to dementia severity. The metabolic and flow reductions correlate with high regional densities of neurofibrillary tangles and evidence for synaptic loss as well as dysfunction. During cognitive or psychophysical stimulation, however, blood flow and metabolism in the affected brain regions can increase to the same extent in mildly demented AD patients as in age-matched controls, despite reduced resting state values. The extent of activation declines with dementia severity and is markedly reduced in severely demented patients. Thus, there appears to be an initial functionally responsive stage in AD that is accompanied by reversible downregulation because of reduced synaptic energy demand of enzymes mediating mitochondrial oxidative-phosphorylation. A later irreversible stage of AD is accompanied by marked synaptic loss, accumulation of intracellular neurofibrillary tangles, reduced general transcriptional capacity, and death of neurons.

Patients with AD at the early stage present with memory decline and impairments of language and visuospatial functions. However, some AD patients occasionally show frontal lobe dysfunctions in the early stage that are known to emerge only at an advanced stage. This subtype of AD is called a frontal variant of AD. In these patients, hypometabolism in frontal cortex as well as temporoparietal regions was shown on FDG-PET scans (Fig. 11.2). The visual variant of AD with prominent visual symptoms and metabolic impairment in occipital cortex has also been reported.

While structural imagings may show a cerebral atrophy in the demented patient, this finding is nonspecific and overlaps with results seen in normal elderly subjects. Patients in whom the diagnosis of AD can be confirmed by PET may be given the opportunity to participate in established or experimental therapy programs. Since prognosis varies among the untreatable dementias, active diagnostic information is useful in planning future medical and family needs. In addition, it is possible that PET could be used to screen and provide predictive information and genetic counseling to individuals and high-risk groups, such as members of familial AD pedigrees. Longitudinal studies of patients with presumed AD have demonstrated a pattern of parietotem-

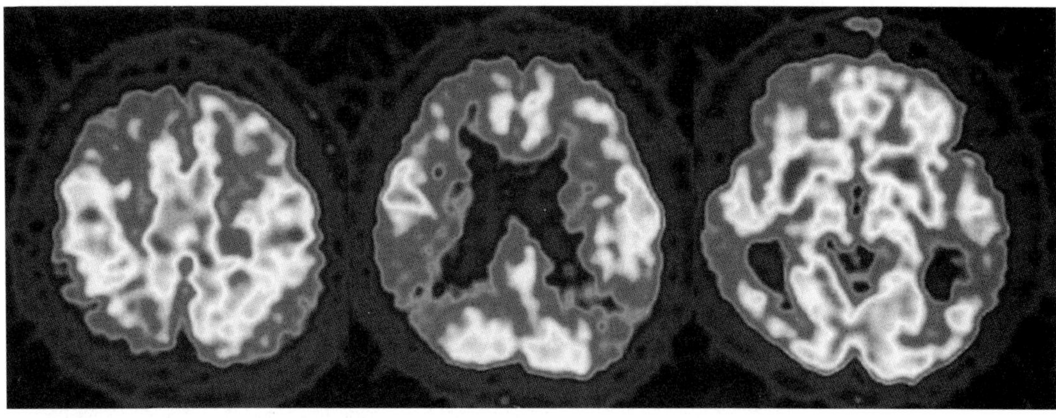

FIGURE 11.2. Selected axial PET images of the brain in a patient with frontal variant of Alzheimer's disease, showing hypometabolism with decreased uptake of ^{18}F-FDG in frontal cortex as well as temporoparietal regions.

poral hypometabolism predicting the ultimate diagnosis 13 months prior to the clinical diagnosis of "probable" AD.[42]

PET and SPECT measures of metabolism and CBF can be used to assess the functional effects of therapeutic drugs in AD. Under resting conditions acute cholinergic stimulation with physostigmine does not affect CBF in healthy control subjects, but it increases CBF in the most affected regions in AD patients.[43,44] Increases in CBF in AD patients have also been reported after acute and fairly short periods of treatment with cholinesterase inhibitors such as tacrine and velnacrine, and with the acetylcholine releaser linopirdine.[45] Similarly, SPECT studies have shown increases in CBF after treatment with the cholinesterase inhibitor donepezil.[46,47] Increases in brain metabolism have been reported after long periods of treatment with cholinergic-enhancing drugs[48] but not after short periods.[33]

The magnitude and extent of hypometabolism correlate with the overall severity of dementia in AD. Correlations also exist between the sites of maximum hypometabolism and the predominant clinical dysfunction exhibited by the patient. For example, left parietotemporal hypometabolism is associated with predominant language dysfunction, while right parietal hypometabolism correlates with abnormalities in visuospatial skills.[49–51] When these cases are followed up over time, glucose metabolism diminishes as cognitive function declines.[51]

In a patient with the appropriate clinical presentation, a specific diagnosis for dementia can be determined from a PET study without the need for extensive additional testing (Fig. 11.3). In demented patients without signs or symptoms of motor dysfunction, abnormal sites of relative hypometabolism include parietal temporal association cortices in AD and frontal temporal association cortex in frontotemporal dementia.[25] In patients who have signs and symptoms of motor dysfunction, PET patterns of hypometabolism include biparietal temporal hypometabolism in some patients with Parkinson's disease, prefrontal

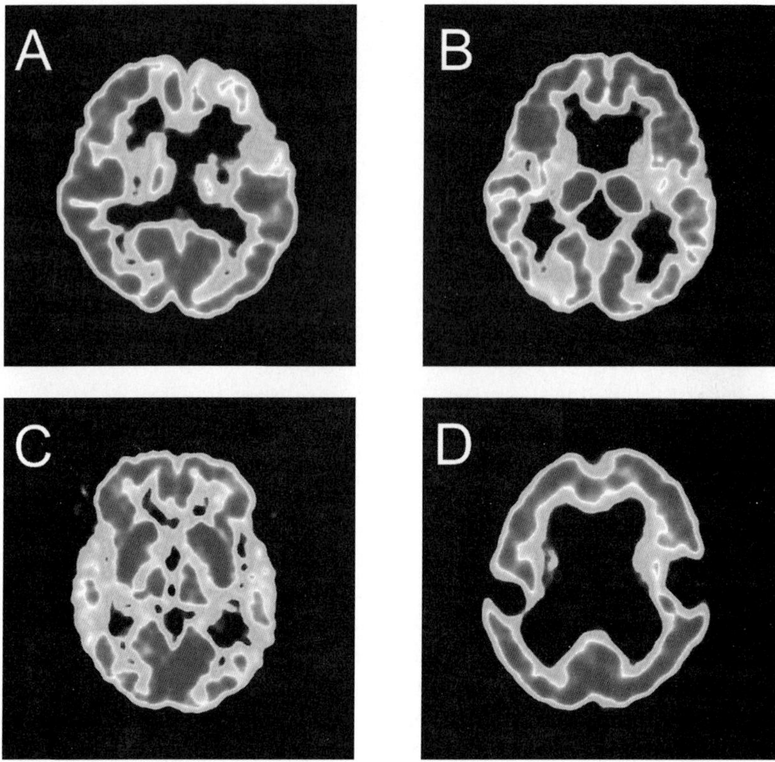

FIGURE 11.3. Selected axial PET images of the brain in patients having frontotemporal dementia with decreased uptake of ^{18}F-FDG in the left frontal cortex (A), Huntington's disease with decreased activity in bilateral striatum and parietal cortices (B), Parkinson's disease and dementia with decreased activity in bilateral parietotemporal cortices (C), and normal pressure hydrocephalus with enlarged lateral ventricles (D).

hypometabolism in progressive supranuclear palsy,[29,30] striatal hypometabolism in Huntington's disease,[26–28] lenticular hypometabolism in Wilson's disease, and random cortical and subcortical zones of hypometabolism in multiinfarct dementia.[31]

The magnitude of the health problem resulting from dementing illnesses is great in terms of medical practice, economics, and family hardship. The ability to diagnose AD early in its course, noninvasively and reliably with PET, will have significant impact on these medical and economic realities.

Neurochemical Imaging

Behavioral studies provide evidence that acetylcholine participates in complex functions such as attention, memory, and cognition. Clinical studies suggest the cognitive deterioration seen in AD and the memory loss associated with normal aging. Recent developments in radiochemistry make it possible to evaluate noninvasively the cholinergic system in the human brain using PET and SPECT. PET and SPECT studies have been performed to evaluate various elements involved with cholinergic neurotransmission in normal aging and dementia, including vesicular acetylcholine transporter, acetylcholinesterase, and muscarinic and nicotinic acetylcholine receptors.[15,17,45]

Cholinergic neuronal integrity can be mapped using radiotracers for acetylcholinesterase and vesicular acetylcholine transporter, and these biochemical markers have been shown to have a good correspondence with choline acetyltransferase (ChAT).[6] Acetylcholinesterase, an enzyme that catalyzes the hydrolysis of acetylcholine to choline and acetic acid, is consistently reduced in the brain of AD patients. The activity of acetylcholinesterase can be measured with PET using labeled acetylcholine analogs that serve as substrates for acetylcholinesterase and hydrolyze to a hydrophilic product that is trapped in the cell.[48] Another method is to use radioligands that bind to acetylcholinesterase. ^{11}C-physostigmine, ^{11}C-*N*-methyl-4-piperidyl acetate, and *N*-^{11}C-methylpiperidin-4-yl propionate (MPP) have been used in PET studies to measure the acetylcholinesterase in brains of healthy volunteers.[17,52] PET studies of the acetylcholinesterase activity using ^{11}C-MPP, a selective substrate for acetylcholinesterase, showed no changes in acetylcholinesterase with normal aging and a reduction of 30% in patients with mild to moderate AD. The smaller reductions reported by this PET study as compared with the postmortem studies (90–95%) most likely reflect the fact that postmortem studies are mostly from patients with very advanced disease.[17] A progressive loss of cortical acetylcholinesterase activity has been observed in AD patients with cognitive decline.[13,15] PET measurement of the acetylcholinesterase activity also allows assessing the efficacy of the various acetylcholinesterase inhibitors that are used therapeutically and determining the doses required to achieve optimal inhibition. It can also help identify patients in whom the concentration of acetylcholinesterase may be too low for acetylcholinesterase inhibitors to be effective.

Vesicular acetylcholine transporters are localized in the acetylcholine terminals and carry acetylcholine from the cytoplasm into the vesicles. ^{123}I-iodobenzovesamicol (IBVM), an analog of vesamicol that binds to the vesicular acetylcholine transporter, has been used to image the living human brain.[17] A SPECT study showed that cortical binding of ^{123}I-IBVM in normal subjects declined only mildly with age (3.7% per decade), but it was markedly reduced in AD patients in whom the reductions predicted dementia severity.[35] The binding levels also differed according to age of onset. With an onset age of less than 65 years, binding was reduced severely throughout the entire cerebral cortex and hippocampus (about 30%), but with an onset age of 65 years or more, binding reductions were restricted to the temporal cortex and hippocampus. This most likely reflects the greater cholinergic loss in early-rather than late-onset AD.[15] Studies of the vesicular acetylcholine transporter are likely to be particularly useful for assessing neuroprotective treatments and may be of use in the detection of early disease.

From postmortem studies it appears that nicotinic receptors are markedly reduced in the brain of AD patients, whereas muscarinic receptors are much less affected.[10] Several radiotracers have been developed for mapping muscarinic receptors.[48] In accordance with postmortem findings, imaging studies have shown a reduction in muscarinic receptors due to aging.[48] Studies in AD subjects have shown reductions as well as no changes in receptor levels.[15]

The neuronal nAChRs are involved in functional processes in brain including cognitive function and memory. A severe loss of the nAChRs has been detected in brain of patients with AD. There is great interest in imaging nAChRs noninvasively for detection of receptor impairments even at a presymptomatic stage of AD as well for monitoring the outcome of drug treatment. ^{11}C-nicotine has been used to study nicotinic receptors in both normal and AD brains by PET.[48] The labeling of the two enantiomers of nicotine, (S)(−) and (R)(+), which predominantly bind to the low- and high-affinity nicotinic sites, respectively,[12] allowed the separate assessment of nicotinic receptor subtypes.[10] Nicotine's binding to nicotinic receptors is quite selective and is predominantly seen at the $\alpha_4\beta_2$ nicotinic receptor subtype. A significant decrease in ^{11}C-nicotine binding was measured in the temporal cortex, frontal cortex, and hippocampus of AD patients. The changes in ^{11}C-nicotine binding were associated with cognitive function and interpreted as reflecting reductions in nicotinic receptors in AD. These studies also showed a lower binding of the (R)(+) enantiomer of nicotine relative to the (S)(−) one in the AD brain, which was interpreted as reflecting a predominant loss of high affinity for nicotinic receptors.

However, the binding of ^{11}C-nicotine is highly influenced by CBF and is limited by its rapid dissociation from the receptor and low specific-to-nonspecific binding ratio.[13] This has also led to the search for new radiotracers with a higher affinity for nAChR. A ligand with a selectivity for the $\alpha_4\beta_2$ nAChRs would be particularly preferable because the $\alpha_4\beta_2$ has been recognized as the predominant subtype that is deficient in AD.[13,15] Recently, several azetidine analogs have been labeled. The azetidine analogs 2-^{18}F-fluoro-3-(2(S)-azetidinylmethoxy)pyridine (2-^{18}F-fluoro-A-85380), 6-^{18}F-fluoro-A-85380, and 5-^{125}I-iodo-A-85380 represent promising imaging agents for noninvasive in vivo studies of $\alpha_4\beta_2$ nicotinic acetylcholine receptors, because of their favorable kinetic properties, high specific-to-nonspecific binding ratio, low in vivo toxicity, and high selectivity for $\alpha_4\beta_2$ nAChRs. Several epibatidine analogs have also been developed. PET studies with analogs of epibatidine such as ^{18}F-norchlorofluoroepibatidine (^{18}F-NFEP) (±)-exo-2-(2-^{18}F-fluoro-5-pyridyl)-7-azabicyclo[2.2.1]heptane (^{18}F-FPH), and *N*-methyl ^{18}F-NFEP (^{18}F-methyl-NFEP) showed very high specific-to-nonspecific binding ratios in the nonhuman primate.[53] However, it is still uncertain whether the epibatidine analogs can be applied in humans due to risk of toxicity.

PET studies of nAChR can be useful for monitoring the outcome of drug treatment. Long-term treatment with tacrine (80 mg daily for 3 months) increased binding of ^{11}C-nicotine in the temporal cortex of AD patients, which was interpreted as reflecting a restoration of nicotinic receptors.[48] These results are in agreement with preclinical data showing that cholinergic stimulation leads to upregulation of nicotinic receptors.[16] Tacrine also decreased the differences in the binding of the (R)(+) enantiomer of nicotine relative to the (S)(−) one, suggesting a preferential effect on high-affinity sites.[10] The changes in synaptic acetylcholine concentration after interventions can be measured using an nAChR radioligand ^{18}F-NFEP, which is sensitive to competition with endogenous acetylcholine.[53] Because of the toxicity of ^{18}F-NFEP, these studies have been limited to nonhuman primates and have shown that the acetylcholinesterase inhibitor physostigmine (0.03 mg/kg intravenously) significantly increases a synaptic acetylcholine concentration in the striatum, as reflected by decreased binding of ^{18}F-NFEP in the striatum. The measure of extracellular acetylcholine is particularly promising for the evaluation of pharmacologic treatments since most drugs are targeted to enhance a cholinergic function by increasing extracellular acetylcholine.

Amyloid Plaque Imaging

Confirmation of the clinical diagnosis of AD is based on the detection of amyloid plaques and neurofibrillary tangles in the brain. Unfortunately, such measures, until recently, could only be done postmortem. However, recent developments in radiotracers may now allow for the measurement of amyloid plaques and neurofibrillary tangles in the brain in vivo. Several strategies have been proposed for use with PET[52] or SPECT[54] that are based on labeling analogs of congo red, a dye that is used to stain an amyloid in postmortem tissue. PET studies with 2-(1-{6-[(2-^{18}F-fluoroethyl)(methyl)amino]-2-napthyl}ethylene)malononitrile (^{18}F-FDDNP) have shown good uptake in the human brain but greater accumulation and slower clearance of ^{18}F-FDDNP in AD patients than in control subjects. The accumulation in AD patients was greater in the hippocampal region and was detected even in patients with mild AD. The areas with high ^{18}F-FDDNP retention were the ones with low glucose metabolism.[52] The binding of ^{18}F-FDDNP to amyloid plaques was confirmed in postmortem studies. Amyloid plaque imaging will be of use not only in the diagnosis of AD but also in the investigation of the temporal relationship among amyloid deposition, neuronal loss, and cognitive decline, and assessment of the effects of drugs in disease progression. This imaging technique may help to treat AD patients early in their disease when response to treatment is usually better.

Vascular Dementia and Cerebrovascular Disease

Vascular dementia is the second most common cause of dementia in the elderly, accounting for 15% to 30% of all cases.[2] There are various types of underlying damage to tissue and vessels in vascular dementia, including single or multiple infarcts that involve association and limbic cortices (multiinfarct dementia), small subcortical infarcts disrupting corticosubcortical circuits (lacunar-type subcortical vascular dementia), and white matter lesions (Binswanger-type subcortical vascular dementia). Vascular dementia develops when a threshold of total brain tissue destruction has been exceeded, or when critically located infarctions disrupt multiple cognitive functions (strategic infarct dementia). Damage to the mesial frontal region (anterior cerebral artery territory infarction), the angular gyrus or the dorsolateral prefrontal region (middle cerebral artery territory infarction), the inferomedial temporo-occipital region (posterior cerebral artery territory infartion), and the subcortical structure such as basal ganglia and thalamus can cause a strategic infarct dementia.

PET studies in vascular dementia show global reductions in cerebral metabolism with additional focal and asymmetric areas of hypometabolism that are not limited to specific cortical or subcortical brain regions. This metabolic pattern differs from that in AD, with hypometabolism affecting the association areas and relative sparing of subcortical structures. Metabolic impairment seen in PET is often more widespread than that shown by CT, MRI, or even neuropathologic techniques, suggesting that single lesions may have extensive and distant metabolic sequelae. These remote metabolic effects have been attributed to degeneration of fiber tracts with disconnection of distal structures and to microscopic infarcts not apparent on gross examination but manifested as hypometabolic regions. Increasing severity of dementia correlates with global hypometabolism (i.e., the total volume of hypometabolic regions rather than the quantity of tissue destruction) and increasing involvement of the frontal cortex.[55] SPECT in vascular dementia reveals diffusely diminished CBF with superimposed focal areas of more severe hypoperfusion. Vascular dementia could produce any pattern, but the presence of one or more scattered perfusion defects, either unilateral or bilateral, with an asymmetric distribution is most suggestive of vascular dementia.

The clinical picture of vascular dementia varies, and the role of functional brain imaging of CBF and metabolism would be expected to be different among subtypes of vascular dementia. In multiinfarct dementia (cortical infarcts), PET and SPECT are of value in detecting regions at risk, but the role would be supplementary in clinical evaluation of patients. Subcortical small infarcts that disrupt corticosubcortical circuits result in cognitive dysfunction. Small infarcts involving the thalamus, caudate, and globus pallidus, which are central components of the corticosubcortical circuits, are classified into strategic lesions. Disruption of the frontal-subcortical circuits leads to cognitive impairment with striking frontal lobe features, and disruption of the memory-related circuits leads to amnesia. In this type of vascular dementia, apart from detecting regions at risk, the role of PET and SPECT would be to prove functional deprivation of remote cortices. Frontal involvement is a definitive functional brain imaging feature of subcortical strategic lesions leading to dementia. In white matter lesions, documenting the presence of chronic ischemias and then illustrating a functional deprivation of cortices would be the most important roles of PET and SPECT. However, this needs to be determined in further studies.

Cerebrovascular disease is a vascular abnormality resulting in abnormal CBF. Its most common cause is progressive narrowing of the major arteries supplying blood to the brain, resulting in thrombogenic disease or sudden occlusion of blood flow, which, if large enough, results in eschemic stroke. Stroke is caused by a variety of pathologic changes that affect either the intracranial or extracranial blood vessels, producing a focal reduction in blood flow or multifocal regions of perfusion compromise. In most of these cases, the end result is cerebral infarction due to reduced CBF and inadequate delivery of oxygen and glucose. ^{133}Xe dynamic SPECT is a quantitative and sensitive measure of cerebrovascular status and hemodynamic constraints in both spared and affected brain, providing evidence for reorganization and cerebral plasticity. ^{18}F-FDG-PET and ^{31}P MR spectroscopy can show a reorganization in the contralateral hemisphere after stroke, with parallel changes in glucose and high-energy phosphate metabolism related to poststroke recovery.

Cerebrovascular disease and AD are common in the elderly, and both frequently coexist. In addition to the features of dementia typical for AD and the accentuated atrophy in the parietal and medial temporal lobes demonstrated on MRI, temporoparietal and posterior cingulate abnormality indicates an involvement of Alzheimer pathology. When frontal abnormality is lacking, the effects of subcortical infarcts on cortical function would be negligible.

A longitudinal analysis of regional cerebral glucose metabolism in vascular dementia showed that the progression of dementia can be delayed by the adenosine uptake blocker propentofylline and that neuropsychological and metabolic changes are closely related.

Dementia with Lewy Bodies

Dementia with Lewy bodies (DLB) is a common form of dementia, accounting for 15% to 20% of all dementia in old age.[56,57] The disorder shares clinical and pathological features with both AD and Parkinson's disease. The differentiation of DLB from these other disorders therefore poses diagnostic difficulties. Lewy bodies are neuronal inclusions composed of abnormally phosphorylated, neurofilament proteins aggregated with ubiquitin and α-synuclein. In Parkinson's disease, Lewy body formation and neuron loss in brainstem nuclei, particularly the substantia nigra, lead to movement disorder. In DLB, significant Lewy body formation also occurs in paralimbic and neocortical structures, and extensive depletion of acetylcholine neurotransmission in neocortical areas occurs as a result of the degeneration in the brainstem and basal forebrain cholinergic projection neurons. Dementia is usually, but not always, the presenting feature; a minority of patients present with parkinsonism alone, some with psychiatric disorder in the absence of dementia, and others with orthostatic hypotension, falls or transient disturbances of consciousness.[5,58] The most frequent clinical misdiagnosis of DLB is AD.

Structural brain imaging in DLB reveals a generalized cerebral atrophy, although 40% of patients show a preservation of medial temporal lobe structures, unlike in AD. There is no difference from AD in terms of degree of ventricular enlargement, frontal lobe atrophy, or presence of white-matter changes on MRI.[59]

FDG-PET studies have shown that among widespread cortical regions showing glucose hypometabolism in DLB, the metabolic reduction is most pronounced in the occipital cortex compared to that in AD, which is consistent with the pathologic findings.[60] Measures of the glucose metabolism in the occipital cortex may be an informative diagnostic aid to distinguish DLB from AD.

In DLB there is a considerable degeneration of nigral neurons with depletion of striatal dopamine as well as cortical neuronal loss. In contrast, AD is not associated with significant changes in dopamine metabolism. Using SPECT, a significant reduction in striatal uptake of a dopamine transporter ligand ^{123}I-2-carbomethoxy-3-(4-iodophenyl)-*N*-(3-fluoropropyl)nortropane was seen in DLB but not in AD, indicating dopaminergic degeneration in DLB.[61] This may prove to be a useful diagnostic test for distinguishing DLB from AD in vivo.

Frontotemporal Dementia

Frontotemporal dementia (FTD) is the most common form of primary degenerative dementia after AD that affects people in middle age, accounting for up to 20% of presenile dementia cases. The salient clinical characteristic is a profound alteration in character and social conduct, occurring in the context of relative preservation of instrumental functions of perception, spatial skills, praxis, and memory. Parkinsonian signs of akinesia and rigidity develop with disease progression and may be marked in a proportion of patients. A minority of patients with frontotemporal dementia develop neurologic signs of motor neuron disease. Postmortem pathologic examination reveals bilateral atrophy of the frontal and anterior temporal lobes and degeneration of the striatum. Only a minority of patients exhibit Pick-type histologic changes, hence the term *frontotemporal dementia* is preferred to Pick's disease.

PET and SPECT studies have consistently shown anterior distribution of functional impairment in FTD. Reductions in glucose metabolism and blood flow in the frontal and anterior temporal cortices with frequent asymmetric patterns are seen (Fig. 11.4). Metabolic or flow reduction in parietal and striatal areas has also been shown. The reduction in the binding of the dopamine transporter ligand ^{11}C-WIN 35,428 (2β-carbomethoxy-3β-(4-fluoro-phenyl)tropane) in the striatum of FTD patients was shown and related to the severity of extrapyramidal symptoms of the patients.[62]

Dementia with Basal Ganglia Disorders

Functional neuroimaging can aid in the diagnosis of basal ganglia disorders associated with dementia. Imaging studies in Huntington's disease, progressive supranuclear palsy, Wilson's disease, and corticobasal degeneration are described.

Huntington's Disease

Huntington's disease (HD) is an autosomal, dominantly inherited neurodegenerative disorder that is caused by an unstable and abnormally

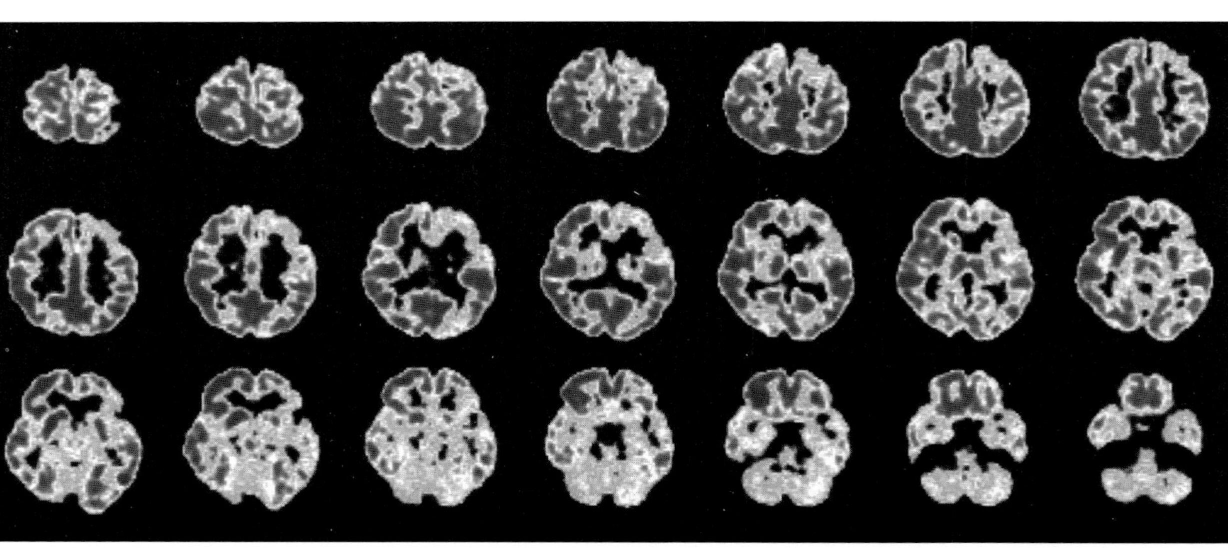

Figure 11.4. Axial FDG-PET images of the brain in a patient with frontotemporal dementia, showing asymmetric hypometabolism in the frontotemporal regions.

expanded trinucleotide [cysteine-alanine-glycine (CAG)] repeat in the *IT15* gene on chromosome 4. The three main clinical features of HD are movement disorder, progressive frontostriatal dementia, and psychiatric disturbance. HD results from the loss of specific sets of cholinergic and γ-aminobutyric acid (GABA)ergic neurons in the striatum.

CT/MRI reveals diminished volume of the caudate nuclei with loss of the convex bulge of the nucleus into the lateral aspects of the frontal horns of the lateral ventricles. The bicaudate index (width of both lateral ventricles divided by distance between the outer tables of the skull at the same level) distinguishes HD from other disorders with cerebral atrophy. FDG-PET studies show reduced striatal glucose metabolism (Fig. 11.3). Clinical scores of functional capacity, bradykinesia, rigidity, and dementia correlate with caudate hypometabolism; scores of chorea and eye-movement abnormalities correlate with putamen hypometabolism; and scores of dystonia correlate with thalamic hypermetabolism. FDG-PET measures of cortical metabolism are normal in preclinical disease, but patients later develop extensive hypometabolism in prefrontal and inferior parietal areas. Additionally, several studies have demonstrated that a proportion of relatives at risk for HD have significantly reduced striatal glucose metabolism. Resting rCBF, like glucose metabolism, is reduced in the striatum and cortex of patients with established HD.

The earliest histopathologic change seen in HD is the loss of medium spiny neurons from the striatum. These GABAergic projection neurons express dopamine receptors. Accordingly, severe loss of striatal D_1 and D_2 receptor binding in HD has been demonstrated at postmortem as well as in vivo using PET and SPECT. Postmortem reductions in D_2 binding have also been found in the frontal cortex, and in vivo studies using PET have reported reduced D_1 binding in frontal and temporal cortices in HD. PET has demonstrated that ~50% of at-risk asymptomatic adults and mutation carriers have reduced striatal D_1 and D_2 receptor binding.

Progressive Supranuclear Palsy

Progressive supranuclear palsy (PSP), also designated Steele-Richardson-Olszewski syndrome, is clinically characterized by early postural instability and falls, supranuclear gaze palsy, parkinsonism, pseudobulbar palsy, and frontal lobe signs such as impairment of executive functions, forgetfulness, and slowing of thought processes. Pathologically, patients have neuronal loss, gliosis, intraneuronal neurofibrillary tangle formation, and granulovacuolar degeneration that are most marked in the midbrain.

CT reveals atrophy of the midbrain, with less severe volume loss of the pons, cerebellum, and cerebral hemispheres. PET studies reveal a global decrease in cerebral glucose metabolism and blood flow, but the decrease is more marked in the frontal cortex. Decreased activity in the striatum, thalamus, and midbrain is also seen. Frontal metabolism was significantly correlated with disease duration, intellectual deterioration, and frontal neuropsychological scores. Reduced frontal metabolism could be due to anatomic and/or functional impairment of subcortical structures, despite the well-recognized specific cortical pathology in PSP, predominating in the posterior frontal cortex. Striatal and thalamic hypometabolism is most likely a consequence of functional changes in the basal neural circuitry, since these structures are usually spared on neuropathologic examination of PSP patients. In contrast, midbrain hypometabolism could preferentially reflect the severe neuronal loss reported at that level.

PET studies demonstrated equally severe impairment of ^{18}F-fluorodopa uptake in the caudate, anterior putamen, and posterior putamen of patients with PSP, unlike Parkinson's disease patients who showed severe impairment in the posterior putamen with relative sparing of the anterior putamen and caudate.[63] Similar results were obtained in a PET study with dopamine transporter ligand ^{11}C-WIN 35,428.[64] These findings suggest that there is progressively more extensive nigral involvement in PSP than in Parkinson's disease. Also, the severity of decrease in striatal ^{18}F-fluorodopa uptake in PSP patients paralleled the degree of reduction in frontal CBF.[65] This suggests that the impairment of cerebral function in PSP is determined to a large extent by brainstem pathology.

Wilson's Disease

Wilson's disease is an inherited defect in the copper-carrying serum protein ceruloplasmin, resulting in abnormal copper deposition in the basal ganglia, liver, and cornea. Neurologically, patients demonstrate dysarthria, dystonia, rigidity, cerebellar abnormalities, tremor, gait and postural disturbances, and mild dementia. PET reveals globally diminished cerebral metabolism with relatively more marked changes in the lenticular nuclei. ^{18}F-fluorodopa PET demonstrates diminished uptake in the striatum of symptomatic patients with Wilson's disease.[66]

Corticobasal Degeneration

Corticobasal degeneration (CBD) is an increasingly recognized neurodegenerative disease with both motor and cognitive dysfunction. The most characteristic initial motor symptoms are akinesia, rigidity, and apraxia. Dystonia and alien limb phenomena are frequently observed. There is often a parkinsonian picture with failure or lack of efficacy of dopaminergic medical therapy. Cognitive decline, prompting the diagnosis of dementia, may be the most common presentation of CBD that is misdiagnosed. Pathology is characterized by an asymmetric frontoparietal neuronal loss and gliosis with ballooned, achromatic cortical neurons, nigral degeneration, and variable subcortical involvement. Structural imaging reveals asymmetric atrophy in the frontoparietal cortex contralateral to the dominantly affected limb. Statistical parametric mapping analysis of FDG-PET images comparing CBD to controls showed a metabolic decrease in premotor, primary motor, supplementary motor, primary sensory, prefrontal, and inferior parietal cortices, and also striatum and thalamus contralateral to the more affected limb.[67–69]

^{18}F-fluorodopa uptake also was reduced asymmetrically in both the caudate nucleus and the putamen.[67]

Normal Pressure Hydrocephalus

Normal pressure hydrocephalus (NPH) is an obstructive communicating hydrocephalus that classically produces the clinical triad of dementia, gait disturbance, and urinary incontinence. It is caused by obstruction of cerebrospinal fluid (CSF) absorption in the superior sagittal sinus. NPH may be idiopathic and may occur as a manifestation of the late decompensation of compensated congenital hydrocephalus, or may follow head trauma, subdural hematoma, subarachnoid hemorrhage, meningitis, or encephalitis.

Structural imaging reveals enlarged ventricles and is crucial to the identification and differential diagnosis of NPH. Ventricular enlargement in NPH is characterized by greater dilatation of the anterior horns (frontal and temporal) of the lateral ventricles than of the posterior horns. Usually disproportionate enlargement of the ventricles and relatively modest sulcal dilatation, if any, are seen, but atrophy of the cortical mantle occurs in the course of normal aging. The presence of some degree of peripheral atrophy does not exclude consideration of NPH.

SPECT reveals diffusely reduced CBF, more pronounced posteriorly than anteriorly. SPECT may aid in identifying patients who are likely to respond to shunting. It has been reported that patients with higher anterior than posterior blood flow were less likely to improve following surgery than patients who had equal flow anteriorly and posteriorly or greater posterior flow. PET reveals diffusely reduced glucose metabolism in hydrocephalus. Restoration of normal metabolic rates after successful shunt surgery has been reported.

Infectious Dementias

Creutzfeldt-Jakob disease (subacute spongiform encephalopathy) is a prion infection of the brain that is rapidly progressive and usually fatal within 1 year. Clinically, dementia, ataxia, myoclonus, and muscle rigidity are characteristic. Neuropathologic alterations include spongiform changes, nerve cell loss, and marked gliosis. SPECT and PET imaging reveal diffuse and multifocal reductions in gray matter CBF and metabolism. These imaging techniques may be most useful in selecting areas for diagnostic brain biopsy.

Acquired immune deficiency syndrome (AIDS) dementia complex is a progressive dementing illness caused by infection with the human immunodeficiency virus (HIV). Between 70% and 90% of AIDS patients develop neuropsychological impairment that is characterized by inattention, mental slowing, loss of spontaneity, reduced motor performance, and incoordination. At autopsy, mild to moderate cerebral atrophy is seen, and neuropathology is found primarily in subcortical structures, particularly the basal ganglia and thalamus. CT and MRI studies reveal general atrophy, atrophy of the basal ganglia, and white matter lesions that appear to increase in severity with progression of the HIV infection. SPECT shows multifocal cortical and subcortical areas of hypoperfusion. PET studies have demonstrated relative subcortical hypermetabolism in AIDS and early AIDS dementia complex, while more advanced AIDS dementia complex is associated with hypometabolism in cortical and subcortical gray matter and in the temporal lobe. In addition, PET and SPECT have been shown to be sensitive to reversal or improvement of abnormalities brought about by drug treatment, reflecting clinical improvement in neurologic and cognitive deficits.

Depressive Pseudodementia

A considerable proportion of geriatric depression patients show a cognitive decline that is comparable to primary degenerative dementia in severity. However, this condition is differentiated from primary dementia by its reversibility. This reversible dementia syndrome of geriatric depression has been called a depressive pseudodementia. PET studies show a decreased blood flow in the left anterior medial frontal lobe in depressive pseudodementia patients, while noncognitively impaired depressed patients have a decreased blood flow in the left anterior lateral prefrontal areas.[70] A SPECT study in elderly depressive pseudodementia patients revealed decreased blood flow in the temporoparietal region, a finding similar to that of AD and different from that of depression without cognitive impairment.[71] This functional image finding may have a relevance to the report that elderly depressed patients with cognitive impairment that improves with treatment carry an increased chance of developing an irreversible dementia in the future when compared to age-matched patients with depression alone.[72]

References

1. Aronson MK, Ooi WL, Geva DL, et al. Dementia: age-dependent incidence, prevalence, and mortality in the old. Arch Intern Med 1991;151:989–992.
2. Canadian Study of Health and Aging Working Group. Canadian study of health and aging: study methods and prevalence of dementia. Can Med Assoc J 1994;150:899–913.
3. Clarfield AM. The reversible dementias: do they reverse? Ann Intern Med 1988;9:476–486.
4. Kukull WA, Larson EB, Reifler BV, et al. The validity of three clinical diagnosis criteria for Alzheimer's disease. Neurology 1990;40:1364–1369.
5. McKeith IG, Perry RH, Fairbairn AF, et al. Operational criteria for senile dementia of Lewy body type (SDLT). Psychol Med 1992;22:911–922.
6. Mesulam MM, Mufson EJ, Levey AI, et al. Cholinergic innervation of cortex by the basal forebrain: cytochemistry and cortical connections of the septal area, diagonal band nuclei, nucleus basalis (substantia innominata), and hypothalamus in the rhesus monkey. J Comp Neurol 1983;214(2): 170–197.
7. Coyle JT, Price DL, DeLong MR. Alzheimer's disease: a disorder of cortical cholinergic innervation. Science 1983;219:1184–1190.

8. Bierer LM, Haroutunian V, Gabriel S, et al. Neurochemical correlates of dementia severity in Alzheimer's disease: relative importance of the cholinergic deficits. J Neurochem 1995;64:749–760.
9. Boller F, Lopez OL, Moossy J. Diagnosis of dementia: clinicopathological correlations. Neurology 1989;39:76–79.
10. Nordberg A. Neuroreceptor changes changes in Alzheimer disease. Cerebrovasc Brain Metab Rev 1992;4;303–328.
11. Flynn DD, Ferrari-DiLeo G, Levey AI, et al. Differential alterations in muscarinic receptor subtypes in Alzheimer's disease: implications for cholinergic based therapies. Life Sci 1995;56:869–876.
12. Court JA, Perry EK. Distribution of nicotinic receptors in the CNS. In: Stone TW, ed. CNS Neurotransmitters and Neuromodulators. London: CRC Press, 1995:85–104.
13. Kellar KJ, Wonnacott S. Nicotinic cholinergic receptors in Alzheimer's disease. In: Wonnacott S, Russell MAH and Stolerman IP, eds. Nicotine Psychopharmacology: Molecular, Cellular and Behavioural Aspects. Oxford, UK: Oxord University Press, 1990:341–373.
14. Davies P, Feisullin S. Postmortem stability of α-bungarotoxin binding sites in mouse and human brain. Brain Res 1981;216:449–454.
15. Sugaya K, Giacobini E, Chiappinelli VA. Nicotinic acetylcholine receptor subtypes in human frontal cortex: changes in Alzheimer's disease. J Neurosci Res 1990;27:349–359.
16. Norberg A. The effect of cholinesterase inhibitors studied with brain imaging. In: Giacobini E, ed. Cholinesterases and Cholinesterase Inhibitors. London: Martin Dunitz, Ltd 2000:237–247.
17. Frey KA, Minoshima S, Kuhl DE. Neurochemical imaging of Alzheimer's disease and other degenerative dementias. Q J Nucl Med 1998;42:166.
18. Langlais PJ, Thal L, Hansen L, et al. Neurotransmitters in basal ganglia and cortex of Alzheimer's disease with and without Lewy bodies. Neurology 1993;43:1927–1934.
19. Perry EK, Marshall E, Perry RH, et al. Cholinergic and dopaminergic activities in senile dementia of Lewy body type. Alzheimer Dis Assoc Disord 1990;4:87–95.
20. Perry E, Goodchild R, Griffiths M, et al. Clinical neurochemistry: developments in dementia research based on brain bank material. J Neural Transm 1998;105:915–933.
21. Homer AC, Honavar M, Lantos PL, et al. Diagnosis dementia: do we get it right? BMJ 1988;297:894–896.
22. Jellinger K, Danielxzyk W, Fisher P, et al. Clinicopathological analysis of dementia disorders in the elderly. J Neurol Sci 1990;95:239–258.
23. Gilleard CJ, Kellett JM, Coles JA, et al. The St. George's dementia bed investigation: a comparison of clinical and pathological diagnosis. Acta Psychiatr Scand 1992;85:265–269.
24. Crystal H, Dickson MD, Fuld P, et al. Clinicopathological studies in dementia: non-demented subjects with pathologically confirmed Alzheimer's disease. Neurology 1988;38:1682–1687.
25. Kamo H, McGeer PL, Harrop R, et al. Positron emission tomography and histopathology in Pick's disease. Neurology 1987;37:439–445.
26. Kuhl DE, Phelps ME, Markham CH, et al. Cerebral metabolism and atrophy in Huntington's disease determined by F-18 FDG and computed tomographic scan. Ann Neurol 1982;12:425–434.
27. Hayden MR, Martin WRW, Stoessl AJ, et al. Positron emission tomography in the early diagnosis of Huntington's disease. Neurology 1986;36:888–894.

28. Mazziotta JC. Huntington's disease: studies with structural imaging techniques and positron emission tomography. Semin Neurol 1989;9:360–369.
29. D'Antona R, Baron JC, Samson T, et al. Subcortical dementia: frontal cortex hypometabolism detected by positron tomography in patients with progressive supranuclear palsy. Brain 1985;108:785–799.
30. Foster NL, Gilman S, Berent S, et al. Cerebral hypometabolism in progressive supranuclear palsy studies with positron emission tomography. Ann Neurol 1998;104:754–778.
31. Benson DF, Kuhl DE, Hawkins RA, et al. The F-18 fluorodeoxyglucose scan in Alzheimer's disease and multi-infarct dementia. Arch Neurol 1983;40: 711–714.
32. Minoshima S, Giordani B, Berent S, et al. Metabolic reduction in the posterior cingulate cortex in very early Alzheimer's disease. Ann Neurol 1997; 42:85–94.
33. Szelies B, Herholz K, Pawlik G, et al. Cerebral glucose metabolism in presenile dementia of the Alzheimer type: follow-up of therapy with muscarinergic choline agonists. Fortschr Neurol Psychiatr 1986;54:364–373.
34. Ishii K, Sasaki M, Kitagaki H, et al. Reduction of cerebellar glucose metabolism in advanced Alzheimer's disease. J Nucl Med 1997;38:925–992
35. Johnson KA, Jones BL, Holman JA, et al. Preclinical prediction of Alzheimer's disease using SPECT. Neurology 1998;50:1563–1571.
36. Gomez-lsla T, Price TL, McKeel DW, et al. Profound loss of layer II entorhinal cortex neurons occurs in very mild Alzheimer's disease. J Neurosci 1996;16:4491–4500.
37. Welsh KA, Butters N, Hughes JP, et al. Detection and staging of demential in Alzheimer's disease: use of the neuropsychological measures developed for the consortium to establish a registry for Alzheimer's disease. Arch Neurol 1992;49:448–452.
38. Ohnishi T, Hoshi H, Nagamachi S, et al. High-resolution SPECT to assess hippocampal perfusion in neuropsychiatric diseases. J Nucl Med 1995;36: 1163–1169.
39. Julin P, Lindqvist J, Svensson L, et al. MRI-guided SPECT measurements of medial temporal lobe blood flow in Alzhemer's disease. J Nucl Med 1997;38:914–919.
40. Rodriguez G, Nohili F, Copello F, et al. ^{99m}Tc-HMPAO regional cerebral blood flow and quantitative electroencephalography in Alzheimer's disease: a correlative study. J Nucl Med 1999;40:522–529.
41. Braak H, Braak E. Neuropathological staging of Alzheimer related changes. Acta Neuropathol 1991;82:239–256.
42. Perry RJ, Hodges JR. Attention and executive deficits in Alzheimer's disease. A critical review. Brain 1999;122:383–404.
43. Geaney DP, Soper N, Shepstone BJ, et al. Effect of central cholinergic stimulation on regional cerebral blood flow in Alzheimer disease. Lancet 1990; 335:1484–1487.
44. Gustafson L, Edvinsson L, Dahlgren N, et al. Intravenous physostigmine treatment of Alzheimer's disease evaluated by psychometric testing, regional cerebral blood flow (rCBF) measurement, and EEG. Psychopharmacol Berl 1987;93:31–35.
45. van Dyck CH, Lin CH, Robinson R, et al. The acetylcholine releaser linopirdine increases parietal regional cerebral blood flow in Alzheimer's disease. Psychopharmacol (Berl)1997;132:217–226.
46. Staff RT, Gemmell HG, Shanks MF, et al. Changes in the rCBF images of patients with Alzheimer's disease receiving Donepezil therapy. Nucl Med Commun 2000;21:37–41.

47. Warren S, Hier DB, Pavel D. Visual form of Alzheimer's disease and its response to anticholinesterase therapy. Neuroimaging 1998;8:249–252.
48. Nordberg A. PET studies and cholinergic therapy in Alzheimer's disease. Rev Neurol Paris 1999;155(suppl 4):S53–S63.
49. Foster NL, Chase TN, Fedio P. Alzheimer's disease: focal cortical changes shown by positron emission tomography. Neurology 1983;33:961–965.
50. Friedland RP, Budinger TF, Koss E, et al. Alzheimer's disease: anterior-posterior hemispheric alterations in cortical glucose utilization. Neurosic Lett 1985;53:235–240.
51. Haxby JV, Grady CL, Koss E, et al. Longitudinal study of cerebral metabolic asymmetries and associated neuropsychological patterns in early dementia of the Alzheimer type. Arch Neurol 1990;47:753–760.
52. Barrio JR, Huang SC, Cole G, et al. PET imaging of tangles and plaques in Alzheimer disease with a highly hydrophobic probe. J Labelled Cpd Radiopharm 1997;42(1):5194–5195.
53. Ding YS, Logan J, Bermel R, et al. Dopamine receptor-mediated regulation of striatal cholinergic activity: positron emission tomography studies with norchloro F-18 fluoroepibatidine. Neurochemistry 2000;74(4):1514–1521.
54. Bornebroek M, Verzijlbergen JF, Haan J, et al. Potential for imaging cerebral amyloid deposits using 123I-labelled serum amyloid P component and SPECT. Nucl Med Commun 1996;17:929–933.
55. Bench CJ, Dolan RJ, Friston KJ, et al. Positron emission tomography in the study of brain metabolism in psychiatric and neuropsychiatric disorders. Br J Psychiatr 1990;157(9):82–95.
56. Weiner MF. Dementia associated with Lewy bodies. Arch Neurol 1999;56: 1441–1442.
57. Holmes C, Cairns N, Lantos P, et al. Validity of current clinical criteria for Alzheimer's disease, vascular dementia with Lewy bodies. Br J Psychiatry 1999;174:45–50.
58. Byrne E J, Lennox G, Lowe J, et al. Diffuse Lewy body disease: clinical features in 15 cases. J Neurol Neurosurg Psychiatry 1989;52:709–717.
59. Barber R, Scheltens P, Gholkar A, et al. White matter lesions on magnetic resonance imaging in dementia with Lewy bodies, Alzheimer's disease, vascular dementia, and normal aging. J Neurol Neurosurg Psychiatry 1999;67:66–72.
60. Imamura T, Ishii K, Sasaki M, Kitagaki H, et al. Regional cerebral glucose metabolism in dementia with Lewy bodies and Alzheimer's disease: a comparative study using positron emission tomography. Neurosci Lett 1997; 235(1–2):49–52.
61. Walker Z, Costa DC, Inca P, et al. In-vivo demonstration of dopaminergic degeneration in dementia with Lewy bodies. Lancet 1999;354:646–647.
62. Rinne JO, Laine M, Kaasinen V, et al. Striatal dopamine transporter and extrapyramidal symptoms in frontotemporal dementia. Neurology 2002; 58(10):1489–1493.
63. Brooks DJ, Ibanez V, Sawle GV, et al. Differing patterns of striatal F-18 dopa uptake in Parkinson's disease, multiple system atrophy, and progressive supranuclear palsy. Ann Neurol 1990;28(4):547–555.
64. Ilgin N, Zubieta J, Reich SG, et al. PET imaging of the dopamine transporter in progressive supranuclear palsy and Parkinson's disease. Neurology 1999;52(6):1221–1226.
65. Leenders KL, Frackowiak RS, Lees AJ. Steele-Richardson-Olszewski syndrome. Brain energy metabolism, blood flow and fluorodopa uptake measured by positron emission tomography. Brain 1988;111(33):615–630.
66. Snow BJ, Bhatt M, Martin WR, et al. The nigrostriatal dopaminergic path-

way in Wilson's disease studied with positron emission tomography. J Neurol Neurosurg Psychiatry 1991;54(1):12–17.
67. Laureys S, Salmon E, Garraux G, et al. Fluorodopa uptake and glucose metabolism in early stages of corticobasal degeneration. J Neurol 1999;246(12): 1151–1158.
68. Garraux G, Salmon E, Peigneux P, et al. Voxel-based distribution of metabolic impairment in corticobasal degeneration. Mov Disord 2000;15(5): 894–904.
69. Lutte I, Laterre C, Bodart JM, et al. Contribution of PET studies in diagnosis of corticobasal degeneration. Eur Neurol 2000;44(1):12–21.
70. Dolan RJ, Bench CJ, Brown RG, et al. Regional cerebral blood flow abnormalities in depressed patients with cognitive impairment. J Neurol Neurosurg Psychiatry 1992;55(9):768–773.
71. Cho MJ, Lyoo IK, Lee DW, et al. Brain single photon emission computed tomography findings in depressive pseudodementia patients. J Affect Disord 2002;69(1–3):159–166.
72. Alexopoulos GS, Meyers BS, Young RC, Mattis S, Kakuma T. The course of geriatric depression with "reversible dementia": a controlled study. Am J Psychiatry 1993;150:1693–1699.

12

Cardiology

Dong-Soo Lee, Jin-Chul Paeng, Myung-Chul Lee, and E. Edmund Kim

The glucose analog ^{18}F-fluorodeoxyglucose (FDG) provided, for the first time, the ability to noninvasively probe and characterize the regional metabolism of glucose as a major fuel substrate of the heart. Positron emission tomography (PET) became a tool for demonstrating the metabolic processes directly in the myocardium. Clinical studies showed the dependency of the heart's substrate selection on circulatory levels of glucose, free fatty acid, and insulin. Regional ^{18}F-FDG uptake markedly in excess of myocardial blood flow in dysfunctional myocardium after infarction, with chronic coronary artery disease or with ischemic cardiomyopathy, became recognized as a hallmark of myocardial viability or potentially reversible contractile dysfunction. Defined as a blood flow metabolism mismatch (Fig. 12.1), the regional glucose uptake pattern identifies patients as being at high risk of cardiac events and identifies patients who will benefit most from surgical revascularization. The patterns predict a postrevascularization improvement in global left ventricular function, in symptoms related to congestive heart failure, and in long-term survival.

Myocardial PET has been used in the evaluation of absolute myocardial blood flow, metabolism, and other measures in vivo. Several PET tracers have been used for this purpose and the widely used ones are ^{82}Rb, ^{13}N-ammonia, and ^{15}O-water as perfusion tracers, and ^{11}C-acetate, ^{18}F-FDG as metabolism tracers.[1] Recently, various tracers have been used for imaging of the cardiac nervous system or myocardial receptors.

Perfusion assessment using ^{82}Rb is simple, for it is taken up by myocardium in proportion to blood flow like Tl 201 in myocardial single photon emission computed tomography (SPECT). ^{13}N-ammonia and ^{15}O-water, however, need more complicated dynamic imaging and analysis. Tracer kinetics using a compartment model are essential to understand PET assessment using these tracers.

^{18}F-FDG-PET is usually used for the assessment of myocardial viability in the ischemic myocardial dysfunction. The evaluation of myocardial viability is essential in the decision to intervene for revascularization, and has been a major concern in using PET cardiology.

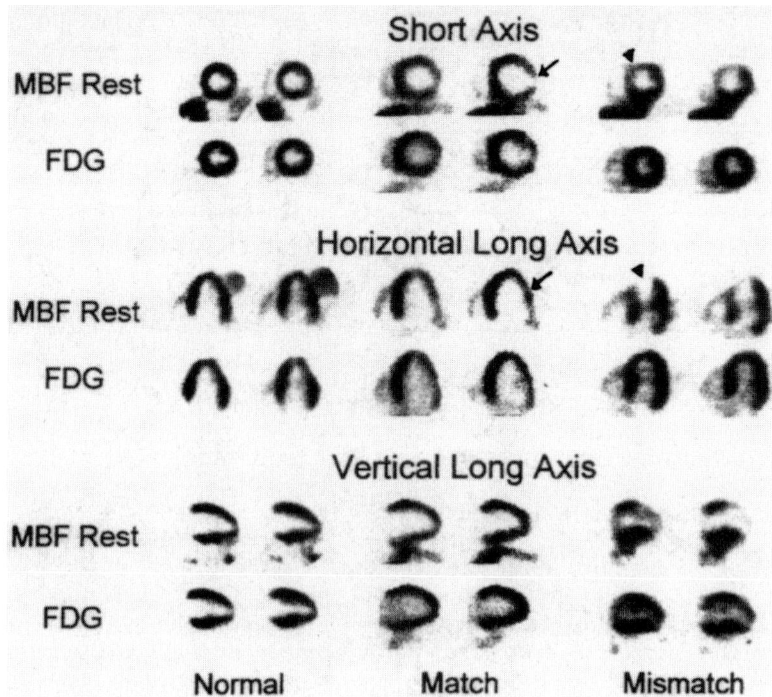

FIGURE 12.1. Patterns of myocardial blood flow with ^{13}N-ammonia and metabolism with ^{18}F-FDG uptake in patients with ischemic cardiomyopathy on the short axis, and the horizontal and vertical long axes PET images. Note the normal ammonia and FDG uptake in patient A (*left panel*) with the hypokinetic anterior wall of the left ventricle, the decreased perfusion in the lateral wall (*arrows*) of patient B (*center*) with concordantly reduced glucose uptake (*match*), and the reduction of blood flow in patient C (*right panel*) while FDG uptake is preserved in the anterior and anteroseptal walls (*arrowheads*) (*mismatch*). (From Schelbert,[1] with permission.)

^{18}F-FDG-PET

^{18}F-FDG is a tracer for glucose metabolism. A perfusion-decreased myocardium is considered viable if the glucose metabolism is preserved. ^{18}F-FDG is an analog for deoxyglucose and it is taken up by myocardium through the glucose transporter. ^{18}F-FDG uptake depends on both the glucose transport and phosphorylation activity by hexokinase, which is the phosphorylate 6-position carbon of deoxyglucose.[1,2]

^{18}F-FDG uptake can be analyzed by using the three-compartment model (Fig. 12.2). C_P^* and C_E^* are concentrations of FDG in plasma and tissue, respectively. C_M^* is the concentration of phosphorylated substrates. From this model, changes in the concentration of FDG and FDG-6-P can be calculated as

$$\frac{dC_E^*(t)}{dt} = K_1C_P^*(t) - k_2C_E^*(t) - k_3C_E^*(t) + k_4C_M^*(t)$$

$$\frac{dC_M^*(t)}{dt} = k_3C_E^*(t) - k_4C_M^*(t)$$

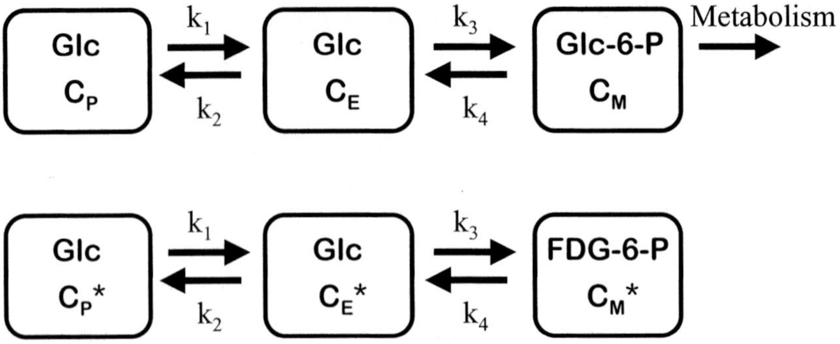

Glc C_P $\underset{k_2}{\overset{k_1}{\rightleftarrows}}$ Glc C_E $\underset{k_4}{\overset{k_3}{\rightleftarrows}}$ Glc-6-P C_M $\xrightarrow{\text{Metabolism}}$

Glc $C_P{}^*$ $\underset{k_2}{\overset{k_1}{\rightleftarrows}}$ Glc $C_E{}^*$ $\underset{k_4}{\overset{k_3}{\rightleftarrows}}$ FDG-6-P $C_M{}^*$

k_1: Substrate transport rate from plasma to tissue

k_2: Substrate transport rate from tissue to plasma

k_3: Phosphorylation rate in tissue

k_4: Dephosphorylation rate in tissue

FIGURE 12.2. Metabolism of glucose (Glc) and fluorodeoxyglucose (FDG) in the three-compartment model. C_P and C_E are concentrations of FDG in plasma and tissue, respectively. C_M is the concentration of phosphorylated substrates. Regional metabolic rate (rMRglu) and lumped constant (LC) are calculated.

By solving these differential equations, the concentration of FDG can be derived as

$$C_E{}^*(t) = \frac{K_1}{a_2 - a_1}((k_4 - a_1)e^{-a_1 t} + (a_2 - k_4)e^{-a_2 t}) \otimes C_P{}^*(t)$$

$$C_M{}^*(t) = \frac{K_1 k_3}{a_2 - a_1}(e^{-a_1 t} - e^{-a_2 t}) \otimes C_P{}^*(t)$$

$$a_{1,2} = \frac{k_2 + k_3 + k_4 \mp \sqrt{(k_2 + k_3 + k_4)^2 - 4k_2 k_4}}{2}$$

PET cannot discriminate metabolized from unmetabolized FDG; therefore, the radioactivity on FDG-PET is the total amount of FDG in the tissue. Thus,

$$C^*_{\text{tiss}} = \frac{K_1}{a_2 - a_1}((k_3 + k_4 - a_1)e^{-a_1 t} + (a_2 - k_3 - k_4)e^{-a_2 t}) \otimes C^*_P(t)$$

From this equation, k_1, k_2, k_3, and k_4 are calculated by linear regression, and regional metabolic rate of glucose (rMRglu) is calculated as

$$\text{rMRglu} = \frac{1}{\text{LC}} \cdot \frac{k_1 k_3}{k_2 + k_3} C_P \qquad \text{LC} = \frac{\left(\dfrac{k_1 k_2}{k_2 + k_3}\right)_{\text{FDG}}}{\left(\dfrac{k_1 k_2}{k_2 + k_3}\right)_{\text{Glu}}}$$

In this equation, the lumped constant (LC) corrects the difference between the metabolic rates of glucose and FDG. Although 0.67 was usually used for LC in myocardium, a calculating method was recently suggested:

$$LC = R_p + (R_t - R_p)\frac{k_3}{k_2 + k_3} \qquad (R_p = 0.43,\ R_t = 2.26)$$

Myocardial Perfusion PET

^{13}N-ammonia is a widely used PET tracer for the assessment of myocardial perfusion. The initial distribution of ^{13}N-ammonia demonstrates the perfusion status of myocardium. Because ^{13}N has a short half-life of 10 minutes, ^{18}F-FDG-PET can be performed in a short time for the assessment of the glucose metabolism. ^{13}N-ammonia PET can also be performed in the rest and stress conditions such as SPECT. The delayed uptake of ^{13}N-ammonia was reported to demonstrate myocardial retention, and consequently a kind of myocardial metabolism. ^{82}Rb is also used as a tracer for perfusion due to its short half-life of 75 seconds and its availability to perform repetitive studies such as stress–rest protocol.

^{13}N-ammonia is present in plasma as a form of NH_4^+ or NH_3, and taken up in tissue as the form of ^{13}N-glutamine through the glutamate-glutamine reaction. This process is demonstrated by the two-compartment model (Fig. 12.3). C_a and C_E represent unmetabolized free ammonia in artery and tissue, respectively, and C_M represents metabolized ^{13}N compounds. V is the volume of distribution for free ammonia, and the constant of 0.8 is usually used.

When considering the spillover effect from the blood pool to the myocardial area, the total radioactivity demonstrated on PET images is given as:

$$C_{tiss}(t) = C_E(t) + C_M(t) + Sp \cdot C_a(t)$$

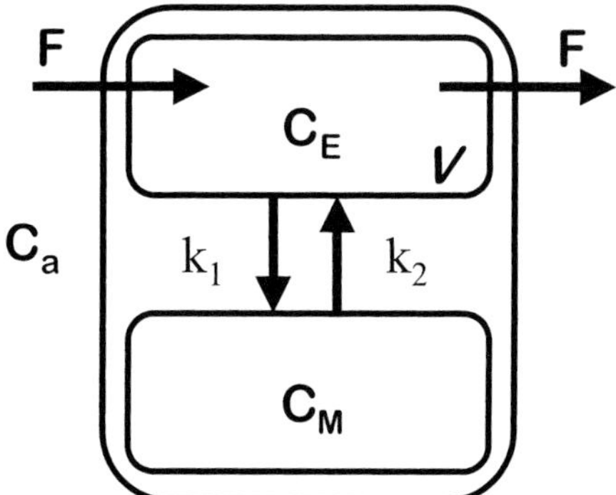

FIGURE 12.3. Metabolism of ammonia in the two-compartment model. C_a and C_E represent unmetabolized free ammonia in artery and tissue, respectively, and C_M represents metabolized ^{13}N compounds. V is the volume of distribution for free ammonia.

By the results of the differential equation for C_E and C_M, where τ = dummy variable, F = flow, Sp = spillover fraction, t = time, it is calculated with the assumption of $k_2 = 0$ as

$$\frac{C_{tiss}(t)}{C_a(t)} = K \cdot \frac{\int_0^t C_a(\tau)d\tau}{C_a(t)} + \frac{F^2 V}{(F + K_1)^2} + \mathrm{Sp}$$

In this equation, K is a slope of a first-order function and it can be acquired by the linear regression method. Subsequently, the regional myocardial blood flow can be calculated by the relationship between K and blood flow, F:

$$K = F \cdot (1 - 0.607e^{1.25/F})$$

^{15}O-water PET can also be used as a tracer for perfusion, as the water is taken up in the myocardium by free diffusion. Therefore, the single-compartment model can be adopted for the assessment of myocardial perfusion. As in the protocol for stress–rest SPECT, stress and rest perfusion can be assessed. The perfusible tissue index (PTI) can be calculated from the single-compartment model and the constant of the partial volume effect. The PTI has been reported in another study to demonstrate myocardial viability and heterogeneity of perfusion.

As water diffuses freely into tissue, the Kety-Schmidt model can be used (Fig. 12.4). In this model, C_t is expressed as

$$\frac{dC_t(t)}{dt} = F \cdot C_a(t) - F \cdot C_V(t)$$

This differential equation can be solved by assuming that tracer concentrations in tissues and veins are in an instantaneous equilibrium:

$$C_t(t) = F \cdot C_a(t) \otimes e^{\frac{-F \cdot t}{\lambda}} = F \cdot \int_0^t C_a(\tau)e^{\frac{-F}{\lambda}(t-\tau)}\, d\tau$$

where λ is the partition coefficient and is usually set as 0.92. This equation can be written using correction parameters for partial volume effect (F_{MM}) and spillover:

$$C_t(t) = F_{MM} \cdot F \cdot C_a(t) \otimes e^{\frac{-F \cdot t}{\lambda}} + \mathrm{Sp} \cdot C_a(t)$$

^{11}C-Acetate PET

The myocardial oxygen consumption rate (MVO_2) can be measured by an invasive method in which arterial and venous hemoglobin con-

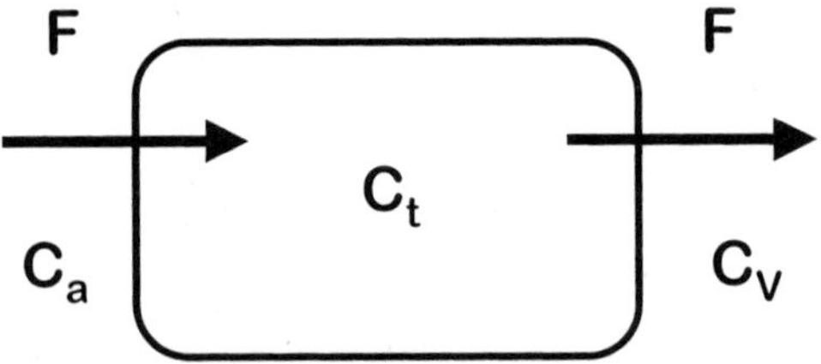

FIGURE 12.4. The Kety-Schmidt model for the calculation of the perfusible tissue index (PTI). Water diffuses freely into tissue.

centration, oxygen saturation, and blood flow are measured. This method is the gold standard for measurement of MVO_2; however, it is invasive due to catheterization and it cannot measure regional MVO_2. ^{11}C-acetate PET can be used for noninvasive evaluation of oxygen consumption.[3]

In a cell, acetate accesses the mitochondrial matrix immediately, where it makes an ester bond with coenzyme A (CoA). This results in acetyl-CoA being oxidized in the Krebs cycle, in which a form of carbon dioxide is removed at the lung by exhalation. ^{11}C-acetate has the same physiologic pathway as that of acetate, and therefore is a tracer for myocardial oxidative metabolism. The half-life of ^{11}C is 20 minutes. It is appropriate to measure uptake and clearance of ^{11}C acetate, which is taken up maximally within 2 to 5 minutes and cleared with a half-life of 20 minutes.

In various heart models, such as the Langendorf model of an isolated rabbit heart and open/closed canine heart models, clearance of ^{11}C-acetate demonstrated a linear correlation with myocardial oxygen consumption in a wide range of blood flow. Human data also support this relationship; that is, the clearance of ^{11}C-acetate measured by PET showed a good correlation with the oxygen consumption rate measured by the invasive method. The clearance of ^{11}C-acetate on PET demonstrates the myocardial aerobic metabolism that produces energy for myocardial contraction, and consequently demonstrates a performance of the Krebs cycle, with the assumption that the pool of acetate and acetyl-CoA is not varied. This finding is based on the fact that ^{11}C-acetate is easily fluxed into the Krebs cycle as a substrate, and that this influx is usually not influenced by the substrate condition. ^{11}C-acetate PET is not interfered with easily by other factors, whereas ^{17}F-FDG-PET is considerably influenced by the competitive mechanisms of free-fatty acid and glucose, plasma glucose level, and insulin sensitivity/resistance of the tissue. The myocardium with preserved ^{11}C-acetate clearance is more likely to be viable. ^{11}C-acetate clearance has been reported to be a better predictor than ^{18}F-FDG uptake.[3]

Other Miscellaneous Tracers

^{11}C-palmitate is another tracer for the metabolism of fatty acid. It is cleared from the blood rapidly, and the clearance is correlated with regional blood flow. In the myocardium it is cleared by biexponential kinetics. The faster one is correlated with the clearance of ^{11}C carbon dioxide, and is considered to represent beta-oxidation. The slower one represents its subsequent oxidization in the Krebs cycle. Although ^{11}C-palmitate is a representative fatty acid tracer, it has several disadvantages. The major one is the short time of oxidation. As ^{11}C-palmitate is very rapidly degraded by beta-oxidation, there is only a short time to analyze the tracer. Moreover, as palmitate can leave a cell without full oxidation and the resultant iodinated or phenylated derivatives can be retained in the myocardium, it makes the analysis of the metabolism more complicated.

As future perspectives, several new tracers are now in trials. New trials include perfusion, metabolism tracers, and receptor or neurotransmitter images. The most widely used ones at present are imaging tracers for the cardiac nervous system. Several ^{11}C- or ^{18}F-labeled catecholamines and their analogs are used for imaging of the sympathetic nervous system. The assessment of the cardiac nervous system is reported to have a correlation with the prognosis in ischemic heart disease, congestive heart failure, and other cardiomyopathy.

Myocardial Viability

Noninvasive assessment of viable myocardium is essential for the determination of reperfusion therapy such as coronary artery bypass graft (CABG) or percutaneous transluminal coronary angioplasty (PTCA). The term *viability* usually means that the function of the myocardium can be recovered by revascularization. Therefore, the gold standard for viability is a functional assessment after revascularization.

As the viability is more problematic in the myocardium with persistent decrease of perfusion, the assessment of perfusion only is not enough to discriminate viable myocardium from scarred myocardium. In this point of view, the finding of cellular energy production or preserved metabolism is important information for viability. Myocardium uses almost all kinds of substrate according to the cellular condition. In normal aerobic conditions, fatty acids are usually the main energy sources, while in the postprandial state the high plasma level of glucose and insulin induces myocardium to use glucose as the main energy source. The large amount of energy produced by aerobic substrate catabolism can provide enough energy for myocardial contraction. However, anaerobic catabolism using glucose is the main energy source in the ischemic condition, which can afford only basal cellular metabolism. Therefore, the assessment of myocardial perfusion and various metabolisms using PET can reveal myocardial viability.[4]

The aerobic substrate metabolism provides most of the energy for myocardial contraction. The main substrates for aerobic metabolism in myocardium are fatty acids and glucose metabolized by beta-oxidation and glycolysis, respectively. And finally, they undergo the Krebs cycle. The amount of adenosine triphosphate (ATP) made in the Krebs cycle is the same as in glucose and fatty acids.

Substrate conversion occurs in an ischemic condition from fatty acids to glucose, in which glucose is metabolized by the anaerobic pathway, resulting only in the increase of glucose uptake in ischemic myocardium. The energy made from the sole anaerobic metabolism is not enough to maintain myocardial function and is used just to preserve cellular integrity. Scarred myocardium after infarction performs basal metabolism of fibroblasts. Ischemic myocardium can be considered viable when it shows increased uptake of glucose because this is evidence of the preservation of the intact myocardium that produces the energy for the survival and repair of the cells. ^{18}F-FDG-PET is the best method for the assessment of glucose uptake.

Stunning refers to the dysfunction in spite of preserved blood flow, and *hibernation* refers to the dysfunction of adaptation in response to the decreased blood supply. These factors decrease oxygen consumption physiologically and inhibit contraction. Stunned myocardium recovers function spontaneously with time, and hibernating myocardium recovers function only by revascularization.[5] Increased uptake of glucose following increased energy production demonstrates a higher likelihood of preserved cellular integrity and functional recovery after revascularization. Therefore, increased uptake of ^{18}F-FDG in ischemic area (perfusion–metabolism mismatch) is a sign of myocardial viability (Fig. 12.5).[6]

Perfusion–metabolism mismatch is not only a sign for viability, but also a sign for poor prognosis in the case without adequate treatment. The myocardium with perfusion–metabolism mismatch shows 50% of the annual cardiac event rate.[7] Therefore, in cases of perfusion–metabolism mismatch in ischemic myocardium, the risk of conservative therapy is significantly higher than that of revascularizing intervention.

Comparison of ^{18}F-FDG-PET, Myocardial Perfusion SPECT, and Dobutamine Echocardiography

It has been studied whether it is possible to diagnose viable myocardium by the assessment of perfusion. Viability assessment by perfusion status was based on the facts that myocardial perfusion is a nutrient flow, perfusion–metabolism coupling is maintained in most of the myocardium, and perfusion and contraction are usually in a linear relationship in most cases.

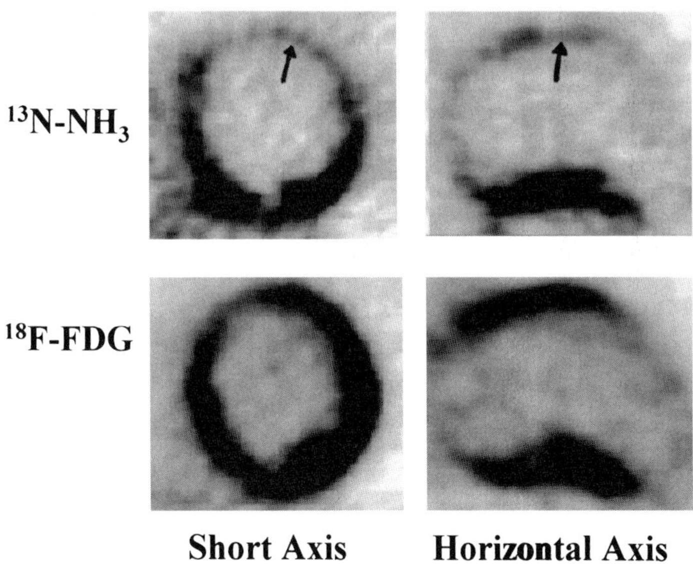

FIGURE 12.5. Perfusion–metabolism mismatch. Uptake of ^{18}F-FDG for metabolism (*lower row*) is preserved in the anterior wall of the left ventricle, while uptake of ^{13}N-ammonia for blood flow is markedly reduced (*arrows*) (*upper row*).

The most widely used tool in assessing myocardial blood flow is a perfusion SPECT using Tl 201– or technetium (Tc-99m)–labeled agents.[8] Viable myocardium usually demonstrates a higher uptake of perfusion tracers than that of scarred myocardium, although it is significantly decreased when compared with that of normal myocardium. Because Tl 201 can be taken up through Na-K adenosine triphosphatase (ATPase) and Tc-99m methoxy-isobutyl-isonitrile (MIBI) can show the retention by sustained mitochondrial membrane potential, uptake of these agents can be related with the viability of myocardium.

Tl 201 has the characteristic redistribution. Segments with the rest perfusion defect usually show increased uptake at 4- or 24-hour delayed images. About 15% to 56% of resting perfusion defect is improved at the delayed image. Tl 201 uptake at 24-hour delayed image demonstrates maximal potential of myocardial uptake. A segment with Tl 201 redistribution is considered to have higher probability of viability. Although reinjection of Tl 201 is an alternative for delayed image, there is some limitation in that reinjection image demonstrates a mixed status of rest uptake and redistribution.

^{18}F-FDG-PET has a positive predictive value of 80% to 90% for viability.[9] High predictive values were acquired when perfusion and glucose metabolism were compared quantitatively. As low as 60% of the positive predictive value was reported when semiquantitative analysis of glucose uptake was used without information about perfusion.

There is an echocardiographic method for viability assessment. Contractile reserve induced by an inotropic agent is a major concern for viability in this method. When ^{18}F-FDG and dobutamine-stress echocardiography are compared as tools for viability assessment, ^{18}F-FDG-PET has higher sensitivity, while dobutamine-stress echocardiography has higher specificity.[8] However, there are several disadvantages of echocardiography in that it is dependent on the experience of the operators, and quantitative analysis is not available at present.

^{18}F-FDG also has minor limitations. For adequate assessment of myocardial viability, the perfusion status should be assessed and compared. ^{18}F-FDG is not interpretable in cases of acute myocardial infarction or diabetes because uptake is influenced by the substrate condition.

^{18}F-FDG SPECT and Camera-Based PET

With the advantage of low cost, a SPECT camera equipped with a high-energy collimator or coincidence detection circuit has been used for positron imaging.[10] For this purpose, collimators should have thick septa and sufficient thickness. Because an annihilation gamma ray has high energy of 511 keV, it is not affected by attenuation as much as a conventional gamma ray image using Tc-99m. However, camera-based PET using a coincidence detection circuit is enormously affected by attenuation and is not interpretable without attenuation correction. For simultaneous evaluation of myocardial perfusion and metabolism, dual-isotope simultaneous imaging or consecutive imaging has been suggested.

^{18}F-FDG-SPECT has the same mechanism for detection of viability. When compared with ^{18}F-FDG-PET, ^{18}F-FDG-SPECT has been reported to have a similar sensitivity in spite of a slightly lower specificity. ^{18}F-FDG-SPECT also shows predictive value for hard or soft cardiac events.[11]

References

1. Schelbert HR. F-18 deoxyglucose and the assessment of myocardial viability. Semin Nucl Med 2002;27:60–69.
2. Sandler MP, Bax JJ, Patton JA, et al. Fluorine-18-fluorodeoxyglucose cardiac imaging using a modified scintillation camera. J Nucl Med 1998;39: 2035–2043.
3. Porenta G, Cherry S, Czernin J, et al. Noninvasive determination of myocardial blood flow, oxygen consumption and efficiency in normal humans by carbon-11 acetate positron emission tomography imaging. Eur J Nucl Med 1999;26:1465–1574.
4. Auerbach MA, Schoeder H, Hoh C, et al. Prevalence of myocardial viability as detected by positron emission tomography in patients with ischemic cardiomyopathy. Circulation 1999;99:2921–2926.
5. Bax JJ, Wijns W, Cornel JH, et al. Accuracy of currently available techniques for prediction of functional recovery after revascularization in patients with left ventricular dysfunction. J Am Coll Cardiol 1997;30:1452–1460.
6. Srinivasan G, Kitsiou AN, Bachrach SL, et al. [18F] Fluorodeoxyglucose single photon emission computed tomography. Can it replace PET and thallium SPECT for the assessment of myocardial viability? Circulation 1998;97:843–850.
7. Di Carli M, Davidson M, Little R, et al. Value of metabolic imaging with positron emission tomography for evaluating prognosis in patients with coronary artery disease and left ventricular dysfunction. Am J Cardiol 1994;73:527–533.
8. Bax JJ, Cornel JH, Visser FC, et al. Comparison of fluorine-18-FDG with rest-redistribution thallium-201 SPECT to delineate viable myocardium and predict functional recovery after revascularization. J Nucl Med 1998; 39:1481–1486.
9. Bax JJ, Cornel JH, Visser FC, et al. Prediction of improvement of contractile function in patients with ischemic ventricular dysfunction after revascularization by fluorine-18 fluorodeoxyglucose single-photon emission computed tomography. J Am Coll Cardiol 1997;30:377–383.
10. Dietlein M, Knapp WH, Lauterbach KW, Schicha H. Economic evaluation studies in nuclear medicine. Eur J Nucl Med 1999;26:553–580.
11. Patterson RE, Eisner RL, Horowitz SF. Comparison of cost-effectiveness and utility of exercise ECG, single photon emission computed tomography, positron emission tomography, and coronary angiography for diagnosis of coronary artery disease. Circulation 1995;91:54–65.

13

Infectious and Inflammatory Diseases

Kyung-Han Lee and June-Key Chung

Positron emission tomography (PET) with fluorine-18-fluoro-2-deoxy-D-glucose (FDG) is a powerful tool to diagnose, stage, and monitor cancer patients. While this technique exploits the fact that enhanced glucose utilization leading to high FDG uptake is characteristic for a variety of cancers, FDG is not a tumor-specific agent. Infectious or inflammatory lesions with high concentrations of activated leukocytes and/or macrophages also show significantly elevated levels of FDG accumulation. Such lesions can be mistaken for malignancy in patients undergoing PET studies for cancer evaluation, which may lead to false-positive interpretation. However, in patients with known or suspected infectious or inflammatory lesions, FDG-PET can be used to quantify the pathologic increase in glucose metabolism of inflammatory processes and may be a powerful clinical tool for the diagnosis of monitoring inflammatory activity. FDG-PET thus may be useful for evaluating such diseases caused by infections from a variety of bacteria, mycobacteria, virus, and fungi, and also infectious or inflammatory processes.

Nonisotope radiologic imaging for evaluating infectious and inflammatory foci, such as computed tomography (CT) and magnetic resonance imaging (MRI), are frequently used for the delineation of many types of infectious disease. In particular, the evaluation of soft tissue infections, including cellulitis, myositis, fasciitis, abscess, and septic arthritis, is often aided by MRI or CT due to their excellent anatomic resolution and soft tissue contrast.[1] However, these methods are not very specific in diagnosing and monitoring treatment response of infectious lesions. Difficulties frequently arise in differentiating active from indolent lesions, and also in evaluating patients with previous surgical intervention.

In contrast, radiotracer imaging methods are often valuable for judging inflammatory activity or physiologic alterations associated with disease. Most infectious or inflammatory lesions can be visualized with radiolabeled autologous leukocytes or gallium 67 citrate. However, leukocyte scan suffers from shortcomings such as laborious preparation and risk of blood handling. Gallium scans have the disadvantage of delayed images. These scintigraphic modalities also have the limited diagnostic accuracy depending on the disease, such as low gallium scan sensitivity for abdominal lesions due to substantial background uptake,[2] or low sensitivity of leukocyte scan for detecting infection of the vertebrae.

PET has superior spatial resolution and allows excellent anatomic localization of pathologic lesions with high FDG uptake. Infectious lesions are known to be capable of high FDG uptake levels, and standard uptake values (SUVs) exceeding 6 or 7 have been reported.[3] Moreover, since the FDG accumulation is rapidly increased with high target to background ratios, PET imaging can provide diagnosis within a couple of hours. But the requirement for a few hours of patient fasting, the potential lower sensitivity for diabetic patients, and the problem of differentiating infection from tumor lesions are limitations. The high sensitivity and specificity of FDG-PET may allow its use as a single nuclear medicine imaging procedure without the need for combining additional scans, as are often utilized for detecting an infection. Other advantages of FDG-PET include high interobserver agreement for interpretation, possible high sensitivity for low-grade infections, and applicability to patients with neutropenia, as well as those with metal implants. FDG-PET increasingly becomes accepted as a cost-effective and efficient modality, and an adjunct or alternate to other imaging methods for the evaluation of infectious diseases.

Glucose Uptake in Leukocytes

The mechanism of enhanced FDG accumulation has been well investigated in tumor cells, but much less so in infection and inflammation. FDG accumulation into infectious lesions is due mostly to uptake by inflammatory cells, such as leukocytes and macrophages, and by granulation tissue.[4] Quiescent inflammatory cells do not generally exhibit high levels of glucose utilization in comparison to cancer cells. During inflammation, however, activated leukocytes and macrophages utilize glucose as an energy source for chemotaxis and phagocytosis, thereby exhibiting a dramatic influx of glucose concomitant with high metabolic activity.[5]

Neutrophils stimulated with n-formyl-methionyl-leucyl-phenylalanine have been shown to increase FDG uptake more than 200% over unstimulated cells.[6] Such dramatic enhancement of FDG uptake in activated leukocytes has been considered to reflect the well-described phenomenon of respiratory burst in these cells. However, in a recent study by Jones et al,[7] a temporal dissociation between stimulated respiratory burst activity and deoxyglucose uptake in neutrophils was demonstrated. It was also noted that neutrophil priming without stimulation of respiratory burst could induce an identical increase in deoxyglucose uptake. These results demonstrate that, contrary to previous belief, stimulation of respiratory burst activity is not an essential requirement for enhanced FDG uptake in activated neutrophils.[7] A similar finding has been reported for monocytic cells where enhanced FDG uptake following activation with interferon persisted despite inhibition of respiratory burst activity.[8]

The mechanism for increased FDG uptake in inflammation is explained by the finding that activated inflammatory cells also have an increased expression of glucose transporters. Chakrabarti et al[9] examined T-cell–enriched human lymphocytes and observed undetectable levels of glucose transporter GLUT-1 in unstimulated cells. GLUT-1 stimulation became detectable at 24 hours, peaked at 48 hours, and disappeared at 96 hours.[9] Similarly, immunostaining of experimental infectious and tumor tissues have shown high expression levels of GLUT-1 and GLUT-3 in infectious and inflammatory lesions, although GLUT-1 expression level was higher in the tumor tissue.[10]

There are several reports that inflammatory lesions demonstrate a decrease of uptake after 60 minutes postinjection.[11,12] Such behavior of FDG uptake in inflammatory lesions may be explained by dephosphorylation of FDG-6-phosphate due to significant levels of glucose-6-phosphatase within inflammatory cells.[13]

Although, false-negative findings due to elevated blood glucose concentrations are a well-recognized problem for FDG-PET imaging in tumor patients, there is some evidence that FDG uptake in infectious or inflammatory lesions is less affected by hyperglycemia compared to tumor tissue,[14] although there also have been contrary reports.[15,16] While awaiting further clarification of this relationship, it is presently recommended that serum glucose levels do not exceed 11 mmol/L during FDG-PET studies for infection, as is done for oncology patients.

Clinical Applications

Chronic Osteomyelitis

In contrast to acute osteomyelitis, chronic osteomyelitis secondary to trauma or surgery is often difficult to diagnose. Since lesions may remain indolent for a long time only to become reactivated many years later, and clinical symptoms, laboratory parameters, and radiologic findings are uncharacteristic in many cases, the diagnosis of chronic osteomyelitis often remains a clinical challenge. The suspected presence of infectious bone lesions can be investigated with CT and MRI, which offer excellent anatomic delineation of disease extent. Although MRI provides sensitive visualization of bone marrow lesions, the findings are often nonspecific.[17] Moreover, MRI is frequently of limited value in patients with infection of small bones, diabetic or immunocompromised patients, and those with previous trauma, surgery, or preexisting marrow conditions. Therefore, combined radionuclide scintigraphy becomes useful in complicated situations.[18]

Several nuclear medicine imaging methods can be used for evaluating chronic osteomyelitis. Three-phase bone scans offer sensitive detection of lesions (Fig. 13.1), but procedures that are more specific to inflammation are usually utilized. Gallium scan has a better specificity

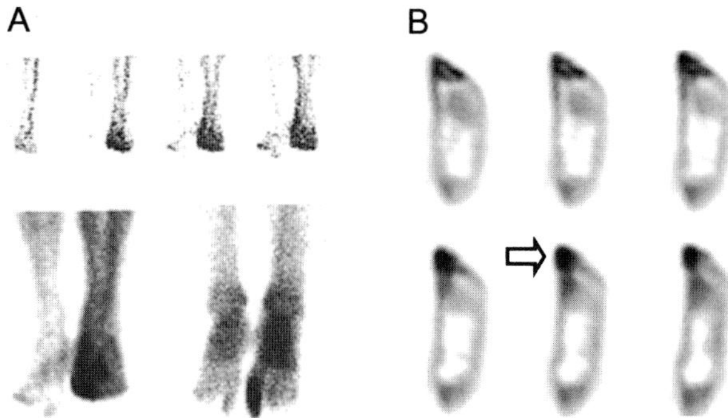

FIGURE 13.1. A: Three-phase bone scintigraphy. Dynamic flow study (*upper row*) over bilateral feet with technetium (Tc)-99m methylene diphosphanate (MDP) shows an increased blood flow to the left foot. Blood pool (*left*) and static delayed (*right*) images of the feet (*lower row*) show increased vascularity (*closed arrow*) and markedly increased activity (*arrowhead*) in the great toe of the left foot with chronic osteomyelitis. B: Transaxial PET images of left foot show markedly increased uptake of ^{18}F-FDG in the great toe with chronic osteomyelitis.

than bone scans and often provides useful information, but the accuracy in patients suspected of osteomyelitis has been shown to be only 70% to 80%.[19] Moreover, false-positive results are seen in patients with fracture healing or uninfected endoprostheses.[20,21] Leukocyte scans have a reasonable accuracy for detecting chronic osteomyelitis, but the false-negative rate is relatively high.[22] Scintigraphic imaging of leukocyte accumulation is particularly unreliable for osteomyelitis that occurs in the axial skeleton, where granulocytes are naturally present. For detection of chronic osteomyelitis in the central skeleton, the leukocyte scan attains sensitivities only in the range from 53% to 76%.[23,24] In addition, it is sometimes difficult with these methods to differentiate between osteomyelitis and soft tissue infections surrounding the bone.

It has been shown that FDG-PET is highly sensitive for the detection of soft tissue and bone infections,[25] and that it can correctly distinguish chronic osteomyelitis from a healing lesion.[26] FDG-PET appears to be particularly useful in suspected chronic osteomyelitis patients when other imaging modalities are negative, or when infection of the axial skeleton is suspected. Guhlmann et al[27] prospectively examined FDG-PET in 31 patients suspected of chronic osteomyelitis (28 confirmed to have osteomyelitis) and found a sensitivity of 100% and specificity of 92%. In another study of 51 patients suspected of chronic osteomyelitis in the peripheral or central skeleton, the sensitivity and specificity were 97% to 100% and 95%, respectively, with FDG-PET, compared to 86% to 92% and 77% to 82%, respectively, with combined bone scanning and antigranulocyte imaging.[28] De Winter et al[29] investigated 60 patients with suspected chronic musculoskeletal infection and found that FDG-PET correctly identified all 25 cases with infection. Of the four false-positive findings, two cases had surgery less than 6 months prior to the study. The sensitivity, specificity, and accuracy were 100%, 88%, and 93%, respectively, for the whole group, and 100%, 90%, and 94%, respectively, for patients with suspected infection of the central skeleton.[29]

An important finding in these studies is that PET was particularly superior to other scintigraphic methods for detecting osteomyelitis within the central skeleton. These are areas where leukocyte scans or antigranulocyte antibody imaging frequently present osteomyelitis lesions as nonspecific photopenic areas. De Winter et al,[30] specifically investigating FDG-PET accuracy in 83 patients suspected of chronic vertebral infections, found that PET had a sensitivity, specificity and accuracy of 100%, 74%, and 90%, respectively. The specificity rose to 91% when patients who were operated within 6 months were excluded. Thus FDG-PET is highly accurate and has great promise in the diagnosis of chronic osteomyelitis, especially in the central skeleton within active bone marrow.

FDG-PET has also been shown to be able to assess the process of inflammatory activity in tuberculous spondylitis.[31,32] The high FDG uptake in tuberculous spondylitis lesions appears to decrease or become normalized after tuberculostatic treatment.[33]

Because of the extremely high sensitivity of PET imaging in detecting infection, a negative study essentially rules out osteomyelitis.[34,35] This can be important when bone anatomy and structure have been altered by trauma, surgery, or soft tissue infection, which often makes exclusion of chronic osteomyelitis difficult with radiologic imaging. However, because of frequent nonspecific accumulation, caution is required in order to avoid false-positive results when interpreting localized areas of FDG uptake on PET.

Prosthesis-Associated Infection

Arthroplasty-related pain is common in patients with lower limb prosthesis, and accurate identification of infection in such patients is clinically important since prompt and active treatment is required. However, differentiating aseptic loosening from prosthesis-associated infection is well recognized as a difficult task. An MRI is limited in specificity for the differential diagnosis in painful arthroplasty patients due to the presence of violated bone. Bone scintigraphy is very sensitive for detecting infection and has a high negative predictive value, but results are not specific enough to reliably differentiate prosthesis infection from loosening.[36] Gallium scan in combination with bone scan has shown an improved specificity of 81%, but this is achieved at the expense of decreased sensitivity to 66%.[37,38] Leukocyte scintigraphy has been found to have better accuracy for diagnosing infected prosthesis, and the reported sensitivity, specificity, and positive and negative predictive values for leukocyte scan combined with bone marrow scan are 77%, 86%, and 54% and 95%, respectively.[39]

FDG-PET is an effective modality for detecting postarthroplasty infection (Fig. 13.2), and in contrast to CT or MRI, is not affected by the presence of metal implants. FDG-PET is particularly useful in patients

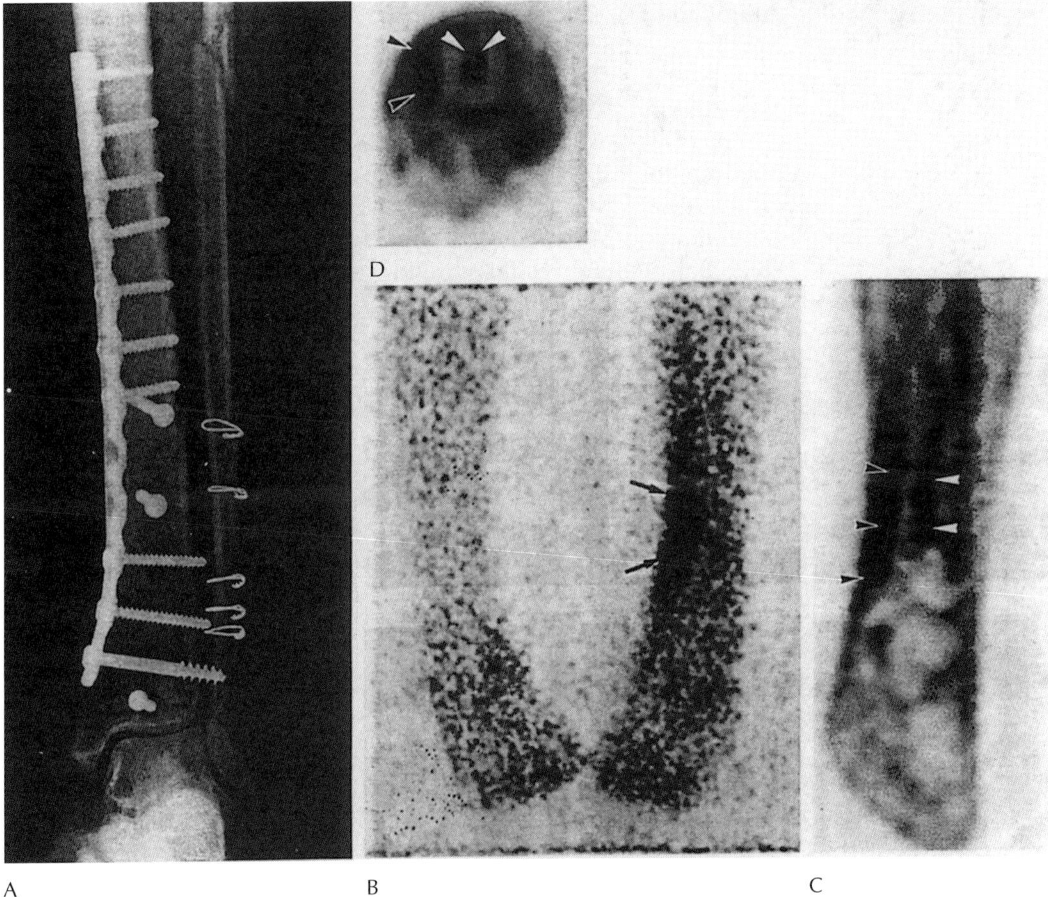

FIGURE 13.2. Images of left lower leg in a patient with a titanium implant in the left tibia after open fracture. A: Frontal radiograph shows a central osteopenia in the distal tibia with multiple screws and suture lines. B: Anterior status image using In 111 antigranulocyte antibody shows an increased activity (*arrows*) at the medial side of left calf. Coronal (C) and axial (D) selected PET images show intense uptake of ^{18}F-FDG in the soft tissue (*black arrowheads*) medial to the osteosynthetic plate of the left calf as well as vertical linear increased intramedullary activity in the distal left tibia, corresponding to soft tissue infection with tibial osteomyelitis. (From Temmerman et al,[40] with permission).

with clinical and laboratory signs of infection but with indistinct signs on the bone scan and radiographs.[40] Based on a study of 74 prostheses in 62 patients in whom infection was suspected, the sensitivity, specificity, and accuracy of FDG-PET for detecting hip prostheses infection were 90%, 89%, and 90%, respectively.[41] Diagnosis of infection in knee prostheses from the same study showed a sensitivity of 91%, specificity of 72%, and accuracy of 78%. Another study showed a similar specificity for detecting infection in total knee arthroplasties with FDG-PET. In this study, 21 patients suspected of knee prostheses infection prospectively underwent technetium (Tc)-99m-HMPAO leukocyte single photon emission computed tomography (SPECT) and FDG-PET, which demonstrated specificities and sensitivities of 53% and 100%, respectively, for leukocyte SPECT, and 73% and 100%, respectively, for PET.[42]

Although FDG-PET is useful for detecting infections associated with lower limb arthroplasty, nonspecific increased FDG uptake after arthroplasty persists for longer periods than the usual 6 months for most other surgical procedures on the bone. False-positive cases showing high FDG uptake on uninfected loosened prosthesis are not uncommon. Thus, caution should be applied in interpreting any increased periprosthetic activity compared to adjacent tissue as infection, since this would lead to very low diagnostic specificity.[43] It has been suggested that positive results should be reserved for lesions with increased FDG uptake present along the interface between prosthesis and bone.[44] It appears that FDG-PET is more accurate for detecting infections associated with hip prostheses than with knee prostheses. The diagnostic criteria in the latter patients are not as optimal as in those with hip prostheses, owing to relatively high false-positive rates. The reason for the lower accuracy for diagnosing painful knee prostheses is not clear, but it has been proposed that attenuation correction can lead to false-positive interpretation from introduction of artifacts for PET imaging of prosthetic knees.[45]

Vasculitis

Vasculitis is a rare group of diseases characterized by inflammation in the blood vessels, and its severity can vary greatly from mild diseases to severe, life-threatening multisystem diseases. Different types of primary systemic vasculitis include giant cell arteritis, Takayasu arteritis, polyarteritis nodosa, Wegener's granulomatosis, and Kawasaki disease. As with any rare disease, its diagnosis or management is often difficult.[46] Doppler sonography, CT, and MRI allow a noninvasive approach to vasculitis, partially replacing angiography by allowing simultaneous evaluation of luminal and vascular wall changes.[47]

Nuclear medicine has several roles in the management of patients with systemic vasculitis. Scintigraphic imaging of the inflammatory process may help diagnose patients presenting with nonspecific symptoms and equivocal serology, define the distribution of inflammatory lesions, monitor the response of inflammatory lesions to treatment, and improve our understanding of the pathophysiology of vasculitic diseases. Imaging with radiolabeled leukocytes in vasculitis patients has shown focal areas of increased soft tissue neutrophil uptake and abnormalities of granulocyte kinetics involving the lung and spleen.[48,49] Reuter et al[50] retrospectively investigated leukocyte imaging in the management of 50 patients with systemic vasculitis. The authors found that leukocyte imaging was useful for detecting unsuspected sites of disease and monitoring disease activity, and that scintigraphy was superior to conventional radiography or CT for detecting vasculitic involvement of the respiratory tract. There appears to be a significant relationship between Wegener's granulomatosis and nasal uptake on leukocyte scans.[50] However, since leukocyte scans more effectively visualize pyogenic rather than chronic inflammations, their utility may be limited in vasculitic diseases with chronic inflammation and, thus, variable neutrophilic content.

With high accumulation of FDG in granulomatous lesions, FDG-PET has potential usefulness in the diagnosis of vascular inflammation. Giant cell arteritis and polymyalgia rheumatica are closely related disorders that affect the elderly and cause substantial morbidity. The diagnosis is made by clinical signs and confirmed by pathologic findings characterized by chronic granulomatous inflammation of the walls of large and medium-sized arteries. It is a multisymptom disease that often presents with challenging issues and diagnostic dilemmas.[51] Although steroids are the mainstay of therapy, they have numerous side effects, particularly in the elderly.[52] Patients with giant cell arteritis or polymyalgia rheumatica show increased FDG uptake in the wall of affected vessels.[53] Blockmans et al[54] evaluated FDG-PET in five patients with polymyalgia rheumatica and six patients with temporal arteritis. Four of six patients with giant cell arteritis and four of five patients with polymyalgia had increased FDG uptake in their thoracic vessels. The increased FDG has been shown to normalize after successful steroid therapy.[55] Thus, it is suggested that FDG-PET findings in vasculitis patients may aid in diagnosis as well as evaluation of disease extent, therapy response, and disease recurrence.

In contrast to giant cell arteritis, Takayasu arteritis is a rare form of chronic large vessel vasculitis mostly affecting young females in Asian and Latin American countries. The disease mainly involves the aorta and its main branches as well as the coronary and pulmonary arteries, causing stenosis or obstruction of the involved arteries. Because symptoms and signs of Takayasu arteritis are nonspecific at an early stage, the diagnosis is usually made at a relatively late stage. Suppression of inflammation and preservation of vascular competence are the aims of treatment. Demonstration of a patient with FDG accumulation on affected vessels has shown that FDG-PET can detect Takayasu arteritis at an early stage, thus permitting early treatment and possible prevention of progression to the occlusive stage of this disease.[56]

Fever of Unknown Origin

Fever of unknown origin (FUO) is defined as recurrent fever of 38.3°C or greater, lasting 2 to 3 weeks or longer, and undiagnosed after 1 week of appropriate evaluation. It is a diagnostic challenge because the cause of such fever is manifold. Infection accounts for only 20% to 40% of FUOs, and the majority of patients have collagen vascular disease or neoplasm, which are responsible for about 50% to 60% of all cases. Although leukocyte scans have a high diagnostic accuracy in the detection of granulocytic pathology, they are of only limited value in FUO due to the low prevalence of purulent processes in these cases.[57] Ga 67 citrate imaging shows acute, chronic, granulomatous, and autoimmune inflammation and also various malignant diseases. Therefore, Ga 67 citrate is currently considered to be the tracer of choice in the diagnostic workup of FUO.[58] However, gallium scans' low resolution, delayed imaging, and physiologic intestinal distribution of gallium reduce its specificity for detecting abdominal lesions.

FDG-PET with high sensitivity may be useful for detecting foci as an origin of the fever in FUO patients. Dreyer et al[59] reported that FDG-PET performed on 10 pediatric FUO patients revealed pathologic uptakes in 11 of 13 exams, nine of which were later proven to be true positive results. Lorenzen et al[60] performed FDG-PET following negative findings on common imaging methods in FUO patients, and found that PET was able to detect abnormal lesions in four of four patients who were confirmed to have tuberculosis, *Pneumocystis carinii* pneumonia, chronic inflammatory hematoma, and aortitis. In a later study, the authors described FDG-PET findings in 16 patients with FUO in whom conventional diagnostics had not been conclusive. Nonphysiologic accumulations of FDG led to the final diagnosis in 11 of 12 patients. Of the four FDG-PET negative patients, two had rheumatic fever, and the origin of fever was unrevealed in the remaining two patients.[61] Blockmans et al[62] investigated FDG-PET in 58 consecutive cases of FUO and found 24 of 46 abnormal FDG-PET scans were helpful in diagnosis and the remaining 22 were noncontributory. In a subgroup of 40 patients, the administration of both FDG-PET and gallium scintigraphy, FDG-PET and gallium scintigraphy were helpful in diagnosis in 35% and 25%, respectively. All foci of abnormal gallium accumulation were also detected by FDG-PET. The authors concluded that FDG-PET is a valuable second-step technique in patients with FUO and compares favorably with gallium scintigraphy. Meller et al[63] prospectively evaluated coincidence FDG imaging and gallium SPECT in 20 FUO patients. FDG imaging was positive and essentially contributed to the final diagnosis in 11, and had a sensitivity and specificity of 84% and 86%, respectively. For the 18 patients who received both exams, FDG imaging had a sensitivity of 81% and specificity of 86%, while gallium SPECT yielded a sensitivity and specificity of 67% and 78%, respectively. These studies suggest that FDG imaging has respectable accuracy in the setting of FUO and appears to be a promising diagnostic tool in patients with FUO in whom conventional diagnostics are unsuccessful.

Abdominal Inflammation

Inflammatory bowel disease (IBD) is a group of diseases that cause the small and/or large bowel to become inflamed. Crohn's disease and ulcerative colitis are the best-known forms of IBD. Because the chronic unpredictability of IBD makes it a difficult disease to treat, early detection is essential in developing patient confidence and cooperation. Imaging techniques may aid in the diagnosis of IBD, which is essentially one of exclusion. Determining disease activity can be clinically important for making appropriate treatment plans.

Radiolabeled leukocyte scans are useful in IBD and can be effective in evaluating disease activity. The test, however, is time-consuming, and obtaining sufficient blood for labeling can be difficult. Because activated inflammatory cells use more glucose, active inflammatory lesions in Crohn's disease or ulcerative colitis also have increased glucose consumption, allowing visualization by FDG-PET. Bicik et al[64] prospectively performed endoscopy and FDG-PET in six patients with Crohn's disease or ulcerative colitis and found high glucose uptake in histologically confirmed areas of inflammation, which was higher with clinically active disease. For children, FDG-PET may be a useful adjunct to colonoscopy and barium studies. Skehan et al[65] investigated FDG-PET in 18 young patients with IBD, and seven with nonspecific abdominal pain or diarrhea. The overall sensitivity of PET for detecting IBD was 81% and specificity was 85%. On a segment-by-segment basis, PET correctly identified active disease in 76% of individual bowel segments with a sensitivity and specificity of 71% and 81%, respectively. Thus, FDG-PET can be used to identify an active inflammation in IBD. Since the magnitude of FDG accumulation correlates well with the disease activity index, FDG-PET may also be useful for long-term monitoring or assessment of therapeutic efficacy.[64,66]

FDG has been reported to accumulate in other forms of intestinal inflammation as well, examples of which include *Clostridium difficile*–associated diarrheal illness[67] and acute enterocolitis.[68,69] In view of the physiologic intestinal FDG activity seen in subjects without abdominal disease, however, care is warranted to avoid potential false-positive interpretation of bowel activity.

Lung Infection and Sarcoidosis

Intense FDG uptake lesions in the lung are sometimes seen in active infection or inflammation, which can often lead to the false-positive interpretation of malignant disease. When the lesions appear as intense focal or multifocal FDG uptake lesions, they are difficult to distinguish from pulmonary metastases. Infectious lesions appear as apical, segmental, or lobar patterns, which may be differentiated from malignant tumors.[70] Pneumonia typically appears on PET as segmental or lobar lesions with high FDG uptake (Fig. 13.3).[71–73] While these lesions generally have FDG uptakes less intense than that of cancer, bacterial pneumonia lesions have been reported with markedly elevated FDG uptake.[74]

In endemic regions, pulmonary histoplasmosis[75] and tuberculosis[76] also appear as lesions with high FDG accumulation. Liu et al[77] investigated FDG-PET in 28 patients with suspected pulmonary tuberculosis and found that active FDG uptake lesions of SUV levels exceeding 2.5 had a sensitivity of 100% and specificity of 44% for diagnosing active tuberculosis (Figs. 13.4 and 13.5). FDG-PET may be useful in the assessment of lesion activity in infectious lung disease, and acute active lesions have been shown to have higher FDG uptakes than chronic active or healing lesions.[78]

Sarcoidosis is a chronic systemic disorder of unknown cause that most frequently affects the lung, although virtually any organ can be involved. Thoracic sarcoidosis lesions demonstrate significant FDG uptake when evaluated with PET.[79–81] While PET does not presently appear to have a major role in diagnosing sarcoidosis, it may be useful for assessing inflammatory activity and treatment effect in known patients. Evidence that FDG uptake levels may reflect disease activity has been

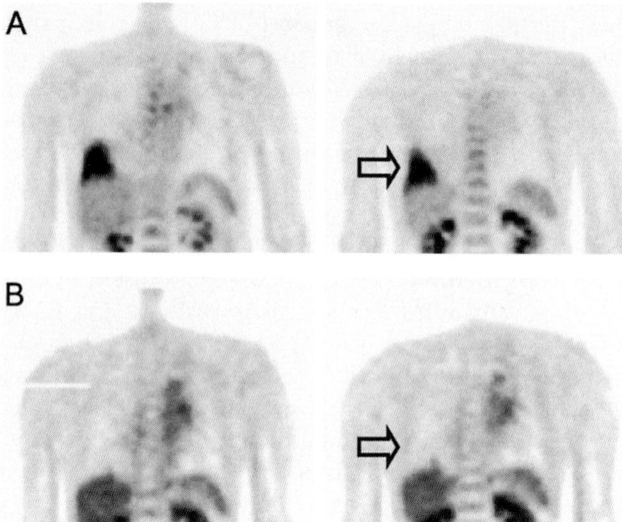

FIGURE 13.3. Selected coronal PET images of the chest demonstrate markedly increased uptakes of ^{18}F-FDG in the lateral-basal segment of right lower lung (*open arrow*) with acute bacterial pneumonia before the antibiotic therapy (A). Note almost complete resolution of the abnormality on follow-up study after therapy (B).

provided by Brudin et al,[82] who found that increased FDG uptake in sarcoidosis lesions normalized after high-dose steroid treatment. In a study investigating FDG and ^{11}C-methionine PET findings in sarcoidosis patients, Yamada et al[83] observed that patients with higher FDG-to-methionine uptake ratios in mediastinal and hilar lymph nodes had a considerably higher rate of improvement, suggesting this may be a useful index. FDG-PET is also able to discriminate between active and in-

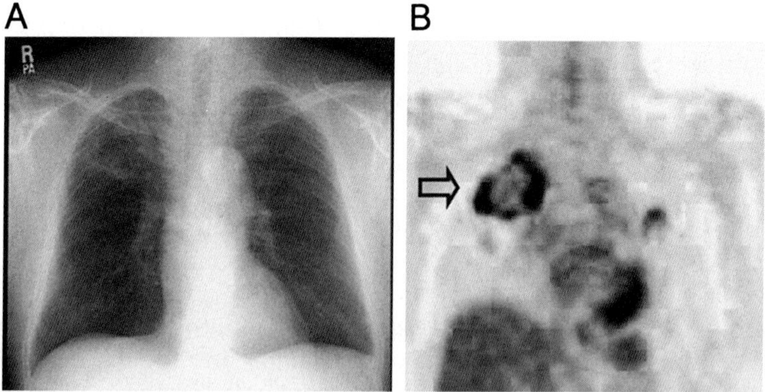

FIGURE 13.4. Frontal view of the chest x-ray (A) shows irregular infiltrations outlining cavity in the right upper lung with active tuberculosis. Selected coronal PET image of the chest (B) shows a markedly increased uptake of ^{18}F-FDG in the periphery of the cavitary lesion (*arrow*) in the right upper lung.

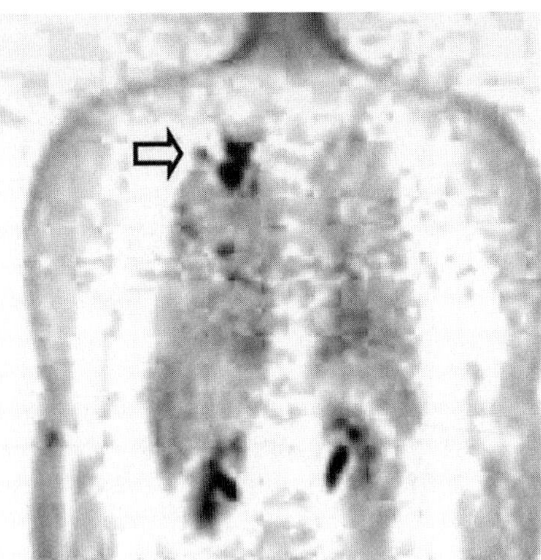

FIGURE 13.5. Selected coronal PET image without attenuation correction for the examination of nodules in the right upper lung shows two focal areas of markedly increased uptake of ^{18}F-FDG. Biopsy revealed active tuberculomas.

active lesions in children with chronic granulomatous disease, which are difficult to discriminate with CT studies.[84]

Acquired Immunodeficiency Syndrome

Because of the variety of the types of infection that occur in patients with acquired immunodeficiency syndrome (AIDS), it is essential to determine the nature of the underlying infection before effective therapy is instituted. FDG-PET can be used to detect opportunistic infections and malignancies in AIDS patients. A major role of FDG-PET is to detect the correct location for initiating further procedures such as biopsy, aspiration, or other diagnostic modalities. FDG-PET has been shown to successfully localize infection sites caused by pseudomonas, mycobacteria, and cryptococcal and staphylococcal microorganisms in AIDS patients. The overall sensitivity and specificity for detecting infectious or malignant lesions was 92% and 94%, respectively.[85] It has been cautioned, however, that lymph node uptake in patients with generalized lymphadenopathy should not be mistaken for lymphoma.

The incidence of primary central nervous system (CNS) lymphomas is increased several thousandfold in AIDS patients. These are B-cell malignancies consistently associated with Epstein-Barr virus that typically occur late in the course and are associated with a very short survival. However, both CNS lymphoma and toxoplasmosis appear as ring-enhancing lesions on MRI and CT and are difficult to distinguish, thereby remaining a problem for accurate diagnosis.[86] As lymphomas characteristically show high FDG accumulation, FDG-PET can detect lymphomas with high sensitivity, highlighting more lesions than with CT. Generally, confirmation of lymphoma would still require tissue biopsy, since high FDG uptake is not specific for lymphoma. However, in the case of AIDS, FDG imaging has been proposed to differentiate

CNS lymphoma from opportunistic infections. As lymphomas are metabolically more active, their lesions have higher FDG uptakes and can be distinguished from toxoplasmosis lesions, which have lower FDG accumulation.[87–89] Thus, FDG-PET is a promising noninvasive diagnostic procedure that may obviate the need for brain biopsy in AIDS patients with suspected CNS lymphoma.

Conclusion

FDG-PET has rapidly evolved from a purely research modality to a clinical necessity. In addition to its important utility for evaluating cancer patients, FDG-PET imaging more recently has been shown to be very sensitive in the detection and localization of a variety of infectious and inflammatory diseases. PET has theoretical and practical advantages over other scintigraphic methods such as leukocyte or gallium scintigraphy. It becomes more and more evident that FDG-PET imaging can play a major role in the evaluation of patients with suspected infection or inflammation in whom other imaging modalities are inconclusive. PET has been shown to be particularly valuable in the evaluation of chronic osteomyelitis, infected prostheses, sarcoidosis, and fever of unknown origin. PET imaging to detect and characterize infection and inflammation will increasingly contribute to our understanding of these disorders and may well become a major clinical indication in the day-to-day practice of medicine.

References

1. Ma LD, Frassica FJ, Bluemke DA, et al. CT and MRI evaluation of musculoskeletal infection. Crit Rev Diagn Imaging 1997;38(6):535–568.
2. Alazraki NP. Gallium-67 imaging in infection. In: Early PJ, Sodee DB, eds. Principles and Practice of Nuclear Medicine, 2nd ed. St. Louis: Mosby-Year Book, 1995:702–713.
3. Sugawara Y, Braun DK, Kison PV. Rapid detection of human infections with fluorine-18 fluorodeoxyglucose and positron emission tomography: preliminary results. Eur J Nucl Med 1998;25(9):1238–1243.
4. Kubota R, Yamada S, Kubota K et al. Intratumoral distribution of fluorine-18-fluorodeoxyglucose in vivo: high accumulation in macrophages and granulation tissues studies by microautoradiography. J Nucl Med 1992; 33:1972–1980.
5. Weisdorf DJ, Craddock PR, Jacob HS. Glycogenolysis versus glucose transport in human granulocytes: differential activation in phagocytosis and chemotaxis. Blood 1982;60:888–893.
6. Lehmann K, Behe M, Meller J, et al. F-18-FDG uptake in granulocytes: basis of F-18-FDG scintigraphy for imaging infection. J Nucl Med 2001;42: 1384(abstr).
7. Jones HA, Cadwallader KA, White JF, et al. Dissociation between respiratory burst activity and deoxyglucose uptake in human neutrophil granulocytes: implications for interpretation of ^{18}F-FDG PET images. J Nucl Med 2002;43(5):652–657.
8. Paik JY, Lee KH, Choe YS, et al. Increased ^{18}F-FDG uptake in human monocytic U937 cells stimulated with interferon-γ. J Nucl Med 2000;41(5):321(abstr).

9. Chakrabarti R, Jung CY, Lee TP, et al. Changes in glucose transport and transporter isoforms during the activation of human peripheral blood lymphocytes by phytohemagglutinin. J Immunol 1994;152(6):2660–2668.
10. Mochizuki T, Tsukamoto E, Kuge Y, et al. FDG uptake and glucose transporter subtype expressions in experimental tumor and inflammation models. J Nucl Med 2001;42(10):1551–1555.
11. Yamada S, Kubota K, Kubota R, et al. High accumulation of fluorine-18-fluorodeoxyglucose in turpentine-induced inflammatory tissue. J Nucl Med 1995;36:1301–1306.
12. Nakamoto Y, Higashi T, Sakahara, et al. Delayed FDG-PET scan for the differentiation between malignant and benign lesions. J Nucl Med 1999;40: 247 p.
13. Paik J-Y, Lee K-H, et al. Usefulness of insulin to improve F-18 FDG labeling and retention for in vivo PET imaging of monocyte trafficking. Nucl Med Commun 2002;23(6):551–557.
14. Zhuang HM, Loman JC, Cortes-Blanco A, et al. Hyperglycemia does not adversely affect FDG uptake by inflammatory and infectious lesions in FDG PET imaging. J Nucl Med 2000;41:1396(abstr).
15. Zhao S, Kuge Y, Tsukamoto E, et al. Effects of insulin and glucose loading on FDG uptake in experimental malignant tumours and inflammatory lesions. Eur J Nucl Med 2001;28(6):730–735.
16. Zhao S, Kuge Y, Tsukamoto E, et al. Fluorodeoxyglucose uptake and glucose transporter expression in experimental inflammatory lesions and malignant tumours: effects of insulin and glucose loading. Nucl Med Commun 2002;23(6):545–550.
17. Seeger LL, Dungan DH, Eckardt JJ, et al. Nonspecific findings on MR imaging. The importance of correlative studies and clinical information. Clin Orthop 1991;(270):306–312.
18. Tehranzadeh J, Wong E, Wang F, et al. Imaging of osteomyelitis in the mature skeleton. Radiol Clin North Am 2001;39(2):223–250.
19. Merkel KD, Brown ML, Dewanjee MK, et al. Comparison of indium-labeled leukocyte imaging with sequential technetium-gallium scanning in the diagnosis of low-grade musculoskeletal sepsis. J Bone Joint Surg 1985; 67A:465.
20. Al-Sheik W, Sfakianakis GN, Mnaymneh W, et al. Subacute and chronic bone infections: diagnosis using In-111, Ga-67 and Tc-99m MDP bone scintigraphy, and radiology. Radiology 1985;155:501–506.
21. Plestro JP. The current role of gallium imaging in infection. Semin Nucl Med 1994;24:128–141.
22. Datz FD. Indium-111 labeled leukocytes for the detection of infection: current status. Semin Nucl Med 1994;24:92.
23. Datz FL, Thorne DA. Cause and significance of cold bone defects on indium-111-labeled leukocyte imaging. J Nucl Med 1987;28(5):820–823.
24. Palestro CJ, Kim CK, Swyer AJ, et al. Radionuclide diagnosis of vertebral osteomyelitis: indium-111-leukocyte and technetium-99m-methylene diphosphonate bone scintigraphy. J Nucl Med 1991;32(10):1861–1865.
25. Stumpe KD, Dazzi H, Schaffner A, et al. Infection imaging using whole-body FDG-PET. Eur J Nucl Med 2000;27(7):822–832.
26. Sugawara Y, Braun D, Kison P, et al. Rapid detection of human infections with fluorine-18 fluorodeoxyglucose and positron emission tomography. Preliminary results. Eur J Nucl Med 1998;25:1238.
27. Guhlmann A, Brecht-Krauss D, Suger G, et al. Chronic osteomyelitis: detection with FDG PET and correlation with histopathologic findings. Radiology 1998;206(3):749–754.

28. Guhlmann A, Brecht-Krauss D, Suger G, et al. Fluorine-18-FDG PET and technetium-99m antigranulocyte antibody scintigraphy in chronic osteomyelitis. J Nucl Med 1998; 39(12):2145–2152.
29. de Winter F, van de Wiele C, Vogelaers D, et al. Fluorine-18 fluorodeoxyglucose-positron emission tomography: a highly accurate imaging modality for the diagnosis of chronic musculoskeletal infections. J Bone Joint Surg 2001;83A(5):651–660.
30. de Winter F, van de Wiele C, Gennel F, et al. ^{18}F FDG PET in the diagnosis of chronic vertebral infections. J Nucl Med 2002;43(5):132(abstr).
31. Schmitz A, Kalicke T, Willkomm P, et al. Use of fluorine-18 fluoro-2-deoxy-D-glucose positron emission tomography in assessing the process of tuberculous spondylitis. J Spinal Disord 2000;13(6):541–544.
32. Ho AY, Pagliuca A, Maisey MN, et al. Positron emission scanning with ^{18}F-FDG in the diagnosis of deep fungal infections. Br J Haematol 1998; 101(2):392–393.
33. Kalicke T, Schmitz A, Risse JH, et al. Fluorine-18 fluorodeoxyglucose PET in infectious bone diseases: results of histologically confirmed cases. Eur J Nucl Med 2000;27(5):524–528.
34. Zhuang H, Duarte PS, Pourdehand M, et al. Exclusion of chronic osteomyelitis with F-18 fluorodeoxyglucose positron emission tomographic imaging. Clin Nucl Med 2000;25(4):281–284.
35. Chacko TK, Zhuang HM, Alavi A. FDG-PET is an effective alternative to WBC imaging in diagnosing and excluding orthopedic infections. J Nucl Med 2002;43(5):126(abstr).
36. Smith SL, Wastie ML, Forster I. Radionuclide bone scintigraphy in the detection of significant complications after total knee joint replacement. Clin Radiol 2001;56(3):221–224.
37. Merkel KD, Brown ML, Fitzgerald RH Jr. Sequential technetium-99m HMDP gallium-67 citrate imaging for the evaluation of infection in the painful prosthesis. J Nucl Med 1986;27:1413–1417.
38. Kraemer WJ, Saplys R, Waddell JP, et al. Bone scan, gallium scan, and hip aspiration in the diagnosis of infected total hip arthroplasty. J Arthroplasty 1993;8(6):611–616.
39. Scher DM, Pak K, Lonner JH, et al. The predictive value of indium-111 leukocyte scans in the diagnosis of infected total hip, knee, or resection arthroplasties. J Arthroplasty 2000;15:295–300.
40. Temmerman OP, Heyligers IC, Hoekstra OS, et al. Detection of osteomyelitis using FDG and positron emission tomography. J Arthroplasty 2001;16(2):243–246.
41. Zhuang H, Duarte PS, Pourdehand M, et al. The promising role of 18F-FDG PET in detecting infected lower limb prosthesis implants. J Nucl Med 2001;42(1):44–48.
42. Van Acker F, Nuyts J, Maes A, et al. FDG-PET, 99mtc-HMPAO white blood cell SPECT and bone scintigraphy in the evaluation of painful total knee arthroplasties. Eur J Nucl Med 2001;28(10):1496–1504.
43. Marwin SE, Tomas MB, Palestro CJ. Improving the specificity of 18F-FDG imaging of painful joint prosthesis. J Nucl Med 2002;43(5):126(abstr).
44. Zhuang H, Alavi A. 18-fluorodeoxyglucose positron emission tomographic imaging in the detection and monitoring of infection and inflammation. Semin Nucl Med 2002;32(1):47–59.
45. Heiba SI, Luo JQ, Sadek S, et al. Attenuation correction induced artifact in F-18 FDG PET imaging following total knee replacement. Clin Positron Imag 2000;3:237–239.
46. Johnston SL, Lock RJ, Gompels MM. Takayasu arteritis: a review. J Clin Pathol 2002;55(7):481–486.

47. Angeli E, Vanzulli A, Venturini M, et al. The role of radiology in the diagnosis and management of Takayasu's arteritis. J Nephrol 2001;14(6):514–524.
48. Peters M. Nuclear medicine in vasculitis. Rheumatology 2000;39:463–470.
49. Jonker N, Peters AM, Gaskin G, et al. A retrospective study of granulocyte kinetics in patients with systemic vasculitis. J Nucl Med 1992;33: 491–497.
50. Reuter H, Wraight EP, Qasim FJ, et al. Management of systemic vasculitis: contribution of scintigraphic imaging to evaluation of disease activity and classification. Q J Med 1995;88:509–516.
51. Ussov WY, Peters AM, Savill J, et al. Relationship between granulocyte activation, pulmonary granulocyte kinetics and alveolocapillary barrier integrity in extrapulmonary inflammatory disease. Clin Sci 1996;91:329–335.
52. Gurwood AS, Malloy KA. Giant cell arteritis. Clin Exp Optom 2002;85(1): 19–26.
53. Blockmans D, Stroobants S, Maes A, et al. Positron emission tomography in giant cell arteritis and polymyalgia rheumatica: evidence for inflammation of the aortic arch. Am J Med 2000;108(3):246–249.
54. Blockmans D, Maes A, Stroobants S, et al. New arguments for a vasculitic nature of polymyalgia rheumatica using positron emission tomography. Rheumatology 1999;38(5):444–447.
55. Turlakow A, Yeung HW, Pui J, et al. Fluorodeoxyglucose positron emission tomography in the diagnosis of giant cell arteritis. Arch Intern Med 2001;161(7):1003–1007.
56. Hara M, Goodman PC, Leder RA. FDG-PET finding in early-phase Takayasu arteritis. J Comput Assist Tomogr 1999;23(1):16–18.
57. Meller J, Becker W. Nuclear medicine diagnosis of patients with fever of unknown origin. Nuklearmedizin 2001;40(3):59–70.
58. Peters AM. The use of nuclear medicine in infections. Br J Radiol 1998; 71(843):252–261.
59. Dreyer M, Borgwardt L, Reichnitzer C, et al. The role of whole body FDG-PET in pediatric patients with fever of unknown origin. J Nucl Med 2001;42:142.
60. Lorenzen J, Buchert R, Bleckmann C, et al. A search for the focus in patients with fever of unknown origin: is positron-emission tomography with F-18-fluorodeoxyglucose helpful? Rofo Fortschr Geb Rontgenstr Neuen Bildgeb Verfahr 1999;171(1):49–53.
61. Lorenzen J, Buchert R, Bohuslavizki KH. Value of FDG PET in patients with fever of unknown origin. Nucl Med Commun 2001;22(7):779–783.
62. Blockmans D, Knockaert D, Maes A, et al. Clinical value of [^{18}F]fluoro-deoxyglucose positron emission tomography for patients with fever of unknown origin. Clin Infect Dis 2001;32(2):191–196.
63. Meller J, Altenvoerde G, Munzel U, et al. Fever of unknown origin: prospective comparison of [^{18}F]FDG imaging with a double-head coincidence camera and gallium-67 citrate SPECT. Eur J Nucl Med 2000;27(11): 1617–1625.
64. Bicik I, Bauerfeind P, Breitbach T, et al. Inflammatory bowel disease activity measured by positron-emission tomography. Lancet 1997;350(9073): 262.
65. Skehan SJ, Issenman R, Mernagh J, et al. ^{18}F-fluorodeoxyglucose positron tomography in diagnosis of pediatric inflammatory bowel disease. Lancet 1999;354(9181):836–837.
66. Jacobson K, Mernagh JR, Green T, et al. Positron emission tomography in the investigation of pediatric inflammatory bowel disease. Gastroenterology 1999;116:A742(abstr).

67. Hannah A, Scott AM, Akhurst T, et al. Abnormal colonic accumulation of fluorine-18-FDG in pseudomembranous colitis. J Nucl Med 1996;37(10): 1683–1685.
68. Meyer MA. Diffusely increased colonic FDG uptake in acute enterocolitis. Clin Nucl Med 1995;20(5):434–435.
69. Kresnik E, Mikosch P, Gallowitsch HJ, et al. F-18 fluorodeoxyglucose positron emission tomography in the diagnosis of inflammatory bowel disease. Clin Nucl Med 2001;26(10):867(abstr).
70. Bakheet SM, Saleem M, Powe J, et al. F-18 fluorodeoxyglucose chest uptake in lung inflammation and infection. Clin Nucl Med 2000;25(4):273–278.
71. Jones HA, Clark RJ, Rhodes CG, et al. Positron emission tomography of 18FDG uptake in localized pulmonary inflammation. Acta Radiol Suppl 1991;376:148.
72. Yoon SN, Park CH, Kim MK, et al. False-positive F-18 FDG gamma camera positron emission tomographic imaging resulting from inflammation of an anterior mediastinal mass in a patient with non-Hodgkin's lymphoma. Clin Nucl Med 2001;26(5):461–462.
73. Goswami GK, Jana S, Santiago JF, et al. Discrepancy between Ga-67 citrate and F-18 fluorodeoxyglucose positron emission tomographic scans in pulmonary infection. Clin Nucl Med 2000;25(6):490–491.
74. Kapucu LO, Meltzer CC, Townsend DW, et al. Fluorine-18-fluorodeoxyglucose uptake in pneumonia. J Nucl Med 1998;39(7):1267–1269.
75. Croft DR, Trapp J, Kernstine K, et al. FDG-PET imaging and the diagnosis of non-small cell lung cancer in a region of high histoplasmosis prevalence. Lung Cancer 2002;36(3):297–301.
76. Goo JM, Im JG, Do KH, et al. Pulmonary tuberculoma evaluated by means of FDG PET: findings in 10 cases. Radiology 2000;216(1):117–121.
77. Liu RS, Shei HR, Feng CF, et al. Combined ^{18}F FDG and ^{11}C acetate PET imaging in diagnosis of pulmonary tuberculosis. J Nucl Med 2002; 43(5):127(abstr).
78. Ichiya Y, Kuwabara Y, Sasaki M, et al. FDG-PET in infectious lesions: the detection and assessment of lesion activity. Ann Nucl Med 1996; 10(2):185–191.
79. Gotway MB, Storto ML, Golden JA, et al. Incidental detection of thoracic sarcoidosis on whole-body 18-fluorine-2-fluoro-2-deoxy-D-glucose positron emission tomography. J Thorac Imag 2000;15(3):201–204.
80. Pitman AG, Hicks RJ, Binns DS, et al. Performance of sodium iodide based ^{18}F-fluorodeoxyglucose positron emission tomography in the characterization of indeterminate pulmonary nodules or masses. Br J Radiol 2000; 75(890):114–121.
81. Pitman AG, Hicks RJ, Kalff V, et al. Positron emission tomography in pulmonary masses where tissue diagnosis is unhelpful or not possible. Med J Aust 2001;175(6):303–307.
82. Brudin LH, Valind SO, Rhodes CG, et al. Fluorine-18 deoxyglucose uptake in sarcoidosis measured with positron emission tomography. Eur J Nucl Med 1994;21(4):297–305.
83. Yamada Y, Uchida Y, Tatsumi K, et al. Fluorine-18-fluorodeoxyglucose and carbon-11-methionine evaluation of lymphadenopathy in sarcoidosis. J Nucl Med 1998;39(7):1160–1166.
84. Gungor T, Engel-Bicik I, Eich G, et al. Diagnostic and therapeutic impact of whole body positron emission tomography using fluorine-18-fluoro-2-deoxy-D-glucose in children with chronic granulomatous disease. Arch Dis Child 2001;85(4):341–345.
85. O'Doherty MJ, Barrington SF, Campbell M, et al. PET scanning and the human immunodeficiency virus-positive patient. J Nucl Med 1997;38(10): 1575–1583.

86. Flinn IW, Ambinder RF. AIDS primary central nervous system lymphoma. Curr Opin Oncol 1996;8(5):37357–37366.
87. Heald AE, Hoffman JM, Bartlett JA, et al. Differentiation of central nervous system lesions in AIDS patients using positron emission tomography (PET). Int J STD AIDS 1996;7(5):337–346.
88. Villringer K, Jager H, Dichgans M, et al. Differential diagnosis of CNS lesions in AIDS patients by FDG-PET. J Comput Assist Tomogr 1995;19(4): 532–536.
89. Hoffman JM, Waskin HA, Schifter T, et al. FDG-PET in differentiating lymphoma from nonmalignant central nervous system lesions in patients with AIDS. J Nucl Med 1993;34(4):567–575.

14

Brain Tumors

Franklin C.L. Wong and E. Edmund Kim

Basic Considerations

In 2003, it is estimated that 18,300 new cases of primary brain and nervous system tumors will occur, with 13,100 deaths.[1] Every year approximately 35,000 adult Americans develop primary or metastatic brain tumors.[2] Central nervous system (CNS) tumors are the most prevalent solid tumors in children under 15 years of age, the second leading cancer-related cause of death after leukemia in children, and the third leading cancer-related cause of death in adolescents and adults between the ages of 15 and 35 years.[2] The majority of intracranial tumors occur in patients over the age of 45 years, and evidence suggests that the incidence of malignant gliomas among the elderly is increasing.[3]

About 16% of patients with brain tumors have a family history of cancer,[2] and various genetic disorders can predispose people to brain tumors. Chromosomal abnormalities include an increased number of copies of chromosome 7 or 22, and nonrandom losses associated with chromosomes 9p, 10p, 10q, and 17p.[4] Loss of chromosome 17p with or without *p53* gene alteration is seen in lower grades of astrocytoma,[5] loss of 9p appears to represent an intermediate event that occurs in most higher grade astrocytomas,[6] and loss of a portion of chromosome 10 is a late event seen primarily in glioblastoma multiforme tumors.[7] Patients with multifocal gliomas are more likely than other glioma patients to have germline cell *p53* mutations, to have a second malignancy, or to have other family members with cancer.[8]

Multiple deletions of chromosome 22 have been associated with meningiomas.[9] It has been postulated that such chromosomal losses may result in the deletion of tumor suppressor genes that normally inhibit tumorigenesis. In addition to chromosomal abnormalities, cytokine and receptor aberrations are also seen in brain tumors. Of cells that produce tumor growth factor, α cells are more often demonstrated in high-grade and more aggressive astrocytomas. Likewise, increased levels of epidermal growth factor receptors are seen in high-grade astrocytomas.[7]

Symptoms of intracranial tumors are produced primarily by the tumor mass itself, the surrounding edema, or the infiltration and destruction of normal tissue. The symptoms are headache, nausea and vomiting, behavioral and personality changes, slowing of psychomotor function, visual changes, and speech disturbances. Seizures are the presenting symptoms in only about 20% of patients. In most primary spinal axis tumors, symptoms and signs do not arise from parenchymal invasion, but from spinal cord and nerve root compression. Motor weakness is dominant with impairment of function at the affected levels. Radicular spinal syndrome presents as a sharp pain in the distribution of a sensory nerve root. Local paresthesia, impaired sensations of pain and touch, weakness, and muscle wasting are common. Intramedullary spinal tumors also produce syringomyelic dysfunction, destroying lower motor neurons, resulting in segmental muscle weakness, wasting, and loss of reflexes. Pain and temperature sensations are lost, but the sense of touch is preserved.

Pathology, Grading, Classification, and Diagnosis of Brain Tumors

Gliomas include astrocytomas, oligodendrogliomas, ependymomas, and mixed-type tumors. Astrocytomas are the most common type of malignant brain tumor in adults, accounting for 75% to 90% of such lesions. Histologically, astrocytomas are categorized as low-grade astrocytoma, mid-grade anaplastic astrocytoma, or high-grade glioblastoma multiforme.

Cell density, pleomorphism, anaplasia, nuclear atypia, mitoses, endothelial proliferation, and necrosis are used to grade astrocytomas.[10] The presence of necrosis differentiates anaplastic astrocytomas from glioblastoma multiforme.[11] Necrosis was found to be a significant predictor of short survival time.[12]

Low-grade gliomas constitute about 10% to 20% of all adult primary brain tumors. The majority are astrocytomas; approximately 5% are oligodendrogliomas or mixed oligoastrocytomas. They are well differentiated and lack all the cellular features (high cellularity, pleomorphism, mitoses, vascular endothelial proliferation, and necrosis) that characterize anaplastic glioma.

Much less common than the astrocytic tumors, oligodendrogliomas have a somewhat even peak incidence in people between the ages of 25 and 49 years. They tend to infiltrate the cerebral cortex more than do astrocytomas.[13] Clinically, these tumors present in the typical fashion of hemispherical astrocytomas in the frontal or temporal lobe. Ependymomas are tumors arising from cells of ependymal lineage. Sixty percent of intracranial ependymomas are infratentorial, and the fourth ventricle is the most common site.[14] Of the supratentorial ependymomas, 50% are primarily intraventricular.

Intraventricular tumors frequently cause increased intracranial pressure and hydrocephalus. As a result, most patients present with headache, nausea, vomiting, papilledema, and ataxia.

Medulloblastomas most likely originate from germinative neuroepithelial cells in the roof of the fourth ventricle. Most (50–60%) medulloblastomas occur in children 1 to 10 years old, with a peak between ages 5 and 9 years. Childhood medulloblastoma typically arises in the cerebellum, mostly in the midline and posterior veins. In adults, it typically arises in a cerebellar hemisphere. The risk of metastasis within the craniospinal intradural axis is relatively high.[15] Up to 30% of cases have positive cytology or myelographic evidence of spinal metastasis. Extra-CNS metastases occur in less than 5% of cases, and most metastases are to long bones. The overall disease-free 5-year survival rate for medulloblastoma is approximately 50%.[16]

Meningiomas arise from arachnoidal cells in the meninges. The majority of meningiomas are differentiated, with low proliferative capacity and limited invasiveness. Less commonly, meningiomas are more anaplastic, have a higher proliferative capacity, and are invasive. On CT and MRI scans, meningiomas are well-defined lesions that are easily enhanced with the contrast agent.[17] The major tumors occurring in the cerebellopontine angle are the acoustic nerve tumors and meningiomas. Acoustic neuromas or neurilemomas can originate on the cranial nerve VIII. Neurilemomas can compress cranial nerves V, VII, IX, and X. Acoustic schwannomas are more common among people in the fifth decade of life, but can occur earlier when they are associated with familial neurofibromatosis. Auditory and vestibular branch involvement occurred in 98% of the cases, facial weakness with disturbances of taste in 56%, and gait abnormality in 41%.[18]

Only about 1% of all non-Hodgkin's lymphomas are primary CNS lymphomas. Increased incidence of CNS lymphoma is correlated with the disappearance of intermediate-grade histology, suggesting a shift in the biology of the tumors.[19] Both AIDS-related and non–AIDS-related primary CNS lymphomas are frequently B-cell lymphomas of the histiocytic type. CNS lymphomas most often occur in men. It has been found that 52% of cases were supratentorial, 34% were multiple, 12% were cerebellar, 2% were in the brainstem, and less than 0.5% were spinal.[20] The contrast-enhanced computed tomography (CT) and magnetic resonance imaging (MRI) appearance of these lesions is sometimes distinctive. Multiple lesions and homogeneous enhancement or signal is suggestive of CNS lymphoma. Brain metastases occur in 25% to 35% of all cancer patients, of which approximately 15% are symptomatic. Eighty percent of brain metastases are supratentorial.[21] Most cerebral metastases originate from lung, melanoma, kidney, colon, soft tissue sarcoma, breast, and non-Hodgkin's lymphoma.

Meningeal carcinomatosis is found in 5% to 8% of patients with solid tumors.[22] The most common tumors to metastasize to the leptomeninges are lung, breast cancers, non-Hodgkin's lymphoma, melanoma, and genitourinary cancer. Mode of spread is via hematogenous seeding of the arachnoid. Direct examination of the spinal fluid (SF) for tumor cells is a common way to make a diagnosis, and MRI with gadolinium diethylenetriamine pentaacetic acid (Gd-DTPA) is helpful in the diagnosis.

MRI of Brain Tumors

Imaging studies play an important role in the diagnosis and anatomic localization of intracranial tumors and provide information about the morphology and pathology of these lesions. The advent of MRI scanning, with its multiplanar imaging capabilities, high inherent contrast sensitivity for normal neural tissue and pathologic processes, and availability of Gd-DTPA to characterize intracranial lesions further, has made this the primary imaging modality for assessing suspected brain tumors.[23]

Glioblastoma multiforme has a predilection for the white matter of the cerebral hemispheres, especially the frontal lobes, and frequently infiltrates extensively into adjacent lobes and deep structures. Invasion of the cortex, leptomeninges, and dura also occurs. The tumor is typically heterogeneous with focal areas of necrosis and hemorrhage centrally and often one or more cysts. There is usually a rim of viable tumor and extensive perifocal edema. The tumor on MRI[24] is usually large and often heterogeneous in intensity, producing hypointensity on T1-weighted images and hyperintensity on T2-weighted images (Fig. 14.1). Focal areas of acute hemorrhage or hemosiderin deposition are often best seen on gradient echo images, but may produce areas of marked hypointensity on T2-weighted images (less commonly hyperintensity on T1-weighted images). There are vasogenic edema and microscopic tumor infiltration of white matter tracts. These tumors usually demonstrate moderate heterogeneous contrast enhancement, but irregular thick rim or nodular enhancement is also seen (Fig. 14.1A). In tumors clinically in remission, the white matter changes seen on T2-weighted images are much more extensive than the volume of any residual tumor. In recurrent tumors, the abnormal signal intensity on T2-weighted images has been correlated with tumor extent.[25]

On MRI, low-grade diffuse fibrillary astrocytomas typically have well-defined margins and little associated edema or mass effect. They are usually superficial in location, and involvement of gray matter may be identified as thickening of the cortical mantle. They are fairly homogeneous, isointense to hypointense on T1-weighted images, and mildly hyperintense on T2-weighted images, with no necrosis or hemorrhage. Contrast enhancement patterns are variable.[24] Low-grade gliomas may present as discrete focal masses with smooth margins. Atypical (cystic) meningiomas may mimic low-grade gliomas on MRI. Gliomas may also mimic vasogenic edema or encephalomalacia when they infiltrate white matter tracts. Anaplastic astrocytomas are often heterogeneous with areas of necrosis and cystic formation. There is usually vasogenic edema of adjacent white matter, and more intense irregular contrast enhancement. MRI, with its high sensitivity for parenchymal lesions, detects more multifocal gliomas with the same signal characteristics as solitary tumors of similar grade. Gliomatosis cerebri is an extreme form of diffuse glioma characterized by diffuse glial overgrowth.[26]

Oligodendrogliomas are usually heterogeneous in signal intensity but predominantly isointense to gray matter on T1-weighted images

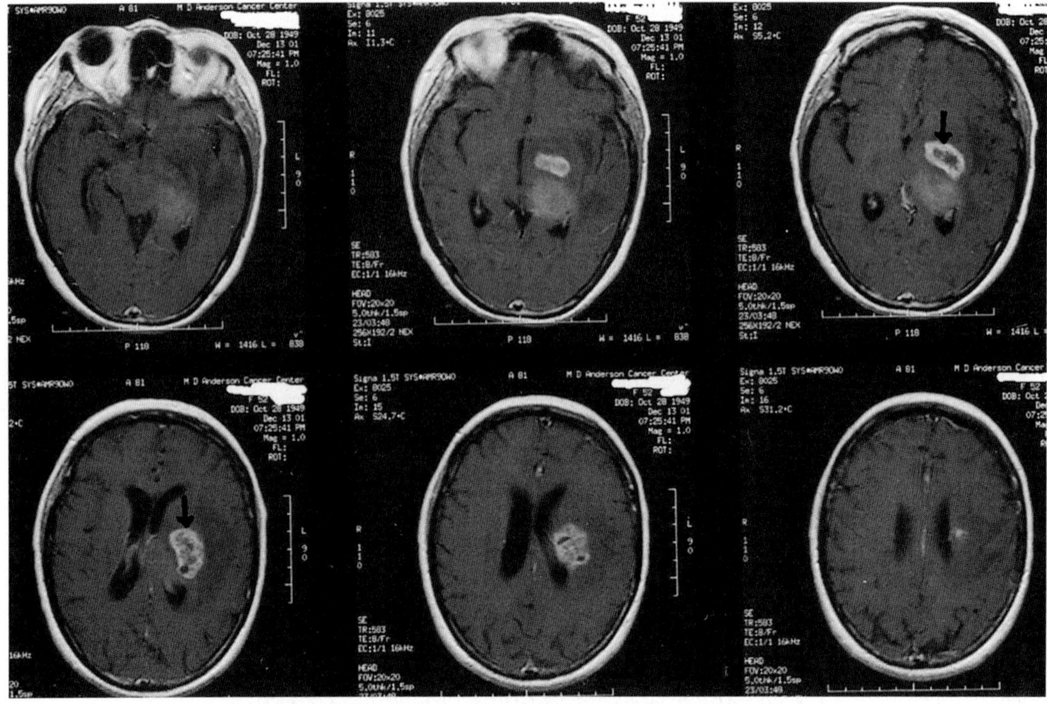

A

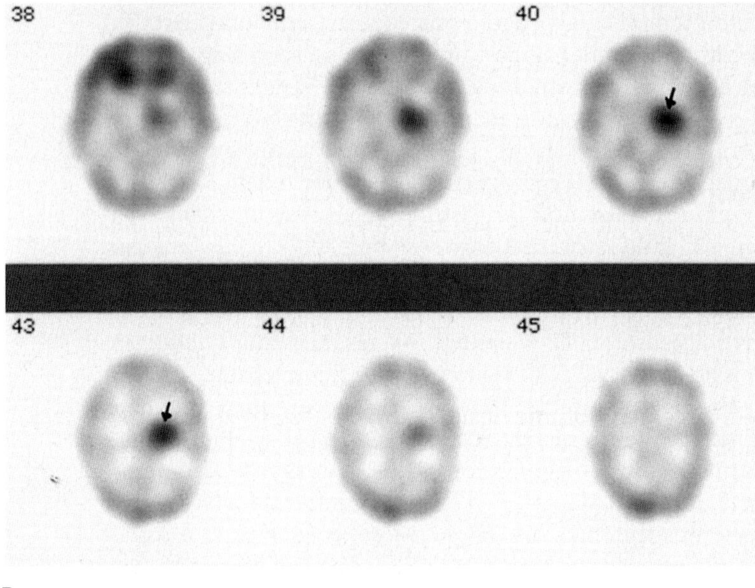

B

FIGURE 14.1. Transaxial MRI, Tl 201 SPECT, and FDG-PET images of the brain in a patient with glioblastoma multiforme. A: MRI of a patient with glioblastoma multiforme showing a large lesion in the left caudate with enhancement (*arrows*). B: Tl 201 SPECT scan showing markedly elevated uptake of Tl 201 in the left caudate (*arrows*), while there is mimimal uptake in the rest of the brain. C: ^{18}F-FDG-PET showing faintly increased uptake in the left caudate area (*arrows*), while other parts of the brain show variable and high uptake.

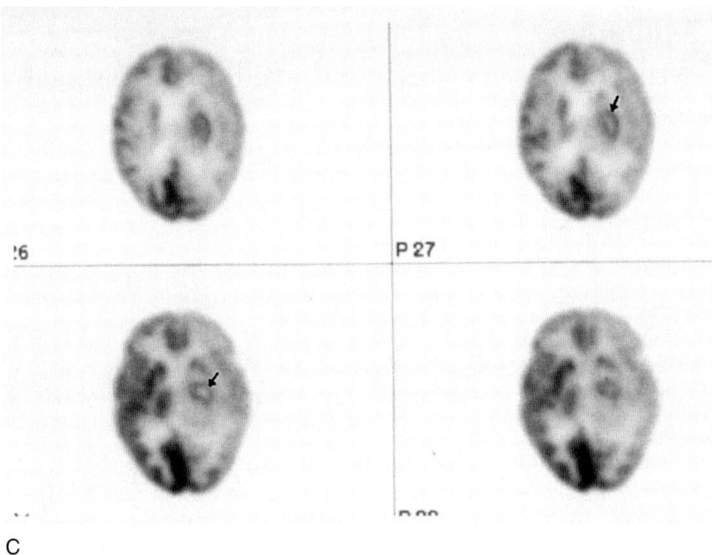

C

FIGURE 14.1. (continued)

and hyperintense on T2-weighted images. The heterogeneity reflects cystic change, blood products, and tumoral calcification. On MRI, choroid plexus papillomas are usually homogeneous and slightly hypointense to normal white matter on T1-weighted images and slightly hyperintense on T2-weighted images. These tumors are generally hyperdense on CT. Meningiomas tend to be nearly isotense to gray matter on all pulse sequences on MRI; 30% to 40% are mildly hypointense in T1-weighted images and mildly hyperintense on T2-weighted images. The presence of a dural tail shown as homogeneously enhancing dural thickening is highly suggestive. As with CT, enhancement of meningiomas is usually homogeneous and intense.

Lesions of primary CNS lymphoma tend to be hypointense to gray matter on T1-weighted images and hyperintense on T2-weighted images. There is a variable zone of abnormal high signal intensity on T2-weighted images surrounding the lymphomatous mass consisting of edema and infiltrating tumor cells. There is usually intense and homogeneous enhancement of the lesions on T1-weighted images.[27] Epidural metastases tend to be hypointense to brain on T1-weighted images and hyperintense on T2-weighted images. They usually demonstrate homogeneous enhancement. The blood–brain barrier does not exist for metastatic lesions because they elaborate their own vascular supply.[28] Contrast-enhanced MRI is the most sensitive method for assessing the cerebral metastasis.[29] On MRI, metastases are usually hypointense to isointense on T1-weighted images. On T2-weighted images, the solid components of metastases are usually isointense to gray matter. Hypointensity may be encountered in hemorrhagic or calcified lesions and sometimes in melanoma. The pattern of enhancement on MRI may vary from homogeneous to rim enhancing.

Reperfusion

The advent of rapid techniques greatly improved MRI tissue sensitivity and specificity without sacrificing its high spatial resolution, allowing the measurement of alterations in tissue perfusion and diffusion as well as other functional parameters. Functional MRI can provide information on tissue hemodynamics, water mobility, and diffusion in characterization of pathophysiologic brain conditions. A zone of nonfunctioning, but still viable tissue, surrounding the infarct (penumbra zone) may recover its function if blood flow can be restored.[30] Cell death may cause the demand for oxygen to fall and the oxygen tension to rise, and a biochemical cascade. Whatever the mechanism, reperfusion does not reestablish normal perfusion or blood volume, nor does it involve the normal number of perfused capillaries. In an acute reperfusion stage, blood flow and volume increase.[31] It appears that the greater the extent to which cell death has occurred, the more excessive the reperfusion. During reperfusion, the supply of oxygen often exceeds its demand, and postischemic increases in flow above normal levels may actually lead to increased tissue damage in the form of hemorrhage and edema. Moreover, the release of oxygen free radicals may increase during reperfusion and directly harm the tissue. The reactive hyperemia (increased flow and blood volume) following ischemia is of no immediate relation to cell viability or functional integrity. Diffusion-weighted MRI may be useful for the classification of malignant brain tumors. Microvascular perfusion, cell size, and distribution of water in the extravascular space may have impact on the measured apparent diffusion coefficient (ADC).[32] Diffusion-weighted imaging may prove informative in differentiating epidermoid tumors from extraaxial cysts.[33] Concepts in tumor biology point to the importance of tumor vascularity (angiogenesis) as critical in the regulation of tumor growth and malignant potential.[34] Expression of angiogenic growth factor genes in astrocytomas may contribute to their growth and progression. Measurement of tissue microvascular blood volume appears to be sensitive to the phenotypic expression of angiogenesis, particularly increased microvascular density.

In comparing MRI cerebral blood volume maps with positron emission tomography (PET) using carbon monoxide, the MRI maps were particularly sensitive for the microvasculature and relatively insensitive for larger vessels in the brain (Fig. 14.1B). It is not possible to make a differential diagnosis between high-grade and low-grade gliomas based on the measured ADC due to overlapping diffusion values.[32] The edema surrounding tumors has a higher diffusion coefficient than the surrounding normal brain tissue, while the necrotic areas of gliomas have a higher diffusion coefficient compared with the active tumor area. Low-grade gliomas are typically more homogeneous on MRI. Cerebral blood volume mapping may be useful when evaluating radiation necrosis, showing diminished cerebral blood volume. It also may be useful in guiding optimal sites for stereotactic biopsies.

Magnetic Resonance Spectroscopy

Magnetic resonance spectroscopy (MRS) can noninvasively measure numerous biochemicals and pH. Various pulse sequences have been used for single-voxel techniques, but the most commonly used technique is image-selected in vivo spectroscopy (ISIS).[35] The minimum spatial resolution or volume of interest is determined by signal-to-noise ratio and is about 50 mL. Echo-localized sequences are advantageous compared with the ISIS technique. The commonly used spin-echo technique is called point resolved spectroscopy (PRESS) or proton imaging of metabolites (PRIME).[36,37] Water suppression is typically performed using a water-eliminated Fourier transform (WEFT) or chemical shift selective (CHESS) sequence.[38] The advantage of stimulated-echo acquisition mode (STEAM) over PRESS is that it is technically much easier to acquire spectra. The minimum spatial resolution or volume of interest (VOI) is determined by the signal-to-noise (S/N) ratio and is about 1 mL.[38]

MR spectroscopic imaging combines the advantages of MRI and MR spectroscopy in that spectral information is obtained from multiple volume elements within a designated field of view (FOV).[39] Much pathology in the brain is multifocal, and tumors are not metabolically or anatomically homogeneous.

^{31}P-MRS can provide information concerning tissue energetics, phospholipid metabolism, and intracellular pH. An acute change in the PCr/Pi ratio is a sensitive measure of ischemia. Phosphomonoesters (PMEs) and phosphodiesters (PDEs) represent precursors to membrane synthesis and breakdown products, respectively. Changes in PME and PDE may be useful markers of cell proliferation. The pH can be determined by the chemical shift between Pi and PCr resonances. ^{1}H-MRS can provide information concerning neuronal density, membrane constituents, amino acid metabolism, and glycolysis. *N*-acetylaspartate (NAA) is a neuronal marker and is absent in glial cells.

The most common features of tumor spectra are decreased PDE, PDE/adenosine triphosphate (ATP) ratio, and decreased pH. ^{1}H-MRS has been more reliable, and tumor spectra are easily discerned from normal tissue by decreased NAA and increased Cho.[40] Increased inositols, Ala, Lac, and Lip and decreased Cr have been also reported.[41] Tumor cell death following treatments was characterized by increasing Pi and decreasing PME, PDE, and high-energy phosphates.[42] Lac is a specific marker of mitochondrial damage or relative hypoxia and not overt cell death. Late brain injury after radiation therapy is thought to arise from endothelial damage, which results in reduced regional blood flow to the treated areas. Early radiation damage can be detected by ^{1}H-MRS and may be useful for managing supportive therapies to prevent the progression to fatal injury. Highly depressed levels of NAA, Cho, and Cr with an intense, broad proton peak between 0 and 2 parts per million (ppm) were consistent with tissue necrosis. ^{31}P-MRS also showed depressed levels of all metabolites in the treated tumor region. ^{31}P-MRS of the infectious lesions showed a marked loss of phosphorus signal. The Lac/Cho ratio was also significantly elevated in patients with infection, while the NAA/Cho ratio was significantly depressed in patients with tumors. Multivoxel spectroscopy technique can define the extent of the tumorous tissues and characterize the peritumorous regions in biochemical terms, which may be useful for treatment planning.[43] MR spectroscopic imaging maps generally show that the tumor area has high Cho, low NAA, relatively normal Cr, and increased Lac. Ischemic tumor tissue can be seen on the Lac image. Metastases and glioblastomas had much higher Lac levels. The abnormalities shown by MRS imaging extended beyond the tumor as defined by MRI.

PET Introduction in Brain Tumors

In the study of patients with brain tumors, anatomic changes that are clinically significant occur starting at sizes of millimeters and the pathologic processes occurs at concentrations of submillimolar (mM or 10^{-3} M) levels. In fact, genetic aberrations and early subcellular injuries occur at subpicomolar (pM, or 10^{-12} M) ranges. Before imaging studies become available, the above events are usually identified on autopsy or by surgical biopsy followed by histochemistry and detailed microscopic examination. Imaging studies analyze the chemical signals of the brain and the tumors and display these signals along with their differences in spatial coordinates with good resolution. Evaluation of human brain tumors by imaging techniques therefore requires good spatial resolution of the anatomic details as well as sensitive signals reflecting the pathologic processes occurring at organic, cellular, and subcellular levels.

Traditional structural imaging modalities such as CT and MRI remain the primary study tools of human brain cancer because of their superior resolution, currently at submillimeter levels. The spatial resolution of CT and MRI are one magnitude better than the current PET resolution of 5 to 8 mm. Together with contrast enhancement techniques, CT or MRI provides anatomic as well as gross physiologic aberrations such as tumor mass, edema, and rupture of blood–brain barriers. These anatomic and gross pathologic changes occur at the molar (M) and mM ranges. The use of CT and MRI is limited by their current abilities to detect cellular or molecular alterations at concentrations below mM levels. On the other hand, current PET technologies detect molecular changes from molar (M) to subpicomolar ranges and is the only imaging modality to fill the large void left by CT or MRI, that is, from the cellular and subcellular events at the mM to pM levels. The study of human brain tumor using PET started in the 1970s. Gross pathology at the vascular level such as perfusion abnormalities were reported with ^{15}O-water PET.[44] Breakdown of blood–brain barriers was reported by Ga 68 PET.[45] Differential vascular responses between vessels in tumor versus brain were reported under adenosine pharmacologic stimulation using ^{15}O-water PET.[46] Vascular response to physiologic stimulation in a patient with brain tumor to identify motor or sensory representation in brain parenchyma has been used as a clinical tool for presurgical planning.[47] Down to the cellular level and subcellular level, the study of tumor regional perfusion, oxygen consumption and glucose utilization have been in the literature since the late 1970s.[48] In the 1980s, increased ^{18}F-fluorodeoxyglucose (FDG) uptake in gliomas were correlated with tumor grades.[49] Because of its uptake by the normal cerebral cortex, ^{18}F-FDG has remained the main tracer to study the brains of patients with and without tumors. Despite the popular use of FDG in PET study of brain tumors, the mechanism of FDG uptake remains to be fully understood. Likely explanations include increased hexose kinase activities,[50] increased uptake by surrounding macrophages,[51] and increased levels of glucose transporters.[52]

The search for specific tumor markers in imaging continues, with increasing emphasis on tumor-specific molecules such as essential amino acids (e.g., L-methionine),[53] nucleotides (thymidine),[54] and dopamine D2 receptors[55] and peripheral benzodiazepine receptors.[56] Because of the stringent technical requirements, most of these studies were conducted from a research perspective. The clinical use of this expensive PET technology that is not widely available often demands different considerations.

Clinical Utility of PET in Brain Tumors

Tumor grading and staging remains an important task of the clinical oncologist. There are earlier reports on correlation of glioma grades with ^{18}F-FDG-PET.[49] However, the acceptance of this notion varies. Often PET is not used to grade human brain tumor.

Because of limited availability of the short-lived tracers, which require a nearby cyclotron and rapid synthesis as well as quality assurance, clinical PET is available only to large academic medical centers. Furthermore, because of the inferior spatial resolution, PET is best positioned to study the brain tumor patients for whom CT and MRI offer little help. In fact, owing to the improved early diagnosis and treatment, brain tumor patients have improved survival, and, ironically, they have proved difficult for CT or MRI to evaluate. Since either the tumor or the treatment or both have altered the architecture of normal brain parenchyma, grossly abnormal CT/MRI signals such as contrast enhancement often remain regardless of whether there is recurrent tumor. This is the area in which PET remains most useful in the differentiation of recurrent brain tumor from posttreatment necrosis.

The most frequently used tracer in clinical PET is ^{18}F-FDG. When used to study patients with brain tumor, it poses a technical challenge. The tumor is expected to have higher uptake (and hence contrast) than the surrounding tissue without tumor. However, the gray matter in normal human cerebral cortex already has higher FDG uptake than the white matter and other tissues in the body (Fig. 14.1C). The contrast of the signal from the tumor versus the brain is thus decreased, leading to possibly lowered sensitivity. This problem may be overcome by the following technically simple schemes. First, the location of the hypermetabolic tumor helps identify tumors in the hypometabolic white matter. Second, comparison with prior studies may find a lesion with increasing uptake. Third, co-registration with anatomic imaging such as MRI reveals the exact locations of the lesions. Fourth, presentation of the images in standard uptake value (SUV) or other semiquantitative parameters helps to assess the contrast of the signals.

To be clinically useful, the results of the PET study should have a direct impact on the treatment plans. Most PET studies of brain tumors are concerned with primary brain tumors, for example, gliomas, because the findings may direct the subsequent treatment plans such as continuing chemotherapy, further surgery, or observation. Other tumors such as meningiomas and metastasis have been only scantily reported because the treatment plans are directed by surgery for meningioma. In the case of metastasis, therapy is directed by the treatment of the primary tumor. Furthermore, PET of both meningiomas and metastasis are reported to have variable uptake of FDG.[57] Therefore, the usefulness of FDG-PET in the routine clinical evaluation of brain tumors other than gliomas remains to be established. Although glioma refers to a group of brain tumors of varying grade, and there is an apparent trend of higher uptake with higher grade, there are very few studies further delineating the FDG uptake of the various gliomas.

There is a unique place for PET in the differentiation of recurrent tumor versus posttreatment necrosis because MRI of these posttreatment patients often reveals persistent contrast enhancement. On the other hand, necrotic tissues often have little FDG uptake, while tumor exhibits marked uptake. It has been found that immediately after radiation treatment, FDG uptake by brain and tumor may slightly increase, only to return to normal and then subnormal in a few weeks.[58] Furthermore, surgery and systemic steroids did not produce any significant FDG uptake change during the next few days. Since the chronic effect of radiation treatment on the normal brain is depressed perfusion and metabolism, the posttreatment effects are expected to enhance the tumor contrast on FDG-PET scans. This latter factor adds to the advantage of detecting tumor from the brain that has known high uptake of FDG. There is an argument that there are many micrometastases in a patient with primary glioma, and therefore distinction of tumor versus no tumor may not be very important because they are already in the entire brain, including the posttreatment necrotic tissues. One study has shown that the FDG uptake in a brain tumor tissue correlates with prognosis and survival.[59] Therefore, FDG uptake in the evaluation of posttreatment necrosis versus residual tumor is indeed important for the clinical management of brain tumor patients.

Although ^{11}C-methionine PET is mostly restricted to research studies, it is most promising as an alternative to ^{18}F-FDG-PET because there is minimal background activity in the brain; therefore, the lesions stand out with good contrast (Fig. 14.2). This technology, however, is limited by the requirement of very short synthesis time because of the short half-life of ^{11}C of 20 minutes. Occasionally, posttreatment necrosis also exhibits high uptake of the tracer.

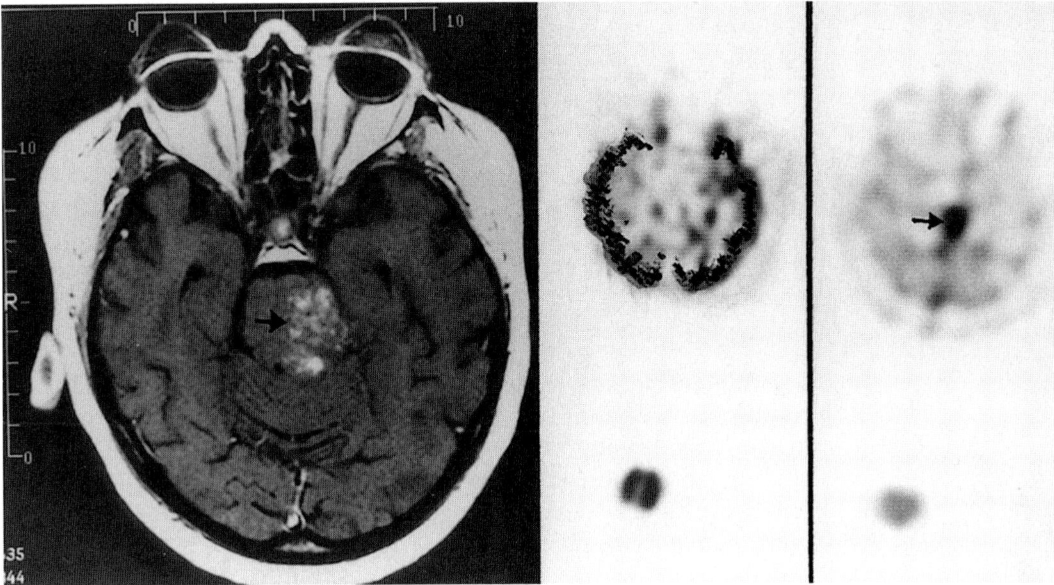

FIGURE 14.2. Transaxial MRI, FDG-PET, and ^{11}C-methionine images of the lower brain in a patient with brainstem glioma. Enhancement is noted on MRI in the left side of the brainstem (*arrow*). Variable and no distinct uptake of ^{18}F-FDG is found in the same area. ^{11}C-methionine PET shows markedly increased activity (*arrow*) in the brainstem confirming the glioma.

Practical Considerations in Clinical Use of PET to Evaluate Brain Tumor Patients

The patient's mental status and mood may be affected by the tumor, and therefore the patient may not understand or comply with instructions. The patient's ambulatory status as well as bowel and bladder control may require special attention. Usually, a PET scan session may not last more than an hour. In special occasions, repeated studies (e.g., with different positron tracers) may require large intervals between scans on the same day to allow for decay of the tracer from the earlier scan. To avoid excessive patient motion or to provide external co-registration with CT/MRI, the patient may be fitted with a thermoplastic mask with openings for the eyes, nose, and mouth. Again, close monitoring of these patients with brain tumor is necessary for a safe and successful scanning session.

To provide PET images useful to clinicians, the images should be available shortly after acquisition and presented in formats readily understood by clinicians. With such time and logistic constraints, some of the optimal theoretical requirements such as attenuation correction and blood sampling may be compromised. There is a current trend to present the PET images with an SUV color-coded format along with a color scale so that the SUV is readily discerned from the images.[60] A recent meta-analysis of FDG-PET indeed has supported the clinical utility in the staging and monitoring of brain tumors (Table 14.1).[61]

Since a sustainable clinical PET operation requires a steady and positive cash flow, payment for PET studies has become one of the major

Table 14.1. Meta-analysis of FDG-PET in the management of brain tumors

Purpose	Studies	Patient	Sensitivity	Specificity
Diagnosis	58	36	0.91	
Staging	31	31	0.86	
Recurrence	403	367	0.79	0.77
Monitor therapy	52	30	0.82	0.83
Others	34	34	0.93	0.67

determinants of its success. Meticulous planning and accurate accounting as well as prescan assurance of payments is crucial. Currently in the United States, PET studies for seven types of cancers (not including primary or secondary brain tumors) are reimbursable. Therefore, success also depends on good documentation and compliance with regulatory requirements.

PET as a Research Tool to Study Human Brain Tumors

The advantages of PET include absolute quantification of the tracers inside the body, or the head, on a pixel-to-pixel basis. With FDG-PET, it is possible to calculate the tracer or metabolite at micromolar concentrations for the region of interest. With other tracers such as ^{11}C-N-methylspiperone (NMSP) for D2 receptors in pituitary adenomas, it is even possible to quantify molecular events at picomolar levels. This level of precision in research requires meticulous attention to protocol details. Furthermore, it is necessary to calibrate the tracer activities measured on the image to the tracer activities measured in blood. For tracers that undergo metabolism during the scan duration, metabolites should also be accurately counted. Therefore, quantification of tracers in human brain tumors may require rigorous procedures such as arterial catheterization, accurate blood collection, readily accessible analytical tools such as high-performance liquid chromatography (HPLC), and labor-intensive computer iterations.

Perfusion PET studies of brain tumors typically involve ^{15}O-water, which has a high extraction coefficient by the brain and tumor tissues. However, because of the wide regional variation of perfusion within the gliomas, perfusion pattern itself is not of great research interest. However, the advantage of ^{15}O-water PET is apparent when repeated studies compare baseline study and studies under pharmacologic or physiologic stimulation.[46] The 2-minute half-life of ^{15}O allows multiple rapid successive testing while the patient is still in the scanner. When exact quantification or repeated scanning is not required, perfusion studies are mostly accomplished by the less expensive and more available SPECT with Tc-99m–labeled hexamethyl propylene amine oxime (HMPAO) or ethyl cysteinate dimer (ECD) as tracers.

For the identification of pathology at subcellular levels, ^{18}F-FDG remains the main thrust in the study of human brain tumors. Exact quantification requires arterial blood sampling to obtain the input function and invariably leads to patient discomfort. Alternatives include monitoring carotid or ventricular activities to estimate the input function. The uptake of FDG by brain or tumor is also affected by the insulin and glucose levels. Therefore, the glucose and postprandial status in patients should be controlled. In fact, the uptake of FDG by the brain has been found to be too large in variation because of technical factors routinely encountered in a clinical setting.[62] Enhanced FDG contrast in brain gliomas has also been reported by suppression of the baseline high cortical uptake under barbiturate coma.[63] Indeed, fasting improved the specificity of diagnosis of meningioma by suppressing gray-matter uptake.[64] Using contrast-enhanced MRI as the gold standard, FDG-PET was able to identify cerebral metastasis with a sensitivity of 75% and a specificity of 83% and a negative correlation with lesion sizes,[65] as demonstrated in Figure 14.3. Even though lesions are obvious on MRI or CT, metastastic tumors to the brain only demonstrate variable amount of FDG uptake and many are not obvious on FDG-PET. For patients with cerebral metastasis, whole-body FDG-PET scan was able to find the primary cancer in the body with a sensitivity of 79%.[66] After gamma-knife

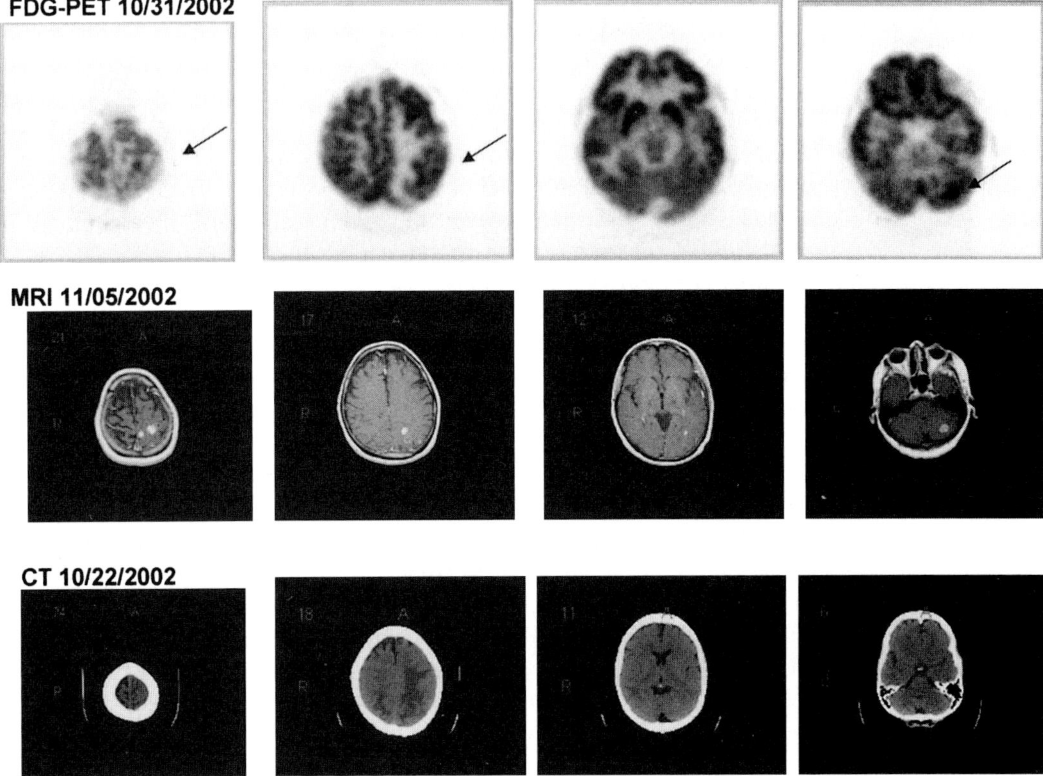

FIGURE 14.3. Transaxial FDG-PET, MRI, and CT images of the brain of a patient with cerebral metastasis from breast cancer. MRI images show multiple enhancing lesions in the left frontal, parietal, occipital, and right parieto-occipital lobes as well as left cerebellum; CT images show multiple areas of edema in corresponding areas; FDG-PET images demonstrate a hypermetabolism with increased activity only in the left parietal and cerebellar metastases (*arrows*).

local irradiation, neither the sensitive (100%) but nonspecific (65%) MRI nor the specific (93%) but nonsensitive (75%) FDG-PET is sufficient to differentiate tumor residuals/recurrence from necrosis.[67]

Some amino acid transporter levels are markedly elevated in tumors. The contrast of tumor to background in ^{11}C-methionine PET is higher than in FDG-PET because of the low uptake by normal brain parenchyma. The uptake of ^{11}C-methionine in tumor and brain tissues is suppressible by oral ingestion of L-phenylalanine. However, high uptake of ^{11}C-methionine has also been reported with radiation necrosis, which is less suppressible by oral L-phenylalanine, therefore providing a basis for distinction from tumors.[68] In fact, parallel study of FDG and ^{11}C-methionine PET has demonstrated concordant increases of these tracers in the anaplstic region of the gliomas but not in regions of necrosis.[69] An ^{18}F-labeled amino acid ^{18}F-α-methylthyrosine (FMT) has been found to culminate in brain tumors with an SUV higher than in normal brain tissues (2.8 versus 1.6).[70] ^{123}I-labeled iodomethyltyrosine, a SPECT tracer, has been shown to exhibit similar biologic characteristics and may prove to be a less expensive and widely available alternative to ^{11}C-methionine.[71]

Tumor tissues require large amount of nucleotides for replication of DNA, while nontumor tissues do not normally divide and do not concentrate nucleotides. ^{11}C-labeled thymidine PET has been reported to show high tumor uptake of the tracer.[54] However, ^{11}C-thymidine undergoes rapid hepatic metabolism and the ^{11}C label is typically cleaved from the molecule to join the general circulation, adding to a rising background activity over a few minutes. The cleavage rate depends to some degree on whether the ^{11}C label is in the 2 position or the 5 position. Nevertheless, multiple compartment kinetic modeling and measurement of metabolites are required for quantification. Iododeoxyuridine (IUDR) is another compound used to detect tumor because of the elevated thymidine kinase. When labeled with I 124, IUDR-PET has demonstrated elevated uptake in human gliomas in a pattern not identical to FDG or thallium SPECT.[72] However, it is also subject to rapid hepatic clearance with a serum half-life of 1.6 minutes. In preparation for Auger electron therapy using IUDR, PET imaging after intratumoral and intracavitary instillation of I 124 IUDR with and without degradation inhibitor into postsurgical glioma sites demonstrates only minimal retention of IUDR into the DNA.[73] Despite disappointing findings, this is an example of how PET can direct patient care and research.

Elevated dopamine D2 receptor has been reported in pituitary adenomas using ^{11}C-NMSP. A nonspecific increase in peripheral benzodiazepine receptor has also been reported using ^{11}C-PK14105.[56] However, the elevation of these receptors are not specific to the tumors and are observed in other cerebral pathologies such as schizophrenia and multiple sclerosis.

Conclusion

PET tracers have proved to be able to detect pathologic processes of brain tumors at the cellular and subcellular levels. This technology has largely remained a research tool. To be a useful clinical tool, PET has to continue to improve to provide speedy and accurate services and be user-friendly for clinicians. With advances from molecular sciences and instrumentation as well as software development, PET will certainly continue to provide useful information as research tools. To make PET a routinely useful clinical tool, efforts still need to be made to convince the public at large of its impact on the care of brain tumor patients.

References

1. Jamal A, Murray T, Samuels A, et al. Cancer statistics, 2003. CA Cancer J Clin 2000;53:5–26.
2. Mahaley MS Jr, Mettlin C, Natarajan N. National survey of patterns of care for brain-tumor patients. J Neurosurg 1989;71:826–836.
3. Grieg NH, Ries LG, Yancik R. Increasing annual incidence of primary malignant brain tumors in the elderly. J Natl Cancer Inst 1990;82:1621–1624.
4. Pershouse MA, Stubblefield E, Hadi A. Analysis of the functional role of chromosome 10 loss in human glioblastomas. Cancer Res 1993;53:5043–5050.
5. Lang FF, Miller DC, Koslow M. Pathways leading to glioblastoma multiforme: a molecular analysis of genetic alterations in 65 histocytic tumors. J Neurosurg 1994;81:427–436.
6. Bigner SH, Mark J, Burger PC. Specific chromosomal abnormalities in malignant human gliomas. Cancer Res 1988;48:405–409.
7. Wong AJ, Zoltick PW, Moscatello DK. The molecular biology and molecular genetics of astrocytic neoplasms. Semin Oncol 1994;21:126–138.
8. Kyritsis AP, Bondy ML, Xiao MI. Germline p53 gene mutations in subsets of glioma patients. J Natl Cancer Inst 1994;86:344–349.
9. Dumanski JP, Rouleau GA, Nordenskjold M. Molecular genetic analysis of chromosome 22 in 81 cases of meningioma. Cancer Res 1990;50:5863–5868.
10. Daumas-Dupont C, Scheithauer B, O'Fallon J. Grading of astrocytomas, a simple and reproducible method. Cancer 1988;62:2152–2157.
11. Bruner JM. Neuropathology of malignant gliomas. Semin Oncol 1994;21: 126–138.
12. Nelson JS, Tsukada Y, Schoenfeld D. Necrosis as a prognostic criterion in malignant supratentorial astrocytic gliomas. Cancer 1983;52:550–555.
13. de la Monte SM. Uniform lineage of oligodendroglioma. Am J Pathol 1989; 135:529–540.
14. Sawyer JR, Sammartino G, Husain M. Chromosome aberrations in four ependymomas. Cancer Genet Cytogenet 1994;74:132–138.
15. Deutsch M. The impact of myelography on the treatment results for medulloblastoma. Int J Radiat Oncol Biol Phys 1984;8:2023–2028.
16. Carrie C, Lasset C, Blay JY. Medulloblastoma in adults. Surgical and prognostic factors. Radiother Oncol 1993;29:301–307.
17. Murtagh R, Linden C. Neuroimaging of intracranial meningioma. Neurosurg Clin North Am 1994;5:217–233.
18. Jackler RK, Pitts LH. Acoustic neuroma. Neurosurg Clin North Am 1990; 1:199–204.
19. Miller DC, Hochberg FH, Harris NL. Pathology with clinical correlations of primary central nervous system non-Hodgkin's lymphoma. Cancer 1994;74:1383–1397.
20. Murray K, Kim L, Cox J. Primary malignant lymphoma of the central nervous system. J Neurosurg 1986;65:600–606.

21. Delathe JY, Krol G, Thaler HT. Distribution of brain metastases. Arch Neurol 1988;45:741–744.
22. Patchell RA, Posner JB. Neurologic complications of systemetic cancer. Neurol Clin 1985;3:729–750.
23. Brant-Zawadzki M, Badami P, Mills CM. Primary intracranial brain imaging. A comparison of magnetic resonance and CT. Radiology 1984;150:435–440.
24. Dean BL, Drayer BP, Bird CR. Gliomas: classification with MR imaging. Radiology 1990;174:411–415.
25. Johnson PC, Hunt SJ, Drayer BP. Human cerebral gliomas: correlation of postmortem MR imaging and neuropathologic findings. Radiology 1989;170:211–217.
26. Spagnoli MV, Grossman RI, Packer RJ. Magnetic resonance imaging of gliomatosis cerebri. Neuroradiology 1987;29:15–18.
27. Roman-Goldstein SM, Goldman DL, Howieson J. MR of primary CNS lymphoma in immunologically normal patients. AJNR 1992;13:1207–1213.
28. Healy ME, Hesselink JR, Press GA. Increased detection of intracranial metastases with intravenous Gd-DTPA. Radiology 1987;165:619–624.
29. Yuh WT, Engelken JD, Muhonen MR. Experience with high dose gadolinium MR imaging in the evaluation of brain metastases. AJNR 1992;13:335–345.
30. Hakim AM. The cerebral ischemic penumbra. Can J Neurol Sci 1987;14:557–559.
31. Crumrine RC, LaManna JC. Regional cerebral metabolites, blood flow, plasma volume and mean transit time in total cerebral ischemia in the rat. J Cereb Blood Flow Metab 1991;11:272–282.
32. LeBihan D, Turner R, Moonen CTW, et al. Imaging of diffusion and microcirculation with gradient sensitization: design, strategy and significance. J Magn Reson Imaging 1991;1:7–28.
33. Tsuruda J, Chew W, Moseley M, et al. Diffusion-weighted MRI of extraaxial tumors. Magn Reson Med 1991;19:316–320.
34. Weidner N, Semple JP, Welch WR, et al. Tumor angiogenesis and metastasis–correlation in invasive breast carcinoma. N Engl J Med 1991;324:1–8.
35. Ordidge RJ, Connelly A, Lohman JAB. Image-selected in vivo spectroscopy (ISIS). A new technique for spatially selective NMR spectroscopy. J Magn Reson 1986;66:283–294.
36. Bottomley PA. Spatial localization in NMR spectroscopy. Ann NY Acad Sci 1987;508:333.
37. Luyten P, Marien AJH, Heindel W. Metabolic imaging of patients with intracranial tumors. H-I MR spectroscopic imaging and PET. Radiology 1990;176:791–799.
38. Frahm J, Bruhn H, Gyngell ML. Localized high-resolution proton NMR spectroscopy using stimulated echoes: initial applications to human brain in vivo. Magn Reson Med 1989;9:79–93.
39. Maudsley AA, Hilal SK, Perman WH. Spatially resolved high-resolution spectroscopy by four-dimensional NMR. J Magn Reson 1983;51:147–152.
40. Alger JR, Frank JA, Bizzi A. Metabolism of human gliomas: assessment with H-1 MR spectroscopy and F-18 fluorodeoxyglucose PET. Radiology 1990;177:633–641.
41. Frahm J, Bruhn H, Hanicke W. Localized proton NMR spectroscopy of brain tumors using short echo time STEAM sequences. J Comput Assist Tomogr 1991;15:915–922.
42. Mattiello J, Evelhoch JL, Brown E. Effect of photodynamic therapy on RIF-1 tumor metabolism and blood flow examined ^{31}p and ^{1}H NMR spectroscopy. Nucl Magn Reson Biomed 1990;3:64–70.

43. Segebarth CM, Baleriaux DF, Luyten PR. Detection of metabolic heterogeneity of human intracranial tumors in vivo by ^{1}H NMR spectroscopic imaging. Magn Reson Med 1990;13:62–76.
44. Ito M, Lammertsma AA, Wise RSJ, et al. Measurement of regional cerebral blood flow and oxygen utilization in patients with cerebral tumors: analytical techniques and preliminary results. Neuroradiology 1982;23:63–74.
45. Yamamoto YL, Thompson CJ, Meyer E, et al. Dynamic positron emission tomography for study of cerebral hemodynamics in a cross section of the head using positron-emitting ^{67}Ga-EDTA and ^{77}Kr. J Comput Assist Tomogr 1977;1:43.
46. Baba T, Fukui M, Takeshita I, et al. Selective enhancement of intratumoral blood flow in malignant gliomas using intra-arterial adenosine triphosphate. J Neurosurg 1990;72(6):907–911.
47. Nariai T, Senda M, Ishii K, et al. Three-dimensional imaging of cortical structure, function and glioma for tumor resection. J Nucl Med 1997;38(10): 1563–1568.
48. Rhodes CG, Wise RJS, Gibbs JM, et al. In vivo disturbance of the oxidative metabolism of glucose in human cerebral gliomas. Ann Neurol 1983;14: 614–626.
49. Di Chiro G, De La Paz RL, Brooks RA, et al. Glucose utilization of cerebral gliomas measured by F-18 fluorodeoxyglucose and PET. Neurology 1982;32:1323–1329.
50. Weber G. Enzymology of cancer cells. N Engl J Med 1997;29:486.
51. Kubota R, Kubota K, Yamada S, et al. Active and passive mechanisms of F-18 fluorodeoxyglucose uptake by proliferating and prenecrotic cancer cells in vivo: a microautoradiographic study. J Nucl Med 1994;35:1067–1075.
52. Fulham MJ, Melisi JW, Nishimiya J, et al. Neuroimaging of juvenile pilocytic astrocytomas: an enigma. Radiology 1994;189(1):221–225.
53. Derlon J-M, Bourdet C, Bustany P, et al. C-11 L-methionine uptake in gliomas. Neurosurgery 1989;25(5):720–728.
54. Conti PS, Hilton J, Wong DF, et al. High performance liquid chromatography of carbon-11-labeled compounds. J Nucl Med 1994;21(8):1045–1051.
55. Yung BCK, Wand GS, Blevins L, et al. In vivo assessment of dopamine receptor density in pituitary macroadenoma and correlation with in vitro assay. J Nucl Med 1993;34(5):133.
56. Pappata S, Cornu P, Samson Y, et al. PET study of carbon-11-PK-11195 binding to peripheral type benzodiazepine sites in glioblastoma: a case report. J Nucl Med 1991;32(8):1608–1610.
57. Lichtor J, Dohrmann GJ. Oxidative metabolism and glycolysis in benign brain tumors. J Neurosurg 1987;67:336–340.
58. Valk PE, Budinger TF, Levin VA, et al. PET of malignant cerebral tumors after interstitial brachytherapy. J Neurosurg 1998;69:830–838.
59. Holzer T, Heerholz K, Jeske J, et al. FDG-PET as a prognostic indicator in radiochemotherapy of glioblastoma. J Comput Assist Tomogr 1993;17(5): 681–687.
60. O'Doherty MJ, Barrington SF, Campbell M, et al. PET scanning and the human immunodeficiency virus-positive patient. J Nucl Med 1997;38(10): 1575–1583.
61. Gambhir SS, Czernin J, Schwimmer J, et al. A tabulated summary of the FDG PET literature. J Nucl Med 2001;32:1S–93S.
62. Camargo EE, Szabo Z, Links JM, et al. The influence of biological and technical factors on the variability of global and regional brain metabolism of 2-F-18-fluoro-2-deoxy-D-glucose. J Cerebral Blood Flow Metab 1992;12: 281–290.

63. Blacklock JB, Oldfield EH, Di Chiro G, et al. Effect of barbiturate coma on glucose utilization in normal brain versus gliomas. J Neurosurg 1987; 67:71–75.
64. Cremerius U, Bares R, Weis J, et al. Fasting improves discrimination of grade 1 and atypical or malignant meningioma in FDG-PET. J Nucl Med 1997;38(1):26–30.
65. Rohren E, Provenzale J, Barboriak, et al. Screening for cerebral metastases with FDG-PET in patients undergoing whole-body staging of non-central nervous system malignancy. Radiology 2003;226(1):181–187.
66. Jeon H-J, Chung J-K, Kim Y-K, et al. Usefulness of whole-body F-18 FDG PET in patients with suspected metastatic brain tumors. J Nucl Med 2002;43(11):1432–1437.
67. Bělohlávek O, Šimonová G, Kantorová I, et al. Brain metastases after stereotactic radiosurgery using the Leksell gamma knife: can FDG PET help to differentiate radionecrosis from tumour progression? Eur J Nucl Med 2003;30:96–100.
68. O'Tuama LA, Phillips PC, Strauss LC, et al. Two-phase C-11 L-methionine PET in childhood brain tumors. Pediatr Neurol 1990;6(3):163–170.
69. Goldman S, Levivier M, Pirotte B, et al. Regional methionine and glucosse uptake in high-grade gliomas: a comparative study on PET-guided stereotactic biopsy. J Nucl Med 1997;38:1459–1462.
70. Inoue T, Shibasaki T, Oriuchi N, et al. F-18 a-methyl tyrosine PET studies in patients with brain tumors. J Nucl Med 1999;40(3):399–405.
71. Weber W, Bartenstein P, Gross MW, et al. Fluorine-l8-FDG PET and iodine-123-IMT SPECT in the evaluation of brain tumors. J Nucl Med 1997;38(5):802–808.
72. Tjuvajev JG, Macapinlac HA, Daghighian F, et al. Imaging of brain tumor proliferative activity with iodine-131-iododeoxyuridine. J Nucl Med 1994; 35(9):1407–1417.
73. Roelcke U, Hausmann O, Merlo A, et al. PET imaging drug distribution after intratumoral injection: the case for I-124 iododeoxyuridine in malignant gliomas. J Nucl Med 2002:43(11):1444–1451.

15

Head and Neck Tumors

Franklin C.L. Wong and E. Edmund Kim

In the United States, head and neck cancers account for 3.0% (39,400) of all new cancers and 2.0% (11,200) of cancer deaths.[1] The disease is more common in many developing countries. The incidence of head and neck cancer increases with age; most patients are older than age 50. The male-to-female ratio is approximately 3:1, and the African-American population has experienced a significant increase.[2] The greatest risk factor is tobacco use. It has been shown that heavy smokers have a five- to 25-fold higher risk of head and neck cancer than nonsmokers. The use of smokeless tobacco is strongly associated with the formation of premalignant oral lesions (hyperkeratosis, epithelial dysplasia), at rates ranging from 16% to 60%.[3] Dietary factors seem to play a role in the risk of oral and pharyngeal cancers. Epidemiologic studies have shown an increased risk of cancer in individuals whose diets lack sufficient quantities of nutrients. Mutagen sensitivity has been shown to be a strong independent risk factor for the development of head and neck cancer and seems to have a multiplicative interaction with smoking. Epstein-Barr virus (EBV) is associated with nasopharyngeal carcinoma (NPC). The EBV viral genome has been found in NPC tissue. Most patients with NPC show evidence of an elevated serum titer of immunoglobulin G (IgG) and IgA antibodies against viral capsid antigen.[4] The association of NPC and EBV is particularly strong in patients with endemic undifferentiated carcinoma.[5] Human papilloma virus, especially types 16 and 18, and herpes simplex virus type I have been detected in the sera and tumor tissues of patients with head and neck cancer.[6]

Multiple independent tumor cells may arise and progress in the same patient in a process known as field cancerization. Metachronous second primary tumors develop at a constant rate of 4% to 7%.[7] Tumorigenesis in the aerodigestive tract is a multistep process of genetic damage caused by continuous exposure to carcinogens. Specific genetic alterations include the activation of oncogenes, the inactivation or mutation of tumor-suppressor genes, and the amplication of growth factors and their receptors. Multiple allelic abnormalities (3p, 9p, 11q, 13q, and 17p) have been documented, and they appear to have prognostic value.[8] The cyclin *D1* gene, also known as *PRAD-1*, *bcl-1*, or *CCND-1*, is located on chromosome 11g13 and amplified in 30% to 50% of patients with head and neck cancers. Overexpression and amplification of cyclin *D1* has also been associated with more advanced disease, more rapid and frequent recurrence of disease, and shortened survival.[9] Mutations and overexpression of the tumor-suppressor gene *p53*, located on the short arm of chromosome 17, occur in 40% to 60% of cancer patients and have been associated with a poor prognosis.[10] Tumors with *p53* mutations recurred at a median time of 6 months, compared with a median time to recurrence of 17.4 months for tumors without mutations.[11] Thirty-eight percent of the patients with *p53*-positive margins relapsed, compared with none of the 12 patients found by polymerase chain reaction to have all tumor margins free of *p53* mutations.[12] Mutation of *p53* has been associated with tobacco and alcohol use, found in 58% of cigarette smokers who also used alcohol. Among patients who smoked but did not drink alcohol, 33% had mutations, whereas only 17% of the patients who neither smoked nor drank alcohol showed mutations of the *p53* gene.[13] Epidermal growth factor receptor (EGFR) is a staging criterion for head and neck cancers based on the tumor-node-metastasis (TNM) system, and primary (T) tumor staging is complex, varying with each primary subsite.

Epidermal growth factor receptor is a cellulose oncogene likely to play a role in head and neck tumorigenesis. Its genetic amplification and overexpression have been demonstrated in preinvasive and invasive lesions.[14] Anti-EGFR monoclonal antibodies upregulate EGFR and may prove useful in enhancing chemotherapeutic efficacy. Proliferating cell nuclear antigen (PCNA) is a nuclear protein whose expression, associated with DNA synthesis, increased 4- to 10-fold as tissue progressed from adjacent normal epithelium to squamous cell carcinoma.[15] Similarly, a high expression of transforming growth factor alpha was also documented to be a strong mitogenic factor, capable of inducing epithelial proliferation.

More than two thirds of patients with head and neck cancer present with stage III or IV disease. For patients with early-stage (I or II) disease, surgery or radiotherapy is used with curative intent. In patients with stage III disease and most patients with stage IV disease, surgery followed by radiation therapy is considered standard care. Despite optimal local therapy, more than 50% of patients with stage III and IV disease develop local or regional recurrence, and nearly 30% develop distant metastases. Chemotherapy is under intense study in locally advanced disease, with promising results.

Cancers of the head and neck include a great variety of tumors, specifically those involving the upper aerodigestive tract. Head and neck cancers originate in the area under the base of the skull to just below the larynx in a cephalocaudal orientation and by the nasal cavity and vermilion border of the lips, anteriorly, to the pharynx, posteriorly. Greater than 90% of head and neck cancers are squamous carcinomas. There are three histopathologic subtypes of nasopharyngeal cancer (NPC): type 1, differentiated squamous cell carcinoma; type 2, nonkeratinizing squamous cell carcinoma; and type 3, undifferentiated or lymphoepithelioma.[16] About 50% to 75% of NPCs in the United States are type 1 or 2, whereas in Asian and African areas, type 3 NPC predominates.

Most patients present with symptoms and signs of locally advanced disease that vary according to the subsite in the head and neck. Sinusitis, unilateral nasal airway obstruction, and epistaxis may be early symptoms of cancer of the nasal cavity and paranasal sinus. Persistent hoarseness demands visualization of the larynx. Otitis media that remains unresponsive to antibiotics may indicate a nasopharyngeal tumor. Chronic dysphagia or odynophagia may be the presenting symptom of oropharyngeal or hypopharyngeal cancer. Supraglottic laryngeal tumors rarely present early symptoms. The location of adenopathy provides clues to the specific subsite of head and neck primary tumors. Subdigastric adenopathy suggests primary cancer of the oral tongue or oropharynx, and posterior cervical adenopathy is a frequent result of regional spread of a nasopharyngeal tumor. Leukoplakia and high-risk erythroplakia are the common premalignant lesions in the head and neck. Up to 40% of cases of dysplastic oral leukoplakia transform into invasive carcinoma. Epstein-Barr virus (EBV) DNA is found in nasopharyngeal carcinoma, and identification of EBV DNA in the lymph node may suggest a tumor of nasopharyngeal origin.[17] Patients who present with a suspicious neck mass should undergo a flexible fiberoptic nasopharyngoscopy or indirect laryngoscopy. A panendoscopy is the definitive diagnostic and staging procedure. Multiple biopsies of any visualized abnormalities or blind biopsies of random areas are performed to define the extent of the disease. If no primary site is found, fine-needle aspiration of the lymph node is performed to establish the diagnosis.

Staging criteria for head and neck cancers are based on the tumor-node-metastasis (TNM) system, and primary tumor (T) staging is complex, varying with each primary subsite.

Prognosis of head and neck cancers is influenced by many factors including tumor grade, size, site, vascularity, lymphatic drainage, host immune response, patient age, sex, national origin, and performance status. Differentiation grade has not been consistently accurate in reflecting the biologic aggressiveness of squamous cancer.[18] Better-differentiated tumors that produce more keratin are thought to be less likely to metastasize. Englarged, hyperchromatic nuclei are associated with less differentiated tumors. Enlarged nuclear size and staining presumably reflects chromosomal abnormalities and increased DNA content. Increased frequency of mitoses in 50% to 70% of squamous cancers has been associated with poor prognosis.[19] Features reflecting aggressive cancer include lymphatic invasion, perineural invasion, lymph node metastases, and penetration of tumor through the capsule of involved lymph nodes. Extracapsular spread has been associated with high rates of distant metastasis.

Diagnosis of Head and Neck Tumors

Two to 5 days after laryngoscopy with anesthesia, magnetic resonance imaging (MRI) should be performed to produce images ranging from the oral cavity to the caudal thyroid border. MRI is a highly sensitive and specific imaging technique for laryngeal and hypopharyngeal tumor staging.[20] Any soft tissue between the cricoid cartilage and the airway may represent subglottic carcinoma or extension. Thyroid adenomas may appear brighter than normal thyroid tissue on T1-weighted images, possibly related to hemorrhagic degeneration. Thyroid carcinomas show T1 and T2 prolongation, and MRI tissue characterization is useful in distinguishing posttreatment fibrosis with short T2 relaxation time from recurrent cancer. Parathyroid adenomas tend to have longer T2 relaxation times than thyroid adenomas. Discrimination between adenomas and hyperplasia is not possible by MRI.[21] Metastatic nodes at times show contrast enhancement in the rim. MRI has an advantage over computed tomography (CT) in the differentiation of lymphadenopathy with various slice orientations and gradient echo techniques revealing vessels.[22] MR angiography allows excellent depiction of the carotid vessels, and is indicated to evaluate vascular displacement or compression by tumor growth, and tumor perfusion.

Early experience with in vivo magnetic resonance spectroscopy (MRS) has shown its potential for obtaining biochemical information, thus enhancing the diagnostic sensitivity of MRI studies.[23] The mean in vitro proton MRS Cho/Cr ratio was significantly higher in tumor than in normal tissue. All in vivo tumor Cho/Cr ratios were greater than the calculated mean in vitro tumor ratio, whereas six of seven volunteers had no detectable Cho and Cr resonance. The data also revealed that a variety of amino acids have a significantly greater likelihood of being detected in tumor than in normal tissues.[24]

PET in Head and Neck Tumors

Head and neck tumors, either primary or metastatic, have been studied with positron emission tomography (PET) using ^{18}F-fluorodeoxyglucose (FDG) for viability, ^{11}C-methionine for amino acid transport, ^{11}C-thymidine for proliferation, as well as ^{18}F-fluoromisonidazole for hypoxia. The apparent advantages of these agents are that the background tracer uptake is usually low and they provide higher specificity. The use of ^{18}F-FDG is the most common because FDG is relatively easier to obtain from cyclotron facilities, and there are well-established quick synthetic procedures.

FDG-PET

The issue of heterogeneous tumor uptake continues to affect the interpretation of FDG-PET because FDG uptake has been correlated with cytometric proliferation indexes to various degrees but not with the perfusion rate of the tumor.[25] In a recent meta-analysis of studies published between 1993 and 1994, the sensitivity of FDG-PET for the detection of primary tumors was 96%. For the detection of lymph node and metastasis, the sensitivity and specificity were 88% and 93%, respectively, and for the differentiation of recurrent tumor from posttreatment changes, 94% and 82%, respectively.[26] The accuracy of FDG-PET is better than that of either CT or MRI in all of the above

TABLE 15.1. **Meta-analysis of FDG-PET in the management of head and neck cancers**

Purpose	Studies	Patient	Sensitivity	Specificity
Diagnosis	193	298	0.93	0.70
Staging	468	591	0.87	0.89
Recurrence	426	511	0.93	0.83
Monitor therapy	128	169	0.82	0.95

applications. Prospective studies of FDG-PET of primary head and neck tumor found sensitivity and specificity of 67% and 100%, respectively, while CT or MRI was accurate in seven of 13 patients.[27] A more detailed analysis of the different applications of FDG-PET in the management of head and neck cancer is given in Table 15.1.[28]

A study of 13 patients with unknown primary head and neck tumors found four of five tumors, failed to detect one, and correctly excluded tumors in eight patients.[29] In patients with untreated lymphomas, a higher uptake (differential uptake ratio, DUR) of FDG was correlated with a worse survival rate.[30] These findings are similar to the conclusion of another study in the evaluation of benign versus malignant lesion using a DUR of 4.0 to distinguish the lesions.[31] For the

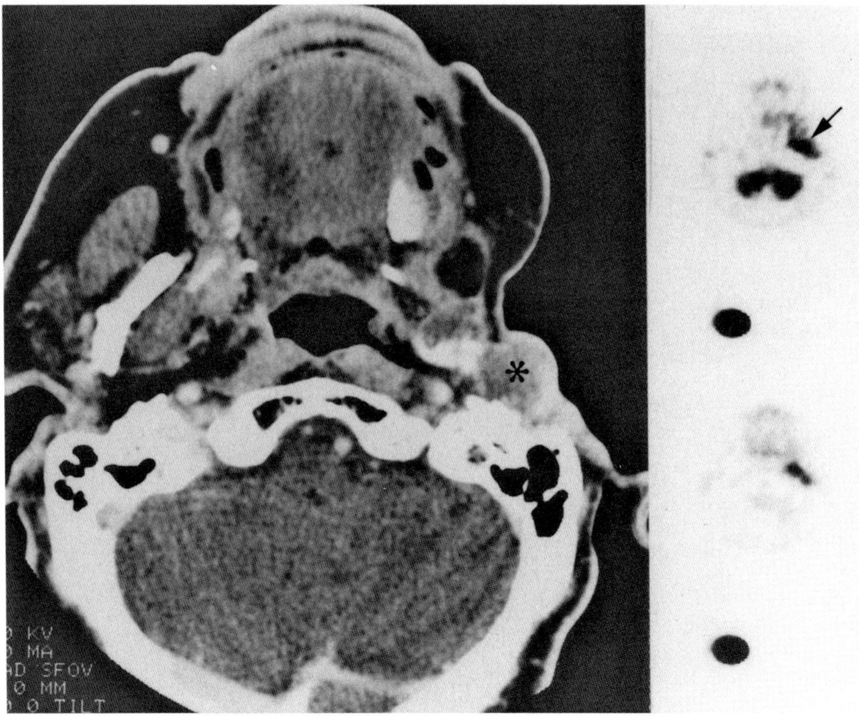

FIGURE 15.1. Selected axial FDG-PET images of the lower head (*right*) demonstrating a hypermetabolism with focal increased activity in the left parotid area of the postsurgical field (*arrow*) after surgical resection and was later confirmed to be recurrent squamous cell carcinoma. Axial CT image of lower head (*left*) shows a nodular enhanced lesion (*).

more difficult case of differentiating recurrent laryngeal tumor from posttreatment changes when clinical observations and conventional imaging (CT/MRI) did not provide a clear-cut distinction, FDG-PET was found to have a sensitivity of 67% and specificity of 57%[32] (Fig. 15.1). More quantitative evaluation will require multiple blood sampling and calculating the regional metabolic rates. In fact, regional metabolic rates indeed detect recurrent head and neck tumors better than the semiquantitative measures such as standard uptake value (SUV) (Figs. 15.2 and 15.3), an analogous index to DUR.[33] When used to study the course of chemotherapy of head and neck tumor, FDG-

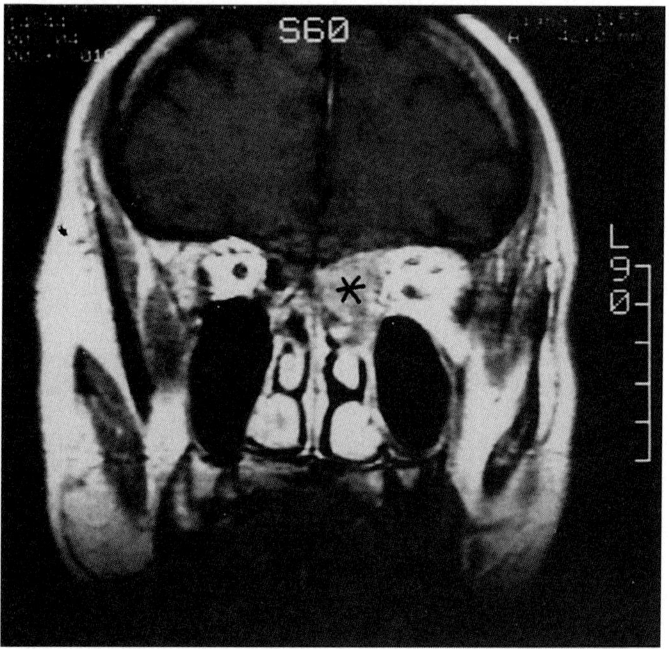

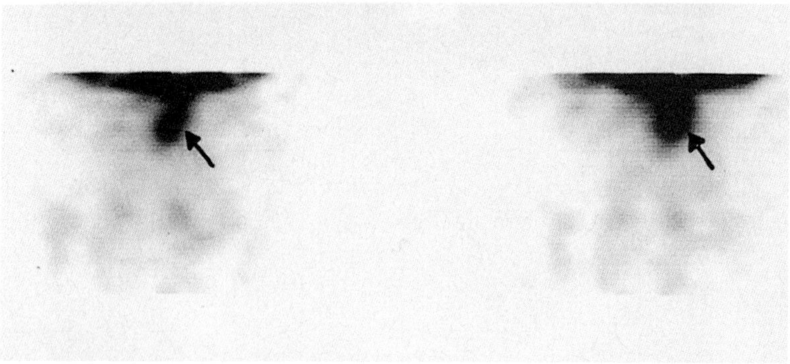

FIGURE 15.2. Selected coronal MRI (*upper*) and FDG-PET images (*lower row*) of the head of a patient with osteosarcoma invading the left sphenoid sinus with contrast enhancement (*) and focal increased uptake (*arrows*), respectively. The maximum standard uptake value (SUV) was 10.9 in the left sphenoidal lesion.

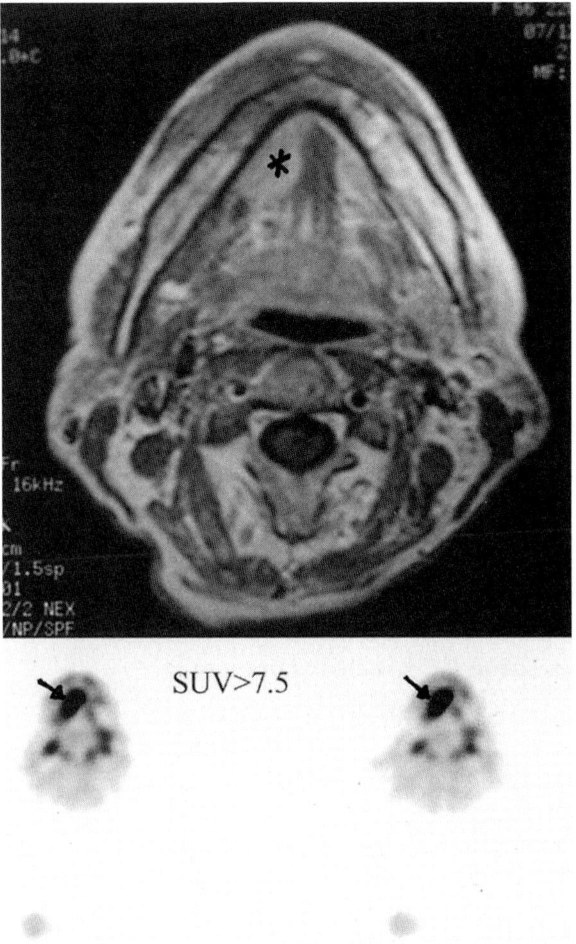

FIGURE 15.3. Selected transaxial contrast images of the floor of mouth showing subtle contrast enhancement (*) on T1-weighted MRI (*upper*) and hypermetabolism with focal increased activity (*arrrows*) on FDG-PET (*lower row*) with a maximum SUV of 7.5 on the right side. The tumor was found to be a squamous cell cancer by biopsy.

PET demonstrates a general trend of decreased uptake after treatment and may be a good indicator to correlate with clinical response.[34] When applied to evaluate cervical lymph nodes of head and neck squamous cell cancer, FDG-PET identifies tumor involvement with a sensitivity of 93% and specificity of 82%.[35] With papillary thyroid cancers, the SUV rises with tumors but remains steady over time with benign lesions.[36] FDG-PET also identifies thyroid cancer metastasis with a sensitivity of 94%, significantly higher than that of thyroglobulin.[37] Even with thyroid cancer patients showing negative ^{131}I thyroid cancer studies, FDG-PET reveals hypermetabolic lesions at a better accuracy, which correlates with a rising thyroglobulin level.[38] The primary head and neck cancer lesions are identified by FDG-PET with sensitivity of

100% and specificity of 89.5%, and the 3-year survival rate is 73% for those with SUVs below the median versus 22% for those below the median SUV of 9.0.[39] As a follow-up study to evaluate combined intraarterial chemotherapy and radiotherapy, FDG-PET has demonstrated a better specificity (89.5% vs 41.2%) to identify residual tumors than MRI has in head and neck cancers.[40]

A more recent development is the co-registration algorithms to correlate anatomic and functional images. In a study of 30 preoperative patients, co-registration of CT or MRI to FDG-PET improves the accuracy to 97% and 100%, respectively. The results are better than with either CT (69%) or MRI (80%) alone, and altered management in seven of the 30 patients.[41] This approach, however, is technically demanding because of the requirement of manipulation of images of different types. Furthermore, the flexible contours of the neck may not permit exact registration of the two types of images, which are typically acquired at different times or on different days. This latter impediment may require the use of thermoplastic molding for the head and neck, which in turn may cause discomfort to these patients who have ailments in the same region.

PET Studies Using ^{11}C-Labeled Compounds

Owing to the short half-life of ^{11}C, clinical studies require close proximity to the imaging facilities and expeditious synthesis. Therefore, these types of PET studies are carried out only in specialized academic centers.

^{11}C-methionine uptake by tumors is presumed to be mediated by neutral amino acid transporters. For tumors larger than 1.0 cm, ^{11}C-methionine PET detected 91% of the malignant head and neck lesions. No correlation was found between the histologic tumor grade and ^{11}C uptake in 30 patients with squamous tumors.[42] The results are comparable to those of FDG in patients who underwent both ^{11}C-methionine PET and FDG-PET.[43] Probably through splanchic shunting and competition at the level of neutral amino acid transporter mechanisms, the tumor uptake of ^{11}C-methionine is subject to significant suppression from food in a nonfasting state.[44] When used to follow the response of head and neck tumor to radiotherapy, ^{11}C-methionine PET shows a markedly lower range of SUV (1.9) in those patients with histologic response, while those with no histologic response had statistically significant higher SUVs (4.1).[45] ^{11}C-methionine is also found to deposit in thyroid gland with SUV of 3.2; with hyperparathyroidism, an SUV of 3.9 is noted in the parathyroid tissues, even though no tumor is identified (Fig. 15.4).[46]

^{11}C-thymidine uptake by tumors has been correlated with the degree of malignancy and the proliferation indexes as well as cells in the S phase during the cell cycle. Depending on the 2 or 5 position of the ^{11}C label, ^{11}C-thymidine undergoes different degrees of rapid metabolism, presumably by the liver, leading to ^{11}C labels released into the general circulation and thus decreasing the signal-to-noise ratio in the tumor. It has been demonstrated that in 13 patients within 10 to 30

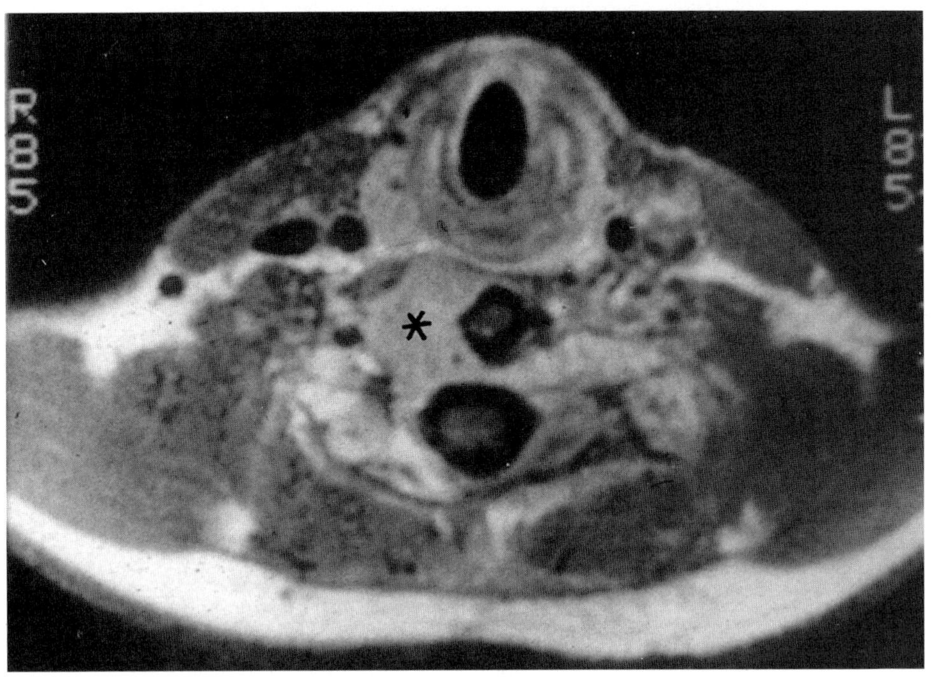

A

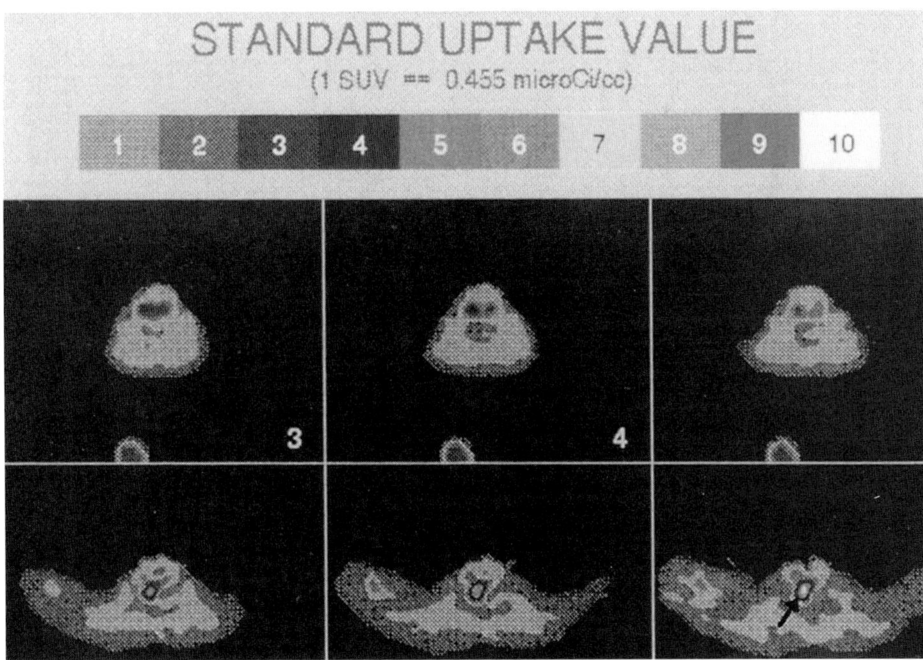

B

FIGURE 15.4. A: Selected transaxial MRI image of the neck in a patient with contrast-enhanced right laryngeal mass (*). B: Selected transaxial PET images of the neck showing a lesion with a focal increased uptake (*arrow*) of ^{11}C-methionine in the right larynx. This lesion was subsequently found to be giant cell tumor.

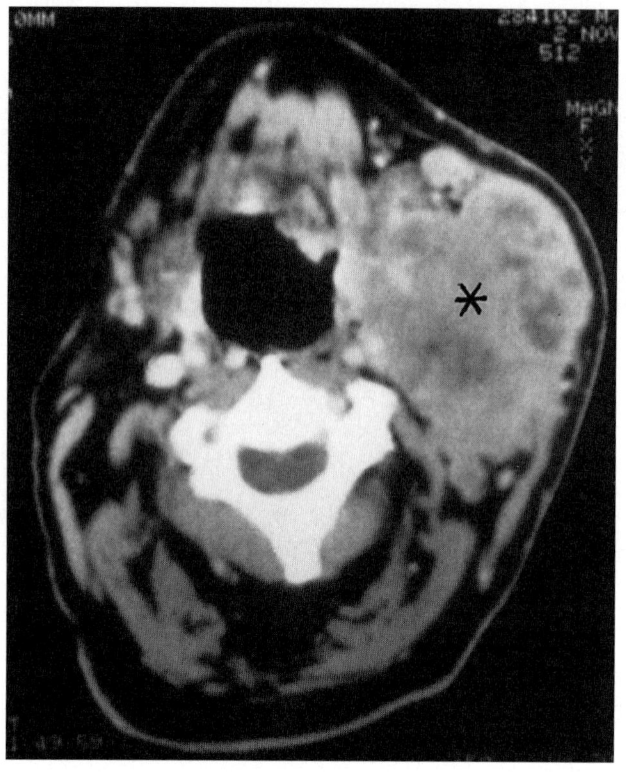

A

B

FIGURE 15.5. A: Transaxial CT image of the neck demonstrating a large necrotizing tumor with irregular contrast enhancement (*) in the left neck. B: Transaxial PET images of the neck show increased fluoromisonidazole (FMISO) uptake (*arrows*) in the lesion with maximum SUV > 4 in the left neck lesion indicating tumor hypoxia.

minutes of PET imaging, the uptake of ^{11}C-thymidine in head and neck tumors remains stable and the kinetic differences are small.[47] On the other hand, in another group of nine patients with squamous cell head and neck carcinomas, between −14% and +40% variations are noted from blood pool ^{11}C activities.[48] Because of rapid hepatic clearance of ^{11}C-thymidine, exact measurement of tumor uptakes requires individual correction for tumor blood volume and poses another technical requirement to measure the blood volume. PET studies of newer agent [N-methyl-^{11}C]α-methylaminoisobutyric acid have found elevated SUVs of about 6.1, which correlated with tumor presence but not with the proliferation index Ki 67.[49]

PET Studies of Tumor Hypoxia

Originally developed as a radiation enhancer, fluoromisonidazole (FMISO) has been labeled with ^{18}F, and the resulting PET images (Fig. 15.5) were suggested to correlate with hypoxic states of head and neck tumors as well as with lung cancers,[50] gliomas,[51] strokes, and myocardial infarctions. The uptake site of FMISO is presumed to be a reductase that is found in metabolically active tumor. The promise of FMISO in oncology is that it may provide an in vivo noninvasive in-

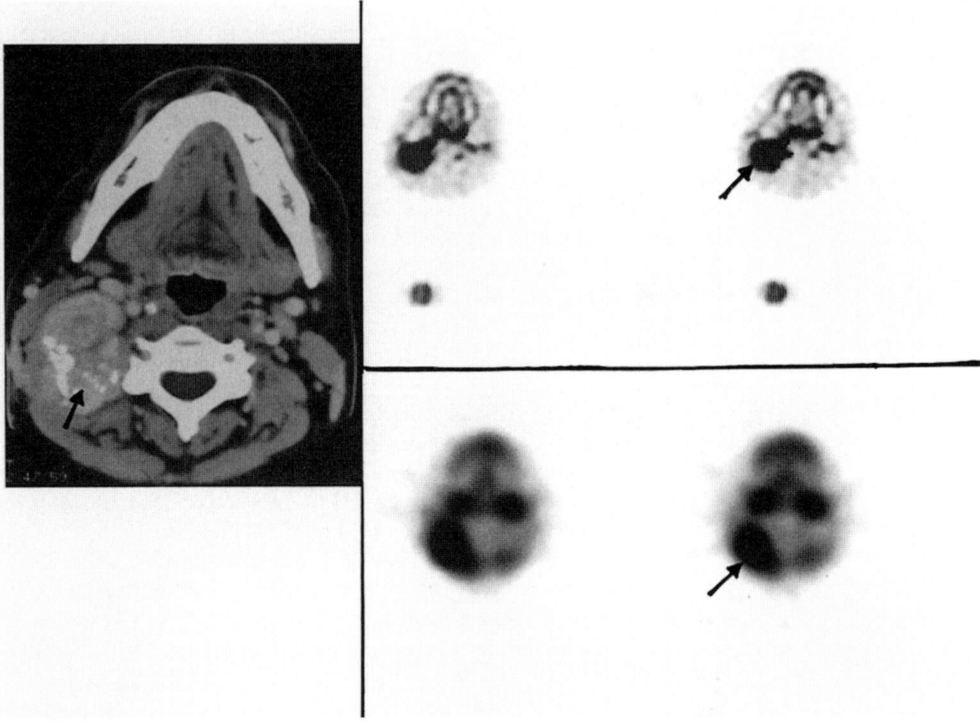

FIGURE 15.6. Selected transaxial CT (*left*), FDG-PET (*right upper row*), and Tc-99m sestamibi SPECT (*right lower row*) images of the upper neck in a patient with synovial sarcoma in the right side of the neck (*arrows*). Focal increased uptakes of ^{18}F-FDG and Tc-99m sestamibi are noted in the corresponding lesion on MRI.

dication of hypoxic states of the tumor and direct radiotherapy plans. However, FMISO-PET suffers from three weaknesses. First, the uptake of FMISO is slow and reaches a plateau at 2 hours with relatively low uptake. Second, the correlation with in vivo measurement of oxygen tension is still to be conclusively demonstrated, although the human dosimetry has been published.[52] Third, the synthesis is not standardized and the quality assurance procedures are not established. Because of these issues, FMISO-PET has remained a research tool available only to a few centers. Another agent, ^{18}F-fluoroerythronitroimidazole, has been studied and shows rising uptake in tumors when tumor-to-plasma ratios are used as indicators.[53]

Besides PET, other scintigraphic modalities such as ^{111}In octreotide and technetium (Tc)-99m sestamibi single photon emission computed tomography (SPECT) (Fig. 15.6) have made good advances and may provide complementary information and less expensive alternatives to PET in the study of human head and neck tumors. Until government payment or reimbursement is secured, PET will remain largely a research tool for the care of patients with head and neck cancers.

References

1. Jamal A, Murray T, Samuels A, et al. Cancer statistics, 2003. CA Cancer J Clin 2003;53:5–26.
2. Spitz MR. Epidemiology and risk factors for head and neck cancer. Semin Oncol 1994;21:281–288.
3. Wray A, McGuire WF. Smokeless tobacco usage associated with oral carcinoma, incidence and treatment outcome. Arch Otolaryngol Head Neck Surg 1993;119:929–933.
4. Hadar T, Rahima M, Kahan E. Significance of specific Epstein-Barr virus IgA and elevated IgG antibodies to vital capsid antigens in nasopharyngeal carcinoma patients. J Med Virol 1986;20:329–339.
5. Liebowitz D. Nasopharyngeal carcinoma. The Epstein-Barr virus association. Semin Oncol 1994;21:376–381.
6. Watts SL, Brewer EE, Paz TL. Human papilloma virus DNA types in squamous cell carcinoma of the head and neck. Oral Surg Oral Med Oral Pathol 1991;71:701–707.
7. Cooper S, Pajak TF, Rubin P. Second malignancies in patients who have head and neck cancer: incidence, effect on survival and implications based on the RTOG experience. Int J Radiat Oncol Biol Phys 1989;17:449–456.
8. Nawroz H, van der Riet P, Hruban RH. Allelotype of head and neck squamous cell carcinoma. Cancer Res 1994;54:1152–1155.
9. Michalides R, van Veelen N, Hart A. Overexpression of cyclin Dl correlates with recurrence in a group of forty-seven operable squamous cell carcinomas of head and neck. Cancer Res 1995;55:975–978.
10. Brachman DG. Molecular biology of head and neck cancer. Semin Oncol 1994;21:320–329.
11. Brachman DG, Grover DE, Voken E. Occurrence of p53 gene deletions and human papilloma virus infection in human head and neck cancer. Cancer Res 1992;62:4832–4836.
12. Brennan JA, Mao L, Hauban RH. Molecular assessment of histopathologic staging. N Engl J Med 1995;332:429–443.

13. Brennan JA, Boyle JO, Koch WM. Association between cigarette smoking and mutation of the p53 gene in squamous-cell carcinoma of the head and neck. N Engl J Med 1995;332:712–717.
14. Kwok TT, Sotherland RM. Enhancement of sensitivity of human squamous carcinoma cells to radiation by epidermal growth factor receptor. J Natl Cancer Inst 1989;81:1020–1024.
15. Shin DM, Voravud N, Ro JY. Sequential increases in proliferation of cell nuclear antigen expression in head and neck tumorigenesis: a potential biomarker. J Natl Cancer Inst 1993;85:971–978.
16. Perez CA. Carcinoma of the nasopharynx. In: Brady LW, Peser C, eds. Principles and Practice of Radiation Oncology. Philadelphia: JB Lippincott, 1992:617–644.
17. Feinmesser R, Miyasaki I, Cheung R. Diagnosis of nasopharyngeal carcinoma by DNA amplification of tissue obtained by fine-needle aspiration. N Engl J Med 1992;326:17–21.
18. Crissman JD, Liu WY, Gluckman J, et al. Prognostic value of histopathologic parameters in squamous cell carcinoma of the oropharynx. Cancer 1984;54:2995–2999.
19. Kokal WA, Gardive RL, Sheibani K, et al. Tumor DNA content as a prognostic indication in squamous cell carcinoma of the head and neck region. Am J Surg 1998;156:276–281.
20. Castelijns JA, Kaiser MC, Valk J, et al. Magnetic resonance imaging of the laryngeal cancer. J Comput Assist Tomgr 1987;11:134–140.
21. Glazer HS, Nimyer JH, Balfe DM. Neck neoplasms: MR imaging. Part II. Radiology 1987;160:349–354.
22. Vogl TJ, Steger W, Balzer J, et al. MRI of the neck, larynx and hypopharynx. In: Hasso AN, Stark DD, eds. Spine and Body MRI. Boston: ARKS, 1991:99–110.
23. Mafee MF, Barany M, Gotsis ED, et al. Potential use of in vivo proton spectroscopy for head and neck lesions. Radiol Clin North Am 1989;27:243–254.
24. Mukherja SK, Schiro S, Gastillo M, et al. Proton MR spectroscopy of squamous cell carcinoma of the extracranial head and neck: in vitro and in vivo studies. Am J Neuroradiol 1997;18:1057–1072.
25. Haberkorn U, Strauss LG, Reisser C, et al. Glucose uptake, perfusion, and cell proliferation in head and neck tumors: relation of positron emission tomography to flow cytometry. J Nucl Med 1991;32:1548–1555.
26. Conti PS, Lilien DL, Hawley K, et al. PET and F-18 FDG in oncology: a clinical update. Nucl Med Biol 1996;23:717–735.
27. Wong WL, Chevretton EB, McGurk M, et al. A prospective study of PET-FDG imaging for the assessment of head and neck squamous cell carcinoma. Clin Otolaryngol 1997;22:209–214.
28. Gambhir SS, Czernin J, Schwimmer J, et al. A tabulated summary of the FDG PET literature. J Nucl Med 2001;42:1S-93S.
29. Braams JW, Pruim J, Kole AC, et al. Detection of unknown primary head and neck tumors by positron emission tomography. Int J Oral Maxillofac Surg 1997;26:112–115.
30. Okada J, Oonishi H, Yoshikawa K, et al. FDG-PET for predicting the prognosis of malignant lymphoma. Ann Nucl Med 1994;8:187–191.
31. Sakamoto H, Nakai Y, Ohashi Y, et al. Positron emission tomographic imaging of head and neck lesions. Eur Arch Otorrinolaringol 1997;suppl 1:S123–126.
32. Austin JR, Wong FC, Kim EE. Positron emission tomography in the detection of residual laryngeal carcinoma. Otolaryngol Head Neck Surg 1995; 113(4):404–407.

33. Lapela M, Grenman R, Kurki T, et al. Head and neck cancer: detection of recurrence with PET and 2-[F-18]-fluoro-2-deoxy-D-glucose. Radiology 1995;197:205–211.
34. Reisser C, Haberkorn U, Dimitrakopoulou-Strauss A, et al. Chemotherapeutic management of head and neck malignancies with positron emission tomography. Arch Otolaryngol Head Neck Surg 1995;121:272–276.
35. Hlawitschka M, Neise E, Bredow J, et al. FDG-PET in the pretherapeutic evaluation of primary squamous cell carcinoma of the oral cavity and the involvement of cervical lymph nodes. Mol Imag Biol 2002;4(1):91–98.
36. Uematsu H, Sadato N, Ohtsubo T, et al. Fluorine-18-fluorodeoxyglucose PET versus thallium-201 scintigraphy evaluation of thyroid tumors. J Nucl Med 1998;39:453–459.
37. Chung J-K, Young S, Lee J-S, et al. Value of FDG PET in papillary thyroid carcinoma with negative I-131 whole-body scan. J Nucl Med 1999;40: 986–992.
38. Schlüter B, Bohuslavizki H, Beyer W, et al. Impact of FDG-PET on patients with differentiated thyroid cancer who present with elevated thyroglobulin and negative I-131 scan. J Nucl Med 2001;42:71–76.
39. Minn H, Lapela M, Klemi PJ, et al. Prediction of survival with F-18-fluorodeoxyglucose and PET in head and neck cancer. J Nucl Med 1997;38(12): 1907–1911.
40. Kitagawa Y, Nishizawa S, Sano K, et al. Prospective comparison of F-18 FDG-PET with conventional imaging modalities (MRI, CT, and Ga-67 scintigraphy) in assessment of combined intraarterial chemotherapy and radiotherapy for head and neck carcinoma. J Nucl Med 2003;44:198–206.
41. Wong WL, Hussain K, Chevretton E, et al. Validation and clinical application of computer-combined computed tomography and positron emission tomography with 2-[18F-fluoro-22-deoxy-D-glucose] head and neck images. Am J Surg 1996;172:628–632.
42. Leskinen-Kallio S, Lindholm P, Lapela M, et al. Imaging of head and neck tumors with positron emission tomography and C-11 methionine in imaging of malignant tumors of the head and neck region. Int J Radiat Oncol Biol Phys 1994;30:1195–1199.
43. Inoue T, Kim EE, Wong FC, et al. Comparison of F-18 fluorodeoxyglucose and C-11 methionine PET in detection of malignant tumors. J Nucl Med 1996;37:1472–1476.
44. Lindholm P, Leskinen-Kallio S, Kirvela O, et al. Head and neck cancer: effect of food ingestion on uptake of C-11 methionine. Radiology 1994;190: 863–868.
45. Lindholm P, Leskinen-Kallio S, Grenman R, et al. Evaluation of response to radiotherapy in head and neck cancer by positron emission tomography and C-11 methionine. Int J Radiat Oncol Biol Phys 1995;32:787–794.
46. Sundin A, Johansson C, Hellman P, et al. PET and parathyroid L-[C-11] methionine accumulation in hyperthyroidism. J Nucl Med 1996;37(11): 1766–1770.
47. Goethals P, van Eijkeren M, Lodewyck W, et al. Measurement of [methyl C-11] thymidine and its metabolites in head and neck tumors. J Nucl Med 1995;36:880–882.
48. van Eijkeren ME, Thierens H, Seuntjens J, et al. Kinetics of [methyl-11C] thymidine in patients with squamous cell carcinoma of the head and neck. Acta Oncol 1996;35:737–741.
49. Sutinen E, Jyrkkiö S, Alanen K, et al. Uptake of [N-methyl-C-11]α-methylaminoisobutyric acid in untreated head and neck cancer studied by PET. Eur J Nucl Med 2003;30:72–77.

50. Rasey JS, Koh WJ, Evans ML, et al. Quantifying regional hypoxia in human tumors with positron emission tomography of F-18 fluoromisonidazole: a pretherapy study of 37 patients. Int J Radiat Oncol Biol Phys 1996; 36:417–428.
51. Valk PE, Mathis CA, Prados MD, et al. Hypoxia in human gliomas: demonstration by PET with fluorine-18-fluoromisonidazole. J Nucl Med 1992; 33:2133–2137.
52. Graham MM, Peterson LM, Link JM, et al. F-18 fluoromisonidazole radiation dosimetry in imaging studies. J Nucl Med 1997;38:1631–1636.
53. Lehtiö K, Oikonen V, Nyman S, et al. Quantifying tumour hypoxia with F-18 fluoroerythronitroimidazole (F-18 FETNIM) and PET using the tumour to plasma ratio. Eur J Nucl Med 2003;30:101–108.

16

Thoracic Cancer

E. Edmund Kim and Franklin C. L. Wong

Lung cancer is the most frequently diagnosed cancer in the world, and the prevalence of lung cancer is increasing globally.[1] It is the leading cause of death from cancer, and the death occurs at a higher frequency in men than in women in most parts of the world.[2] There were 169,400 estimated new cases in 2002. Lung cancer claims approximately 150,900 lives each year in the United States, and 20,000 more women died of lung cancer than breast cancer in 2002.[3] The survival rate is poor, largely because lung cancer is usually diagnosed at an advanced stage. The overall 5-year survival of patients with lung cancer is approximately 14% and has remained unchanged over several decades despite aggressive treatment protocols.[3] Therefore, new diagnostic and treatment strategies are needed if an impact is to be made on the survival of patients with lung cancer. A cure may be achieved by surgery, which is feasible only in patients who present at an early stage. However, even in this early stage, approximately 75% patients will die of recurrent disease.[1,4] Lung cancer is rare before the age of 40, after which age-specific rates rise sharply. The ages with the greatest incidence are between 65 and 79.[1]

There are several extrinsic risk factors. There is general agreement that lung cancer risks are increased by 60% from long-term environmental tobacco smoke exposure, making secondhand smoke a significant added risk factor. Other extrinsic factors include exposure to radon, asbestos, arsenic, and chromium compounds. Radon and asbestos share the distinction of having a synergistic relationship with cigarette smoking. There is increasing evidence that genetic factors can contribute to lung cancer risk. However, research has not yet identified the gene locus or the mechanism.[1,4]

Malignant mesotheliomas are highly aggressive tumors that arise primarily from the surface serosal cells of the pleural, peritoneal, and pericardial cavities. Epidemiologic studies have established that exposure to asbestos fibers is the primary cause of mesothelioma.

Imaging plays a critical role in the initial detection and diagnosis of thoracic malignancies, as well as in pretreatment staging, which is important in identifying patients with localized disease who are likely to benefit from surgical resection.[5] Chest radiography, computed tomography (CT), and magnetic resonance imaging (MRI) are frequently used in patients with suspected lung cancer. These modalities provide anatomic and morphologic information, but they cannot accurately characterize lung, pleural, or lymph node abnormalities as benign or malignant. The diagnosis of lung cancer is usually obtained by sputum cytology, bronchoscopy, percutaneous needle biopsy, thoracoscopy, or open lung biopsy.[6] Since more than 50% of radiographically indeterminate lesions resected at thoracosopy were benign,[1] the accurate method of noninvasively characterizing these lesions could result in the avoidance of unnecessary and expensive procedures that are not always diagnostic. Several radionuclide imaging techniques using Tl 201 chloride, technetium (Tc)-99m sestamibi, Tc-99m P-829 (NeoTect), and ^{18}F-2-fluoro-2-deoxyglucose (FDG) have been proposed to evaluate solitary pulmonary nodules and stage lung cancer. The increased glucose metabolism results from increased expression of glucose transporter messenger RNA, enhanced levels of glucose transporter proteins, Glut-1 and -3, high levels of hexokinase II, and downregulation of glucose-6-phosphatase enzyme.[7] The biochemical differences of FDG between normal and neoplastic tissue have resulted in its routine use for characterizing lesions that are indeterminate by conventional imaging modalities and to stage the tumors.

Pathology of Lung Cancer

Lung cancer arises from epithelial tissue in the lining of the bronchi, bronchioles, alveoli, and trachea. Approximately 90% to 95% of all primary lung cancers are bronchogenic carcinomas. Histologically, approximately 20% of them are small cell carcinomas, and the other 80% are grouped together as non–small cell lung cancers (NSCLCs), which are divided into adenocarcinoma (40%), squamous cell carcinoma (30%), and large cell undifferentiated carcinoma (10%). The classification of lung cancer by the World Health Organization has been accepted worldwide (Table 16.1).[8]

Small cell lung cancer has almost always spread systemically at the time of diagnosis, and chemotherapy is almost always used. Approximately 90% of small cell carcinomas are located centrally and tend to invade longitudinally along submucosal and intramural portions of the bronchial walls and in the supporting tissues and lymphatics.[9] They are often characterized by extensive and bulky mediastinal lymphadenopathy. Small cell and squamous cell carcinomas have a dose-response relationship to increasing tobacco exposure. Adenocarcinoma is increasing worldwide, despite the fact that it does not have a significant dose-response relationship with smoking. This increasing incidence of adenocarcinoma is especially seen in women in the U.S. Most adenocarcinomas are peripheral in origin and arise from alveolar surface epithelium or bronchial mucosal glands. They also can arise as peripheral scar tumors. Squamous cell carcinoma arises most frequently in the proximal segmental bronchi and is associated with squamous metaplasia. It tends to be slow growing and requires 3 to 4 years from

TABLE 16.1. World Health Organization (WHO) classification of epithelial lung tumors

I. Preinvasive lesions
   Carcinoma in situ and squamous dysplasia
   Atypical adenomatous hyperplasia

II. Invasive malignant lesions
   A. Adenocarcinoma
      1. Acinar
      2. Papillary
      3. Bronchoalveolar: nonmucinous (Clara cell) and mucinous (goblet cell) types
      4. Mucus-secreting solid adenocarcinoma
      5. Adenocarcinoma with mixed subtypes
   B. Squamous cell carcinoma
      Variants: papillary, clear cell, small cell, basaloid
   C. Large cell carcinoma
      Variants: neuroendocrine, basaloid, lymphoepithelioma
   D. Small cell carcinoma
   E. Adenosquamous carcinoma
   F. Others
      1. Carcinoid tumors
      2. Adenoid cystic carcinoma
      3. Mucoepidermoid carcinoma
      4. Spindle or giant carcinoma
      5. Unclassified

its onset before clinical detection as an in situ carcinoma. It can be detected early by cytologic examination because its cells exfoliate. Squamous cell carcinomas are located centrally, and are frequently associated with bronchial obstruction. A specific subtype of adenocarcinoma, known as bronchoalveolar carcinoma, presents in three different fashions: a solitary peripheral nodule, multifocal disease, or a progressive pneumonic form spreading from lobe to lobe and affecting the bilateral lungs. Large cell tumors also tend to be peripheral, and many tumors previously characterized as large cell carcinomas are being classified as adenocarcinoma or squamous cell carcinoma with the improved histologic techniques. The prognosis of large cell undifferentiated carcinomas is similar to that of adenocarcinoma.[8]

Adenocarcinomas from primary lung, breast, ovary, stomach, kidney, or prostate cancer frequently metastasize to the pleura and can be extremely difficult to differentiate from epithelial mesothelioma. Metastatic adenocarcinoma with extensive pleural involvement may grossly resemble mesothelioma and has been called pseudomesothelioma.

Diagnosis and Staging of Lung Cancer

Lung cancer growing within the lung parenchymi or the bronchial wall eventually invades the lymphatic channels and vascular structures, resulting in distant metastases. The lymphatic drainage follows the bronchoarterial branching pattern with lymph nodes situated at the origin of these branchings. Lower lobe lymphatics drain into the posterior mediastinum and ultimately to the subcarinal lymph nodes. Right upper lobe lymphatics drain into the superior mediastinum, whereas left upper lobe lymphatics run along the great vessels in the anterior mediastinum and along the main bronchus into the superior mediastinum. Metastatic lymphatic spread of lung cancer follows these lymphatic channels with tumor involving bronchopulmonary (N1), mediastinal (N2–3), and supraclavicular (N3) lymph nodes (Fig. 16.1).[10] Lymphatic spread to the pleural surface can occur in peripheral tumors. Autopsy has revealed lung cancer metastases in every organ system, and the most frequent metastatic sites of NSCLC are bone, liver, adrenal glands, and brain.[8] Revised staging of lung cancer in 1997 by anatomic extent of the primary lung tumor (T), regional lymph nodes (N), and metastases (M) has been used worldwide in the management of lung cancer (Table 16.2). TNM staging (Table 16.3) includes clinical, surgical, and pathologic assessment. Clinical staging typically understages patients compared to the final staging obtained at surgery and pathology. The 5-year survival rate is highly correlated with the stage of lung cancer: 60% to 80% for stage I, 25% to 50% for stage II, 10% to 40% for stage IIIa, and <5% for stage IIIb or IV[8] (Table 16.3). The patient's history and physical examination are very important in evaluating a patient with suspected lung cancer. Sputum cytology (three samples) will be positive in 80% of central tumors, but the yield is less than 20% for small peripheral tumors.[8]

Imaging studies are essential in the evaluation of patients with suspected lung cancer. The detection and diagnosis of lung cancer usually begins with a chest radiograph. The appearance of lung cancer is variable and can range from a subtle finding to the dramatic, depending on location, stage at presentation, and associated findings. In many cases, the major radiographic abnormality is abnormal parenchymal

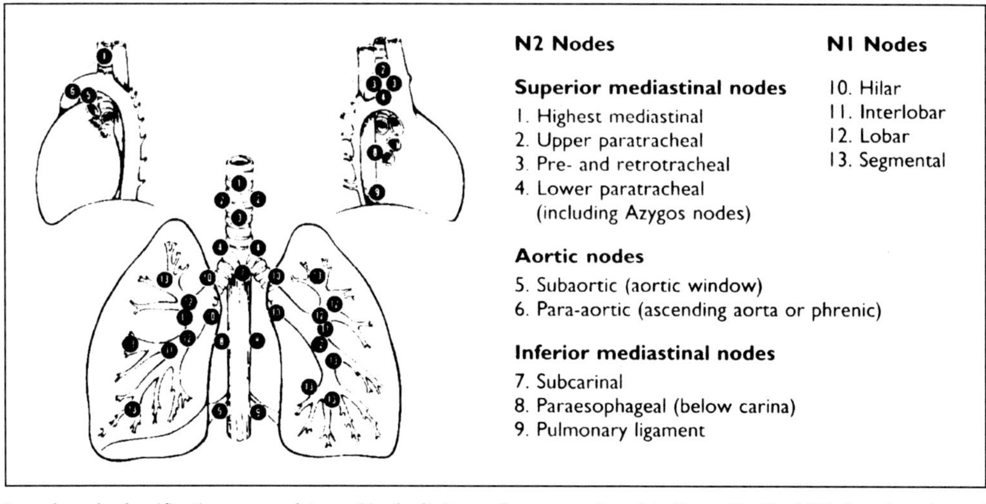

Lymph-node classification nomenclature. Single-digit numbers are assigned to the mediastinal N2, lymph nodes and double-digit numbers to the peribronchial and hilar, N1, lymph nodes.

Figure 16.1. The lymphatic drainage of lung cancer with nomenclature and numbers. (Modified from Mountain et al.[10])

TABLE 16.2. Tumor-node-metastasis (TNM) classification of lung cancer

Primary tumor (T)	
TX	Positive cancer cells but no lesion shown
Tis	Carcinoma in situ
T1	<3 cm in greatest dimension
T2	<3 cm; distal atelectasis
T3	Extension into chest wall, diaphragm; pleura or pericardium; <2 cm from carina or total atelectasis
T4	Invasion of mediastinal organs; pleural effusion
Lymph node (N)	
N0	No involvement
N1	Ipsilateral bronchopulmonary or hilar
N2	Ipsilateral mediastinal, subcarinal, or supraclavicular
N3	Contralateral mediastinal, hilar, or supraclavicular
Distant metastasis (M)	
M0	None
M1	Present

opacification due to atelectasis or postobstructive pneumonitis, which may obscure the central tumor. Central tumors may be visible as an abnormal convexity or density in the hilar region. Often the first indication that a cancer exists is the finding of a solitary pulmonary nodule (SPN), measuring usually <3 cm in diameter. This is seen in up to 1 in 500 chest radiographs, with an estimated malignant rate between 20% and 40%.[11] Lung cancer is most often located in the upper lobes, particularly the right upper lobe, and, not surprisingly, most missed cancers are in the right upper lobe. The right lower lobe is the next common site. Size alone is insufficient for differentiation of benign and malignant lung tumors, although a lesion >3 cm is more likely to be

TABLE 16.3 Current and proposed TNM staging and 5-year survival rate of lung cancer

Staging		5-year survival rate (%)
Current		
I.	T1–2, N0, M0	60–80
II.	T1–2, N1, M0	25–50
III.A	T3, N0–1, M0	25–40
	T1–3, N2, M0	10–30
III.B	T4 or N3, M0	<5
IV.	M1	<5
Proposed (UICC and AJCC)		
I.a	T1, N0, M0	>70
I.b	T2, N0, M0	60
II.a	T1, N1, M0	50
II.b	T2, N1, M0	30
	T3, N0–1, M0	40
III.a	T1–3, N2, M0	10–30
III. b	T4, N3, M0	<5
IV.	M1	<2

AJCC, American Joint Cancer Committee; UICC, Union International Cancer Congress.

malignant. Lamellated or central calcification in granulomas and a popcorn pattern in hamartomas are highy specific, but growing lung cancer may surround a calcified granuloma, and dystrophic calcifications may rarely be seen in primary or metastatic tumor. A minority of carcinoid also calcify. Lobulation of a nodule suggests uneven growth and supports malignancy. Spiculations are thought to represent a desmoplastic response to local tumor extension.[12]

Cavitation is seen in a minority of lung cancer, mostly squamous cell carcinoma, but also occasionally in adenocarcinoma or large cell carcinoma. The cavity wall is usually thick (>5 mm) and may show a nodular internal margin. A maximum wall thickness <4 mm is unlikely to be malignant except for rare cases.[12] Growth correlates with doubling time, which is a measure of volumetric growth, not diameter. Most tumors have a doubling time of between 30 and 490 days (mean value of 120 days). A 9-mm SPN with a doubling time of 100 days will measure 1.1 cm at 3 months and 1.4 cm at 6 months. The absence of growth over a 2-year period is the most reliable indicator of benignity.[4,12]

Cancers arising in the lung apex, known as superior sulcus or Pancoast tumors, are a distinct subgroup with constellation of symptoms. Radiographic findings can be quite subtle and are frequently obscured by overlying musculoskeletal structures, brachiocephalic vessels or pleural thickening. Findings suggestive of malignancy include an apical cap >5 mm, asymmetry of apical caps, apical mass, or adjacent bone destruction.[12] Arm pain secondary to involved brachia plexus or Horner's syndrome (meiosis, ptosis, and anhydrosis) due to involvement of the stellate ganglion are classically associated with Pancoast tumors. Although the most common appearance of bronchoalveolar carcinoma is an SPN (43%), consolidation is the second common pattern (30%) caused by tumor growth along the peripheral airways and alveoli. Air bronchograms and alveolograms are characteristic but not specific. Bronchorrhea (copious white mucoid or watery expectoration) is an unusual and late manifestation. The consolidative pattern has a poorer prognosis than the solitary nodular pattern.[12,13] Hilar or mediastinal adenopathy is sometimes the sole manifestation of lung cancer. Small cell carcinoma tends to show a central adenopathy, but all cell types can have metastatic spread centrally.

Enlargement of the aortopulmonary window, right paratrachial thickening or soft tissue density, double density adjacent to the aortic knob, and abnormal convexity in the azygoesophageal recess are frequent findings of mediastinal metastasis of lung cancer.[12] Pleural involvement usually manifests as a pleural effusion, but a nonmalignant effusion can result from central lymphatic obstruction, pneumonia, congestive heart failure, or pulmonary embolus. Pancoast tumors are often associated with direct extension to ribs or vertebral bodies. Metastatic disease may show destruction or osteolytic lesions in the humerus, sternum, clavicle, or scapula. Lung cancer can also involve the heart by direct extension, or show an enlarging cardiac silhouette by malignant pericardial effusion. Elevation of the diaphragm may indicate phrenic nerve involvement, or be mimicked by a subpulmonic effusion. Hoarseness can be due to tumor involvement of the recurrent laryngeal nerve in the aortopulmonary window.[12]

It is well accepted that CT is the imaging modality of choice for staging lung cancer. Compared with MRI, CT is faster, less expensive, has better spatial resolution, offers superior evaluation of the lung parenchyma, and is more sensitive in detecting calcification. CT plays several vital roles in the evaluation of patients with known or suspected lung cancer. One is to further characterize a suspicious abnormality seen on a chest radiograph. A second and indispensable role is that of pretreatment or preoperative staging. Additionally, CT provides a roadmap for other procedures such as bronchoscopy, mediastinoscopy, video-assisted thoracoscopy, and transthoracic needle biopsy. CT is more accurate in measuring nodular size and quantifying interval growth than chest radiograph. It also can better detect and evaluate calcifications within a nodule. The wall thickness of a cavitary lesion can be measured more accurately with CT. A new technique for the assessment of SPN is based on differential nodular enhancement, as measured with thin-slice CT. Malignant nodules tend to enhance significantly more (20 Hounsfield unit increase) than benign nodules at 2 minutes postinjection of the contrast agent.[14] The CT angiogram sign of branching pulmonary vessels extending >3 cm in the midst of consolidated pulmonary parenchyma has been noted in the majority of bronchoalveolar carcinoma, but can be also seen in pneumonia, infarction, or lymphoma.[15] With CT, the primary tumor is evaluated for initial size and location as well as metastasis to pleura, chest wall, mediastinum, vertebral bodies, adrenal glands, or liver.

The best criterion for diagnosing chest wall invasion is bony destruction. Less reliable signs are pleural thickening, loss of the extrapleural fat plane, an obtuse angle between mass and chest wall, and >3 cm of contact between mass and chest wall. Chest wall invasion does not necessarily exclude resection, but there is increased morbidity and mortality with en bloc resection and chest wall reconstruction.[16] There are CT criteria that distinguish subtle mediastinal invasion from mere mediastinal contiguity. Tumor contact of <3 cm with the mediastinum, <90% of contact with the aorta, and the presence of mediastinal fat between the mass and mediastinal structures suggest technically feasible resectability of the lesion.

Lymph nodes are generally identified as nonenhancing soft tissue densities surrounded by mediastinal fat. A node measuring >1 cm is usually considered abnormal, but enlarged nodes may represent benign reactive adenopathy. Nodes <1 cm in size also may contain microscopic metastases. Central low density can represent fat in a normal node or necrosis in a malignant node. With the advent of helical CT, particularly multidetector-row helical CT, the possibility of accurate mass screening of the at-risk population has been revisited for the prevention of, or delay of developing, lung cancer by means of earlier detection. Current estimates of the prevalence of detectable preclinical lung cancer in at-risk populations based on age 50 to 55, history of smoking, or prior lung cancer range from 2% to 4%.[17] This prevalence results in a positive predictive value of 50% if the screening test is good, with 95% sensitivity and specificity.[17] The cost of lung cancer screening depends on the fee for CT scans, how many false-positive results occur, and how the at-risk population to be screened is defined. Screening could cost more than $39 billion per year, but it may be cost-effective because the cost associated with caring for late-stage lung cancer patients is very high.[18] Most academic radiology societies have suggested that CT screening for lung cancer be reserved for patients enrolled in clinical trials.

MRI may play a complementary role to CT in certain circumstances because of its superior tissue contrast, multiplanar imaging capability, and superb delineation of thoracic vessels. For example, for the evaluation of Pancoast tumors, direct coronal and sagittal imaging with MRI facilitates the assessment of invasion of the chest wall, brachial plexus, subclavian vessels, vertebral bodies, and neural foramina. The superior contrast resolution of MRI suggests an advantage over CT in detecting subtle mediastinal invasion, but its poorer spatial resolution limits this advantage. The replacement of high signal mediastinal fat by lower signal tumor on T2-weighted images suggests the mediastinal invasion. MRI is also believed to be more accurate in establishing superior vena caval potency or obstruction due to thrombus, soft tissue mass, or direct tumor invasion.[19] MRI may also demonstrate chest wall invasion better, and signs include loss of subpleural fat stripe and visualization of soft tissue tumor extension into the chest wall. MRI can differentiate a low-signal benign pleural nodule from high-signal malignant nodules on T2-weighted images.[19] Several studies compared CT and MRI for detection of mediastinal nodal metastases and reported similar sensitivities and specificities of these modalities.

Fluorodeoxyglucose positron emission tomography (FDG-PET) is now being used in the evaluation of patients with focal pulmonary opacities on chest radiographs and in the staging of lung cancer. It is now replacing some of the invasive procedures previously used in the evaluation of lung cancer.

Radionuclide bone scans have been advocated in clinical stage III disease before considering curative therapy. The role of bone scans in asymptomatic patients with early-stage disease is controversial.

Percutaneous fine-needle aspiration (FNA) biopsy of pulmonary nodules is used to obtain tissue for identification of malignancy in pulmonary nodules and other abnormalities detected by CT. It is usually performed using CT guidance, and the positive yield is approximately 95%. A definite benign diagnosis is rarely made by this technique. An indeterminate biopsy must be further evaluated.

Bronchoscopy provides a greater than 90% diagnostic yield when a lesion is identified during the procedure. Peripheral lesions larger than 2 cm in diameter may be reached by brushes, needles, or forceps. It is also useful in staging because of the location of the cancer in the major airway as well as the ability to biopsy enlarged mediastinal lymph nodes.

The most accurate method of staging the superior mediastinal lymph nodes is mediastinoscopy. Anterior mediastinal lymph nodes are evaluated by the extended mediastinoscopic technique, anterior mediastinostomy, or video-assisted thoracoscopy, which also is used to excise peripheral nodules and evaluate pleural disease. Posterior mediastinal nodes can be biopsied by ultrasonograph-guided transesophageal endoscopy.

Thoracotomy is used for diagnosis and staging in less than 5% of patients being evaluated for lung cancer, and unexpected involvement of structures is frequently found, changing the stage of disease at thoracotomy.

FDG-PET

FDG-PET is one of the more recent advances in oncologic imaging that has generated renewed interest in diagnosis, staging, and response to treatment. It allows for the evaluation of the relative level of metabolic activity of a lesion compared with other tissues. It is based on the principle that there is increased utilization of glucose in malignant cells compared with most normal tissues due to the increased number of glucose transporters (I, III) in malignant cells.[20] There is also an increase in the glycolytic rate as a result of increased hexokinase (II) activity. When FDG is administered intravenously, it competes with glucose for transport into cells. Once intracellular, it competes with glucose for phosphorylation by hexokinase to FDG-6-phosphate, which is not a substrate for glycolysis and is not further metabolized. Thus, it becomes trapped in the cancer cells, and the accumulated ^{18}F-FDG-6-phosphate allows for imaging. Malignant lesions demonstrating increased glucose metabolism appear as focal areas of abnormally increased activity.

Technique

FDG-PET is performed on patients in the fasting state to minimize competitive inhibition of FDG uptake by serum glucose. A 4-hour fast is generally recommended, but a 12-hour fast may decrease the myocardial activity to improve the detection of mediastinal metastases. A serum glucose level is routinely obtained at our institution before FDG injection. If the serum level is less than 200 mg/dL, then FDG is administered. If the serum glucose level is greater than 200 mg/dL, the study is delayed with insulin injection as FDG is not advised since it leads to increased activity in skeletal muscle, and thus FDG is less available in tumors. The blood sugar in diabetic patients should be well controlled by oral hypoglycemic agents or insulin before the schedule of FDG-PET.

The FDG dose is 145 μCi (5.4 MBq/kg to a maximum of 20 mCi (740 MBq) for dedicated PET. Smaller doses are required for camera-based PET. Attenuation-corrected whole-body scan provides more accurate detection of small lesions and lesions deep within the body. Ten bed positions are needed for a whole-body scan for a PET scanner with a 15-cm axial field of view. Segmentation of transmission scans in 1 to 2 minutes per bed position reduces the scan time to approximately 100 minutes for whole-body PET. The nonattenuation corrected whole-body scan at eight to 10 bed positions usually takes 32 to 48 minutes of acquisition time. In a patient with lung cancer, ideally a 4-minute brain scan using the three-dimensional (3D) acquisition mode begins 30 minutes after FDG injection. The 3D mode without the septa provides approximately fourfold increased sensitivity for detection of annihilation radiation. There is certainly increased scatter radiation, and improved sensitivity yields better image quality. The scatter radiation in the body is greater than that in the head, and thus 3D acquisition is not currently used for body imaging. After the brain scan, nonattenuation corrected scans are obtained in two-dimensional (2D) acquisition mode for 4 minutes per bed position from the level of the skull base through the mid-thighs, and then an attenuation-corrected chest scan at two bed positions is obtained in the 2D mode using 8 minutes for the emission scan and 10 minutes for the transmission scan at each bed position.[21]

FDG-PET scans are usually interpreted qualitatively. If the FDG uptake in the lesion is greater than that in the mediastinal blood pool, a malignancy is suggested. The semiquantitative parameter, which is an index of glucose metabolism called the standard uptake ratio (SUR) or standard uptake value (SUV) normalizes the amount of FDG uptake in the lesion to the total injected dose and the patient's body weight after the lesion or region of interest (ROI) is outlined on the attenuation-corrected image and the mean activity is measured. The decay-corrected activities are then used to compute the SUV by the following formula:

$$SUV = \frac{Mean\ ROI\ Activity\ (mCi/mL)}{Injected\ Dose\ (mCi)\ Body\ Weight\ (g)}$$

The use of lean body weight and also correction for serum glucose has been suggested, and the time of acquisition also must be standardized since the SUV may change with time after FDG injection.[22]

Solitary Pulmonary Nodules (SPNs)

Focal lung opacities including solitary nodules are usually identified on routine chest radiographs. They are found in approximately 130,000 patients every year in the U.S.[22] Further study to characterize SPN is often performed with chest CT. If the SPN is stable in size for 2 years or longer, it is likely benign. Many lesions are indeterminate as to whether they are benign or malignant by morphologic criteria. Patients may require invasive biopsy, mediastinoscopy, thoracoscopy, or even thoracotomy to determine the nature of the lesion. More than half of radiographically indeterminate lesions that are thoracoscopically resected are found to be benign.[6] FDG-PET has been shown to be an accurate, noninvasive test for the assessment of pulmonary nodules (Figs. 16.2 and 16.3).

A comprehensive meta-analysis by Gould et al[23] of 40 eligible studies, including 1474 focal pulmonary lesions of any size, found the mean sensitivity and specificity for detecting malignancy were 96.0% and 73.5%, respectively. However, in this analysis, there was little data for

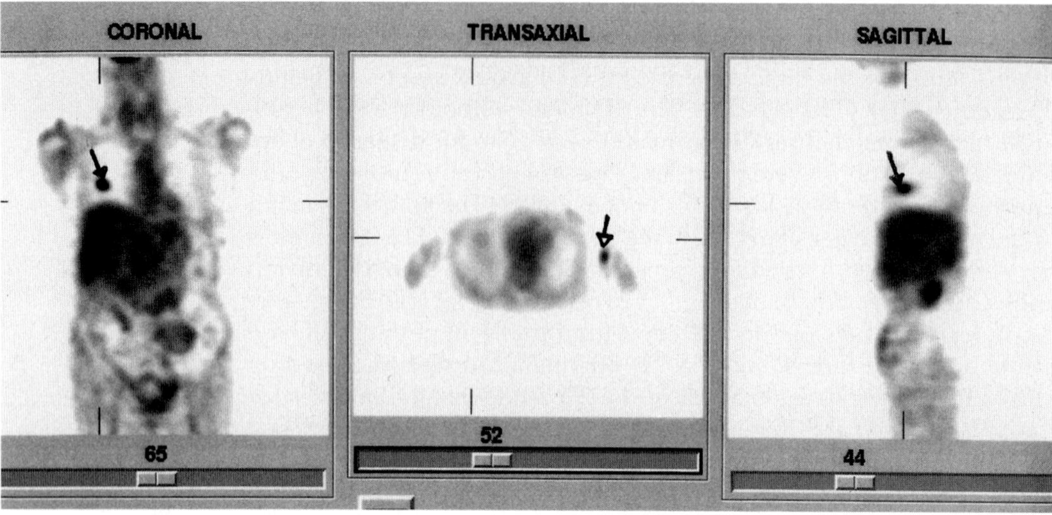

FIGURE 16.2. Selected coronal and sagittal PET images of the axial body as well as an axial image of the lower chest show markedly increased uptake of ^{18}F-FDG in the adenocarcinoma of right lower lung (*closed arrows*). Note focal increased activity in the injection site of left elbow (*open arrow*).

nodules <1 cm in diameter. In a prospective, multicenter study of 89 patients who underwent evaluation of intermediate SPN, FDG-PET had a sensitivity of 92% and a specificity of 90% using the SUV of 2.5 as the cutoff value.[21] Visual analysis of the images demonstrated a sensitivity of 98% and a specificity of 69%, and these results were not significantly different from the results using the SUV data. When the data were evaluated by separating the nodules into those 0.7 to <1.5 cm in diameter and compared with those ≥1.5 cm in diameter, the sensitivity and specificity were not statistically significantly different.

Although there is much excitement about the use of FDG-PET in on-

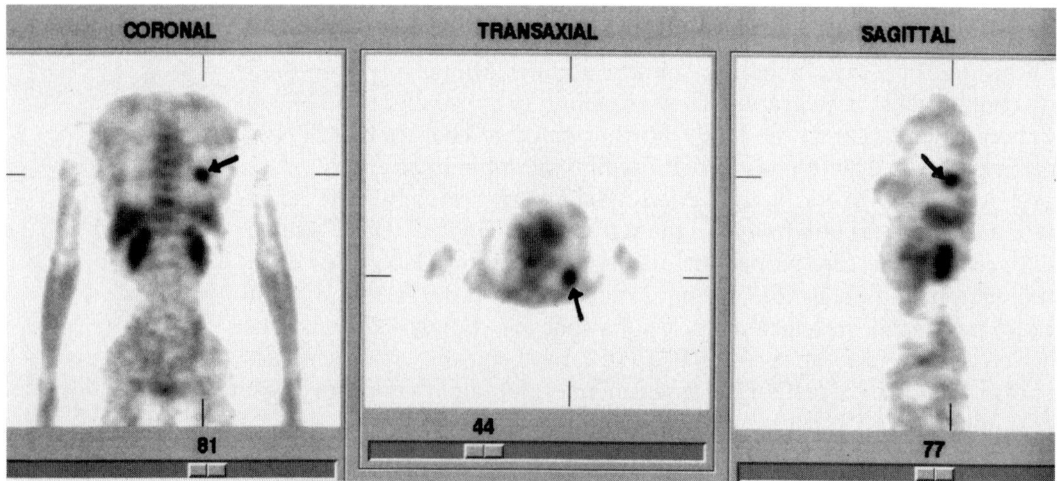

FIGURE 16.3. Selected coronal (*left*) and sagittal (*right*) PET images of the axial body as well as an axial (*middle*) image of the lower chest with ^{18}F-FDG show focal increased activity in the left lower lung with adenocarcinoma (*arrows*).

cology, the technique has its limitations. False-positive FDG-PET can occur with infectious or inflammatory processes. Abnormally increased FDG uptake with the SUV in the abnormal range can be seen with sarcoidosis, tuberculosis, histoplasmosis, cryptococcosis, aspergillosis, and other infections.[21] However, most chronic or indolent inflammatory processes and most acute infectious processes do not have significant FDG accumulation. False-negative FDG-PET has been seen with primary pulmonary carcinoid and bronchoalveolar cell cancer.[21,23] Six of seven carcinoids had SUVs <2.5. The typical carcinoid is slow growing and demonstrates minimal mitotic activity, resulting in less FDG uptake than in NSCLC. Of seven bronchoalveolar lung carcinomas, four were negative by FDG-PET due to less proliferative potential and longer mean doubling time than for other NSCLC.[21,23] False-negative PET is also a problem if the lesion is too small for the resolution of the instrument.

A relationship between prognosis and the amount of FDG uptake in nodules has been documented. Of the 118 patients with SUV <10, a median survival of 24.6 months was found, whereas 37 patients with SUV ≥10 had a statistically significant shorter median survival of 11.4 months. Multivariate analysis demonstrated that the results of a PET scan provided prognostic information independent of other clinical and imaging findings. Nodules with increased FDG uptake require a biopsy for diagnosis, and PET aids in directing the biopsy (Figs. 16.4 and 16.5). FDG-PET precludes the need for invasive biopsy in patients with metabolically inactive lesions. The cost savings of FDG-PET in the evaluation of SPN result from the prevention of unnecessary thoracotomies.

Staging of Lung Cancer

When a lung mass is shown to be malignant, it is important to stage the extent of disease accurately. Appropriate clinical management de-

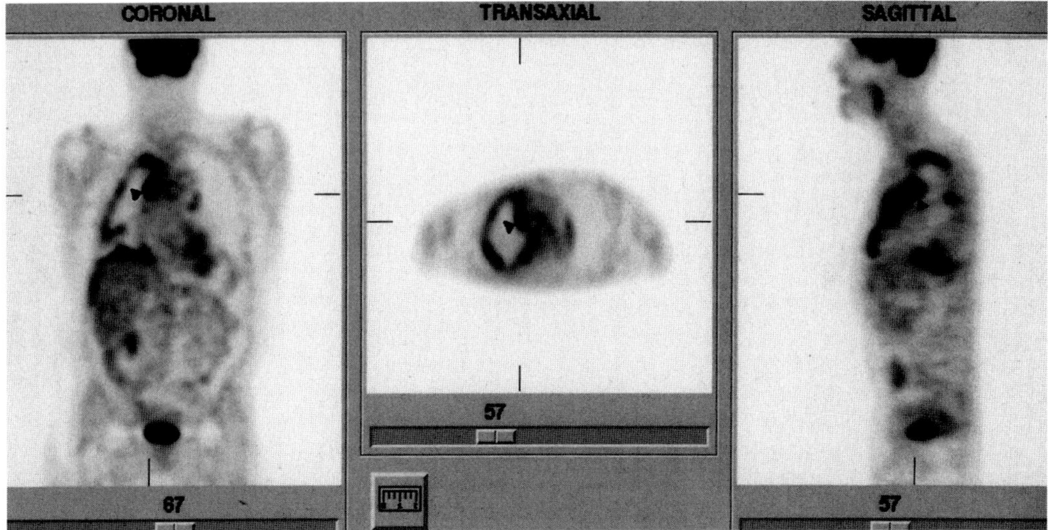

FIGURE 16.4. Selected coronal and sagittal PET images of the axial body and an axial image of the upper chest show markedly increased uptake of ^{18}F-FDG along the right pleura with nodular activity in the upper medial anterior aspect (*arrowhead*) due to mesothelioma.

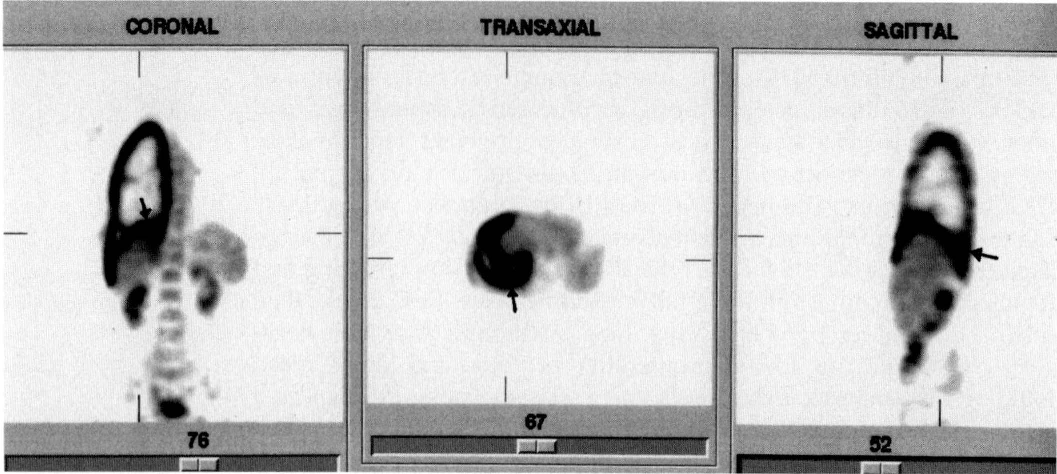

FIGURE 16.5. Selected coronal and sagittal PET images of the axial body as well as an axial image of the lower chest show markedly increased uptake of ^{18}F-FDG along the right pleura with nodular activity along the lung base (*arrows*) due to mesothelioma.

pends on whether there is mediastinal involvement and/or distal disease. Several studies have shown that PET is more accurate than CT for the staging of NSCLC. A tabulated summary of FDG-PET literature about the lung cancer from 1993 through 2000 showed 83% sensitivity and 91% specificity for NSCLC staging, versus 64% and 74%, respectively, for CT.[24] The mediastinum is the most common site for metastases, and PET appears more accurate than CT in detecting metastatic mediastinal lymphadenopathy (Figs. 16.6–16.8). In one retrospective study of 96 patients, 66 with histologically proven malig-

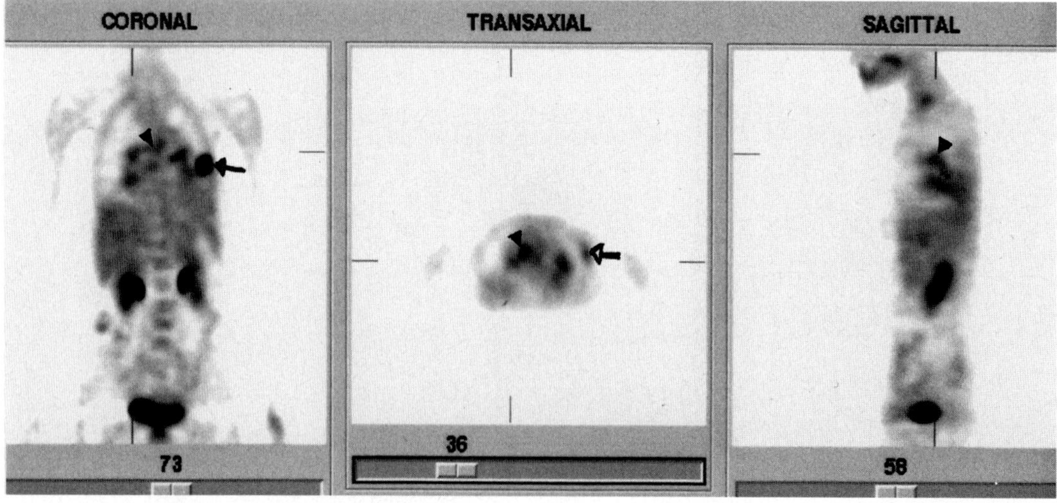

FIGURE 16.6. Selected coronal and sagittal PET images of the axial body as well as an axial image of the mid-chest with ^{18}F-FDG show primary adenocarcinoma in the left lower lung (*closed arrow*) and metastases in the mediastinum (*arrowhead*), perihilar areas, as well as left lower rib (*open arrow*).

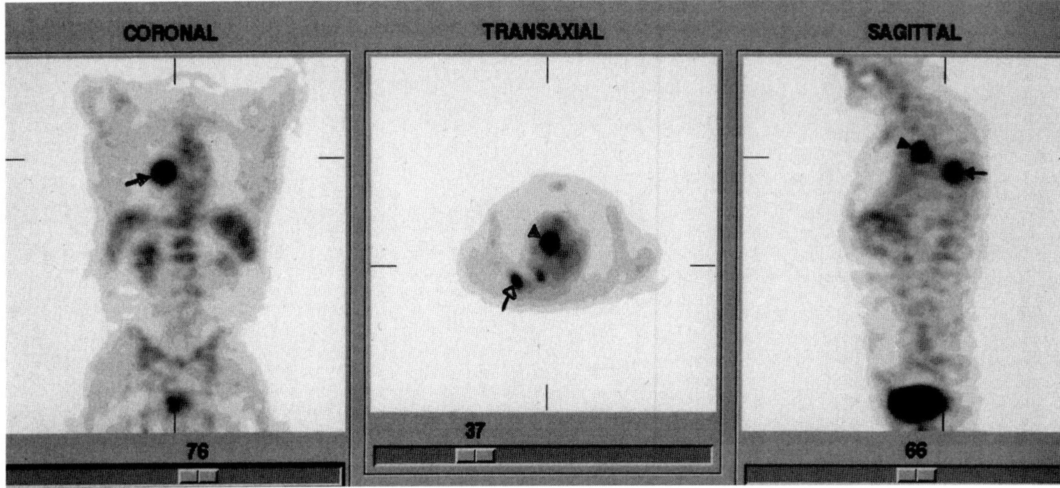

FIGURE 16.7. Selected coronal and sagittal PET images of the axial body and an axial image of the upper chest show markedly increased uptake of ^{18}F-FDG in the primary lung cancer (*closed arrows*), metastatic lesions in the superior mediastinum (*arrowhead*), and right posterior upper ribs (*open arrow*).

nant tumors and 30 with benign masses, the sensitivity and specificity of PET for detecting malignancy was 97% and 89%, respectively. In this study 111 lymph nodes were surgically sampled and the accuracy of FDG-PET in predicting malignancy of nodes was 91% compared with 64% for CT. The sensitivity and specificity of FDG-PET in detecting metastatic mediastinal lymph nodes (Fig. 16.9) was 98% and 94%, respectively.[25]

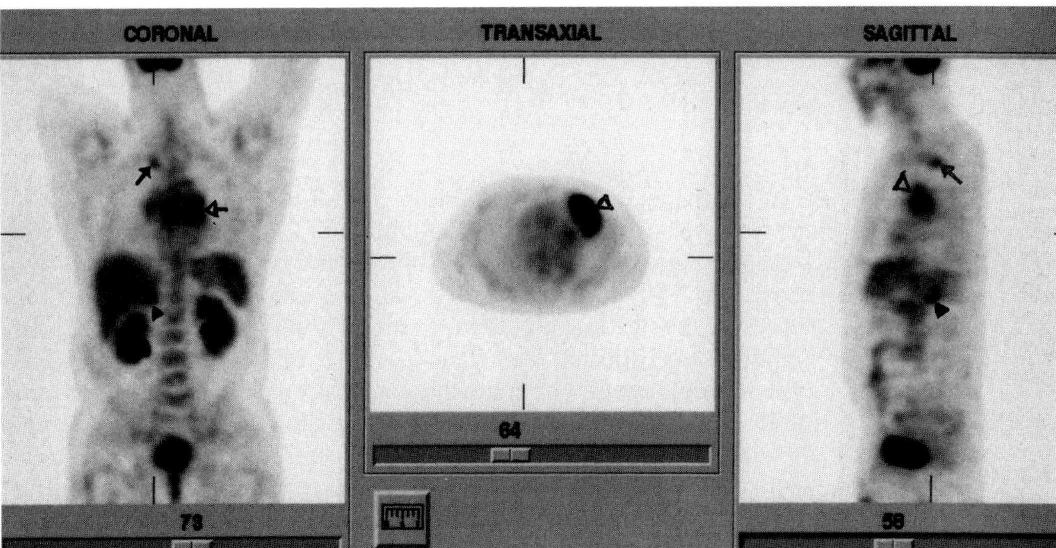

FIGURE 16.8. Selected coronal and sagittal images of the axial body and an axial image of the upper chest with ^{18}F-FDG show markedly increased activity in the primary lung cancer (*open arrowhead*), metastatic lesions in the subcarinal, hilar (*open arrow*), and right paratracheal node (*closed arrows*) as well as right adrenal gland (*closed arrowhead*).

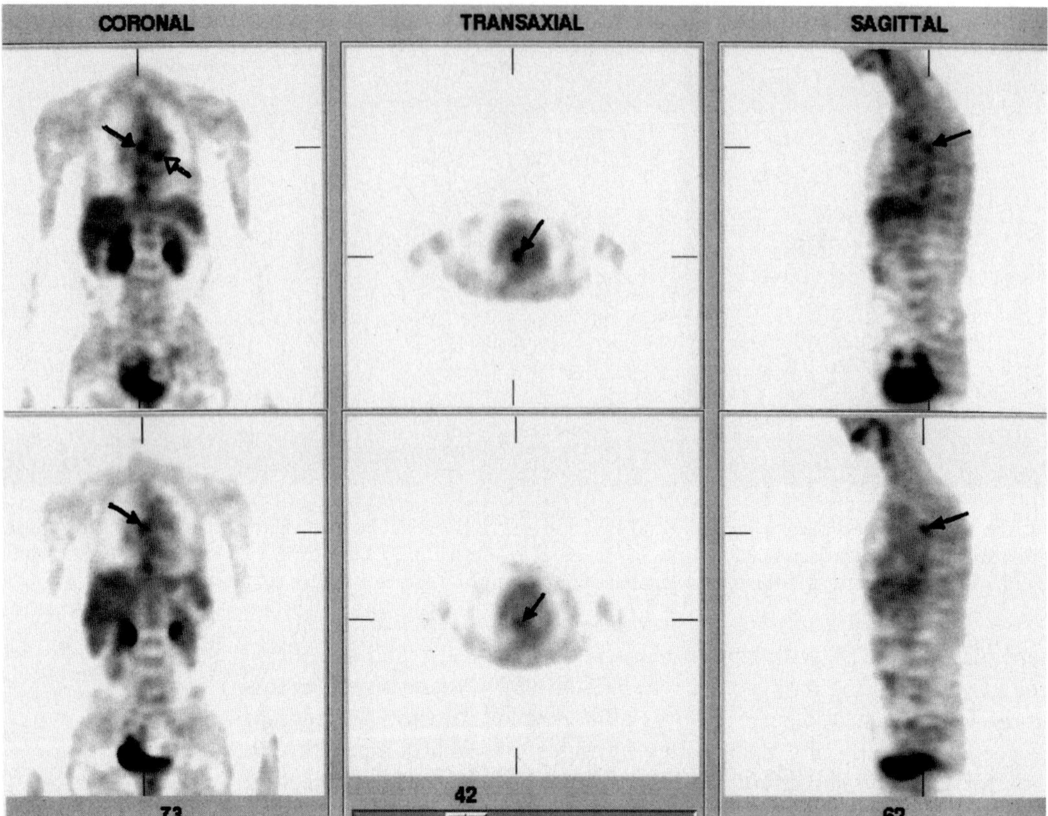

FIGURE 16.9. Selected coronal and sagittal PET images of the axial body as well as an axial image of the mid-chest before (*upper row*) and after (*lower row*) postoperative chemotherapy for lung cancer show a significant metabolic response by decreasing uptake of ^{18}F-FDG in metastatic carinal lymph node (*closed arrows*) and resolution of the focal increased activity in the metastatic left hilar lymph node (*open arrow*).

In a prospective study by Pieterman et al,[26] a logistic regression analysis was used to evaluate the ability of PET and CT to identify malignant mediastinal lymph nodes and distant sites in 102 patients with resectable NSCLC. The sensitivity and specificity of PET for the detection of mediastinal metastases were 91% and 86%, respectively. Detection of unsuspected metastatic disease by PET may permit a reduction in the number of thoracotomies performed for nonresectable disease (Figs. 16.10 and 16.11). For broad groupings of NSCLC stage, 10% of cases were downstaged and 33% upstaged after PET. Stating that incorporated PET provided a more accurate prognostic stratification than did staging with conventional means,[27] PET may reduce the need for mediastinoscopy when the primary NSCLC SUV is <2.5 and the mediastimum is PET negative.[28] The high negative predictive values of PET are benign, biopsy is not needed, and radiographic follow-up is recommended. Some reports have noted that up to 60% of patients with NSCLC develop adrenal metastases, and PET showed 100%

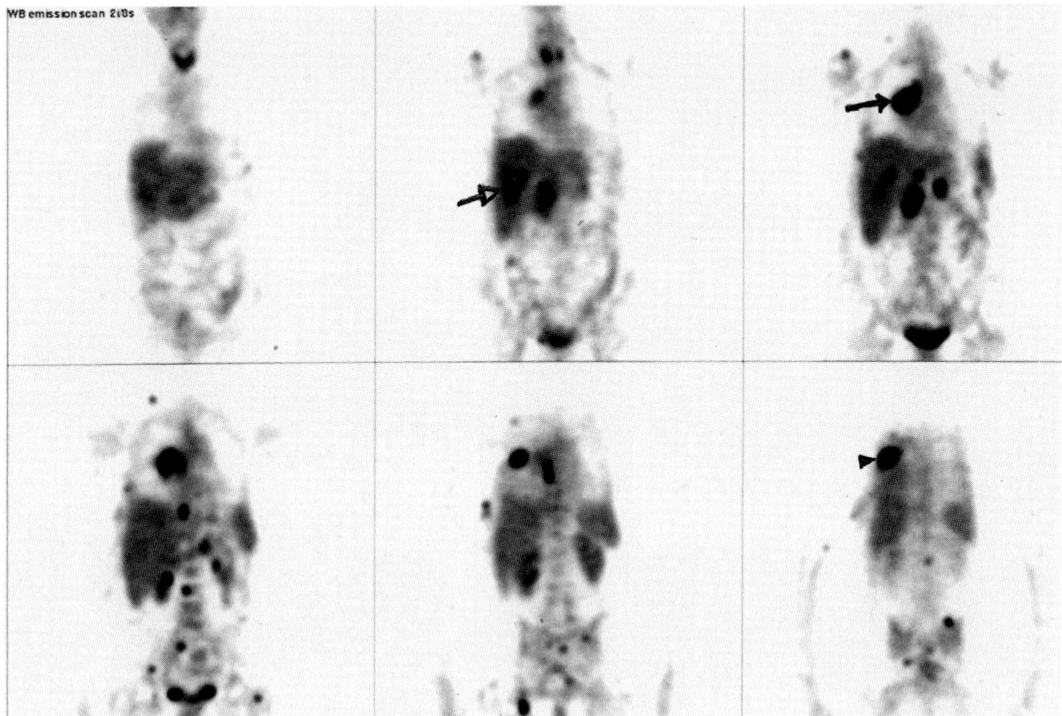

FIGURE 16.10. Coronal PET images of the axial body with ^{18}F-FDG show markedly increased activity in the squamous cell carcinoma of the right hilum (*closed arrow*) and metastases in the right posterior upper lung (*arrowhead*), liver (*open arrow*), and several vertebral bodies, pelvic bones, and the left proximal femur. Note also physiologic activity in the thyroid.

sensitivity and 80% specificity for the diagnosis of adrenal metastasis in CT-detected adrenal lesions between 1 and 9 cm in size.

Detection of Residual or Recurrent Lung Cancer

After potentially curative therapy of NSCLC, abnormalities or symptoms suggesting recurrence can be difficult to characterize. Early detection is important because salvage therapies are available for localized recurrence. PET (Fig. 16.12) better assesses the status of disease and stratifies prognosis than does conventional staging, affects patient management, and should be incorporated into paradigms for suspected recurrence of NSCLC. Lesions with higher tumor-to-muscle ratios responded better to treatment than those with lower ratios. The decrease in FDG uptake after therapy correlated with a partial response to therapy (Fig. 16.13). The relapse rate was higher in tumors with higher uptake ratios before and/or after therapy. The results of a pilot study of the PET use in monitoring response to chemotherapy in 13 patients with primary lung cancer and mediastinal metastases are encouraged. Patz et al[29] studied 43 patients on whom FDG-PET was performed between 4 and 182 months after initial diagnosis and treatment of NSCLC. Thirty-five patients had recurrent or persistent cancer. The median SUV

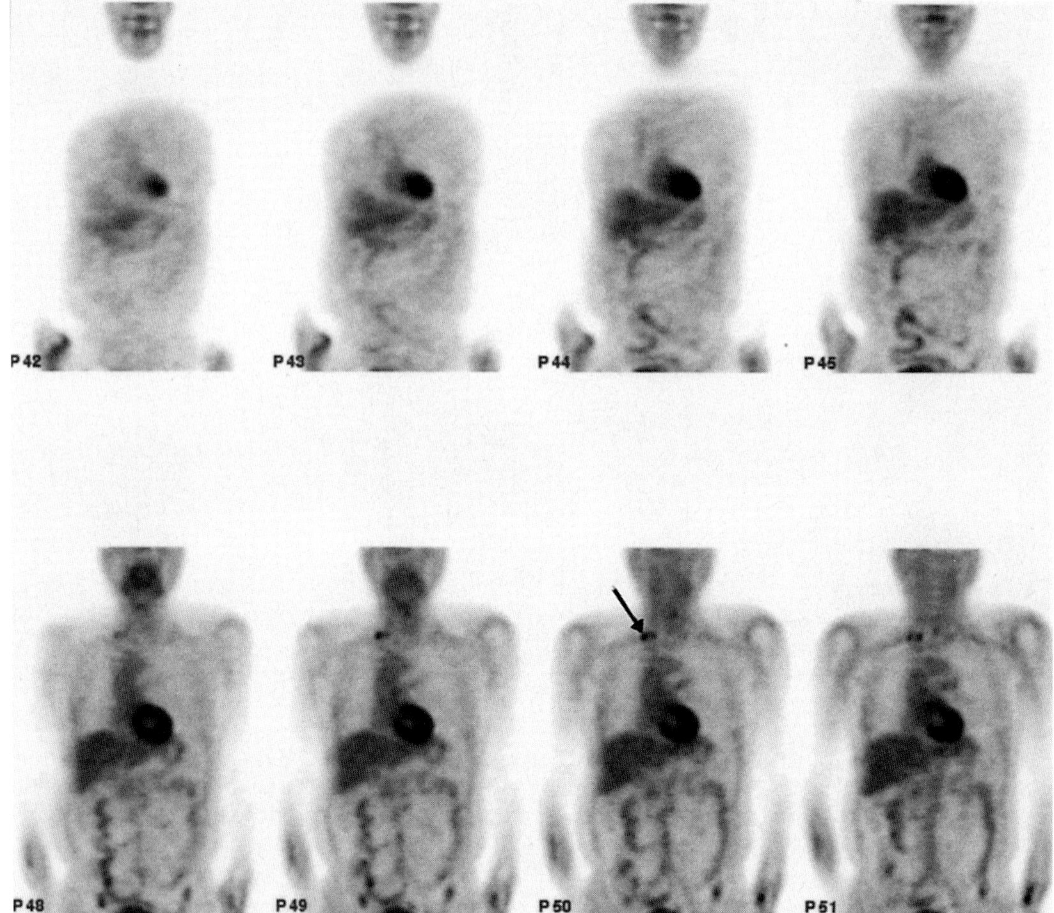

FIGURE 16.11. Coronal PET images of the axial body show small focal areas of ^{18}F-FDG uptake in the metastatic right supraclavicular nodes (*arrow*) of lung cancer.

in the 35 patients who had recurrent or persistent cancer was 7.6 (range 1.9–18), whereas the median SUV in patients who had fibrosis after therapy was 1.6 (range 0.6–2.4). Using an SUV >2.5 to indicate malignancy, FDG-PET had a sensitivity of 97% and a specificity of 100% for the detection of recurrent or persistent disease. In another study of 39 lesions in 38 patients studied by PET after therapy, a sensitivity of 100% and a specificity of 62% were found for the detection of recurrent or persistent lung cancer.[30]

Conclusion

PET (Fig. 16.14) offers an exciting diagnostic tool that can quantify the metabolic activity of a tumor or node, and may reveal additional sites of disease unsuspected on CT, thereby increasing the accuracy of the staging process. Familiarity with the various manifestations of lung

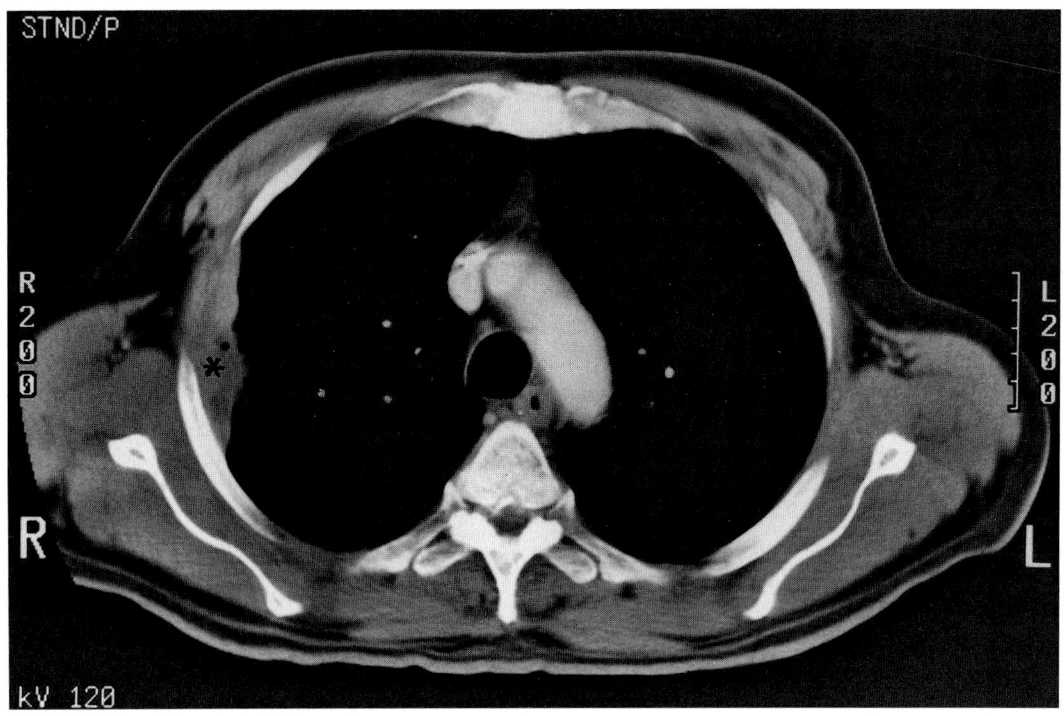

A

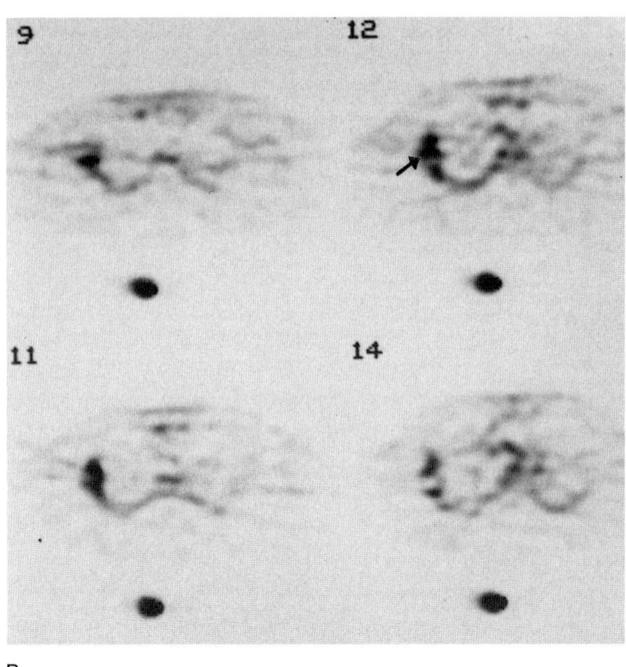

B

FIGURE 16.12. A: Selected follow-up axial CT image of the upper chest show a soft tissue density (*) along the right chest wall. B: Selected axial PET images of the upper chest show increased uptake of ^{18}F-FDG (*arrow*) in the residual cancer following chemoradiation therapy.

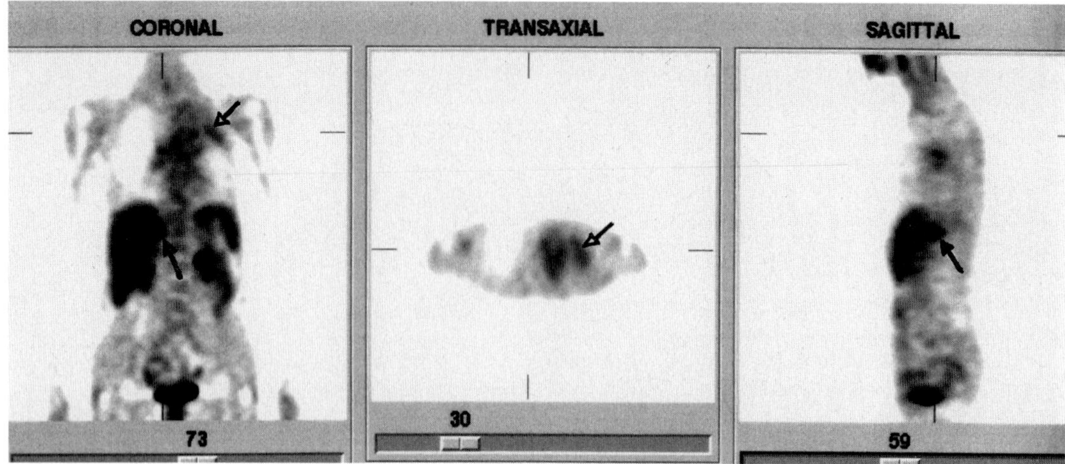

FIGURE 16.13. Selected coronal and sagittal PET images of the axial body as well as an axial image of the upper chest show irregular increased uptake of ^{18}F-FDG in the left upper lung (*open arrow*) and mediastinum due to an inflammatory reaction following radiation therapy. Note also a metastatic lesion (*closed arrow*) in the right adrenal gland.

cancer on chest radiography may help suggest the initial diagnosis. Once a suspicious abnormality is detected, CT is necessary to help confirm the diagnosis by identifying CT findings that would more likely suggest cancer, and to stage the disease. The role of MRI is generally limited to specific problem-solving areas, or when CT findings are equivocal or indeterminate.

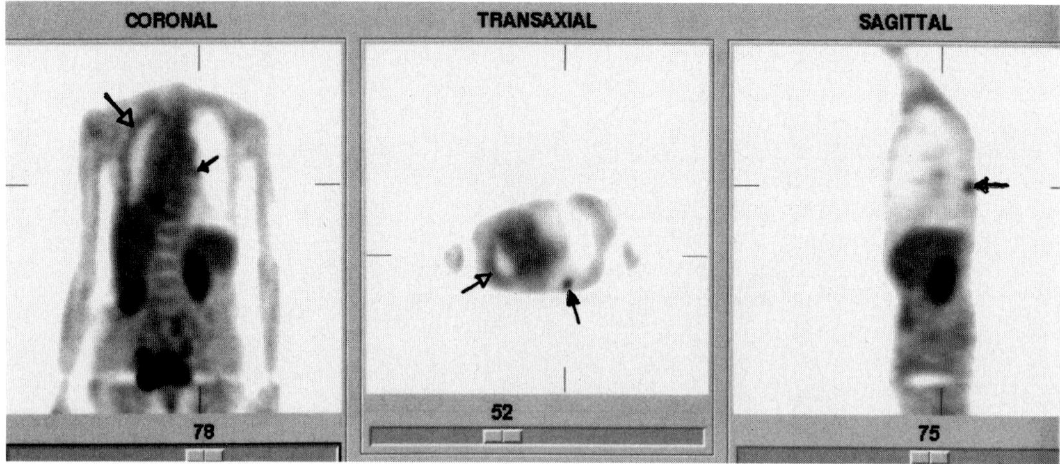

FIGURE 16.14. Selected coronal and sagittal PET images of the axial body as well as an axial image of the mid-chest with ^{18}F-FDG show a significant shift of the mediastinum to the right with slightly increased activity (*open arrow*) along the right chest wall following pneumonectomy for lung cancer. Note the small focal increased activity in the metastatic lesion in the medial posterior aspect of left lower lung (*arrows*).

References

1. Smith RA, Glynn TJ. Epidemiology of lung cancer. Radiol Clin North Am 2000;38:453–470.
2. Magrath I, Litvak J. Cancer in developing countries: opportunity and challenge. J Natl Cancer Inst 1993;85:862–873.
3. Jemal A, Thomas A, Murray T, Thun M. Cancer statistics, 2002. CA Cancer J Clin 2002;52:23–47.
4. Bepler G. Lung cancer epidemiology and genetics. J Thorac Imaging 1999; 14:228–234.
5. Quint LE, Francis IR. Radiologic staging of lung cancer. J Thorac Imaging 1999;14:235–246.
6. Mack MJ, Hazelrigg JR, Landreneau RJ, Acuft TE. Thoracoscopy for the diagnosis of the indeterminate solitary pulmonary nodule. Ann Thorac Surg 1993;56:825–832.
7. Smith TAD. FDG uptake, tumor characteristics, and response to therapy: a review. Nucl Med Commun 1998;19:97–105.
8. Ginsberg RS, Vokes EE, Rosenzweig K. Non-small cell cancer of the lung. In: DeVita VT, Hellman S, Rosenberg SA, eds. Cancer Principles and Practice of Oncology, 6th ed. Philadelphia, Lippincott-Raven, 2002:925–982.
9. Sone S, Sakai F, Takashima S, et al. Factors affecting the radiologic appearance of peripheral bronchogenic carcinomas. J Thorac Imaging 1997;12: 159–172.
10. Mountain C, Libshitz HI, Hermes KE. Lung Cancer: A Handbook for Staging and Imaging. Houston: University of Texas M.D. Anderson Cancer Center, 1992.
11. Yankelevitz DF, Henschke CI. Small solitary pulmonary nodules. Radiol Clin North Am 2000;38:471–478.
12. Romney BM, Austin JH. Plain film evaluation of carcinoma of the lung. Semin Roetgenol 1990;25:45—63.
13. Bouchard EW, Falken S, Molina PL. Lung cancer: a radiologic overview. Appl Radiol 2002;7–19.
14. Swensen SJ, Morin RL, Schueller B, et al. Solitary pulmonary nodule: CT evaluation of enhancement with iodinated contrast material—a preliminary report. Radiology 1992;182:343–347.
15. Schuster MR, Scanlan KA. "CT angiogram sign" establishing the differential diagnosis. Radiology 1991;178:90–95.
16. Park BJ, Louie D, Altorki N. Staging and the surgical management of lung cancer. Radiol Clin North Am 2000;38:545–558.
17. Obuchowski NA, Graham RJ, Baker ME, Powell KA. Ten criteria for effective screening: their application to multislice CT screening for pulmonary and colorectal cancers. AJR 2001;176:1357–1362.
18. Henschke CI, Yankelevitz DF. Screening for lung cancer. J Thorac Imaging 2000;15:21–27.
19. Hatabu H, Syock KW, Sher S, et al. Magnetic resonance imaging of the thorax. Radiol Clin North Am 2000;38:593–616.
20. Flier JS, Mueckler MM, Usher P, et al. Elevated levels of glucose transport and transporter messenger RNA are induced by ras or src oncogenes. Science 1987;235:1492–1495.
21. Coleman RE. PET in lung cancer. J Nucl Med 1999;40:814–820.
22. Lowe VJ, DeLong DM, Hoffman JM, Coleman RE. Optimum scanning protocol for FDG-PET evaluation of pulmonary malignancy. J Nucl Med 1995;36:883–887.

23. Gould MK, Maclean CC, Kuschner WG, et al. Accuracy of positron emission tomography for diagnosis of pulmonary nodules and mass lesions: a meta analysis. JAMA 2001;285:914–924.
24. Gambhir SS, Czernim J, Schwimmer J, et al. A tabulated summary of the FDG-PET literature. N Nucl Med 2001;42(suppl):1S–92S.
25. Graeber GM, Gupta NC, Murray GF. Positron emission tomographic imaging with fluorodeoxyglucose is efficacious in evaluating malignant pulmonary disease. J Thorac Cardiovasc Surg 1999;117:719–727.
26. Pieterman RM,VanPutten JWG, Meuzelaar JJ, et al. Preoperative staging of non-small cell lung cancer with positron emission tomography. N Engl J Med 2000;343:254–261.
27. Hicks RJ, Kalff V, MacManus MP, et al. ^{18}F-FDG-PET provides high-impact and powerful prognostic stratification in staging newly diagnosed non-small cell lung cancer. J Nucl Med 2001;42:1596–1604.
28. Kernstine KH, McLaughlin KA, Menda Y, et al. Can FDG-PET reduce the need for mediastinoscopy in potentially resectable nonsmall cell lung cancer? Ann Thorac Surg 2002;73:394–402.
29. Patz EF Jr, Lowe VJ, Hoffman JM, et al. Persistent or recurrent bronchogenic carcinoma: detection with PET and 2-[F-18]-2-deoxy-D-glucose. Radiology 1994;191:379–382.
30. Inoue T, Kim EE, Komaki R, et al. Detecting recurrent or residual lung cancer with FDG-PET. J Nucl Med 1995;36:788–793.

17

Breast Cancer

E. Edmund Kim and Massashi Yukihiro

In American women, breast cancer is the most frequently diagnosed cancer (212,600 new cases), and the second leading cause of cancer death (40,200 deaths) in 2003.[1] In women aged 40 to 55, breast cancer is the leading cause of all mortality.[1] There has been a slight decline in breast cancer mortality overall,[1] which can be attributed both to the success of early detection and to advanced treatment, particularly systemic therapy. Caucasian women in the United States have a 13.1% lifetime incidence of developing breast cancer, whereas African-American women have a 9.6% lifetime incidence.[1] However, the lifetime risk of dying from breast cancer is 3.4% for both African-American and Caucasian women in the U.S. While the incidence of invasive breast cancer has leveled off, the number of ductal carcinomas in situ (DCIS) has been on the rise, probably a result of the increasing use of screening mammography.

The most common modality for detecting breast cancer is mammography, which is very sensitive but has a low positive predictive value.[2] On ultrasonography it is difficult to distinguish the difference between malignant and benign breast tumors.[3] The sensitivity of magnetic resonance imaging (MRI) is almost 90%, but the specificity is 70%.[3] A reliable noninvasive technique is needed to differentiate benign from malignant breast tumors. Nuclear medicine methods, including positron emission tomography (PET), have been developed for evaluating biochemical and physiologic characteristics of tumors, and they have added unique functional information to the anatomic abnormalities provided by conventional imagings.

Technetium (Tc)-99m hexakis-isobutyl isonitrile (MIBI) is the most popular agent for scintimammography, but Tl 201 chloride and Tc-99m ethylene-bis [bis (2-ethoxyethyl)] phosphine (tetrofosmin) are also used with single photon emission computed tomography (SPECT).[4] ^{18}F-fluorodeoxyglucose (FDG) and ^{11}C-methionine have been also widely used as tumor-seeking agents with PET. Few comparative studies have described the uptake of radiopharmaceuticals as a method of detecting breast cancer. Among SPECT agents, tumor uptake of tetrofosmin was higher than that of MIBI and Tl in mice implanted with MCF-7 breast cancer cells.[4] The order of tumor uptake, from greatest to least, was L-^{18}F-α-methyltyrosine = ^{11}C-methionine > ^{18}F-FDG = tetrofosmin > MIBI = Tl. Tl 201 chloride showed the highest tumor-to-blood ratio (12.8). Tumor-to-muscle ratio, from highest to lowest, was ^{18}F-methyltyrosine = ^{11}C-methionine > ^{18}F-FDG > MIBI > tetrofosmine = Tl.[4] Various radiopharmaceuticals for breast cancer detection have been used for scintimammography and PET.

Although breast cancer is frequently characterized by increased FDG uptake, it displays considerable variation, with many variables affecting the cellular level as well as the microenvironment of tumor masses. Nontumoral tissue such as necrotic and fibrotic tissue may reduce tracer uptake, whereas the presence of inflammatory cells may result in increased FDG accumulation. Like glucose, FDG is a substrate for the first enzyme of glycolysis, hexokinase, and is phosphorylated intracellularly to FDG-6-phosphate. However, because FDG lacks a hydroxyl group in the 2 position, FDG-6-phosphate is not a substrate for either the second enzyme of glycolysis, glucose-6-phosphate isomerase, or for other intracellular metabolic pathways. FDG-6-phosphate is a charged molecule and does not diffuse out of the cell. Because the activity of glucose-6-phosphatase is very low in cancer cells and most normal tissues, the reverse transformation of FDG is relatively slow. Therefore, FDG-6-phosphate remains trapped within the cell, and the cellular level of ^{18}F-activity is related to the rate of glucose uptake and use by the cell. The expression of different types of glucose transporters and hexokinases has been suggested to determine the level of FDG uptake in cancer tissue. PET has attracted considerable attention because of its ability to study a variety of biologic and functional characteristics of breast cancer, such as blood flow, glucose metabolism, and receptor status. Study of tumor blood flow and oxygen utilization does not appear to be clinically relevant.

Staging refers to the grouping of patients according to the extent of their disease, and it is useful in determining the choice of treatment for individual patients, estimating their prognosis, and comparing the results of different treatment programs. Clinical staging includes physical examination, imaging, and pathologic examination of the breast or other tissues to establish the diagnosis of breast carcinoma. The extent of tissue examined pathologically for clinical staging is less than that required for pathologic staging. Appropriate operative findings are elements of clinical staging, including the size of the primary tumor and chest wall invasion, and the presence or absence of local or distant metastasis. Pathologic staging includes all data used for clinical staging, surgical exploration, and resection as well as pathologic examination (Table 17.1).

PET Techniques

Patients must fast for at least 4 to 6 hours before receiving an intravenous injection of 370 to 555 MBq of (10 to 15 mCi) ^{18}F-FDG over 2 minutes so that the serum insulin concentration will be at the basal level and the blood glucose level will be within the normal range (<130 mg/dL). An intravenous cannula is placed in the arm contralateral to

Table 17.1. Staging of breast cancer

Primary tumor (T)	
T0	No evidence of tumor
Tis	Carcinoma in situ
T1	$\leq$2 cm (0.1 < 1a < 0.5, 0.5 < b < 1, 1 < 1c < 2)
T2	2–5 cm
T3	>5 cm
T4	Extension to chest wall (4a), skin (4b), both (4c), or inflammatory carcinoma (4d)
Regional lymph node (N)	
N0	No node metastasis
N1	Movable ipsilateral axillary node
N2	Fixed ipsilateral axillary node
N3	Ipsilateral internal mammary node
Distant metastasis (M)	
M0	No distant metastasis
M1	Metastasis including ipsilateral supraclavicular node
Stage 0	Tis, N0, M0
Stage I	T1, N0, M0
Stage IIA	T0 or T1, N1, M0; T2, N0, M0
IIB	T2, N1, M0; T3, N0, M0
Stage IIIA	T0 or T1, or T2, N2, M0; T3, N1 or N2, M0

the breast tumor, and blood samples are drawn. Patients are positioned supine or prone after comfortable positioning on the scanner table with a foam rubber support and both arms at their sides. A 25-minute transmission study for attenuation correction is performed either before the study or after the completion of the emission study injection, using a connection for emission counts during transmission.

Dynamic imaging of metabolism is performed for 60 minutes after the start of ^{18}F-FDG infusion. The standard clinical protocol is started 60 minutes after tracer injection, and images are acquired over six to eight bed positions and displayed in axial, coronal, and sagittal planes. Transmission scans are obtained with Ge 68 and rod sources, and images are reconstructed using algebraic algorithms. Attenuation correction is required for quantitative or semiquantitative assessment of tracer uptake. Blood flow imaging is performed using 962 to 1998 MBq of ^{15}O-water. Dynamic ^{15}O-water images are collected for 7.75 minutes after injection, and peak total coincidence counting rates do not exceed 700 kilocycles per second (kcps). Background counts from the ^{15}O water study are $\leq$4 kcps at the start of the ^{18}F-FDG studies with a typical ^{18}F-FDG peak counting rate of 80 kcps. Also, 1500 to 2000 mL of 0.45% or 0.9% saline over 1.5 to 2 hours and 20 mg furosemide given over 20 minutes are helpful in facilitating clearance of the activity from the renal collecting system and ureter. A Foley catheter in the bladder is also useful to ensure adequate clearance of bladder activity.

Breast Cancer Diagnosis and Staging by PET

PET of the breast offers physiologic information and therefore it can act as an adjunct to conventional imaging, which provides morphologic information. PET can identify larger breast tumors with high accuracy and has also shown encouraging results in detecting regional lymph node metastases.[5] However, PET is currently restricted by its limited sensitivity in detecting small breast tumors. Partial-volume effects play an important role, but an increase in metabolic activity with tumor growth may also occur. There was no significant relationship between FDG accumulation and tumor size, but a significant difference in FDG uptake was found to be dependent on the microscopic growth pattern of breast cancer.[5] Nodular tumors with clearly visible tumor borders had a higher FDG uptake than did breast carcinomas with diffuse infiltration of surrounding tissue [standard uptake value (SUV) 4.1 ± 2.3 vs. 0.8 ± 0.2)].[5] Invasive lobular carcinomas had significantly lower FDG uptake (SUV 3.8) compared with invasive ductal carcinomas (SUV 5.6).[6] Invasive lobular carcinoma is generally more difficult to diagnose than invasive ductal carcinoma by imaging procedures including mammography, sonography, and MRI.[7]

Tissue heterogeneity is an important factor contributing to the total FDG uptake in tumors. The relative composition of malignant tumors ranges from a few transformed cells to >90% of malignant cells. Because of the limited spatial resolution of PET scanners, the signal derived from tumors represents an average FDG uptake in all tumor components. Components with low metabolic activity, namely, cells containing mucine, connective tissue, and necrosis, may reduce the total FDG uptake in tumors, resulting in a false-negative PET.[8] A weak relationship was found between FDG uptake and the percentage of tumor cells.[5] It has been suggested that the number of tumor cells may gain substantial importance only if the percentage of tumor cells is low (<30%); above this level, the PET signal from tumors reflects primarily the metabolic activity rather than the number of malignant cells. Breast carcinomas consisting of only scattered malignant cells are difficult to identify in PET images.[5] Inflammatory cells may significantly contribute to FDG uptake in tumors. Newly formed granulation tissue around the tumor as well as macrophages in the margins of necrosis show an increased FDG uptake. However, no relationship was found between the presence of inflammatory cells and the intensity of FDG uptake.[5] A weak inverse relationship was found between FDG uptake and the density of microvessels.[5] Under anaerobic conditions, most malignant tumors metabolize glucose primarily to lactate, which results in higher utilization rates for glucose molecules. Hypoxia is present in tumor tissue beyond 100 to 200 μm of functional blood supply and is commonly found in solid tumors. A significant increase in FDG accumulation was found under moderately hypoxic conditions.[9] Studies with ^{15}O-water in human squamous cell carcinoma of the head and neck revealed no correlation between tumor perfusion and FDG uptake.[10]

Recent clinical data indicate that tumor hypoxia negatively affects the therapeutic outcome of both radiotherapy and chemotherapy in various cancers. There was a more than twofold increase in ^{3}H-FDG uptake in MCF7 breast cancer cells under hypoxic conditions, partly due to an increase in glucose transporter activity by reduction of the thiol group in the glucose transport protein.[11] Modulation of hexokinase activity was probably not involved.

Radiodense breasts are found in women undergoing hormone replacement therapy and in those who have had breast augmentation or breast-conserving therapy for breast cancer. Mammographic evaluation of the postbiopsy or postsurgical breast is very difficult because of scar formation or high density of implants. In such situations, FDG-PET (Fig. 17.1) seems to be particularly useful and may obviate the biopsy. FDG-PET can image tumors in the augmented breast without implant displacement and without obvious degradation of image quality by the implant.[12] The potential role of FDG-PET in breast imaging would be for the detection of multicentric or multifocal lesions and thus demonstrate the true extent of breast cancer. The finding of multifocal cancer may alter the therapy from lumpectomy to mastectomy. Another potential role of FDG-PET in detecting occult primary breast cancer in a patient with known metastasis to axillary lymph node has been investigated.

One of the most important roles for FDG-PET is the accurate staging of regional lymph node metastasis (Fig. 17.2). Approximately 60% of patients with breast cancer have regional nodal metastasis at initial diagnosis. The axillary lymph nodes are involved in 40% of patients with breast cancer. The 10-year survival rate is significantly higher in patients with no involvement of nodes (65–80%) than in those with involvement of one to three nodes (38–63%) or more than three axillary nodes (13–27%).[13] The axillary lymph node status is the single most

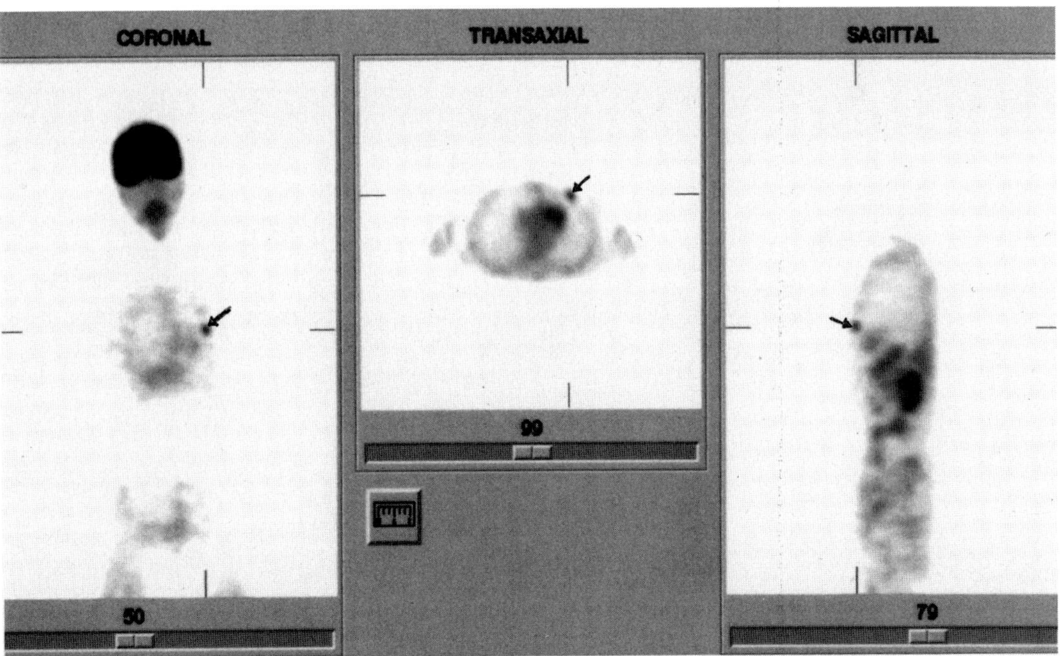

FIGURE 17.1. Selected coronal and sagittal PET images of the whole body as well as an axial image of the lower chest show slightly increased uptake of ^{18}F-FDG in the left breast carcinoma (*arrows*).

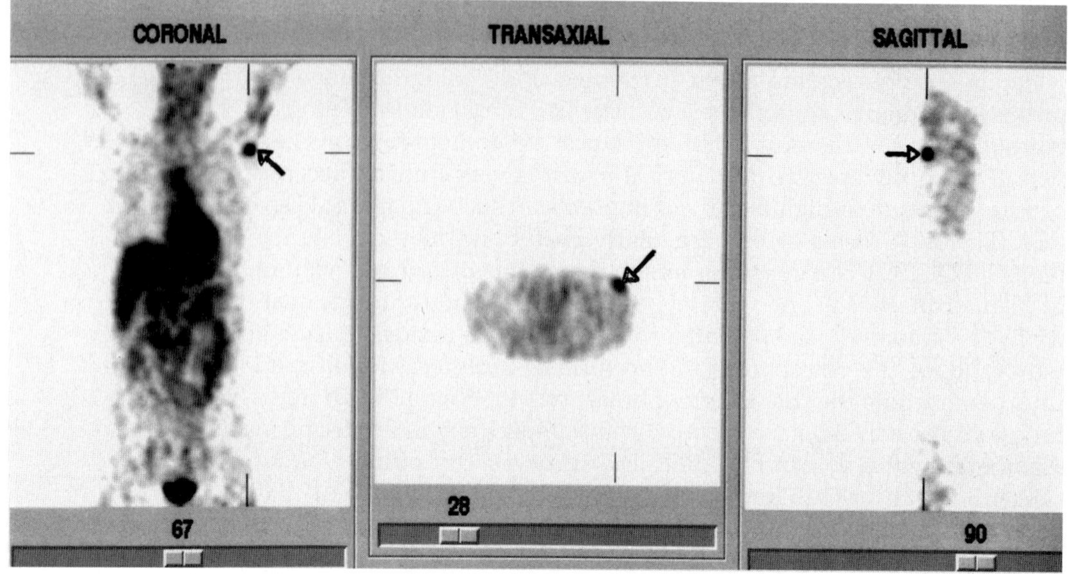

FIGURE 17.2. Selected coronal and sagittal PET images of the axial body as well as an axial image of the upper chest with ^{18}F-FDG show focal increased activity in the left axillary lymph node (*arrows*) due to infiltration of the injection radioactivity intravenously.

important prognostic indicator in breast cancer patients (Figs. 17.3 and 17.4). Avril et al,[14] using qualitative FDG-PET in 51 patients, have reported an overall sensitivity of 79% and specificity of 96% for detection of axillary nodal involvement. However, the sensitivity was only 33% without any change of specificity in patients with tumors <2 cm.

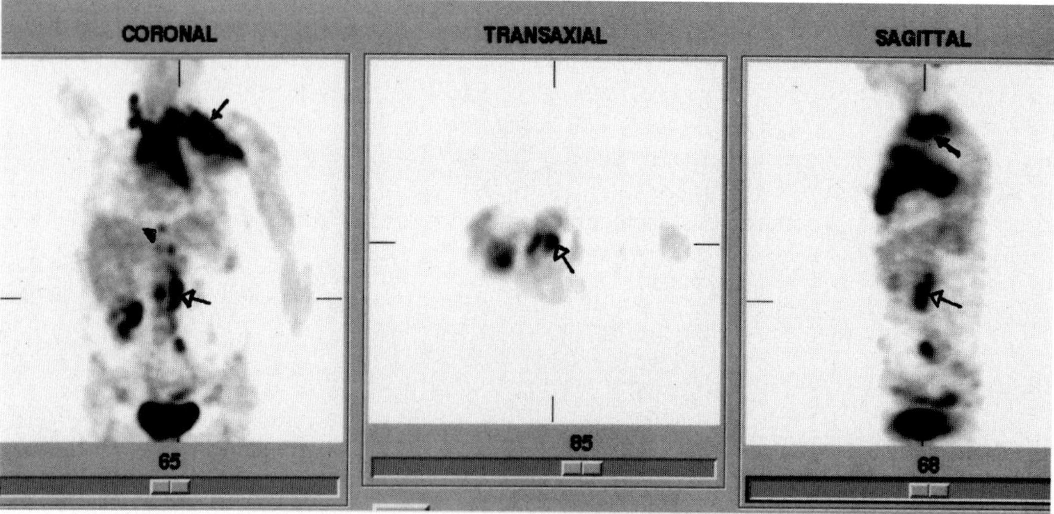

FIGURE 17.3. Selected coronal and sagittal PET images of the axial body and an axial image of the mid-abdomen show markedly increased uptake of ^{18}F-FDG in the right lower jugular, left axillary (*closed arrows*), superior mediastinal, hilar, anterior diaphragmatic (*arrowhead*), bilateral para-aortic (*open arrows*), and left iliac lymphatic chains with metastatic breast cancer.

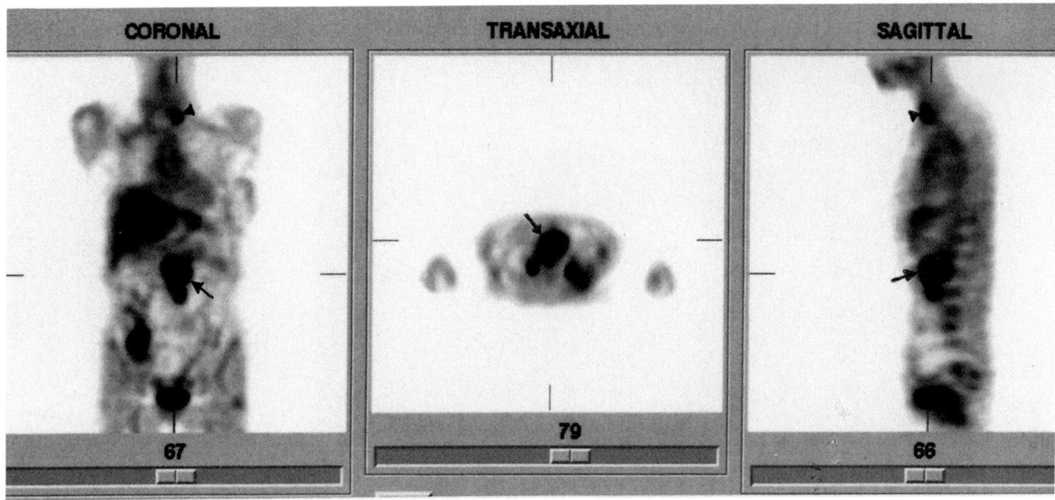

FIGURE 17.4. Selected coronal and sagittal PET images of the axial body and axial image of the upper abdomen with ^{18}F-FDG show markedly increased activity in the left supraclavicular (*arrowheads*) and prevertebral (*arrows*) lymphatic chains with metastatic breast cancers.

In a prospective study of 124 patients, Utech et al,[15] demonstrated a weak correlation between the quantitative FDG uptake in the metastatic axillary nodes and the size and the S-phase fraction of the primary breast tumor in the 44 patients who had axillary nodal involvement. Guided by PET results, axillary dissection might be limited to patients with positive PET studies. However, PET is notable to detect micrometastatic disease to lymph nodes. No imaging technique is routinely used to image internal mammary nodes, and sampling is not routinely performed.

FDG-PET can detect not only the primary breast cancer and nodal metastases, but also bone (Fig. 17.5) and liver (Fig. 17.6) metastases. The overall sensitivity of FDG-PET for the detection of all malignant lesions is reportedly greater than 85%, with a positive predictive value of 94%.[16] Many reports have suggested that PET is more sensitive than conventional staging imaging at detecting the true extent of disease and often reveals unsuspected metastases.

PET for Monitoring Therapy

PET offers the ability to assess tumor metabolic activity quantitatively, and thus may predict tumor behavior and therapeutic response (Fig. 17.7). After therapy, the amount of tumor FDG uptake reflects the number of viable tumor cells present with the glucose metabolic rate of tumor cells (Fig. 17.8).[17] It has been shown that an increase in FDG uptake in breast cancer over time is associated with tumor progression.[18] Semiquantitative and qualitative FDG-PET of primary breast cancers showed a rapid and significant decrease in tumor glucose metabolism shortly after institution of chemohormonotherapy.[19] We have com-

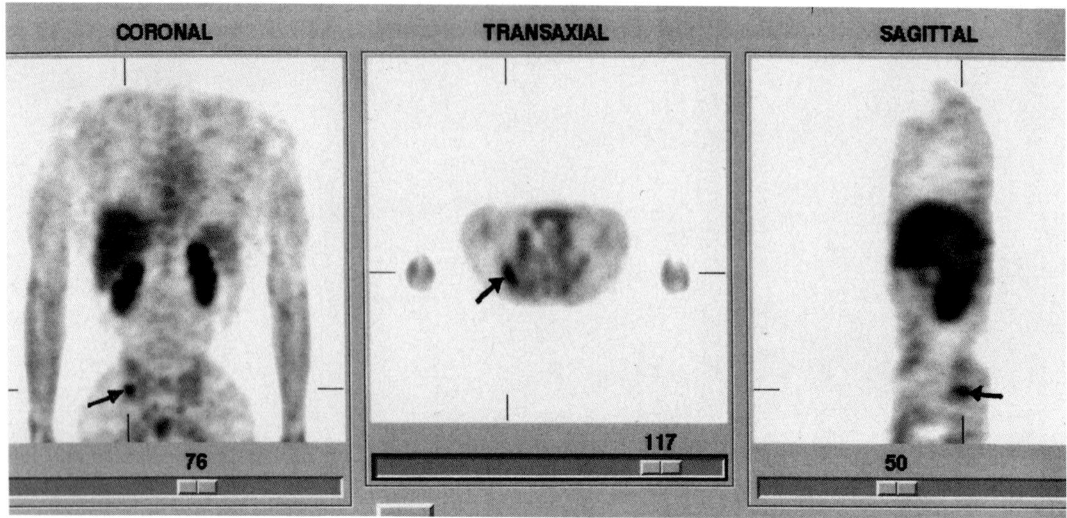

FIGURE 17.5. Selected coronal (*left*) and sagittal (*right*) PET images of the axial body as well as an axial (*middle*) image of the pelvis show focal increased uptake of ^{18}F-FDG in metastatic breast cancer involving the right iliac tuberosity (*arrows*). Note marked physiologic renal activity.

pared FDG-PET with mammography and ultrasonography in 16 patients with locally advanced breast carcinoma who received preoperative chemotherapy. FDG-PET was superior to both mammography and ultrasonography for the detection of primary breast cancer. There was a substantial decrease in tumor metabolism early in the course of effective chemotherapy.[20] These reports suggest that PET could be used to guide changes in treatment regimen early during a course of therapy, based on tumor response at the biochemical level. Recent studies

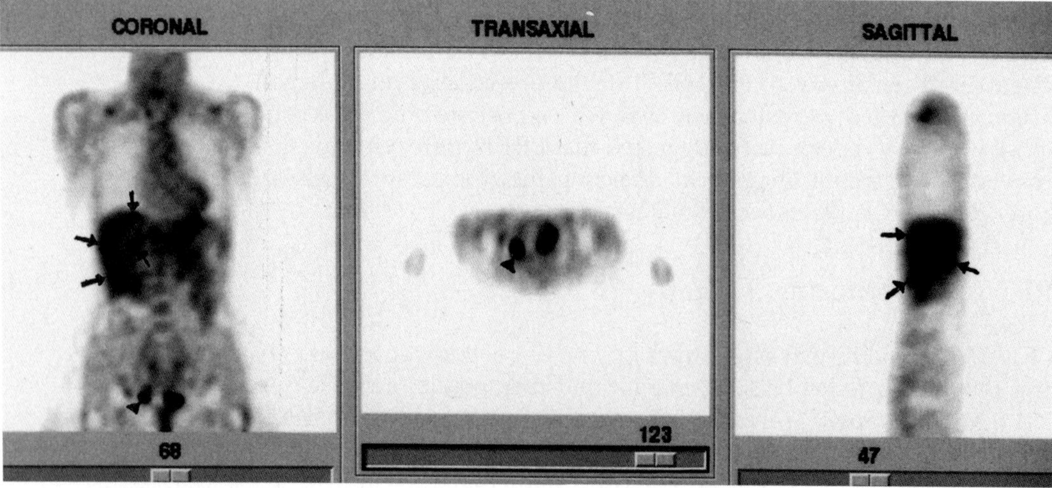

FIGURE 17.6. Selected coronal and sagittal PET images of the axial body and an axial image of the lower pelvis in a patient with breast cancer show markedly increased uptake of ^{18}F-FDG in multiple metastatic lesions in the liver (*arrows*) and also right external iliac lymph node (*arrowhead*). Note physiologic activity in the bilateral anterior neck muscles.

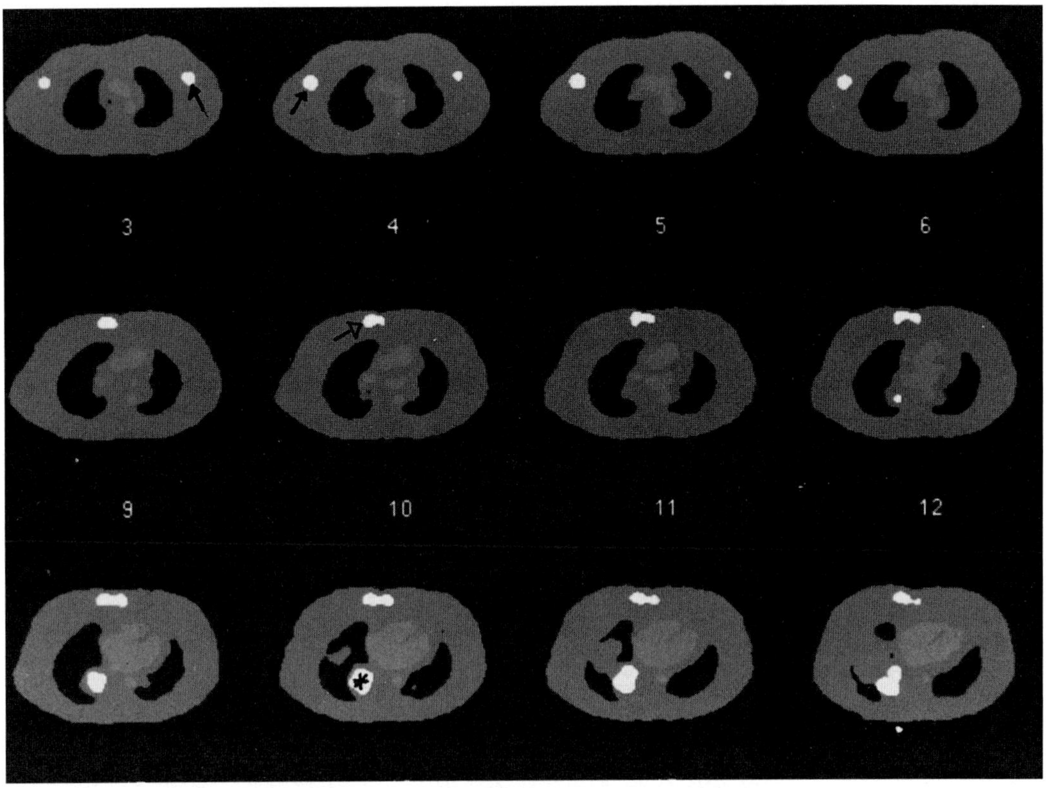

FIGURE 17.7. Superimposed transaxial PET images of the chest in a patient with breast cancer show markedly increased uptake of ^{18}F-FDG in the metastatic axillary nodes (*closed arrows*), sternum (*open arrow*), and right posterior lung base (*). Background activities including heart and liver are ^{15}O-water uptake.

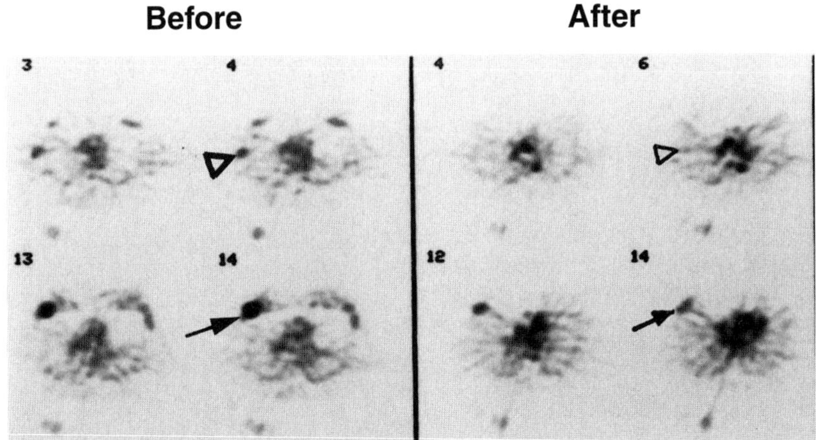

FIGURE 17.8. Selected axial PET images of the chest before and after chemotherapy show a significant metabolic response of the right breast cancer (*arrows*) and metastatic right axillary lymph node (*arrowheads*) with decreasing uptake of ^{18}F-FDG.

also reported that FDG-PET can be used to improve prediction of the clinical outcome of previously treated breast cancer patients relative to what is achievable through conventional imaging alone. The positive and negative predictive values of PET were 93% and 84%, respectively. The prognostic accuracy of single whole-body PET was superior to that of multiple procedures with conventional imaging (90% vs 75%).[21]

Receptor Imaging

The majority of breast cancers are hormone dependent, as shown by increases in the estrogen and progesterone receptors in the tumor. Estrogen receptor (ER)-positive breast cancers are less aggressive than ER-negative ones, and they are likely to respond to hormonal therapy.

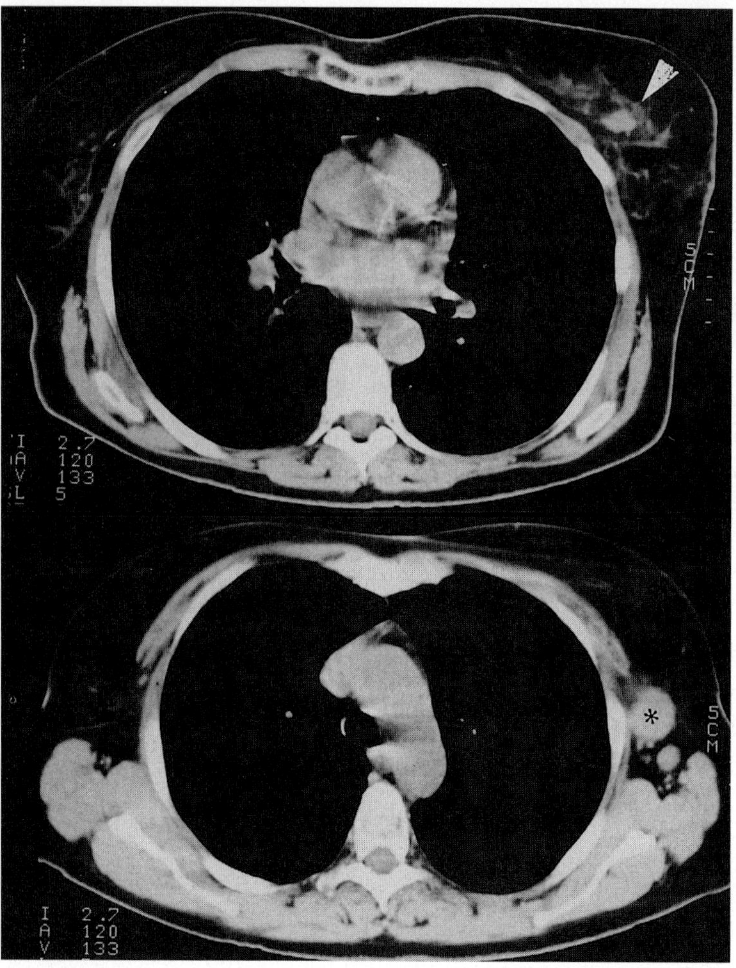

A

FIGURE 17.9. A: Axial computed tomography (CT) images of the chest show a 1.5-cm left breast cancer (*arrowhead*) and 2.5-cm sized left axillary lymph node. B: Selected axial PET images of the chest show minimally increased uptake of ^{18}F-tamoxifen in the left axillary lymph node (*arrows*). Left breast cancer (*arrowheads*) is not identified with significant activity, although estrogen receptor assay was positive.

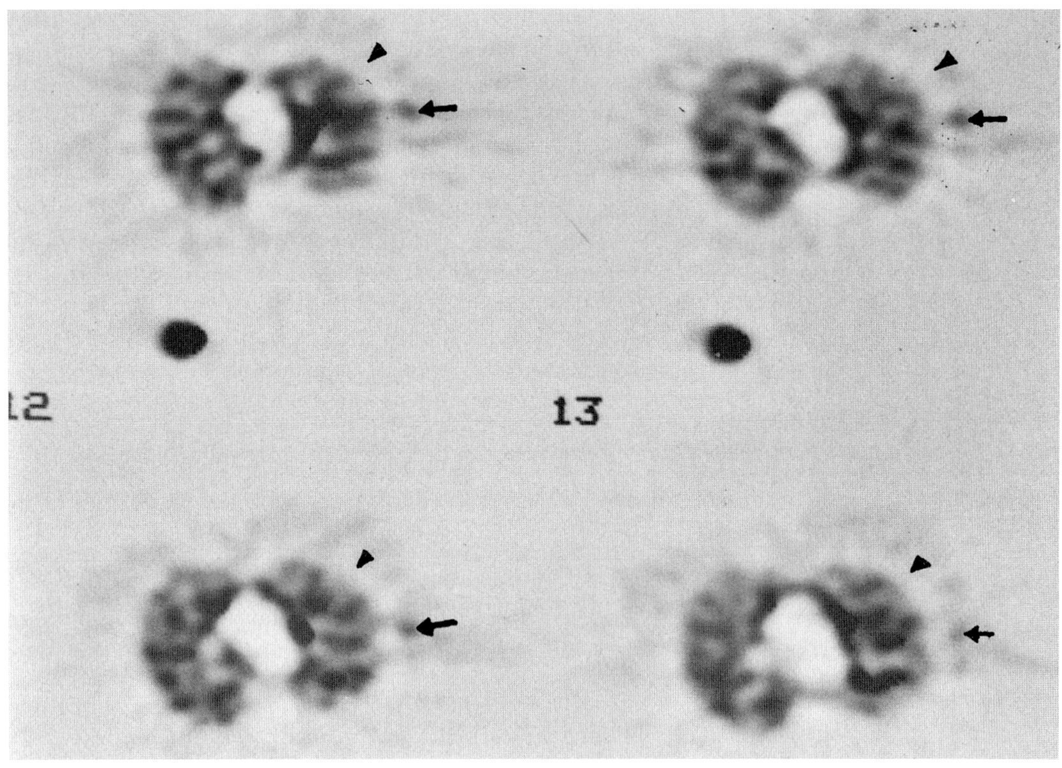

B

FIGURE 17.9. *(continued)*

Quantitative and qualitative assays provide limited information about the functional status of the receptors and responsiveness to hormone therapy: only 55% to 60% of patients with ER-positive breast cancer respond to such treatment.[22] Therefore, a noninvasive method for functional status of receptors would be of critical importance of identifying patients who will benefit from hormone therapy. Various steroidal and nonsteroidal estrogens labeled with ^{77}Br, ^{75}Br, ^{18}F, ^{123}I, and Tc-99m have been synthesized. 16d-^{18}F-fluro-17B-estradiol (FES) has high specific activity and high affinity for ER-positive target tissues. FES-PET has been shown to be highly sensitive (93%) for detection of ER-positive metastatic foci in patients with breast cancer.[23] In addition, FES accumulation within metastatic lesions decreased following institution of tamoxifen therapy.[24] However, there was no significant relationship between FDG uptake and either ER status or FES uptake.[25] The overall rate of agreement between the results of in vitro ER assays and the results of FES PET was 88%.[25] Tumor heterogeneity and ER concordance between primary and metastatic breast cancers have been observed. The information about the intrinsic heterogeneity of receptor expression within individual lesions as well as the concordance or discordance between the primary and metastatic or recurrent lesions may be very useful in selecting the mode of therapy, and the biologic availability of the receptors in vivo may predict more reliably hormone responsiveness than the in vitro assay results (Fig. 17.9). The discordance between primary and metastatic or recurrent lesions has been reported in 20% to 25% of breast cancer patients.[25]

The clinical flare reaction is seen in 5% to 20% of patients with ER-positive metastatic breast cancer and generally occurs within 7 to 10 days after institution of antiestrogen therapy.[26] Clinically and radiographically, the flare reaction is not distinguishable from progression of disease. It is presumably due to temporary agonist effects of the antiestrogen agent on the tumor. It has been shown that tamoxifen and estrogen cause a similar increase in FDG uptakes in ER-rich organs early in the course of therapy.[27] Response to tamoxifen was correctly predicted by the presence of metabolic flare (increased FDG uptake) and the degree of ER blockade (decreased FES uptake) after tamoxifen therapy.[28]

References

1. Jemal A, Thomas A, Murray T, et al. Cancer Statistics, 2002. CA Cancer J Clin 2002;52:23–47.
2. Kopans DB. The positive predictive value of mammography. AJR 1992; 1158:521–526.
3. Stavros AT, Thickman D, Sisney GA, et al. Solid breast nodules: use of sonography to distinguish between benign and malignant lesions. Radiology 1995;196:123–133.
4. Amano S, Inoue T, Tomiyoshi K, et al. In vivo comparison of PET and SPECT radiopharmaceuticals in detecting breast cancer. J Nucl Med 1998; 39:1424–1427.
5. Avril N, Menzel M, Dose J, et al. Glucose metabolism of breast cancer assessed by F-18 FDG-PET: histologic and immunohistochemical tissue analysis. J Nucl Med 2001;42:9–16.
6. Crippa F, Seregini E, Agresti R, et al. Association between F-18 flurodeoxyglucose uptake and postoperative histopathology, hormone receptor status, thymidine labelling index and p53 in primary breast cancer; a preliminary observation. Eur J Nucl Med 1998;25:1429–1434.
7. Paramagul CP, Helvic MA, Adler DD. Invasive lobular carcinoma: sonographic appearance and role of sonography in improving diagnostic sensitivity. Radiology 1995;195:231–234.
8. Brown RS, Leung JY, Fisher SJ, et al. Intratumoral distribution of tritiated fluorodeoxyglucose in breast carcinoma. Are inflammatory cells important? J Nucl Med 1995;36:1854–1861.
9. Clavo AC, Wahl RL. Effects of hypoxia on the uptake of tritiated thymidine, L-leucine, L-methionine and FDG in cultured cancer cells. J Nucl Med 1996;37:502–506.
10. Haberkorn U, Strauss LG, Reisser C, et al. Glucose uptake, perfusion, and cell proliferation in head and neck tumors: relation of positron emission tomography to flow cytometry. J Nucl Med 1991;32:1548–1555.
11. Burgman P, O'Donoghue JA, Humm JL, et al. Hypoxia-induced increase in FDG uptake in MCF7 cells. J Nucl Med 2001;42:170–175.
12. Wahl RL, Helvie MA, Chang AE, et al. Detection of breast cancer in women after augmentation mammoplasty using F-18 fluorodeoxyglucose PET. J Nucl Med 1994;35:872–875.
13. Flanagan FL, Dehdashti F, Siegel BA. PET in breast cancer. Semin Nucl Med 1998;28:290–302.
14. Avril N, Dose J, Jäniicke F, et al. Assessment of axillary lymph node involvement in breast patients with positron emission tomography using ra-

diolabeled 2-(fluorine-18)-fluoro-2-deoxy-D-glucose. J Natl Cancer Inst 1996;88:1204–1209.

15. Utech CI, Young CS, Winter PF. Prospective evaluation of F-18 FDG-PET in breast cancer for staging of the axilla related to surgery and immunocytochemistry. Eur J Nucl Med 1997;23:1588–1593.
16. Hoh K, Hawkins RA, Glaspy JA, et al. Cancer detection with whole-body PET using F-18 FDG. J Comput Assist Tomogr 1993;17:582–289.
17. Haberkorn U, Reinhardt M, Strauss LG, et al. Metabolic design of combination therapy: use of enhanced fluorodeoxyglucose uptake caused by chemotherapy. J Nucl Med 1992;33:1981–1987.
18. Minn H, Soini I. F-18 FDG scintigraphy in diagnosis and follow up of treatment in advanced breast cancer. Eur J Nucl Med 1989;15:61–66.
19. Jansson T, Westlin JE, Ahlström H, et al. PET studies in patients with locally advanced and/or metastatic breast cancer: a method for early therapy evaluation? J Clin Oncol 1995;13:1470–1744.
20. Bassa P, Kim EE, Inoue T, et al. Evaluation of preoperative chemotherapy using PET with F-18 FDG in breast cancer. J Nucl Med 1996;37:931–938.
21. Vranjesevic D, Filmont JE, Meta J, et al. Whole-body F-18 FDG-PET and conventional imaging for predicting outcome in previously treated breast cancer patients. J Nucl Med 2002;43:325–329.
22. Ravdin PM, Green S, Dorr TM, et al. Prognostic significance of progesterone receptor levels in estrogen receptor positive patients with metastatic breast cancer treated with tamoxifen: results of a prospective Southwest Oncology Group study. J Clin Oncol 1992;10:1284–1291.
23. McGuire AH, Dehdashti F, Siegel BA, et al. Positron tomographic assessment of estrogen receptors in breast assays. J Nucl Med 1995;36:1766–1774.
24. Dehdashti F, Mortimer JE, Siegel BA, et al. Positron tomographic assessment of estrogen receptors in breast cancer. Comparison with FDG-PET and in vitro receptor assays. J Nucl Med 1995;36:1766–1774.
25. Butler JA, Trezona T, Vargas H, et al. Value of measuring hormone receptor levels of regional metastatic carcinoma of the breast. Arch Surg 1989;124:1131–1136.
26. Welch MJ, Bonasera TA, Sherman EIC, et al. F-18 FDG and 162-(F-18) fluoroestradiol-17B (FES) uptake in estrogen-receptor (ER)-rich tissues following tamoxifen treatment: a preclinical study. J Nucl Med 1995;36:39–44.
27. Wahl RL, Cody R, Fisher S. Uptake before and after estrogen receptor stimulation: feasibility studies for functional receptor imaging. J Nucl Med 1991;32:1011–1015.
28. Dehdashti F, Flanagan FL, Siegel BA. PET assessment of metabolic flare in advanced breast cancer. Radiology 1997;205:220–225.

18

Esophageal, Gastric, Pancreatic, and Colorectal Cancers

Tomio Inoue, Nobukazu Takahashi, and E. Edmund Kim

Esophageal Cancer

The recent progress in diagnostic and therapeutic methods has changed the clinical management of patients with esophageal cancer. In the field of diagnosis of esophageal cancer, the endoscopic technique using dye or endoscopic ultrasonography (EUS) has increased the diagnostic sensitivity for early esophageal cancer. The prognosis in patients with esophageal cancer has been improved by introducing the lymph node resection of three regions or the superior mediastinum. However, surgery in patients with esophageal cancer is an invasive procedure, and the postsurgical complications are still severe. It requires a cautious treatment decision in patients with esophageal cancer even if the perioperative management has been advanced.[1] Anatomic imaging such as computed tomography (CT), magnetic resonance imaging (MRI), and ultrasonography (US), is the standard examination for investigating tumor extent, tumor invasion to the adjacent organs, and distant metastases. Fluorodeoxyglucose positron emission tomography (FDG-PET) and tumor metabolic imaging can provide supplemental information in conjunction with anatomic imaging (Fig. 18.1).

Staging

To study the extent of the primary tumor, we investigated the relationship between T grade in the tumor-node-metastasis TNM classification of the International Union Against Cancer and the tumor standard uptake value (SUV) of FDG in primary lesions. About 50% of primary lesions of esophageal cancer in the early stage estimated as pT1 (tumor localized within the submucosal layer) were visible on FDG-PET images, while all primary lesions estimated as pT2, pT3, and pT4 were visible. The mean SUV of FDG in pT1 primary lesions was significantly lower than those in pT2, pT3, and pT4. There was a significant linear correlation between the longitudinal diameter of the primary lesion and the SUV of FDG. These results suggest that FDG-PET may provide useful information about the tumor extent of the primary lesion (Fig. 18.2).[2]

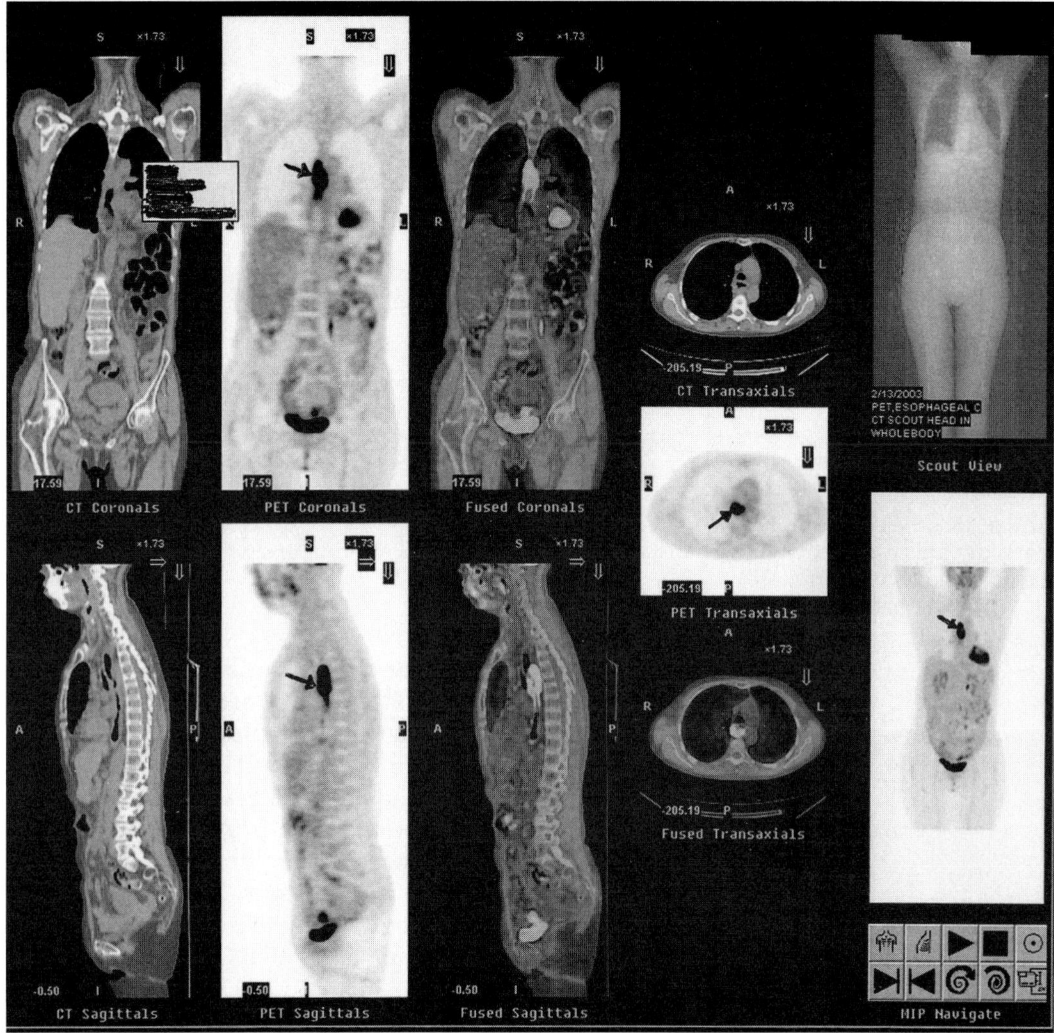

FIGURE 18.1. Selected coronal and sagittal PET and CT images of the axial body as well as an axial image of the mid-chest show markedly increased uptake of ^{18}F-FDG vertically in the posterior mid-chest (*arrows*) located in the mid-esophageal cancer on PET/CT fused images.

Accurate diagnosis of the extent and number of lymph node metastases is important for the management of patients with esophageal cancer, because it relates to the patients' prognosis. In our study, the diagnostic sensitivity, specificity, and accuracy of FDG-PET versus CT for the lymph node metastases were 55% vs 45%, 98% vs 94%, 92% vs 87%, respectively.[2] The sensitivity of FDG-PET and CT was not so high because of the existence of microscopic metastasis. Either intense FDG uptake in the primary lesions or physiologic FDG uptake in the myocardium and stomach may also obscure tracer uptake in the metastatic lesion of the adjacent lymph nodes. Except for the detection of metastases in the abdominal lymph nodes, diagnostic sensitivity for the lymph node metastases of ^{11}C-choline PET was superior to that of

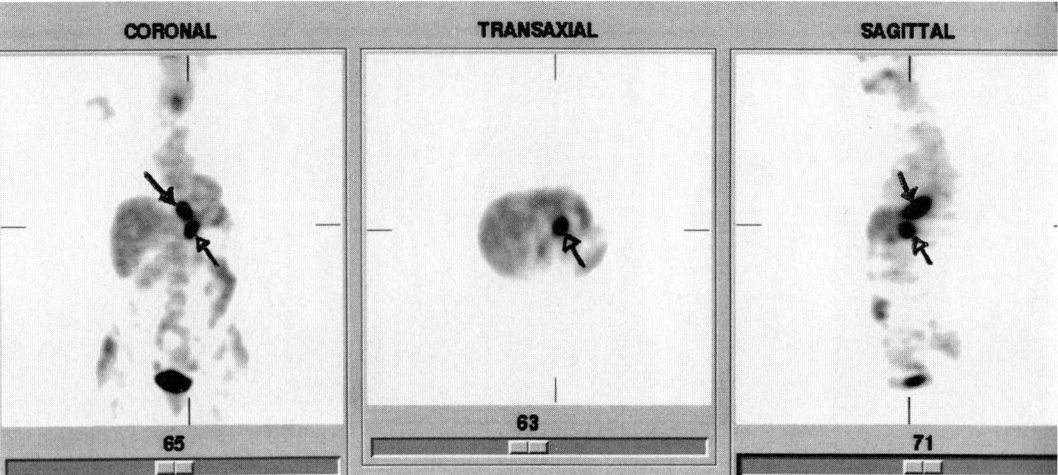

FIGURE 18.2. Selected coronal (*left*) and sagittal PET images of the axial body with ^{18}F-FDG show markedly increased activity in the distal esophageal cancer (*closed arrows*), and a metastatic lesion in the celiac node (*open arrows*).

FDG.[3] The detection by CT of lymph node metastases in the border zone area between the cervical region and the upper mediastinum, such as the supraclavicular and infraclavicular lymph nodes, was difficult in some esophageal cancer cases. In these cases FDG-PET could facilitate the visual interpretation of lymph node metastases. A skip metastasis beyond the adjacent lymph node area is a characteristic phenomenon of metastasis from esophageal cancer. If the range of the field of view of CT or MRI was not sufficient to observe skip lesions, whole-body FDG-PET would be helpful in detecting these skip lesions. FDG-PET, CT, and EUS are probably equivalent in TNM staging accuracy when used independently. When there is nodal FDG uptake in the upper abdomen, differentiating regional lymph node N1 from celiac lymph node M1a is difficult. In these cases, PET/CT would be quite helpful to obtain the accurate TNM staging classification.[4]

Metastases from esophageal cancer are frequently found in the liver, lung, and bone. Lowe et al[4] reported that the greatest contributors to false-positive CT results were nonspecific lesions in the liver and local nodal findings. PET and CT added important M staging information that could not be obtained by EUS.

Monitoring

Wieder et al[5] investigated the time course of tumor glucose utilization in patients with esophageal cancer undergoing preoperative chemoradiotherapy. They measured the SUV of primary lesions prior to chemoradiotherapy at a radiation dose of 14 to 20 Gy, as well as 30 Gy, and 3 weeks after the completion of chemoradiotherapy (immediately preoperatively). The mean SUV at each point was 10.21, 6.83, 3.09, and 3.54, respectively. At a radiation dose of 14 to 20 Gy, the SUV was already significantly decreased. The decrease in tumor SUV at this point was 39.6% in patients with a histopathologic response, whereas it was only 22.3% in patients without a histopathologic response. These results suggest that FDG-PET may be used for early identification of nonresponding tumors and therapy modification.[5]

Case Presentation

A 74-year-old man was diagnosed with advanced esophageal cancer. A double-contrast image of upper GI series revealed a large primary esophageal tumor (Fig. 18.3A). On a coronal view of FDG-PET, intense tumor FDG uptake in the primary lesion (*arrow*) and abnormally increased uptake in the regional lymph nodes were observed (Fig. 18.3B). On a CT image of the upper mediastinum, lymph adenopathy was observed (Fig. 18.3C). On another slice of the coronal view, abnormally increased FDG uptake in the upper mediastinal lymph node and perigastric lymph nodes represented metastatic disease (Fig. 18.3D).

Gastric Cancer

The main diagnostic tool in patients with suspected gastric cancer is an endoscopy. FDG-PET has been widely used in oncology diagnosis, but little in the diagnosis of gastric cancer probably because physiological FDG uptake in the stomach is observed frequently and its contour on tracer uptake is variable and impossible to differentiate from gastric cancer.[6] Physiologic gastric uptake of FDG may be due partly to smooth muscle activity,[7] but the details of the mechanism are still unknown.

Differential Diagnosis and Staging

Yoshioka et al[8] found that FDG-PET demonstrated whole lesions in 42 gastric cancer patients with a sensitivity of 71%, specificity of 74%, and accuracy of 73%. Uptake was high in the primary lesions, liver, lymph node, and lung metastases, but low in the bone metastases, ascites, peritonitis carcinomatosa, and pleuritis carcinomatosa.

The diagnosis of intraabdominal dissemination in patients with gastric cancer is important for determining the indication for surgical resection. Nodules in intraabdominal cavity can be shown on FDG-PET images, but the differentiation from physiologic intestinal FDG uptake is difficult (Fig. 18.4). This diagnostic dilemma may be resolved by the fusion imaging technique of PET/CT.

Monitoring Therapeutic Effect

Stahl et al[9] investigated the predictability of FDG-PET for response to neoadjuvant chemotherapy in patients with gastric cancer. They conducted FDG-PET studies in advanced gastric cancer patients at baseline and 14 days after initiation of cisplatinum-based polychemotherapy. When a reduction of tumor FDG uptake by more than 35% was employed as a criterion for subsequent tumor response, the positive and negative predictive value of FDG-PET for histopathologic response was 77% and 90%, respectively.

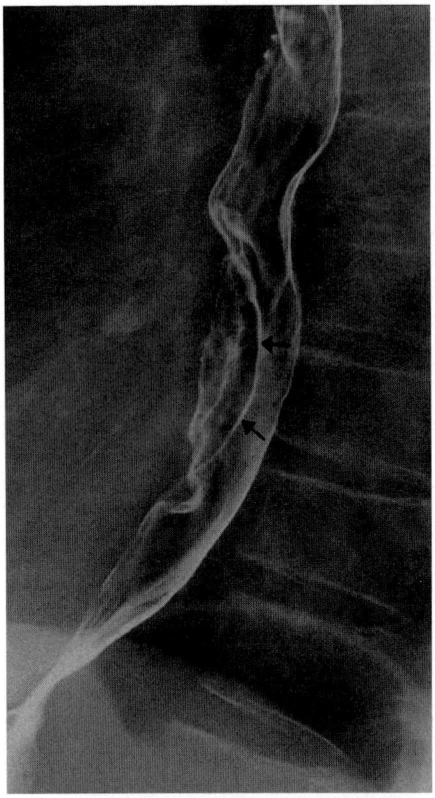

A

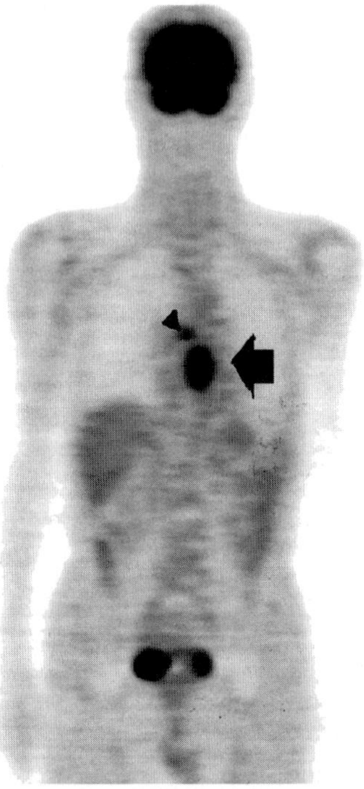

B

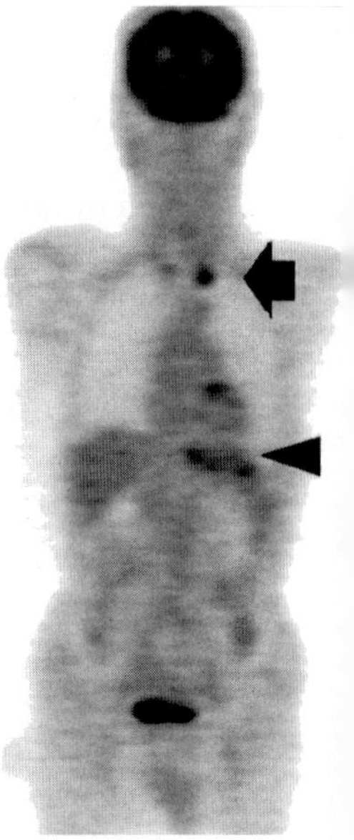

D

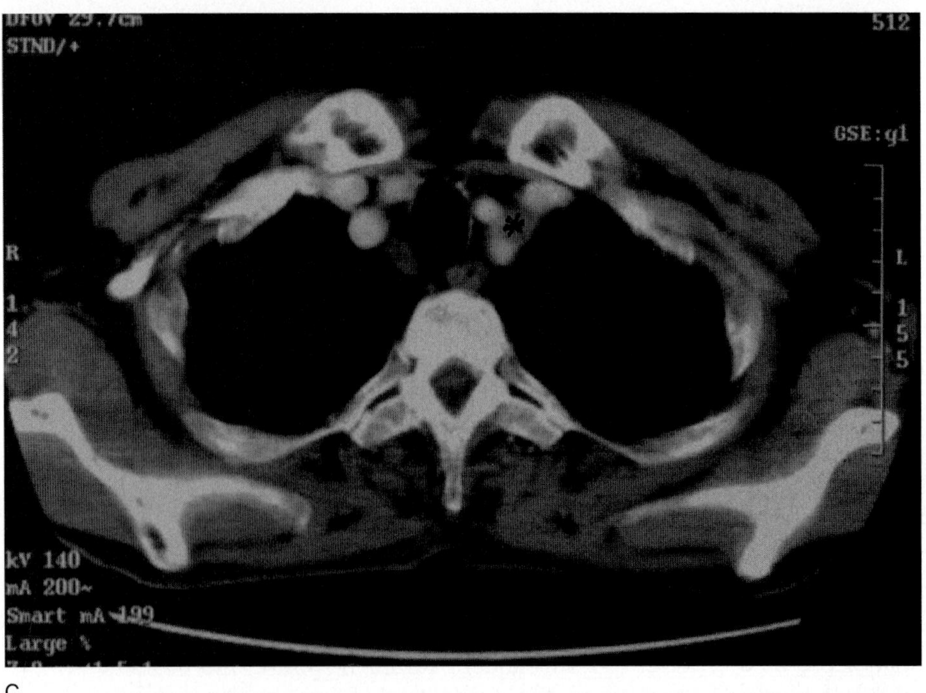

C

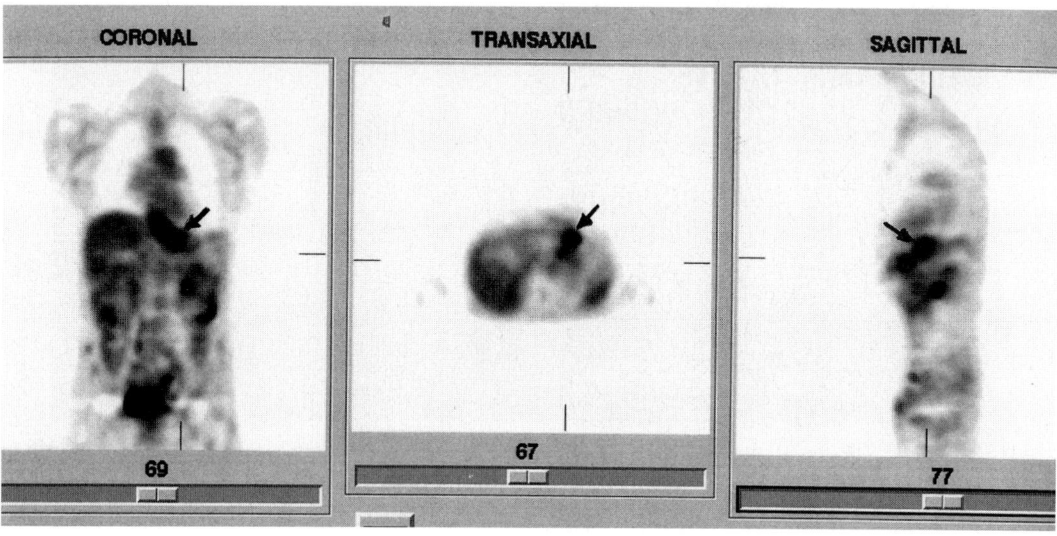

FIGURE 18.4. Selected coronal (*left*) and sagittal (*right*) PET images of the axial body as well as an axial (*middle*) image of the upper abdomen with ^{18}F-FDG show markedly increased activity (*arrows*) in the gastric fundus including the gastroesophageal junction, which has carcinoma.

Case Presentation

A 70-year-old man was diagnosed with advanced gastric cancer. The patient suffered from body weight loss and severe anemia. A bleeding mass near the cardia was found by endoscopic examination, and a poorly differentiated adenocarcinoma was diagnosed histopathologically. CT revealed a diffusely thickened gastric wall (Fig. 18.5A). FDG-PET revealed intense uptake in the primary lesion (*arrowhead*), and metastatic lesions in the retroperitoneal area (*white arrow*) and superior mediastinal area, as well as in the Virchow lymph nodes (*black arrow*) (Fig. 18.5B).

Pancreatic Cancer

FDG-PET is one of the diagnostic modalities expected to improve the diagnostic accuracy for pancreatic tumors, especially in the differentiation between benign and malignant. Generally, FDG-PET reveals high

FIGURE 18.3. A: Double-contrast image of the esophagus shows a large mass of carcinoma with an irregular mucosal pattern in the distal esophagus (*arrows*). B: Selected coronal PET images of the whole body shows markedly increased uptake of ^{18}F-FDG in the distal esophageal carcinoma (*arrow*) and a metastatic lesion in the right subcarinal node (*arrowhead*). C: Axial contrast-enhanced CT image of the upper chest shows a 1-cm left supraclavicular lymph node (*). D: Selected coronal PET image of the whole body, slightly anterior to Fig. 18.1B, shows markedly increased uptake of ^{18}F-FDG in the metastatic esophageal cancer in the left supraclavicular node (*arrow*). Note also moderately increased activity in the metastatic perigastric lymph nodes (*arrowhead*).

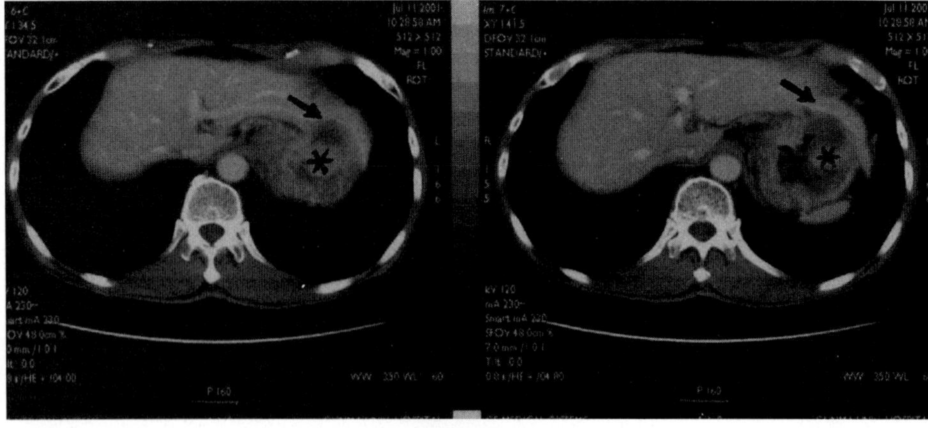

A

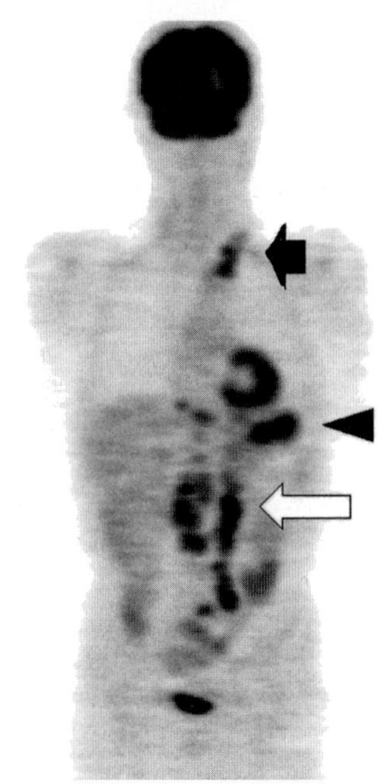

B

FIGURE 18.5. A: Contrast-enhanced axial CT images of the upper abdomen show intraluminal mass (*) and thick wall (*arrows*) of the stomach. B: Selected coronal PET image of the whole body shows increased uptake of ^{18}F-FDG in the gastric cancer (*arrowhead*) and metastatic lesions in the left supraclavicular (*closed arrow*) and para-aortic (*open arrow*) lymph nodes.

uptake of primary and metastatic lesions of pancreatic cancer (Fig. 18.6), while lower FDG uptake occurs in the benign pancreatic lesion such as chronic pancreatitis. Overexpression of the glucose transporter (GLUT) and increased permeability of tumor vessels contributed to the increased FDG uptake in pancreatic cancer.[10,11] Among the subtypes of GLUT, GLUT-1 is especially overexpressed in pancreatic cancer.[10,11]

Differential Diagnosis

In cases of chronic pancreatitis, a postinflammatory mass resulting from formulating pancreatitis mimics malignant pancreatic disease. It

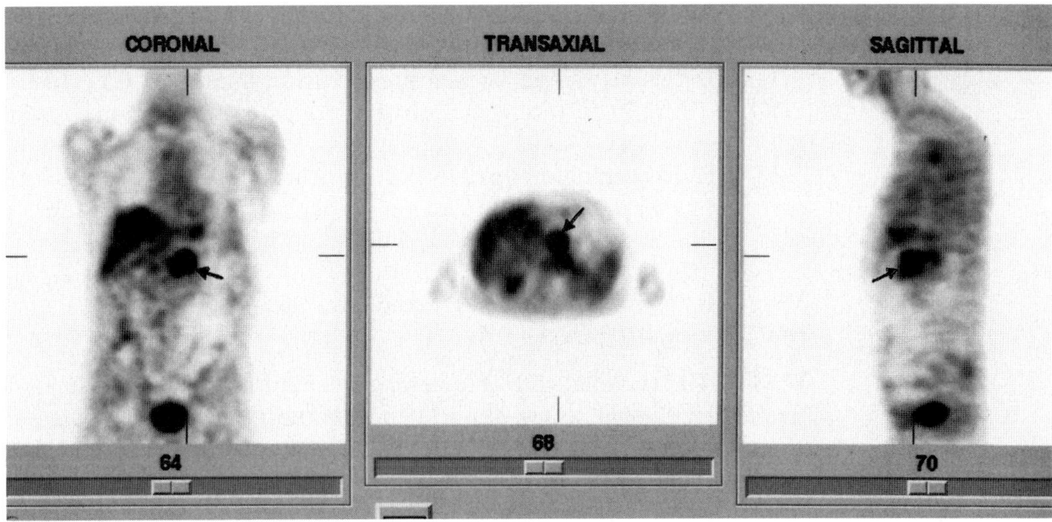

FIGURE 18.6. Selected coronal and sagittal PET images of the axial body and an axial image of the upper abdomen show markedly increased uptake of ^{18}F-FDG in the pancreatic body with carcinoma (*arrows*).

is difficult to have an accurate differential diagnosis between the two diseases. The utility of FDG-PET for the differential diagnosis between benign and malignant disease was reported in a comparative study using CT.[12,13] The sensitivity and the specificity of FDG-PET ranged from 85% to 100% and 77% to 88%, respectively. Overall accuracy ranged from 85% to 95%. These diagnostic results of FDG-PET were superior to those of CT. Objective interpretation of FDG-PET in oncology is based on the semiquantitative index of FDG uptake in lesions, such as the SUV. Many authors found that the average SUV in pancreatic cancer was higher than that of benign pancreatic disease.[12–14] A lesion with an SUV of more than 5.0 is likely to be malignant, while a lesion with an SUV less than 2.5 is likely to be benign. However, the distribution of SUVs overlapped between benign and malignant lesions. As mentioned above, the relatively lower specificity of FDG-PET may be due to FDG uptake in inflammatory cells.

Tumor Detection

Early detection of pancreatic cancer is still difficult despite the recent development of imaging technology such us multi-raw detector CT, fast spin echo MRI, and Doppler US. Higashi et al[15] presented a favorable result for diagnostic sensitivity (74%) of FDG-PET in patients with pancreatic cancers of less than 2 cm in diameter, with a comparative study using other imaging modalities as CT, MRI, endoscopic retrograde cholangiopancreatography (ERCP), and endoscopic US. Many patients with pancreatic diseases suffer from diabetes mellitus, which is a cause of decrease in FDG tumor uptake.

Staging

The identification of primary tumor extent and regional lymph node metastasis with FDG-PET alone is not clinically sufficient because of a lack of spatial resolution. Physiologic intestinal FDG uptake and intense FDG uptake in the primary lesion obscures the faint FDG uptake in adjacent small lymph node lesions. Fusion images of CT/US and FDG-PET help in the interpretation of tumor extent and regional lymph node metastasis.

FDG-PET is useful for the detection of metastatic hepatic lesions from pancreatic cancer. In certain cases of pancreatic cancer, metastatic lesions in the liver invisible on CT/MRI could be visible on FDG-PET.

Diagnosis of Recurrent Disease and Monitoring the Therapeutic Effect

FDG-PET in patients with colorectal cancer and head or neck cancer is useful for clinical follow-up and the diagnosis of recurrent disease, since the good prognosis in patients with these cancers requires long-term follow-up after the initial treatment. On the other hand, recurrent or metastatic lesions in patients with pancreatic cancer occur earlier than those in patients with colorectal and head or neck cancers. There are few reports describing the utility of FDG-PET for the detection of recurrent disease in patients with pancreatic cancer. However, FDG-PET (Fig. 18.7) may be useful for the detection of recurrent lesions after the initial surgical treatment, since postsurgical scars, which interfere with the accurate diagnosis of recurrent disease on CT/MRI, may show faint or no FDG uptake.

Monitoring Therapeutic Effect

The change of tumor FDG uptake derived from PET imaging before and after treatment may be used as an index of therapeutic effect. Patients with higher FDG uptake in a pancreatic tumor tend to have a poor prognosis.

Case Presentation

A 60-year-old man with oral cavity cancer underwent a follow-up FDG-PET study (Fig. 18.8), which accidentally revealed abnormal focal uptake (SUV = 3.0) in the upper abdomen (*arrow*). Focal FDG uptake in a metastatic lesion of the left cervical lymph node was also presented on the coronal section image. CT (Fig. 18.8B) revealed a faint enhanced mass in the pancreas head. A follow-up FDG-PET study was conducted 5 months after the first PET study, and FDG uptake in the left cervical lesion disappeared while it increased in the upper abdomen on the image of the second FDG-PET study (Fig. 18.8C). Unfortunately, we could not conduct a surgical resection of the tumor because of the peritoneal dissemination.

Colon Cancer

Approximately 130,000 new cases of colorectal cancer are diagnosed in the United States every year. Approximately 70% of these patients undergo a radical surgical resection of primary lesions, but only two

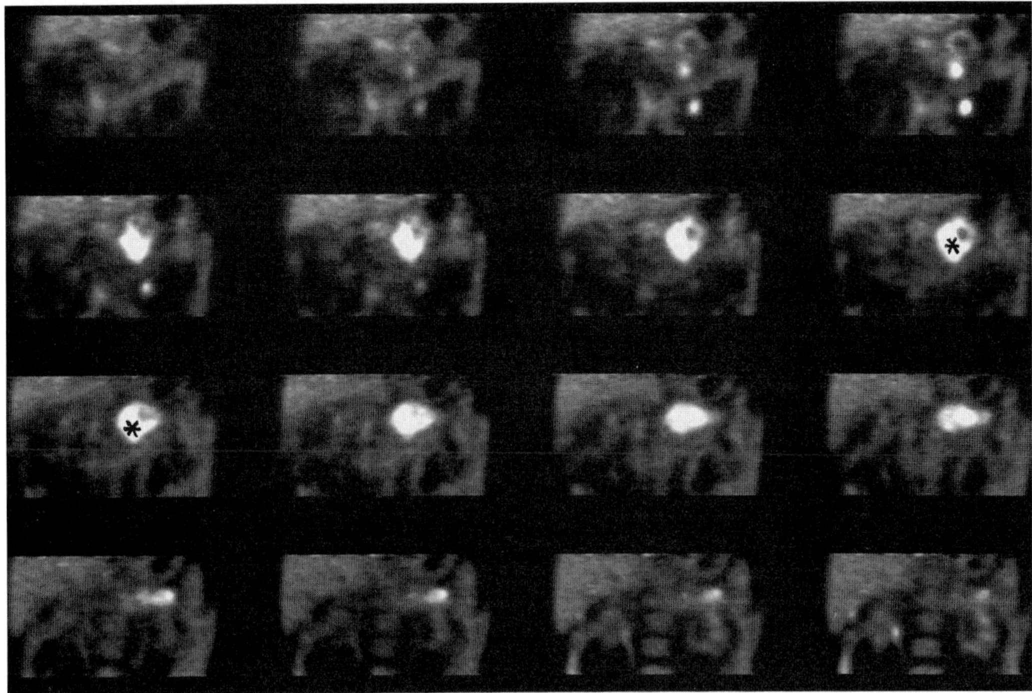
A

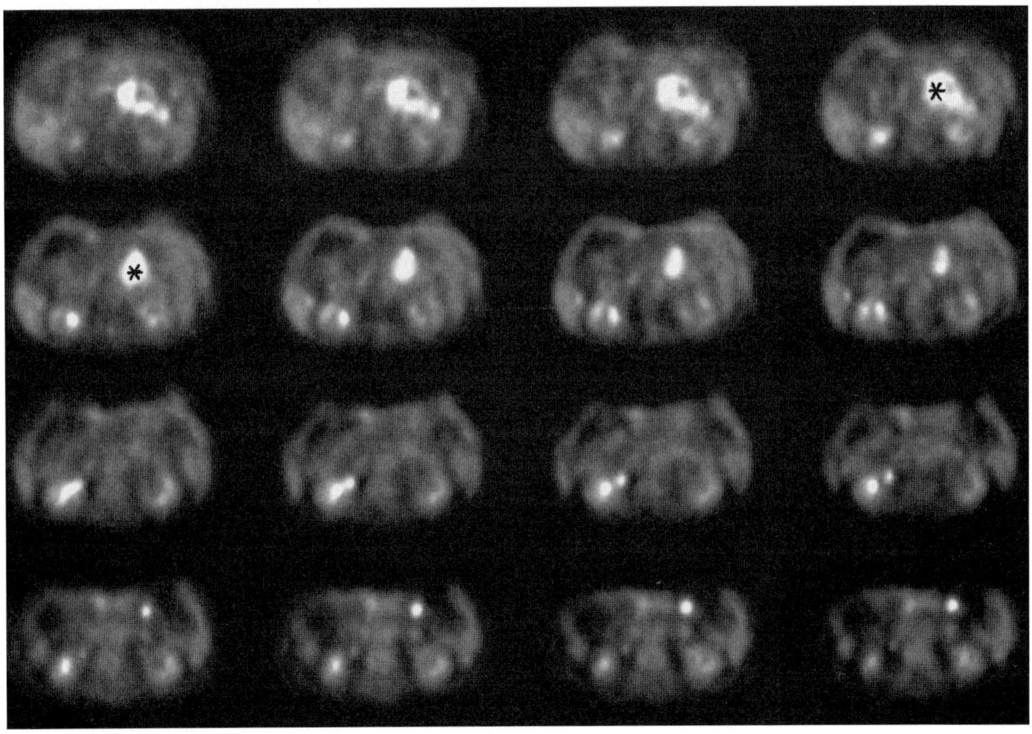
B

Figure 18.7. Coronal (A) and axial (B) PET images of the upper abdomen with ^{18}F-FDG show marked increased activity in the pancreatic body and tail (*) with recurrent carcinoma.

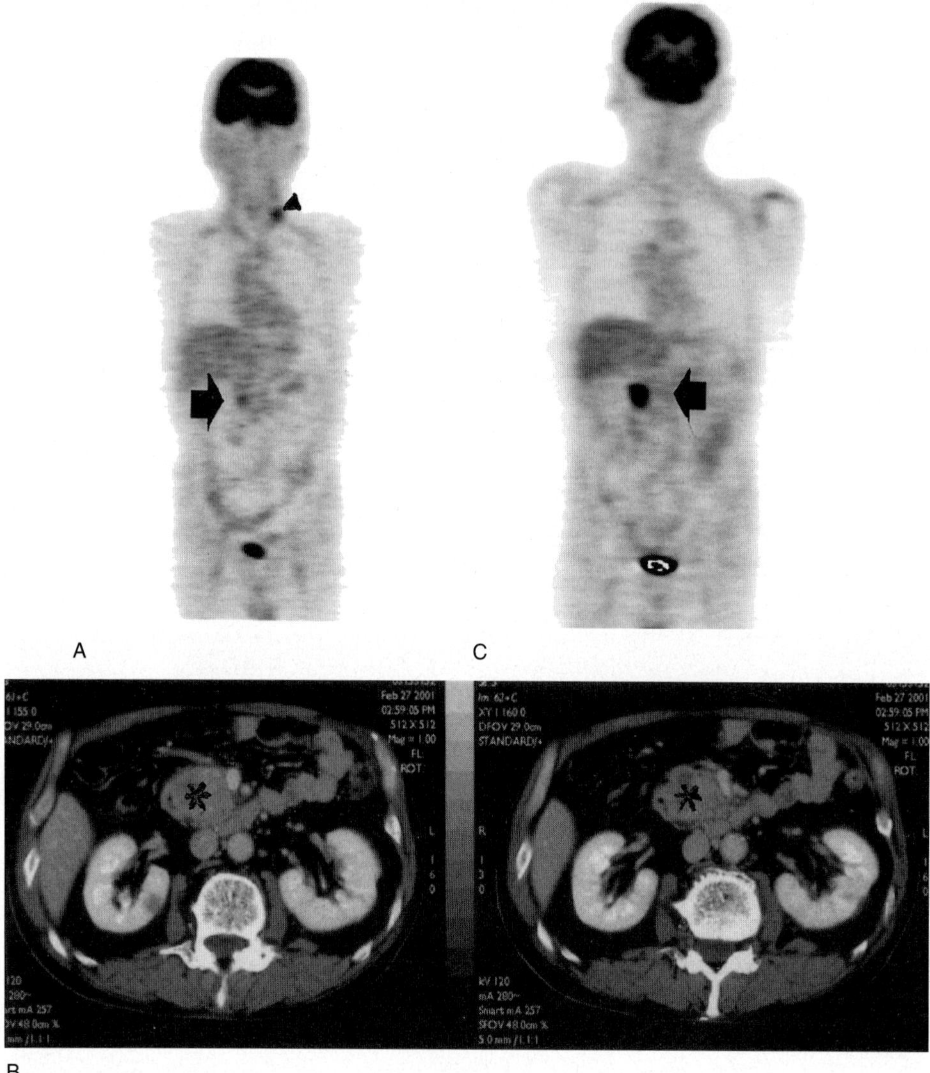

FIGURE 18.8. A: Selected coronal PET image of the whole body shows slightly increased uptake (SUV = 3.0) of ^{18}F-FDG in pancreatic cancer (*arrow*) and a metastatic lesion (*arrowhead*) in the left supraclavicular lymph node. B: Contrast-enhanced axial CT images of the abdomen show 3 × 2 cm pancreatic head carcinoma (*). C: Follow-up coronal image of the whole body shows markedly increased uptake (SUV = 5.5) of ^{18}F-FDG in pancreatic head cancer.

thirds of them are cured. About one third of patients who undergo curative surgical resection of the primary lesion have a recurrence after the initial treatment.[16] After the initial surgical resection of colorectal cancer, the accurate and early detection of potentially respectable metastatic tumors localized in the liver and lung is important in patient management. In cases of rectal cancer and sigmoid colon cancer, the pelvic recurrence that is amenable to resection with curative intent is also important to detect in the course of clinical follow-up after the initial surgical treatment.[17] Diagnosis of recurrence and the appropriate selection of patients for surgery are difficult because of the low sensitivity of CT for early metastasis. Scar formation after resection of rectal cancer, which mimics local recurrence on CT/MRI, may make it difficult to accurately diagnose local recurrence. More accurate preoperative restaging using FDG-PET would reduce the frequency of surgery for nonresectable recurrence, and more sensitive detection of tumor recurrence may increase the rate of resectability at restaging.

Differential Diagnosis and Preoperative Staging

The utility of FDG-PET for initial preoperative staging in patients with colorectal cancer has not been established. Nabi et al[18] reported 100% sensitivity, 43% specificity, 90% positive predictive value, and 100% negative predictive value for FDG-PET in the detection of primary colorectal cancer. Yasuda et al[19] reported that 14 of 59 (24%) patients with colorectal adenoma had positive results on FDG-PET. In cases of colonic adenoma greater than 13 mm in diameter, its sensitivity was 90%. The sensitivity of FDG-PET for lesions localized in the ascending colon, descending colon, and cecum seemed to be higher than that in other sites because of less motion artifact by fixation. The main diagnostic tool for the detection of primary colorectal cancer is a colonoscopy with biopsy or barium enema. Local lymph node metastases are evaluated as part of the surgical procedure. The sensitivity of FDG-PET for the diagnosis of primary lesions and local lymph node metastases at initial diagnosis and initial preoperative staging is of limited clinical importance.

Diagnosis of Recurrent Colorectal Cancer and Preoperative Restaging

The accuracy, sensitivity, and specificity of FDG-PET for the detection of local recurrent tumors were more than 90%.[20] Ito et al[21] compared

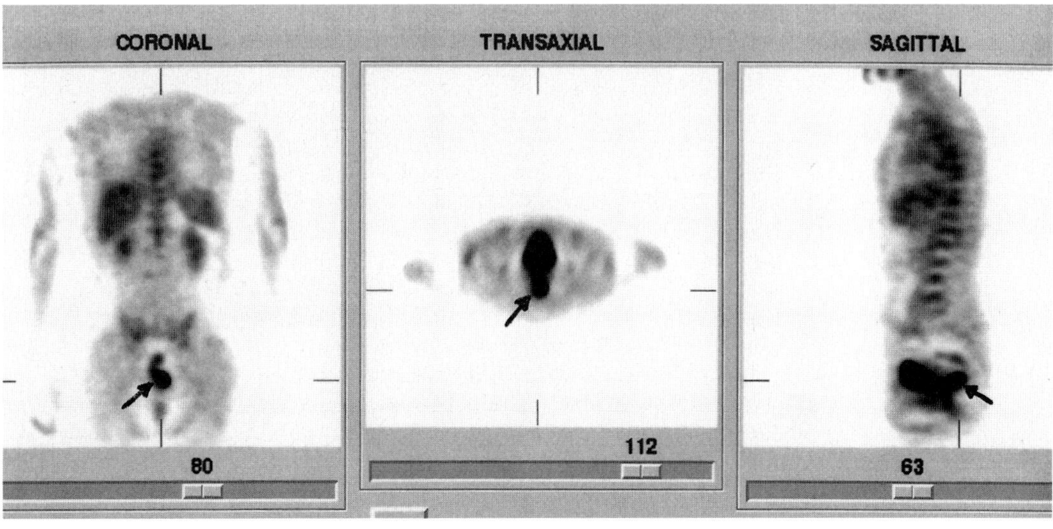

FIGURE 18.9. Selected coronal and sagittal PET images of the axial body and an axial image of the lower pelvis show markedly increased uptake of ^{18}F-FDG in recurrent rectal carcinoma (*arrows*).

findings of FDG-PET and MRI with histopathologic findings, and found that FDG-PET could differentiate a scar from local recurrent tumor. False-negative results on T2-weighted images, on which the lesion is not shown as a high intense area, may be due to the pathologic characteristic of recurrence as fibrotic changes with less tumor cell density.

Whole-body FDG-PET imaging (Fig. 18.9) is valuable for the detection of recurrent tumors in patients who are thought to have possible recurrence on the basis of elevated serum carcinoembryonic antigen (CEA) level.[22] Abouzied et al[23] assessed the usefulness of FDG-PET in 79 patients, including 55 colorectal patients with rising tumor markers and negative/inconclusive conventional imaging modalities, and FDG-

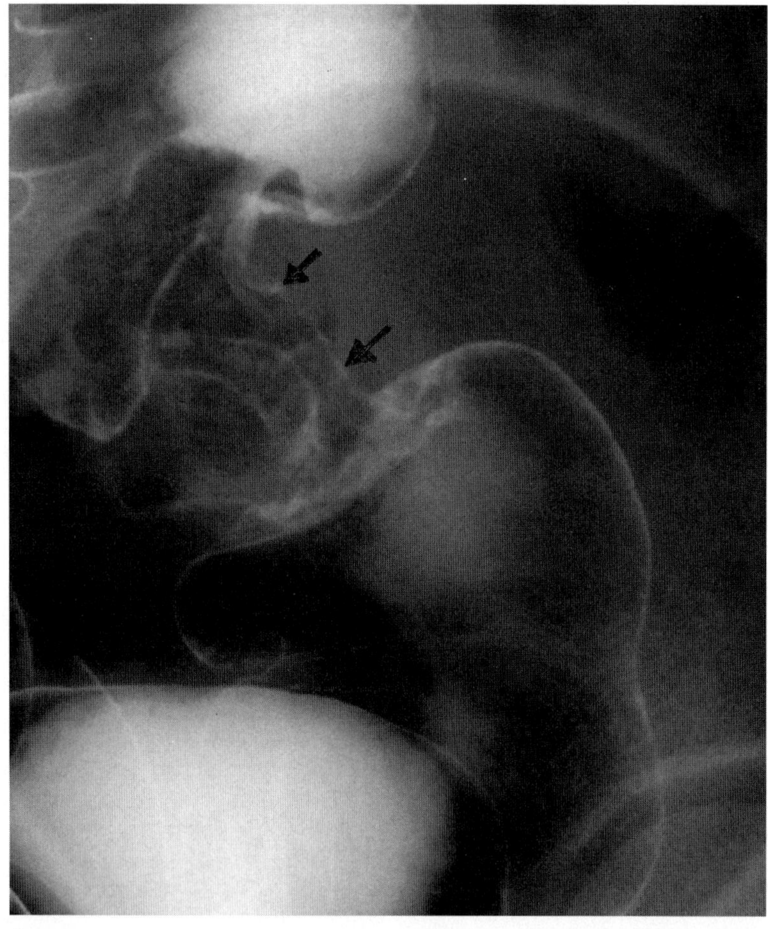

FIGURE 18.10. A: Air-barium double-contrasted colon study shows a carcinoma in the sigmoid colon with the apple-core pattern (*arrows*). B: Axial contrasted CT image of the upper abdomen shows multiple metastatic lesions in the right and left hepatic lobes. C: Selected coronal PET image of the whole body shows markedly increased uptake of ^{18}F-FDG in a colon carcinoma (*closed arrow*) and moderately increased uptake in the metastatic lesions involving the right hepatic lobe (*open arrows*). Note physiologic activity in the gastric fundus (*arrowhead*).

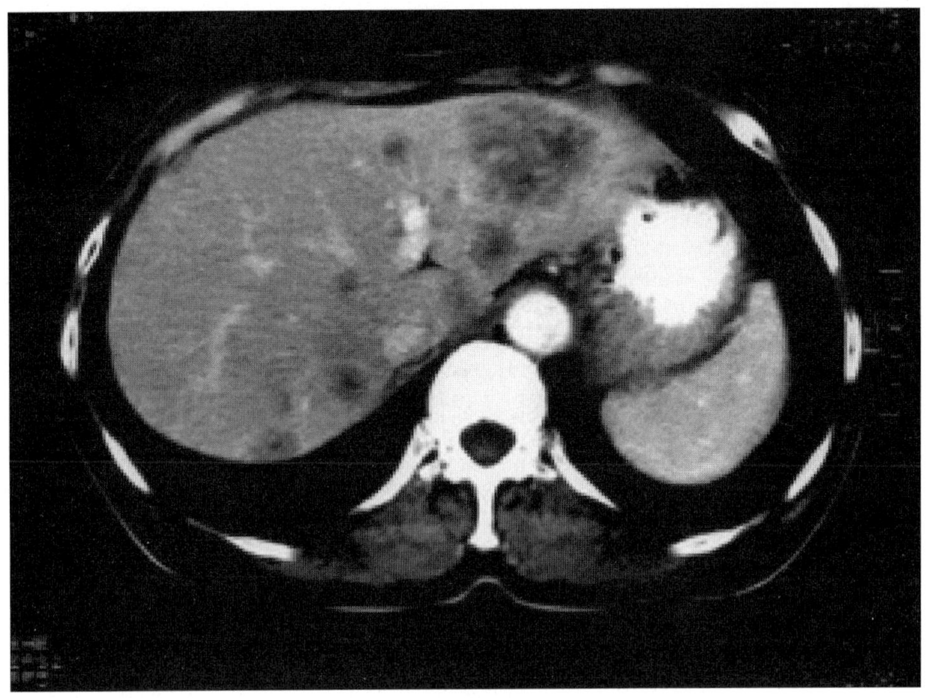

B

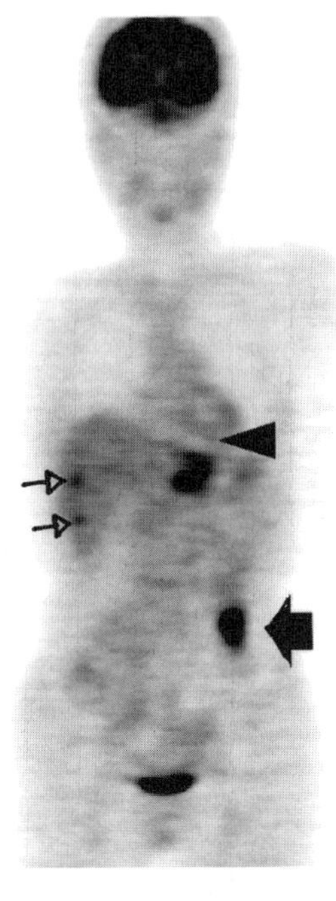

C

FIGURE 18.10. *(continued)*

PET was able to elucidate the responsible lesion of rising tumor markers in 59/79 (75%) and to guide appropriate patient management.

Direct comparison of CT and FDG-PET in a total of 306 patients[20–23] showed for all sites of recurrence, overall sensitivity of 95% for FDG-PET and 66% for CT. Sensitivity for detection of hepatic recurrence was 95% and 83% for PET and CT, respectively, and for pelvic recurrence, 97% and 63%, respectively. FDG-PET seems to be more sensitive than CT, especially in the abdomen and pelvis where about one third of sites that were true positive by FDG-PET were false negative by CT. Delbeke et al[24] compared PET and conventional CT to CT portography, which is more invasive than conventional CT and FDG-PET. Diagnostic accuracy for hepatic recurrence of FDG-PET was more accurate than CT or CT portography (92%, 78%, and 80%, respectively). The sensitivity of CT portography for hepatic recurrence was higher than FDG-PET (97% vs 91%), but FDG-PET had a much higher specificity for hepatic recurrence.[25]

In a recent prospective study of the clinical impact of ^{18}F-FDG in patients with suspected recurrence of colorectal cancer,[25] the management plan for 54 (53%) of 102 patients was altered as a direct result of unexpected PET findings, and planned surgery was abandoned in 26 (60%) of 43 patients with incremental PET findings. The major benefit of FDG-PET may be avoidance of inappropriate local therapies by documentation of widespread disease.

Case Presentation

This is an illustrative case of preoperative staging in a 54-year-old woman with colorectal cancer. Fluoroscopy with barium revealed an advanced primary tumor in the sigmoid colon. The finding indicated

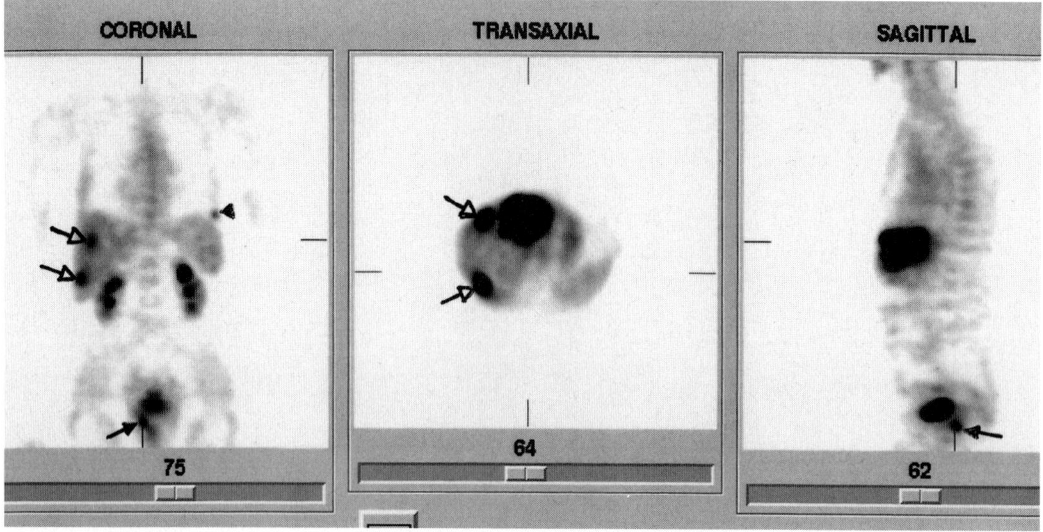

FIGURE 18.11. Selected coronal and sagittal PET images of the axial body as well as an axial image of the upper abdomen show markedly increased uptake of ^{18}F-FDG in the rectal carcinoma (*closed arrows*) and hepatic (*open arrows*) as well as left lower rib (*arrowhead*) metastases.

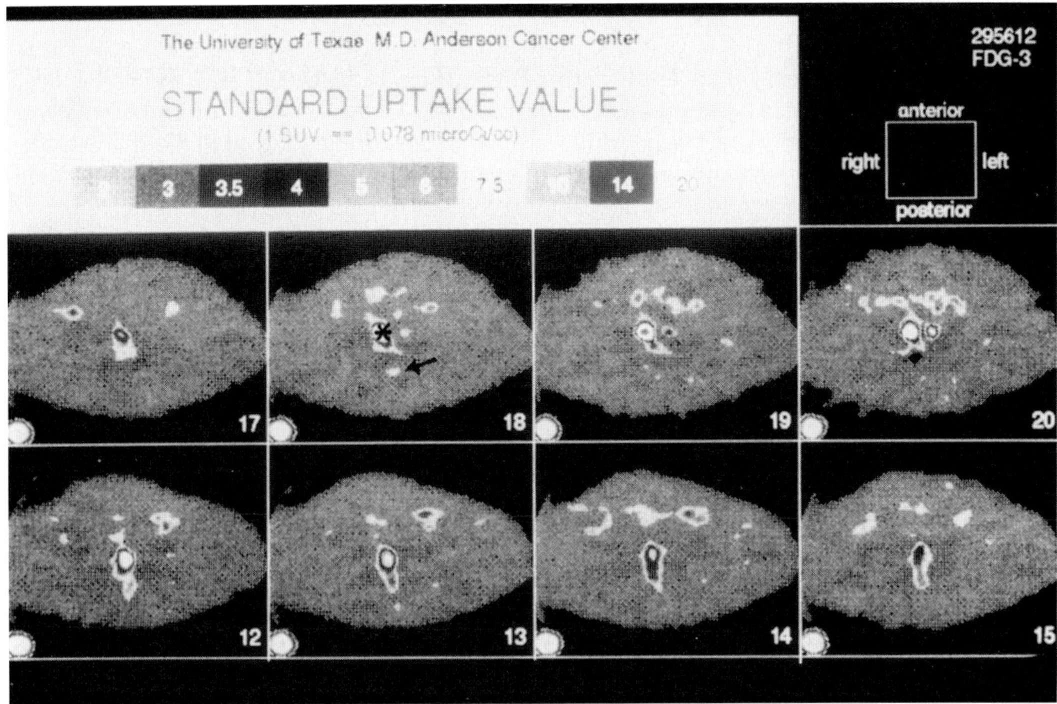

A

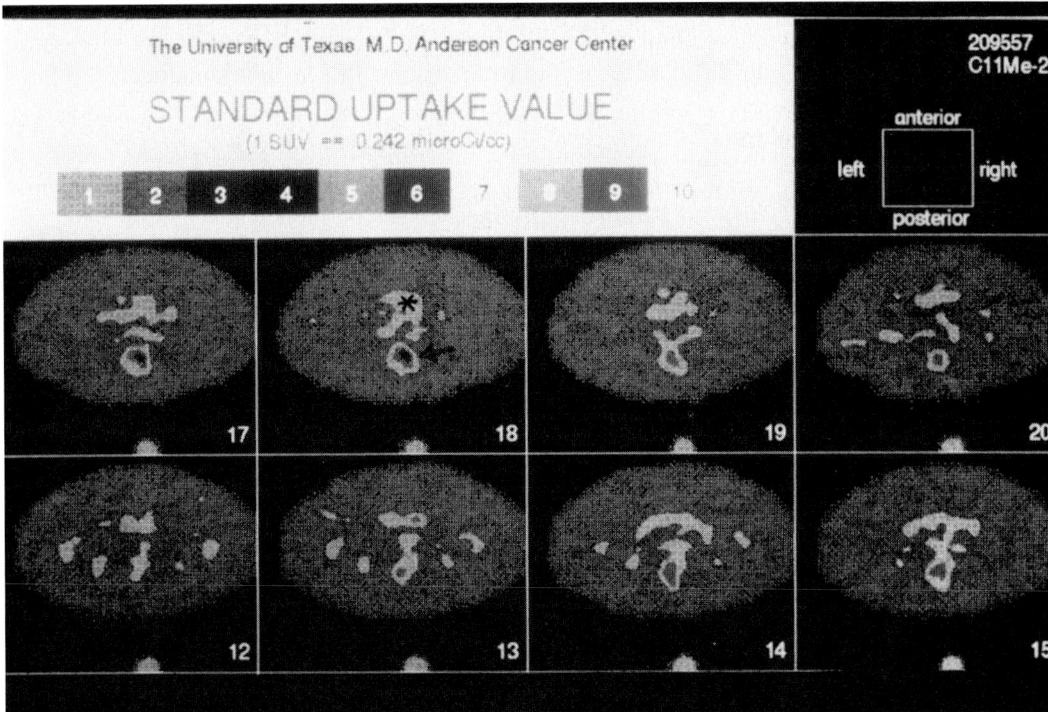

B

Figure 18.12. A: Axial PET images of the lower pelvis show minimally increased uptake of ^{18}F-FDG in a recurrent rectal cancer (*arrow*). Note greater activity in the bladder (*) anterior to the lesion. B: Axial images of the lower pelvis show moderately increased uptake of ^{11}C-methionine in the cancer (*arrow*) and relatively less bladder activity (*) in the same patient.

a so-called apple-core pattern (Fig. 18.10A). CT also showed a large metastatic mass in the left hepatic lobe and other multiple metastatic lesions in the liver (Fig. 18.10B). The coronal view of FDG-PET revealed abnormally increased tracer uptake in the primary lesion (arrow) and a large metastatic lesion in the left hepatic lobe (Fig. 18.10C).

A case involving the evaluation of patients with an elevated CEA level is shown in Fig. 18.11. Whole-body FDG-PET showed recurrent rectal carcinoma metastases in the liver and left rib. Whole-body FDG-PET should be used as the first imaging modality if recurrence of colorectal cancer is suspected (Fig. 18.12). Especially in a case of the following clinical signs, whole-body FDG-PET would be essentially useful for the evaluation of patients: (1) preoperative staging of recurrent tumor, (2) rising serum CEA and negative CT/MRI findings, and (3) equivocal abnormality on CT/MR images.

Although FDG-PET is essentially needed to evaluate patients with suspected recurrent colorectal cancers, we must interpret carefully FDG uptake in the abdomen. We often find intestinal physiologic FDG uptake on the PET image that mimics a colorectal lesion. In general, normal intestinal tracer uptake can be differentiated from abnormal uptake by the visible distribution of activity that is linear and can be shown to follow the expected pattern on the coronal/sagittal view. Since PET/CT imaging can increase the accuracy and certainty of lesion localization in colorectal cancer,[26] the differentiation of physiologic intestinal uptake and pathologic uptake would be more accurate if a PET/CT scan or a two-time-point PET can be obtained.

References

1. Kuwano H, Sumiyoshi K, Sonoda K, et al. Relationship between preoperative assessment of organ function and postoperative morbidity in patients with esophageal cancer. Eur J Surg 1998;164:581–586.
2. Kato H, Kuwano H, Nakajima M, et al. Comparison between positron emission tomography and computed tomography in the use of the assessment of esophageal carcinoma. Cancer 2002;94:921–928.
3. Kobori O, Kirihara Y, Kosaka N, et al. Positron emission tomography of esophageal carcinoma using C-11 choline and F-18 fluorodeoxyglucose: a novel method of preoperative lymph node staging. Cancer 1999:86:1683–1658.
4. Lowe VJ, Mullan BP, Wiersema M, et al. Prospective comparison of PET, CT and EUS in the initial staging of esophageal cancer patients: preliminary results. J Nucl Med 2002;43:66.
5. Wieder H, Zimmermann K, Becker K, et al. Time course of tumor glucose utilization in patients with squamous cell carcinomas of the esophagus undergoing preoperative chemoradiotherapy. J Nucl Med 2002;43:66.
6. Shreve PD, Anzai Y, Wahl RL. Pitfalls in oncologic diagnosis with FDG-PET imaging: physiologic and benign variants. Radiographics 1999;19: 61–77.
7. Cook GJR, Fogelman I, Maisey M. Normal physiological and benign pathological variants of 18-fluoro-2-deoxyglucose positron emission tomography scanning: potential for error in interpretation. Semin Nucl Med 1996; 24:308–314.
8. Yoshioka K, Yamaguchi K, Kubota K, et al. FDG-PET in gastric cancer with metastases or recurrence. J Nucl Med 2002;43:67.

9. Stahl A, Ott K, Becker K, et al. Prediction of response to neoadjuvant chemotherapy in patients with gastric cancer by FDG-PET. J Nucl Med 2002;43:67.
10. Higashi T, Tamaki N, Honda T, et al. Expression of glucose transporters in human pancreatic tumors compared with increased FDG accumulation in PET study. J Nucl Med 1997;38:1337–1344.
11. Reske SN, Grillenberger KG, Glatting G, et al. Overexpression of glucose transporter 1 and increased FDG uptake in pancreatic carcinoma. J Nucl Med 1997;38:1344–1348.
12. Inokuma T, Tamaki N, Torizuka T, et al. Evaluation of pancreatic tumors with positron emission tomography and F-18 fluorodeoxyglucose: comparison with CT and US. Radiology 1995;195:345–352.
13. Delbeke D, Rose DM, Chapman WC, et al. Optimal interpretation of FDG-PET in the diagnosis, staging and management of pancreatic carcinoma. J Nucl Med 1999;40:1784–1791.
14. Zimny M, Bares R, Fass J, et al. Fluorine-18 fluorodeoxyglucose positron emission tomography in the differential diagnosis of pancreatic carcinoma: a report of 106 cases. Eur J Nucl Med 1997;24:678–682.
15. Higashi T, Nakamoto Y, Saga T, et al. Clinical contribution of FDG-PET in evaluating small pancreatic tumors 20 mm in diameter or smaller. Gut 2000; United European Gastroenterology Week abstr.
16. August TA, Ottow RT, Sugarbaker PH. Clinical perspectives on human colorectal cancer metastases. Cancer Metastasis 1984;3:303–324.
17. Turk PS, Wanebo HJ. Results of surgical treatment of nonhepatic recurrence of colorectal carcinoma. Cancer 1993;72:4267–4277.
18. Nabi AH, Doerr RJ, Lamonica DM, et al. Staging of primary colorectal carcinomas with F-18 fluorodeoxyglucose whole-body PET: correlation with histopathologic and CT findings. Radiology 2998:206:755–760.
19. Yasuda S, Fuji H, Nakahara T, et al. F-18 FDG-PET detection of colonic adenoma. J Nucl Med 2001;42:989–992.
20. Huebner RH, Park KC, Shepherd JE, et al. A meta-analysis of the literature for whole-body FDG-PET detection of recurrent colorectal cancer. J Nucl Med 2000;41:1177–1189.
21. Ito K, Kato T, Tadokoro M, et al. Recurrent rectal cancer and scar: differentiation with PET and MR imaging. Radiology 1992;182:549–552.
22. Flangen FL, Dehdashi F, Ogunbiyi OA, et al. Utility of FDG-PET for investigating unexplained plasma CEA elevation in patients with colorectal cancer. Ann Surg 1998;227:319–323.
23. Abouzied MM, Zubeldia JM, Nabi HA. Role of F-18 fluorodeoxyglucose positron emission tomography in the detection of occult recurrent carcinoma presenting with rising tumor markers. J Nucl Med 2002;43:23.
24. Delbeke D,Vitola JV, Sandler MP, et al. Staging recurrent metastatic colorectal carcinoma with PET. J Nucl Med 1997;38:1196–1201.
25. Kalff V, Hicks RJ, Ware RE, et al. The clinical impact of F-18 FDG-PET in patients with suspected or confirmed recurrence of colorectal cancer: a prospective study. J Nucl Med 2002;43:492–499.
26. Cohade D, Osman M, Leal J, et al. Direct comparison of FDG-PET and PET-CT imaging in colorectal cancer. J Nucl Med 2002;43:22.

19

Hepatobiliary Tumors

Byung-Tae Kim and E. Edmund Kim

General Considerations

Cancers of the liver may arise in the parenchymal cells (hepatocellular cancers), or from the intrahepatic bile ducts (cholangiocarcinomas), or metastasize from other organ tumors.

Hepatocellular Carcinoma

Hepatocellular carcinoma (HCC) is the most common cancer in the world among males, especially in the Far East Asian and sub-Saharan African countries, where the annual incidence is up to 500 cases per 100,000 population. In the United States and Western Europe, it is much less common; however, the annual incidence in the United States has increased from 1.4/100,000 in the period 1976 to 1980 to 2.4/100,000 in 1991 to 1995.[1] HCC is up to four times more common in men than in women. The incidence peaks in the fifth to sixth decades of life in Western countries but one to two decades earlier in regions of Asia and Africa with a high prevalence of HCC. The principal reason for the high incidence in parts of Asia and Africa is the frequency of chronic infection with hepatitis B or C viruses, which is an important risk factor. The incidence of this cancer is about 100-fold higher in individuals with evidence of hepatitis B virus (HBV) infection than that in noninfected controls. Any agent or factor that contributes to chronic, low-grade liver cell damage and mitosis makes hepatocyte DNA more susceptible to genetic alterations. Besides chronic viral hepatitis, alcoholic liver disease, α_1-antitrypsin deficiency, hemochromatosis, tyrosinemia, and aflatoxin B_1 are the risk factors for HCC.

As HCC has a less specific clinical appearance, early diagnosis is difficult. The determination of serum levels of α-fetoprotein (AFP) and ultrasonography are suitable diagnostic or monitoring methods for patients with known risk factors. Only biopsy and histologic examination of suspected liver lesions provide definitive diagnosis and grading of HCCs. Imaging procedures to detect liver tumors include ultrasonography, computed tomography (CT), magnetic resonance imaging (MRI), hepatic artery angiography, and technetium scans. Ultrasonography is frequently used to screen high-risk populations and should be the first test if HCC is suspected; it is less costly than CT and MRI and relatively sensitive, and it can detect most tumors greater than 3 cm in diameter. Helical CT and MRI scans with contrast agents are being used with increasing frequency and show higher sensitivities. Percutaneous liver biopsy can be diagnostic if the sample is taken from the area localized by ultrasonography or CT. Because these tumors tend to be hypervascular, percutaneous biopsies should be done with caution.

Staging of HCC is based on tumor size (<50% or ≥50% of the liver), ascites (absent or present), bilirubin (<3 or ≥3 mg/dL), and albumin (<3 or ≥3 g/dL) to establish Okuda stages I, II, and III. The Okuda system predicts clinical course better than the American Joint Cancer Committee (AJCC) tumor-node-metastasis (TNM) system. The natural history of each stage without treatment is stage I, 8 months; stage II, 2 months; and stage III, less than 1 month.

Most patients die within 1 year after diagnosis. Anorexia and cachexia of malignancy are the most frequent causes of death. Although few patients have a resectable tumor at the time of diagnosis because of underlying cirrhosis or distant metastases, surgical resection offers the only chance for cure. The common sites of metastases are lung, brain, bone, and adrenal gland. In patients at high risk for the development of HCC, screening programs have been initiated to identify small tumors when they are still resectable. Because 20% to 30% of patients with early HCC do not have elevated levels of circulating AFP, ultrasonographic screening is recommended.

Liver transplantation may be considered as a therapeutic option, but tumor recurrence and/or metastasis are the major problems. Other approaches include hepatic artery embolization and chemotherapy, alcohol or radiofrequency ablation via ultrasound-guided percutaneous injection, and cryoablation. In patients with resectable tumors, polyprenoic acid (a retinoic acid formulation) and intraarterial ^{131}I-labeled lipiodol have been reported to reduce the rate of recurrence.

A combined occurrence of HCC and cholangiocellular carcinoma has been noted. Fibrolamellar hepatocellular carcinoma is an important variant, which is found in younger patients without liver cirrhosis.

Cholangiocellular Carcinoma

Cholangiocellular carcinoma (CCC) originates from the intra- or extrahepatic bile duct. Adenocarcinoma of the extrahepatic ducts is more common. There is a slight male preponderance (60%), and the incidence peaks in the fifth to seventh decades. Apparent predisposing factors include some chronic hepatobiliary parasitic infestations, congenital anomalies with ectactic ducts, sclerosing cholangitis and chronic ulcerative colitis, and occupational exposure to possible biliary tract carcinogens (nitrosamines, aflatoxins). The lesions of CCCs may be diffuse or nodular. Nodular lesions often arise at the bifurcation of the common bile duct (Klatskin tumors) and are usually associated with a collapsed gallbladder, a finding that mandates cholangiography to view proximal hepatic ducts.

The diagnosis is most frequently made by cholangiography following ultrasound demonstration of dilated intrahepatic bile ducts. Any focal strictures of the bile ducts should be considered malignant until proved otherwise. Endoscopic cholangiography permits obtaining specimens for cytology and insertion of stents for biliary drainage. Survival of 1 to 2 years is possible in some cases. Perhaps 20% of patients have surgically resectable tumors, but 5-year survival is only 10% to 30%. The high recurrence rate limits the value of liver transplantation. Photodynamic therapy (intravenous hematoporphyrin with cholangioscopically delivered light) has been used with promising early results.

Metastatic Tumor

Metastatic tumor of the liver is common. Its size, high rate of blood flow, double perfusion by the hepatic artery and portal vein, and its Kupffer cell filtration function combine to make it the next most common site of metastases after the lymph nodes. In the United States, the incidence of metastatic carcinoma is at least 20 times greater than that of primary carcinoma. At autopsy, hepatic metastasis occurs in 30% to 50% of patients dying from malignant disease. Virtually all types of neoplasms except those primary in the brain may metastasize to the liver. The most common primary tumors are those of the gastrointestinal tract, lung, and breast, as well as melanomas. Less common are metastases from tumors of the thyroid, prostate, and skin.

Most patients with hepatic metastases present with symptoms only to the primary tumor, and the asymptomatic hepatic involvement is discovered in the course of clinical evaluation. Evidence of metastatic invasion of the liver should be sought actively in any patient with a primary malignancy, especially of the lung, gastrointestinal tract, or breast, before resection of the primary lesion. An elevated level of alkaline phosphatase or a mass apparent on ultrasound, CT, or MRI examination of the liver may provide a presumptive diagnosis. Blind percutaneous needle biopsy of the liver results in a positive diagnosis of metastatic disease in only 60% to 80% of cases with hepatomegaly and elevated alkaline phosphatase levels. Serial sectioning of specimens, two or three repeated biopsies, or cytologic examination of biopsy smears may increase the diagnostic yield by 10% to 15%. The yield is increased when biopsies are directed by ultrasonography or CT or obtained during laparoscopy.

Most metastatic carcinomas respond poorly to all forms of treatment, which is usually only palliative. Rarely a single, large metastasis can be removed surgically. Systemic chemotherapy may slow tumor growth and reduce symptoms, but it does not alter the prognosis. Chemoembolization, intrahepatic chemotherapy, and alcohol or radiofrequency ablation may provide palliation.

Positron Emission Tomography

Although many articles have been published on the usefulness of fluorodeoxyglucose positron emission tomography (FDG-PET) for the metastatic cancers of liver, only a few were reported for primary liver tumors. In 1982, Fukuda et al[2] demonstrated increased uptake of fluorine-18-fluoro-2-deoxyglucose (FDG), which is a glucose analog that competes with glucose at transport sites on the cell membrane and in intracellular enzymatic pathways, in the transplantable ascitic hepatoma (AH109A) cells by autoradiography. Yonekura et al[3] also reported a continuous increase of FDG uptake in the metastatic liver tumors from colon carcinoma compared with decrease of FDG uptake in normal liver tissues. In 1985 Paul et al[4] imaged HCC with the Anger camera after FDG injection, and Nagata et al[5] demonstrated an image of recurrent HCC and lymph node metastasis using dedicated whole-body FDG-PET successfully. The metabolism of FDG in the HCC was well studied by Okazumi et al[6] using dynamic PET scan method and hexokinase activity measurement. In their study the rate of glucose inflow from the plasma into the cells was lower for the tumors than that for the surrounding liver tissue, and the rate of phosphorylation by hexokinase was significantly increased in malignant tumors.

In general, glycolysis and glucose utilization are increased in malignant tumors. FDG competes with glucose for phosphorylation by the enzyme hexokinase to FDG-6-phosphate. Phosphohexose isomerase, the enzyme involved in the next step of the glycolytic pathway, cannot act on phosphorylated FDG. The glucose-6-phosphatase, which catalyzes the dephosphorylation of FDG-6-phosphate, is relatively scanty in malignant cells. Thus, more FDG is trapped in malignant tumor cells than in normal cells.

In the normal liver the concentration of glucose-6-phosphatase is high and may clear FDG faster. The differences in the hexokinase/glucose-6-phosphatase ratios and metabolic activity of normal and malignant liver tissue result in visibly increased FDG accumulation in HCC and metastatic tumors on FDG-PET images.

The well-differentiated HCC may retain the properties of normal hepatocytes, and the enzyme activities of glycolytic pathway resemble those of normal hepatocytes. A decrease in differentiation increases glycolytic enzymes and decreases glucose-6-phosphatase levels. The kinetic rate constants and uptake values are significantly higher in poorly differentiated HCC compared with those with higher differentiation. The glucose-6-phosphatase/hexokinase ratios of low-grade HCC have been found to be significantly higher than high-grade HCC. These enzyme activities can be obtained from the rate constants using compartment models in dynamic FDG-PET and have proven to be useful in the characterization of the tumor and monitoring the therapeutic effect. Tumor size, morphology, vascularity, or lipiodol deposits do not influence the quantitative evaluation of viability by glucose metabolism.

Okazumi et al[6] categorized HCC into three types depending on the pattern of accumulation 60 minutes after FDG injection: type 1, greater tumor FDG accumulation compared with surrounding liver tissue; type 2, nearly the same degree of accumulation as the surrounding liver tissue; type 3 (Fig. 19.1), less accumulation than the surrounding liver tissue. In their study of 20 HCC patients, type 1 tumors were

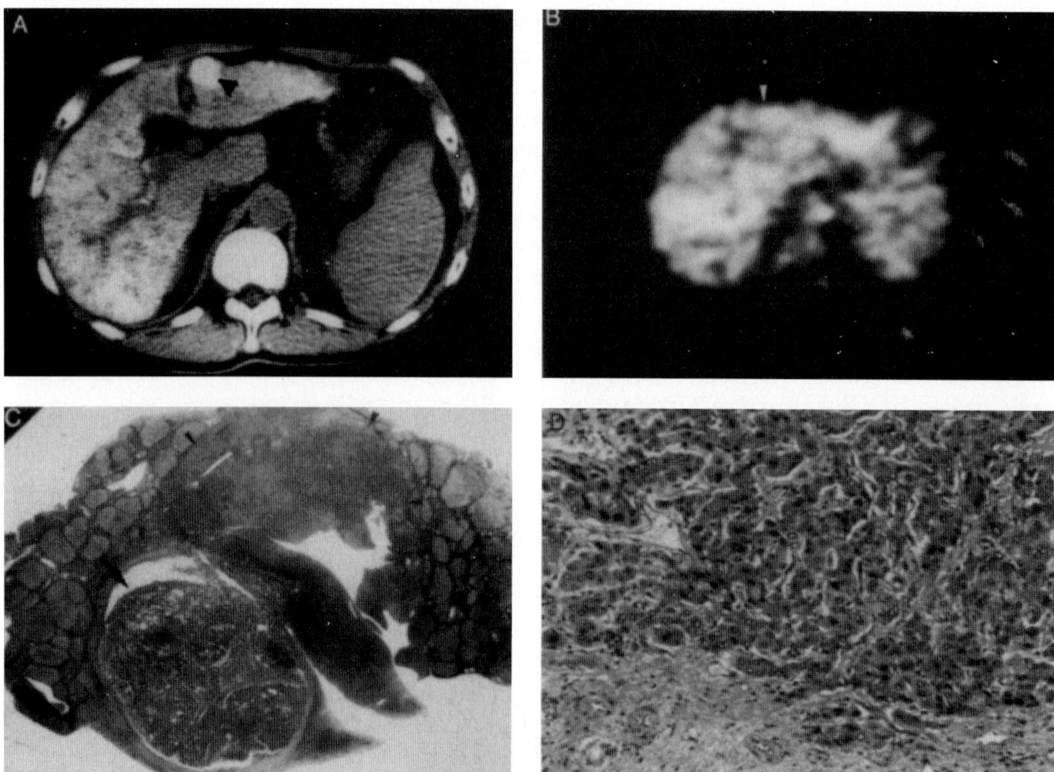

FIGURE 19.1. A: Axial CT image of the upper abdomen shows intratumor lipiodol retention in the lateral segment of left hepatic lobe (*arrowhead*). B: Selected axial PET image of the upper abdomen shows similar uptake of ^{18}F-FDG (*arrowhead*) to the surrounding nontumor region. The SUV was 0.77. C: Low magnification of the tumor shows viable hepatocellular carcinoma (HCC) tissue (*arrowheads*) and necrotic tissue (*arrow*). (D) High magnification of viable HCC tissue (×200). (From Okazumi et al,[6] with permission.)

found in 11 patients (55%), type 2 tumors in six patients (30%), and type 3 tumors in three patients (15%). Three patients with CCC and 10 patients with metastatic liver cancer showed greater tumor FDG accumulation than surrounding liver tissue (corresponding to type 1 HCC).

Torizuka et al[7] evaluated the metabolic activity of the HCC after transarterial chemoembolization therapy in 30 patients using the tumor-to-nontumor ratio of standard uptake value (SUV ratio) and correlated it with the extent of tumor necrosis. They found that increased or similar FDG uptake (SUV ratio ≥0.6) suggests viable residual tumor, whereas decreased or absent FDG uptake (SUV ratio <0.6) indicates effective therapy (necrosis occurred in more than 90% of tumor tissue).

Though the results of these studies are very important in understanding pathophysiology of primary liver tumors, dynamic FDG-PET study is impractical because of its difficulty to perform as a common clinical study.

In 1998 Delbeke et al[8] evaluated the usefulness of static whole-body FDG-PET in the differentiation of benign and malignant hepatic lesions. Their study was a prospective blinded-comparison clinical cohort study in 110 patients with 1 cm or larger hepatic lesions on screening CT. Confirmatory diagnosis was obtained by biopsy or surgery. All 66 liver metastases from adenocarcinoma and sarcoma primaries and eight CCCs showed increased FDG uptake (SUV >3.5 and lesion-to-background ratio >2), whereas only 16 of 23 HCCs had increased FDG uptake. Seven of 23 patients with HCC had poor FDG uptake. All 23 benign hepatic lesions except three abscesses had poor uptake (SUV <3.5 and lesion-to-background ratio <2). One of three abscesses had definitely increased FDG uptake and the others had equivocal uptake. These findings support the results of Okazumi's and Torizuka's studies.

Trojan et al[9] performed whole-body and regional FDG-PET in 14 consecutive patients with HCC and compared the results with ultrasonography, contrast-enhanced helical CT, histologic grading, p53 protein expression, and serum AFP level. Increased FDG uptakes in HCCs of seven patients were indistinguishable from surrounding normal liver tissue in seven other patients. Patients with increased FDG uptakes had larger tumors and higher serum AFP levels than those with indistinguishable FDG uptake from normal tissue. Seven of eight moderately or poorly differentiated HCCs clearly had increased FDG uptake, whereas none of six well-differentiated HCCs were detected. The tumors in patients with strong p53 expression had increased FDG uptake. In this study, tumor size (>5 cm), differentiation, and serum AFP level were major predictors of tumor visualization on FDG-PET. They concluded that static FDG-PET was not a useful method in the early diagnosis of HCC, but it was superior to other imaging methods for detection of extrahepatic spread.

To evaluate the diagnostic usefulness of FDG-PET (Fig. 19.2), Iwata et al[10] also performed it in 48 HCCs, five CCCs, 20 metastatic tumors, two hemangiomas, and three focal nodular hyperplasias. The SUV ratios of multiple HCCs were significantly higher than those of single HCCs. They also compared the SUV and SUV ratio with the Child-Turcotte classification (CTC) score and the Cancer of the Liver Italian Program (CLIP) score. Shiomi et al[11] assessed the usefulness of FDG-PET for predicting outcome in 48 patients with HCC. The tumor volume doubling time correlated significantly with SUV ratio but did not correlate with SUV. The cumulative survival rates of the patients with an SUV ratio greater than 1.5 were significantly lower than those of the patients with an SUV ratio below 1.5. On regression analysis with the Cox proportional hazards model, the SUV ratio and tumor number were significantly related to the survival.

In 1999 Koyama et al[12] acquired PET images twice (1 and 2 hours) after FDG injection in 11 patients with 18 HCCs and four patients with 15 metastatic liver tumors. Tumor to nontumor ratios and tumor to soft tissue ratios on 2-hour images were significantly greater than those on 1-hour images, whereas nontumorous liver tissue to soft tissue ratios were not significantly different and showed no constant tendency.

Morikawa et al[13] demonstrated increased FDG uptake on pretreatment PET in a patient with HCC, decreased FDG uptake after treatment, and reincrease on follow-up, which turned out to be a recur-

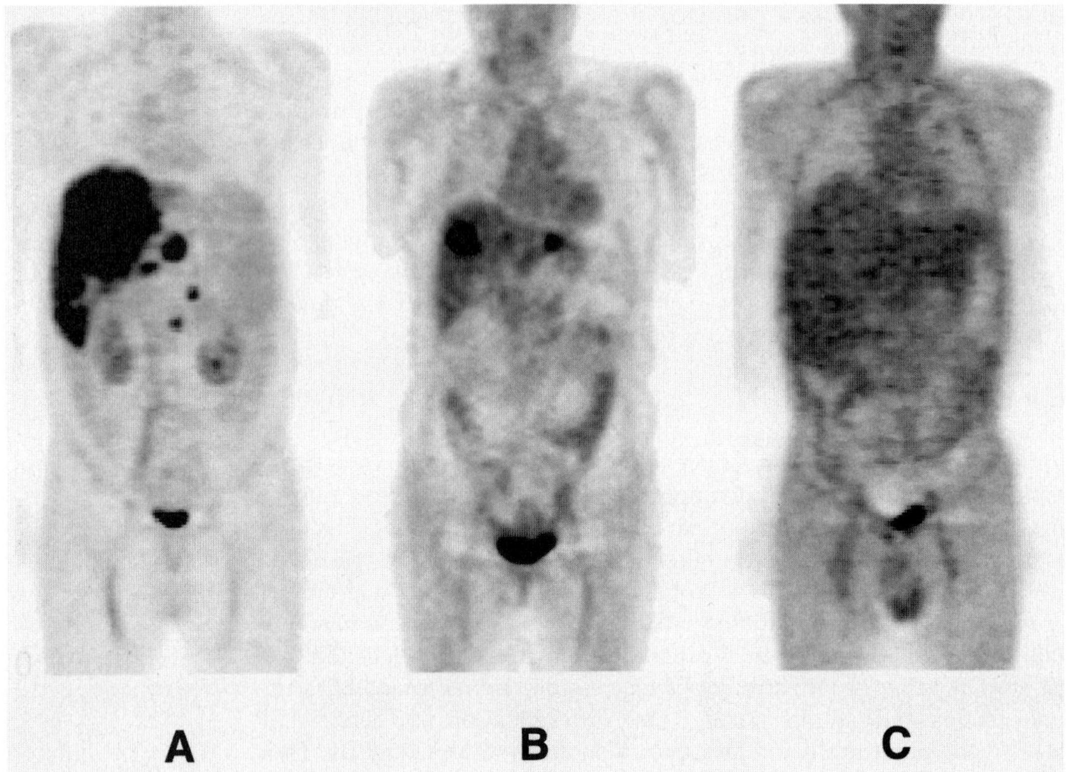

FIGURE 19.2. Selected coronal images of axial body with ^{18}F-FDG show markedly increased activity in the hepatoma involving right and left hepatic lobes as well as probably metastatic lesions in the left para-aortic nodes (A), and two metastatic colon cancers in the right and left hepatic lobes (B). Note slightly heterogeneous activity in the normal liver (C).

rence. They suggested that FDG-PET might be useful in the evaluation of therapy response and recurrence monitoring of HCC.

Although many of the authors already mentioned found that CCC usually showed increased FDG uptake compared with surrounding normal liver tissue, the number of cases was not large enough to analyze statistically. Kluge et al[14] studied the usefulness of FDG-PET in the detection and staging of CCC in 26 adenocarcinomas of the biliary tree, eight benign lesions of the bile ducts, and 20 controls. Twenty-four of 26 CCCs were positive, and all benign lesions as well as 18 of 20 controls were negative. Evaluation by visual means and tumor to nontumor ratio were equally accurate, whereas evaluation by SUV revealed lower accuracy. For the detection of metastatic lesions of CCC, FDG-PET detected seven of 10 distant metastases and only two of 15 regional or hepatoduodenal lymph node metastases. These findings suggest that FDG-PET can be helpful for the detection of distant metastasis but not for the detection of regional lymph node involvement in CCC patients.

Keiding et al[15] tried to detect CCC noninvasively with FDG-PET in patients with primary sclerosing cholangitis (PSC), which predisposes to CCC. Nine patients with PSC, six patients with PSC and CCC, and five controls were included in their study. In each of the PSC plus CCC patients, two to seven hot spots (increased FDG uptake compared with surrounding liver tissue) were seen. No hot spot was seen in the other two groups. The net metabolic clearances (from Gjedde-Patlak plotting) of FDG in CCCs were significantly higher than those of the other two groups. Thus FDG-PET may be useful in the detection of CCC during the follow-up of patients with PSC.

Some authors found that FDG-PET was more accurate than CT and could give more information in detecting hepatic metastases (Fig. 19.3).[16–18] The reported accuracy ranged between 93% and 98%. False-positive results can occur in marked intrahepatic cholestasis, abscess, and lung basal metastases.[19] False-negative results can be obtained

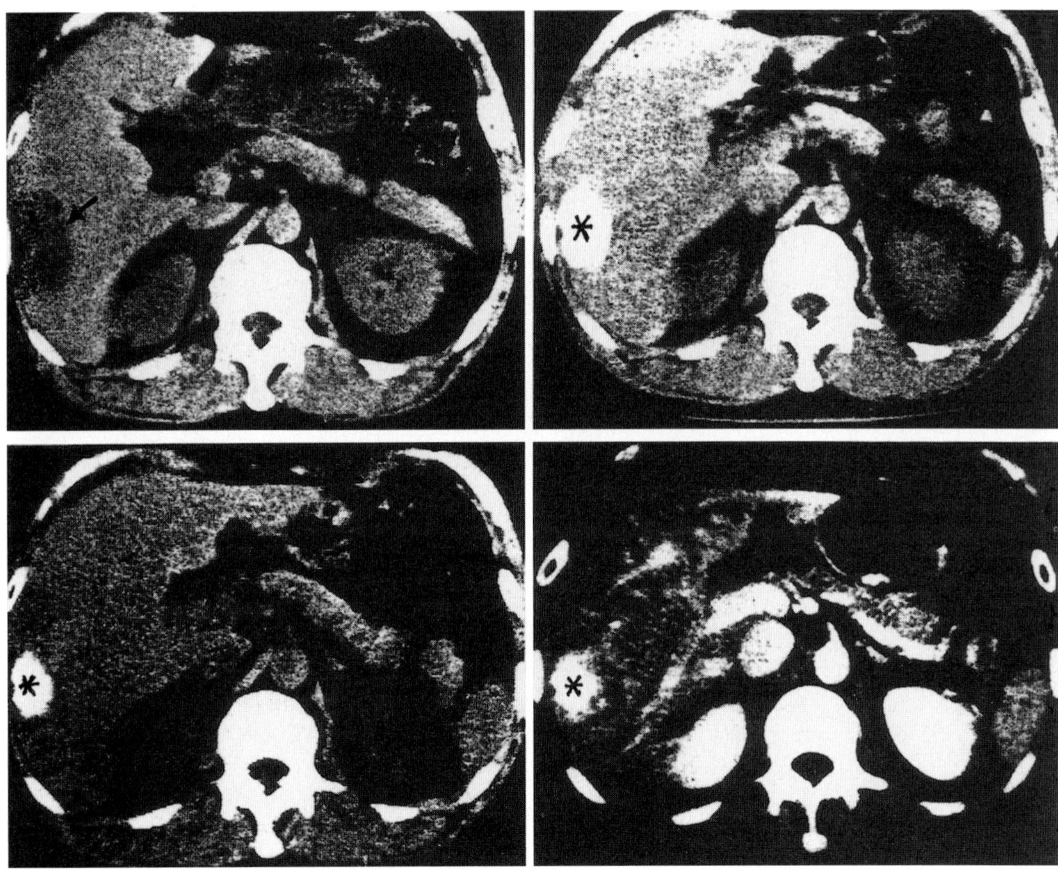

FIGURE 19.3. A: Axial CT images of the upper abdomen (*left upper*) show a low-density lesion in right hepatic lobe (*arrow*) with metastatic rectal adenocarcinoma. Image after arterial embolization (*right upper*) shows a lipiodol accumulation in the tumor (*). Images 4 months (*left lower*) and 8 months (*right lower*) later show a recurrence with developing low density halo around lipiodol uptakes (*). B: Selected axial PET images of the upper abdomen show markedly increased uptake of ^{18}F-FDG in the tumor (*) (*left upper*), and resolution of the abnormality after treatment (*right upper*). Follow-up images at 4 months (*left lower*) and 8 months (*right lower*) show increasing uptake of ^{18}F-FDG in recurrent metastatic rectal cancer (*). (From Imbriaco, et al,[17] with permission.)

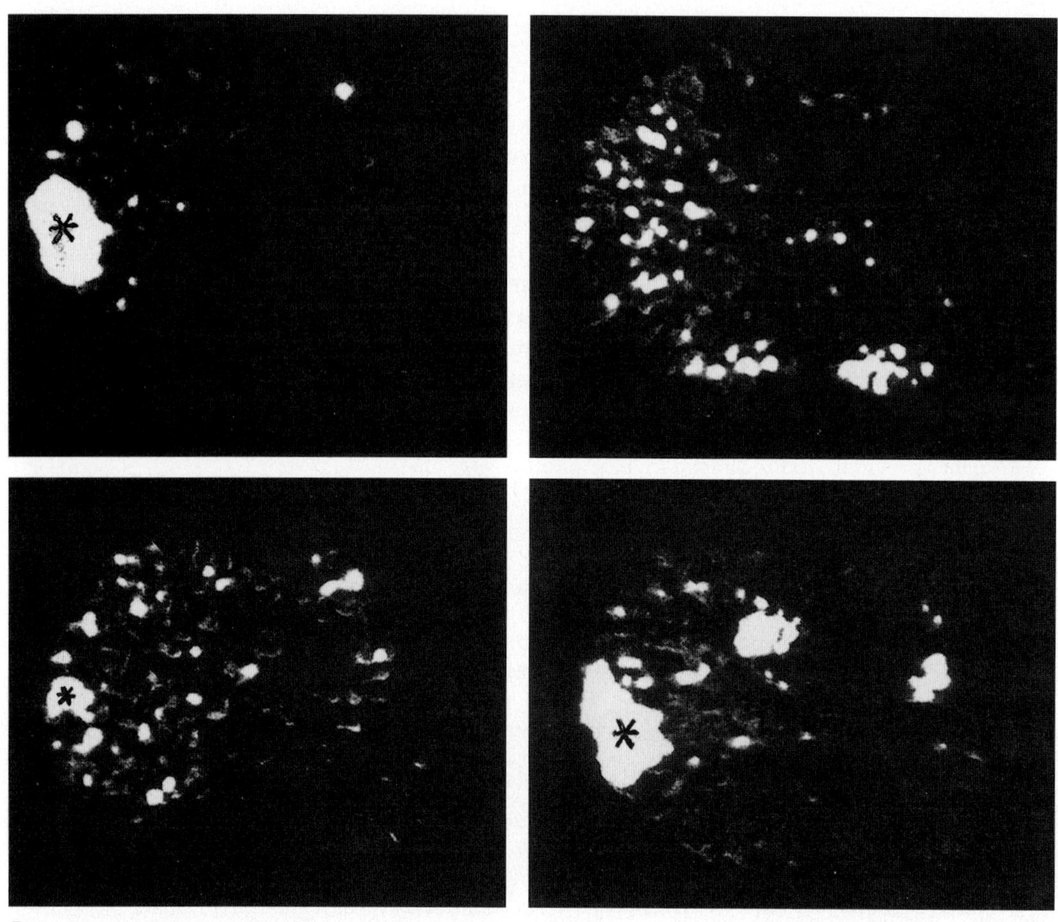

FIGURE 19.3. (*continued*)

when the metastatic lesion is small (less than 1 cm in diameter). The usefulness or diagnostic accuracy of metastatic hepatic tumors is described in the chapters on the primary tumors. Other radiopharmaceuticals, such as ^{13}N-ammonia[20] and ^{11}C-ethanol,[21,22] have been tested in trials to detect liver tumors, but their use is not yet practical.

Outlook

The number of studies on FDG-PET in primary hepatobiliary tumors was to small to establish clear indications. It was probably due to relatively low sensitivity, but FDG-PET can be used in the differentiation of malignant hepatic lesions from benign ones, prediction of prognosis by noninvasive grading of differentiation, and the detection of distant metastases. Nevertheless, further studies are necessary for determining the exact role of FDG-PET in the evaluation and management of patients with hepatobiliary tumors.

References

1. Dienstag JL, Isselbacher K. Tumors of the liver and biliary tract. In: Braunwald E, Fauci AS, Kasper DL, Hauser SL, Longo DL, Jameson JL, eds. Harrison's Principles of Internal Medicine, 15th ed. New York: McGraw-Hill, 1998:588–591.
2. Fukuda H, Matsuzawa T, Abe Y, et al. Experimental study for cancer diagnosis with positron-labeled fluorinated glucose analogs: [^{18}F]-2-fluoro-2-deoxy-D-mannose: a new tracer for cancer detection. Eur J Nucl Med 1982;7:294–297.
3. Yonekura Y, Benua RS, Brill AB, et al. Increased accumulation of 2-deoxy-2-[^{18}F]fluoro-D-glucose in liver metastases from colon carcinoma. J Nucl Med 1982;23:1133–1137.
4. Paul R, Ahonen A, Roeda D, Nordman E. Imaging of hepatoma with 18F-fluorodeoxyglucose. Lancet 1985;1(8419):50–51.
5. Nagata Y, Yamamoto K, Hiraoka M, et al. Monitoring liver tumor therapy with [^{18F}]FDG positron emission tomography. J Comput Assist Tomogr 1990;14:370–374.
6. Okazumi S, Isono K, Enomoto K, et al. Evaluation of liver tumors using fluorine-18-fluorodeoxyglucose PET: characterization of tumor and assessment of effect of treatment. J Nucl Med 1992;33:333–339.
7. Torizuka T, Tamaki N, Inokuma T, et al. Value of fluorine-18-FDG-PET to monitor hepatocellular carcinoma after interventional therapy. J Nucl Med 1994;35:1965–1969.
8. Delbeke D, Martin WH, Martin PS, et al. Evaluation of benign vs malignant hepatic lesions with positron emission tomography. Arch Surg 1998; 133:510–516.
9. Trojan J, Schroeder O, Raedle J, et al. Fluorine-18 FDG positron emission tomography for imaging of hepatocellular carcinoma. Am J Gastroenterol 1999;94:3314–3319.
10. Iwata Y, Shiomi S, Sasaki N, et al. Clinical usefulness of positron emission tomography with fluorine-18-fluorodeoxyglucose in the diagnosis of liver tumors. Ann Nucl Med 2000;14:121–126.
11. Shiomi S, Nishiguchi S, Ishizu H, et al. Usefulness of positron emission tomography with fluorine-18-fluorodeoxyglucose for predicting outcome in patients with hepatocellular carcinoma. Am J Gastroenterol 2001;96:1877–1880.
12. Koyama K, Okamura T, Kawabe J, et al. The usefulness of ^{18}F-FDG PET images obtained 2 hours after intravenous injection in liver tumor. Ann Nucl Med 1999;16:169–176.
13. Morikawa H, Shiomi S, Sasaki N, et al. Hepatocellular carcinoma monitored by F-18 fluorodeoxyglucose positron emission tomography after laparoscopic microwave coagulation therapy. Clin Nucl Med 1999;24:536–538.
14. Kluge R, Schmidt F, Caca K, et al. Positron emission tomography with [^{18}F]fluoro-2-deoxy-D-glucose for diagnosis and staging of bile duct cancer. Hepatology 2001;33:1029–1035.
15. Keiding S, Hansen SB, Rasmussen HH, et al. Detection of cholangiocarcinoma in primary sclerosing cholangitis by positron emission tomography. Hepatology 1998;28:700–706.
16. Gupta N, Bradfield H. Role of positron emission tomography scanning in evaluating gastrointestinal neoplasms. Semin Nucl Med 1996;26:65–73.
17. Imbriaco M, Akhurst T, Hilton S, et al. Whole-body FDG-PET in patients with recurrent colorectal carcinoma. A comparative study with CT. Clin Positron Imaging 2003;3:107–114.

18. Vitola JV, Delbeke D, Sandler MP, et al. Positron emission tomography to stage suspected metastatic colorectal carcinoma to the liver. Am J Surg 1996;171:21–26.
19. Frohlich A, Diederichs CG, Staib L, et al. Detection of liver metastases from pancreatic cancer using FDG PET. J Nucl Med 1999;40:250–255.
20. Hayashi N, Tamaki N, Yonekura Y, et al. Imaging of the hepatocellular carcinoma using dynamic positron emission tomography with nitrogen-13 ammonia. J Nucl Med 1995;26:254–257.
21. Dimitrakopoulou-Strauss A, Gutzler F, Strauss LG, et al. PET-Studien mit C-11-Athanol bei der intratumoralen therapie von hepatozellularen karzinomen. Radiology 1996;36:744–749.
22. Dimitrakopoulou-Strauss A, Strauss LG, et al. Pharmacokinetic imaging of ^{11}C ethanol with PET in eight patients with hepatocellular carcinomas who were scheduled for treatment with percutaneous ethanol injection. Radiology 1999;211:681–686.

20

Gynecologic Cancers

Sung-Eun Kim, June-Key Chung, and E. Edmund Kim

Gynecologic cancers constitute approximately 20% of visceral cancers in women and are divided into three major types: ovarian, cervical, and endometrial. The majority of the gynecologic cancers require surgical removal, along with adjuvant radiotherapy or chemotherapy. The therapeutic option varies with the type and stage of cancer. Therefore, accurate staging is necessary for optimal treatment.

A variety of radiographic techniques are used for evaluating patients with suspected or diagnosed gynecologic malignancies. Unfortunately, morphologic imaging techniques are not optimal for diagnosis, staging, or identifying recurrent disease, while a more or less specific tumor marker, such as serum CA-125, may hold some value for tracking the status and heralding the recurrence in postoperative management.[1,2]

The advent of positron emission tomography (PET) scanning now enables us to detect metabolically active gynecologic cancers with greater accuracy than was possible with anatomic imaging techniques. Moreover, PET scanning is more sensitive for the presence of active cancer than are the tumor markers that are generally available.[3] As in other tumors, ^{18}F-fluorodeoxyglucose (FDG) fluorine is the most commonly used PET agent in gynecologic oncology today.

Ovarian Cancer

Ovarian carcinoma is the leading cause of death among women with gynecologic malignancies. In 1999 there were 25,400 reported new cases of ovarian cancer in the United States, with 14,300 deaths attributed to this disease.[4] Most ovarian tumors are first discovered in the advanced stage. Imaging techniques are relied on to identify the location of suspected lesions and to provide optimal treatment in the hope of reducing mortality. Ovarian cancer commonly seeds the peritoneal surfaces of the abdomen and pelvis and is often seen on the serosal and mesenteric surfaces of the large and small intestine, as well as the liver surface. The right and left hemidiaphragms are also common metastatic sites.

Epithelial ovarian cancer also has the potential to spread through the lymphatics and commonly involves para-aortic lymph nodes without affecting the pelvic nodes. Ovarian cancer rarely metastasizes via the blood to the liver parenchyma, lungs, bones, or brain. The clinical requirements for PET imaging in patients with ovarian cancer are preoperative diagnosis and staging, and differentiation between metastases and nonmalignant pathologic conditions. Although the disease spreads transperitoneally, patients often have tumor seedings that are not visible by conventional techniques such as ultrasound, computed tomography (CT) and magnetic resonance imaging (MRI).

Differential Diagnosis of Adnexal Mass

Although the CA-125 tumor marker is elevated in the majority of patients with advanced ovarian cancer, an established screening procedure for early detection of ovarian cancer is not yet available. A mass lesion of the ovaries is usually detected during gynecologic examination, whereas imaging methods are necessary for evaluating the tumor status and spread.

Chou et al[5] reported quite a high diagnostic accuracy of about 90% for transvaginal color Doppler ultrasonography. CT and MRI are not very reliable in evaluating tumor spread since lymph node metastases and smaller peritoneal implants may be missed. Immunoscintigraphy, which is thought to be the most specific imaging technique, has not been accepted as a routine method. Krag[6] reported the sensitivity and specificity of 69% and 57%, respectively, for immunoscintigraphy and 44% and 79%, respectively, for CT in patients with ovarian cancer.

The values and limitations of FDG-PET for the diagnosis of suspected primary ovarian cancer were described recently. It has been found that most ovarian carcinomas show an increased FDG uptake. However, low glucose metabolism of borderline tumors or early-stage ovarian cancers, together with high FDG uptake in inflammatory lesions, diminishes the sensitivity and specificity of FDG-PET for the diagnosis of primary ovarian cancer.[7]

The first report on ^{18}F-FDG accumulation in ovarian cancer was by Hubner et al,[8] who found a sensitivity of 93% and a specificity of 82% for assessing previous tumors. In the preoperative evaluation of patients with a pelvic mass, PET has been reported to have positive and negative predictive values for malignancy of 86% and 76%, respectively. Zimny et al[9] evaluated ^{18}F-FDG-PET in 26 patients suspected of having ovarian cancer. Quantitative analysis revealed a mean standard uptake value (SUV) of 6.8 ± 2.3 in primary ovarian carcinoma compared to 2.6 ± 1.2 in benign masses. The sensitivity, specificity, and diagnostic accuracy were 88%, 80%, and 85%, respectively.

Grab et al[7] compared the diagnostic accuracy of sonography, MRI and PET in the evaluation of adnexal masses. In a series with 101 patients, sonographic evaluation resulted in correct classification of 11 of 12 ovarian malignancies (sensitivity 92%), but with a specificity of only 60%. With MRI and PET, specificities improved to 84% and 80%, respectively, but sensitivities decreased. When all imaging modalities were combined, sensitivity and specificity were 92% and 85%, respectively, and accuracy was 86%. The combination of ultrasound with MRI and PET may improve accuracy in the differentation of benign from malignant ovarian lesions.

Schroder et al[10] reported the preoperative detectability of ^{18}F-FDG-PET in ovarian carcinoma. Regarding metabolic differentiation of primary ovarian tumors, 85.7% (24/28) of the cases were correctly diagnosed using PET (Fig. 20.1). The only false-positive resulted from an inflammatory adnexal mass. This reading illustrates the limitation of PET in distinguishing malignant from inflammatory processes, which also show an increased glucose metabolism. In a study by Römer et al[11] comprising 24 patients, four of 19 with a primary ovarian mass had an inflammatory adnexal process, which in all cases showed an increased FDG uptake. Thus, FDG-PET in this trial showed a specificity of only 54%, whereas the sensitivity was 83%. Quantitative analysis of the SUV, as recommended by the interdisciplinary consensus meeting, does not improve the diagnostic differentiation of inflammatory adnexal masses from malignant tumors.

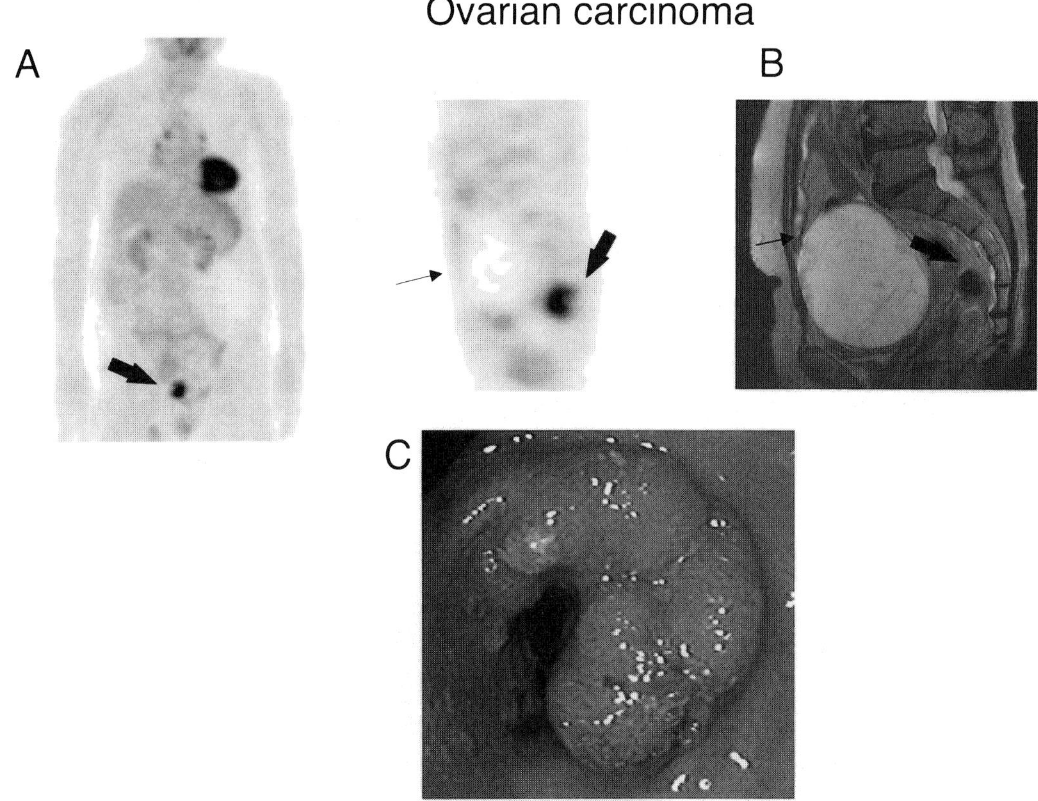

FIGURE 20.1. A: Selected coronal PET image of the axial body and sagittal image of the abdomen and pelvis with ^{18}F-FDG show a focal area of markedly increased activity (*thick arrows*) in the lower presacral space. Note a large ill-defined photopenic area (*thin arrows*) in the anterior pelvis. B: Sagittal T2-weighted MRI of the pelvis shows a large cystic mass (*thin arrow*) and small solid calcific mass (*thick arrow*) in the presacral space. C: Gross specimen from the surgery was a papillary serous cystic adenocarcinoma of the ovary.

Staging

Staging at diagnosis is one of the major prognostic factors in ovarian cancer.[12] At diagnosis, approximately 70% of patients have tumors that have spread beyond the ovary and pelvis to the abdomen (stage III) or beyond (stage IV). Fewer than 20% of patients with advanced ovarian cancer (stage III and IV) live for 5 years after diagnosis.[13]

At present, exploratory laparotomy is the "gold standard" in the staging of ovarian cancer. Staging laparotomy is required for histologic confirmation of the diagnosis, identification of tumor spread, and debulking of tumor masses prior to chemotherapy.

Modern imaging techniques have been introduced for preoperative evaluation of the disease. Ultrasonography, CT, and MRI, however, lack the potential for distinguishing benign reactive changes from cancer infiltration.[14] ^{18}F-FDG-PET can be clinically used for a more complete staging of patients with primary or recurrent ovarian cancer (Figs. 20.2 and 20.3). Schroder et al[10] reported the sensitivity of FDG-PET for the detection of peritoneal carcinomatosis was 72%, which is somewhat lower than optimal, but still higher than the 45% achieved with CT.

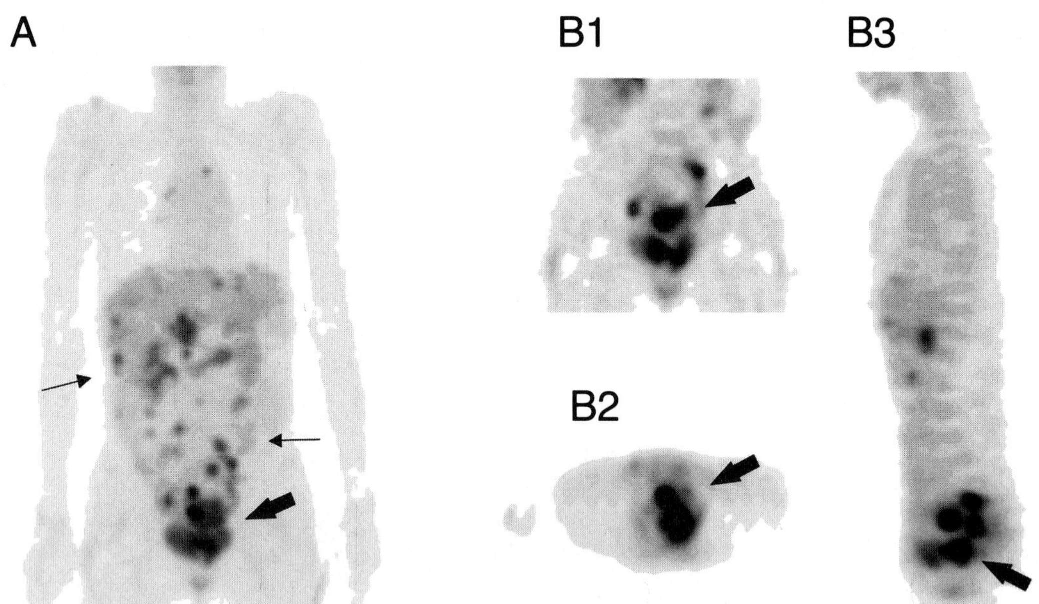

FIGURE 20.2. A: Selected coronal PET image of the axial body with ^{18}F-FDG shows numerous focal areas of slightly to moderately increased activity in the abdomen and pelvis (*arrows*). B: Selected coronal (B1), axial (B2), and sagittal (B3) images of the pelvis show multiple focal areas of markedly increased activity (*thick arrows*). Surgery revealed papillary serous ovarian carcinoma and peritoneal metastasis.

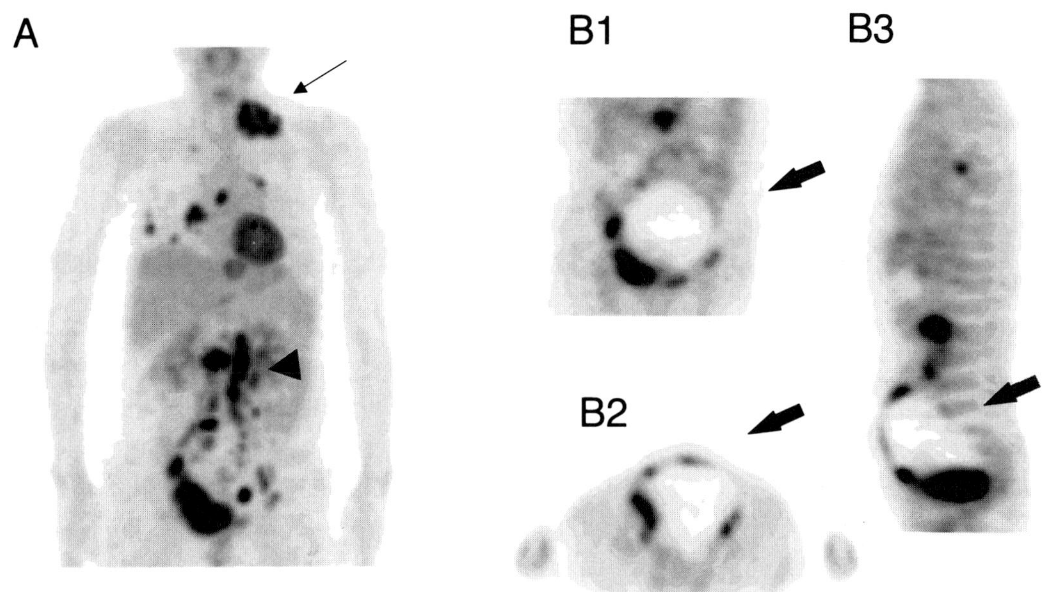

FIGURE 20.3. A: Selected coronal (PET) image of the axial body with ^{18}F-FDG shows metastatic lesions of ovarian cancer in left supraclavicular (*thin arrow*), mediastinal, right hilar, para-aortic (*arrowhead*), and iliac lymphatic chains. Note small metastatic lesions in the right lung. B: Selected coronal (B1), axial (B2), and sagittal (B3) images of the pelvis show a large cystic mass (*thick arrows*) compressing the ureters and bladder.

MRI is not a great improvement over CT, since most metastases in the mesentery and the small intestine remain undetected by both methods. Immunoscintigraphy has a comparable rate of true-positive findings (71%), but its rate of 20% false-positive results is rather high.[6]

Manuel et al[15] evaluated the detectability of FDG-PET prior to surgical exploration and correlated PET image with surgicopathologic findings in primary ovarian cancer. The sensitivity and specificity of FDG-PET were 78% and 86%, respectively. On a regional basis (abdomen and pelvis were divided into five regions of interest) the sensitivity and specificity of PET were 43% and 92%, respectively, while CT or MRI was only 29% sensitive.

PET is of limited value for the detection of microscopic seeding. A typical finding of FDG-PET in cases with peritoneal seeding is diffused and increased uptake around the peritoneal pouch (Fig. 20.4). However, it is sometimes difficult to differentiate abnormal uptake from the normal uptake pattern. Special attention is required to differentiate peritoneal seeding from increased bowel activity, and the clinical value of FDG-PET in primary ovarian cancer still has to be established.[16] Zimny et al[9] reported the sensitivity, specificity, and diagnostic accuracy were 50%, 95%, and 80%, respectively, for evaluating peritoneal

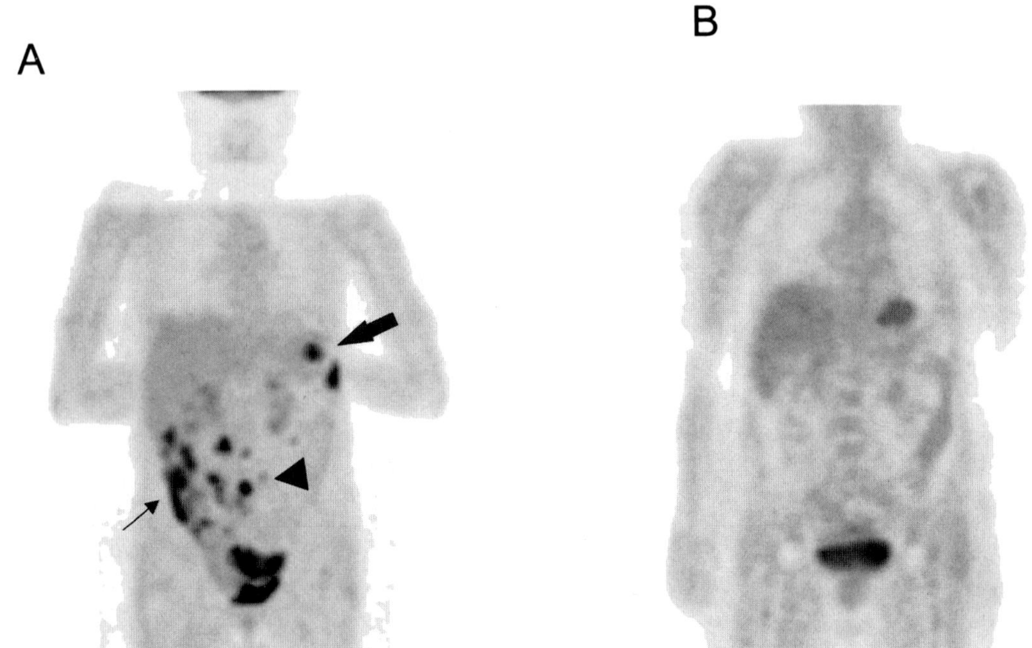

FIGURE 20.4. A: Selected coronal PET image of the axial body with ^{18}F-FDG shows numerous peritoneal metastatic lesions of ovarian cancer. Note curvilinear markedly increased activity (*thin arrow*), ill-defined small focal area of slightly increased activity (*arrowhead*), and focal area of moderately increased activity in the left subdiaphragmatic space for variable patterns of peritoneal lesions. B: Follow-up PET after 6 months of chemotherapy shows no metabolically active lesion.

metastases. In other words, PET misses poorly localized, microscopic-spread disease.[17]

Second-Look Laparotomy

Second-look laparotomy, defined as "a systematic surgical reexploration in asymptomatic patients who have no clinical evidence of tumor following initial surgery and completion of a planned program of chemotherapy for ovarian cancer,"[18] has been used widely to assess response to chemotherapy in clinical trials and standard management of ovarian cancer. However, the second-look laparotomy does not affect survival. In patients with advanced disease, as many as 50% with negative results of second-look operation after combination chemotherapy have experienced a subsequent recurrence. This discouraging statistic suggests that (1) even a thorough exploration does not reveal microscopic residuals in many patients, and (2) this group of patients should be strongly considered for adjuvant chemotherapy.

PET has been evaluated as a substitute for second-look surgery in ovarian cancer patients with a complete clinical, radiographic, and serologic response following primary surgery and chemotherapy.[19]

Casey et al[20] studied the role of PET with second-look laparotomy in seven patients. PET scans were consistent with the presence of tumors in all six patients with residual cancer, even though serum ovarian tumor markers remained below the normal threshold in three of these patients at the time the scans were done. Whole-body PET would provide a sensitive and noninvasive second-look method with little patient discomfort and reasonably fast patient throughput, and at a reasonable cost.

Although PET cannot rule out microscopic persistent or recurrent disease, a negative scan provides prognostic information. It has been shown that patients with a longer relapse-free interval have a higher likelihood of benefiting from surgery. Furthermore, the response rate to retreatment increases with the duration of the treatment-free interval. Patients with a 6-month treatment-free interval have potentially platinum-sensitive disease, and patients with a treatment-free interval of more than 24 months have the greatest likelihood of benefiting from re-treatment. Zimny et al[21] reported that the median relapse-free interval was 20 months for negative PET scans compared to only 6 months for positive scans.

We compared the prognostic value of PET with second-look laparotomy in determining a therapeutic response in patients with advanced ovarian carcinoma following primary chemotherapy. The median duration of survival was 29.6 months with second-look surgery and 30.9 months after PET ($p > .05$). We suggested that whole-body ^{18}F-FDG-PET can be a substitute for second-look laparotomy for following up patients who have had ovarian carcinoma, especially those at high risk for recurrence.[22]

Thus, PET could replace or at least postpone some of the second-look laparotomy in patients who have a suspicious CT scan or rising tumor marker. It remains to be seen, however, whether the most appropriate biopsy site can be localized by PET prior to tissue changes detected by CT or MRI.[23]

Recurrent Ovarian Carcinoma

So far studies have focused on the role of FDG-PET in patients with recurrent ovarian cancer. FDG-PET may be helpful in detecting small recurrent lesions in patients in whom posttherapeutic alterations in anatomy may make it difficult to interpret conventional imaging studies (Fig. 20.5).

In recent reports whole-body ^{18}F-FDG-PET was superior to conventional CT/MRI for detection of recurrent disease.[23–25] The sensitivity was 83% to 91% versus 45% to 91%, and specificity was 66% to 93% versus 46% to 84% for PET and CT/MRI, respectively.[23]

In a study by Zimny et al[21] with 106 scans performed in 54 patients, the overall sensitivity and specificity to detect recurrent ovarian cancer were 83% and 83%, respectively. However, the diagnostic accuracy assessed by Receiver Operating Curve (ROC) analysis varies among the subgroups of patients enrolled in this study. PET was more accurate in patients with suspected recurrence with a diagnostic accuracy

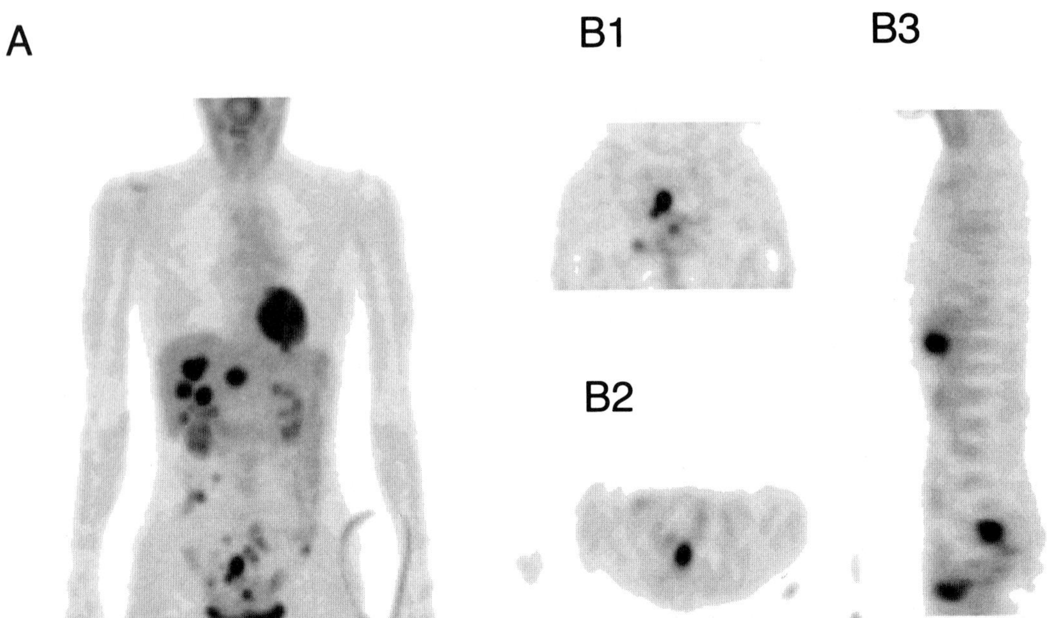

FIGURE 20.5. A: Selected coronal PET image of the axial body with ^{18}F-FDG shows recurrent ovarian cancer in the right pelvis near the midline and several metastatic lesions in the liver. B: Selected coronal (B1), axial (B2), and sagittal (B3) images of the pelvis show a focal area of markedly increased activity in the right presacral space near the midline due to recurrent ovarian carcinoma.

of 93% and sensitivity of 94%, compared to 71% and 65% in patients judged as clinically free of disease.[24] More importantly, the analysis of patients with rising tumor marker CA-125 and negative or nondiagnostic findings of conventional imaging revealed a sensitivity of 96% with only one false-negative scan.[25]

In another report, by Nakamoto et al[17] on patient-based analysis, the overall sensitivity, specificity, and accuracy of conventional imaging modalities were 73%, 75%, and 73%, respectively, and these rates improved to 92%, 100%, and 94%, respectively, by considering both conventional imaging modalities and PET findings.

In conclusion, FDG-PET may provide additional information in the detection of tumor recurrence when conventional imaging methods are negative. The high accuracy of FDG-PET plus CA-125 suggests that the combination may have a significant role in the management of patients with ovarian cancer.

PET/CT Imaging

FDG-PET imaging of the abdomen and pelvis may be difficult due to the physiologic bowel uptake and bladder activity and a lack of anatomic landmarks. A new combined PET/CT scanning provides fused PET and CT images without the problems of organ motion, temporal differences, and patient positioning.[26]

Makhija et al[27] reported the effectiveness of combined PET/CT in confirming and localizing recurrent disease in ovarian cancer in a specifically chosen high-risk subgroup of patients with recurrent ovarian/fallopian tube cancers (n = 8). Seven patients had a negative CT and five patients had lesions that were correctly identified by PET/CT. Blodgett et al[26] evaluated the lesion detectability and effectiveness in patients with recurrent ovarian cancer and compared CT with combined PET/CT. PET/CT identified an additional lesion compared to CT in 12/15 (80%) and changed management in 11/15 (73%) of patients. They emphasized that PET/CT is an important modality for restaging patients with recurrent ovarian carcinoma, especially in patients with rising CA-125 levels.

Cost-Effectiveness

Smith et al[28] evaluated ^{18}F-FDG-PET for detecting and staging recurrent ovarian cancer, when applied in selecting the most appropriate treatment and avoiding second-look surgeries using the Monte Carlo simulation analysis. In this report assumptions in the management pathway were as follows: (1) a positive PET scan led to either laparoscopy or laparotomy, followed by chemotherapy (true-positive PET) or follow-up (false-positive PET); (2) a negative PET scan resulted in continued follow-up (true-negative PET) or laparotomy (false-negative PET); and (3) a laparotomy led to chemotherapy or follow-up. Using PET to manage the diagnostic evaluation, the number of unnecessary laparotomies was reduced from 70% to 5%. Cost savings per patient ranged from $1,941 to $11,766. Therefore, FDG-PET can reduce unnecessary invasive staging procedures and management, and PET in place of second-look surgery would yield substantial cost savings to the patient.

Limitations

Distinguishing Malignant from Benign Lesions

The limitation of FDG-PET is in distinguishing malignant from inflammatory processes, which also show increased glucose metabolism.[15] False-positive cases for a corpus luteum cyst, ovarian endometriosis, and the gestational pouch were reported with a focally raised FDG uptake.[12]

Type of Tumor

False-positive results were seen in benign serous cyst adenoma, endometriosis, and endometrioma, and false-negative PET information was observed in a mesothelioma and a borderline serous tumor.[8]

Tumor Size

Lesions smaller than 1 cm were quite difficult to identify, not only because of the relatively poor spatial resolution but also because of the longer acquisition time of PET. Count recovery from small lesions may not be sufficient because of peristalsis of the alimentary tract and respiratory movement during image acquisition. Thus, even if PET findings are negative, small lesions sometimes may be detected by second-look laparotomy. However, patients typically receive follow-up chemotherapy for recurrence and systemic metastasis. Very small lesions that cannot be detected on PET scans may be sensitive to drugs, while larger lesions are resistant to drugs because of possible penetration barriers. Therefore, if FDG-PET reveals highly accumulated lesions remaining in a patient even after repeated chemotherapy, resection would be recommended. If PET findings are negative, chemotherapy may be proposed because some small lesions may remain. Thus, PET can be useful in the therapeutic decision.[17]

Nonpathologic (Physiologic) Uptake

Physiologic uptake in the stomach, colon, ureter, and bladder is sometimes difficult to differentiate from pathologic lesions. Such accumulation may mask abnormal uptake due to tiny disseminated lesions.[17] The combination of hydration, administration of a diuretic such as furosemide, and use of a Foley catheter with a drainage bag is an effective method of reducing physiologic uptake in the kidneys, ureter, and bladder. But reducing the physiologic uptake in the colon is difficult.[29]

The use of the SUV and SUV ratio may be helpful in distinguishing between physiologic bowel activity and ovarian cancer metastatic to the bowel serosa. Holschneider et al[30] suggested that SUV and SUV ratio (cutoff value of 3.0 for SUV and 1.75 for SUV ratio) were significantly higher in cases of cancer metastasis to the bowel than in patients with no evidence of bowel metastases.

^{11}C-Methionine PET

Tumor imaging in the pelvis may be problematic since normal excreted activity in the urine may interfere with tumor identification. An essential amino acid, methionine, labeled with ^{11}C, has been found to be a valuable tracer for metabolic imaging of human cancer. High uptake of ^{11}C-methionine may correlate with poor histologic grade of differentiation and high cell proliferation, which suggests that tissue uptake of methionine may reflect the biologic aggressiveness of cancer (Fig. 20.6).[32]

Lapela et al[32] showed that it is possible to separate poorly differentiated from well-differentiated tumors. They tried to differentiate benign and malignant ovarian tumors. They reported that benign or borderline malignant tumors did not accumulate ^{11}C-methionine, whereas all carcinomas had significant uptakes. The mean SUV of the primary carcinoma was 7.0 ± 2.2, and the mean K_i was 0.14 min^{-1}.

We found that ^{11}C-methionine PET can be used to differentiate physiologic uptake of FDG from a true lesion (Fig. 20.7).[33] In a series of 16 gynecologic cancers, the higher diagnostic accuracy of the methionine PET [sensitivity = 80% (4/5), specificity = 100% (11/11), and accuracy = 94% (15/16)] than that of FDG-PET [sensitivity = 40% (2/5), specificity = 91% (10/11), accuracy = 75% (12/16)] was found for the detection of recurrent gynecologic cancer in the pelvic region postoperatively.

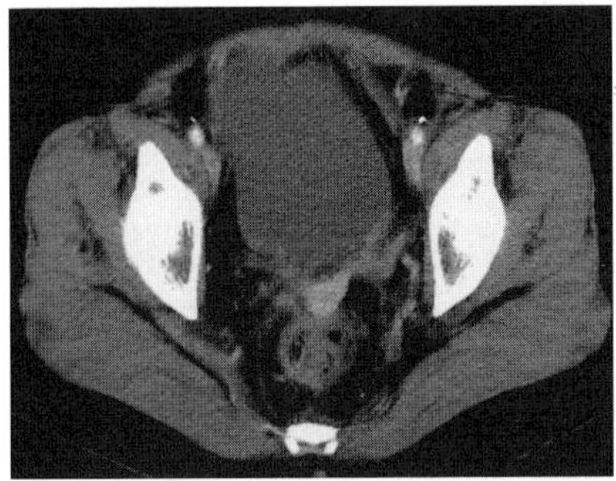

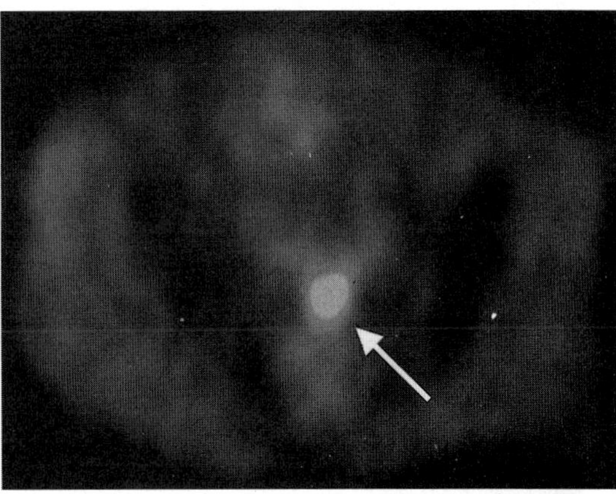

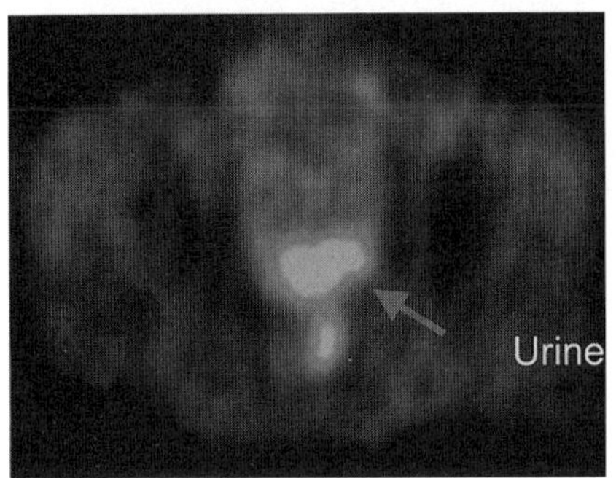

FIGURE 20.6. Transaxial CT image (*upper left*) of the lower pelvis shows a small contrast-enhanced lesion in the midline behind the bladder. Axial PET image (*right*) of the lower pelvis with ^{11}C-methionine shows a focal area of markedly increased activity (*arrow*) in the middle of the pelvis. Slightly lower image (*left lower*) shows a physiologic activity in the bladder. Biopsy revealed a recurrent ovarian carcinoma. This is a true-positive case.

Cervical Cancer

Cancer of the cervix is estimated to be the second most frequently diagnosed cancer in women worldwide. Although the overall mortality from cervival cancer has decreased due to early detection and treatment of preinvasive disease, the mortality of invasive cervical cancer has not changed in the past 30 years. The treatments and prognosis of invasive cervical cancer are determined by the stage of disease, volume of the primary tumor, grade of tumor, and presence of lymph node metastasis. Patients at an early stage of cervical cancer without lymph node metastasis are considered as surgical candidates, whereas radiotherapy is often the preferred treatment when lymph node metastases are present.[34]

Preoperative Staging

Carcinoma of the cervix metastasizes in a predictable pattern. The tumor usually spreads from the primary cervical lesion sequentially to pelvic, para-aortic, and supraclavicular lymph nodes, and then ultimately to nonnodal distant metastatic sites such as the lung, liver, and

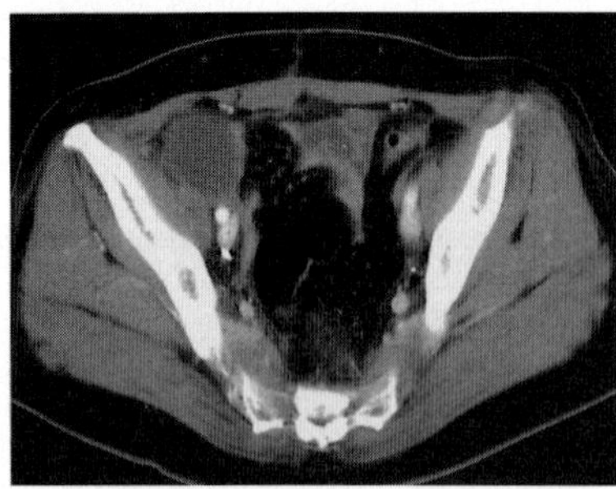

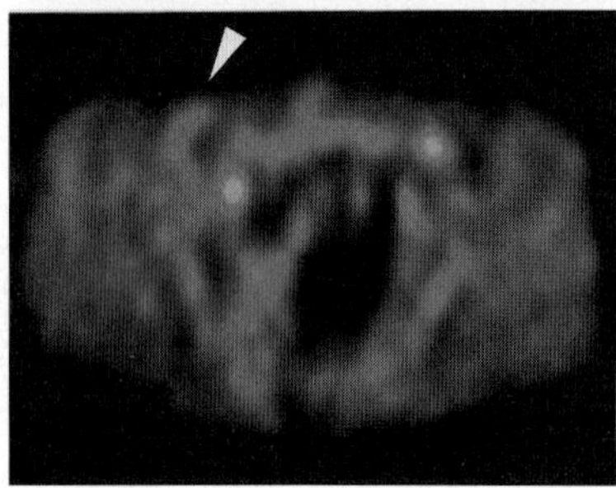

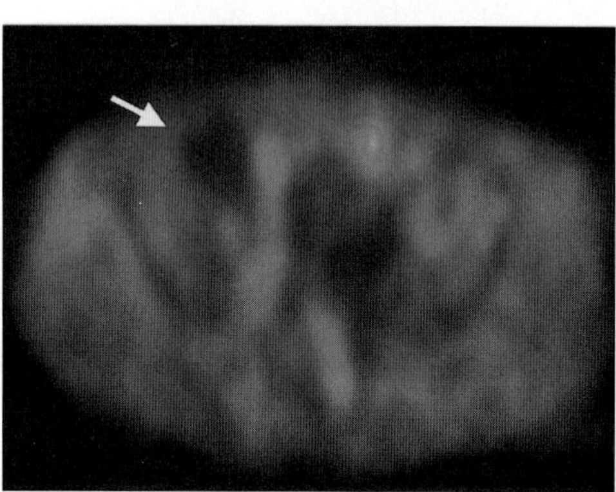

FIGURE 20.7. Axial CT image of the upper pelvis (*left upper*) shows a round cystic lesion with a contrast-enhanced rim in the anterior right pelvis. Axial PET image with ^{11}C-methionine at the comparable level shows no significant uptake (*arrow*) of methionine. Slightly lower level image (*left lower*) shows slightly increased activity in the rim of the lesion or physiologic bowel activity. Surgery revealed a lymphocyst. This is a true-negative case.

bone. Metastasis to para-aortic lymph nodes in the absence of pelvic nodal metastasis is exceptionally uncommon.[34,35]

Cross-sectional imaging modalities such as CT and MRI have proven to be useful for evaluating morphologic risk factor such as tumor size, depth of stromal invasion, stage of disease, and lymph node metastasis. Overall staging accuracy of 58% to 88% has been reported, but low sensitivity (44%) was found. Neither tumor size nor early parametrial invasion can be evaluated reliably. MRI is now considered to be the most accurate imaging method for evaluation of tumor size and parametrial invasion. Overall staging accuracy of 80% to 92%, has been shown, whereas the sensitivity for nodal metastasis is similar to that with CT (50%).[36]

A few reports compared FDG-PET with CT and surgical staging for detecting lymph node metastasis in patients with cervical cancer (Fig. 20.8). Sugawara et al[37] reported an 86% sensitivity of FDG-PET for pelvic and para-aortic lymph node metastasis (Fig. 20.9), as compared with a 57% sensitivity of CT in a study of 21 patients with cervical cancer of stages 1B to 4A. Rose et al[38] reported a sensitivity and specificity of 75% and 92%, respectively, for FDG-PET in depicting para-aortic lymph node metastasis in more advanced stages (2B to 4A) before a surgical staging lymphadenectomy was done (Fig. 20.10). They observed a higher sensitivity of FDG-PET for pelvic (100%) than for para-

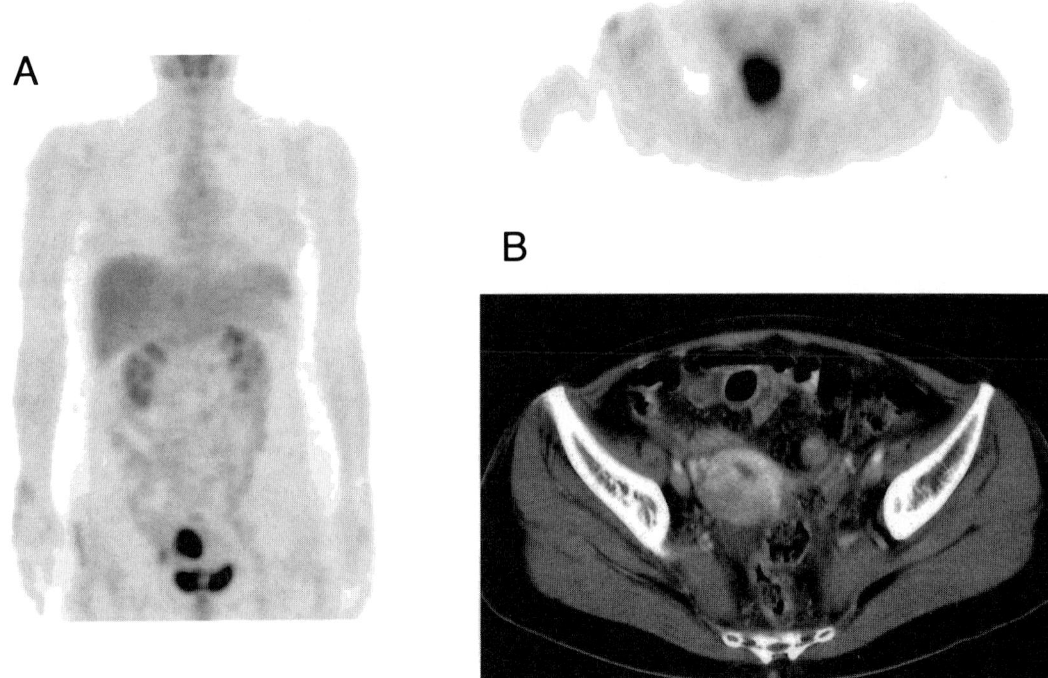

FIGURE 20.8. A: Selected coronal PET image of the axial body with ^{18}F-FDG shows a focal area of markedly increased activity in the right pelvis. B: Selected axial PET image of the pelvis (*right upper*) shows markedly increased uptake of FDG, corresponding to the contrast-enhanced lesion in the uterine cervix seen on axial CT (*right lower*). Surgery revealed a cervical carcinoma.

aortic (75%) lymph node metastases. Grigsby et al[39] reported that FDG-PET detects abnormal lymph node regions more often than does CT (Fig. 20.11). In 101 patients, CT demonstrated abnormally enlarged pelvic lymph nodes in 20 (20%) and para-aortic lymph nodes in seven (7%). PET demonstrated abnormal FDG uptake in pelvic lymph nodes in 67 (67%), in para-aortic lymph nodes in 21 (21%), and in supraclavicular lymph node in eight (8%).

Reinhardt et al[40] reported that node staging resulted in sensitivities of 91% with FDG-PET and 73% with MRI and specificities of 100% with PET and 83% with MRI. The positive predictive value (PPV) of PET was 100%, and that of MRI 67%. The metastatic involvement of lymph node sites was identified on PET with a PPV of 90%, and on MRI 64% ($p < .05$).

Thus, FDG-PET is a reliable alternative to conventional imaging for lymph node staging in patients with cervical cancer.

Recurrence

The recurrence rate of uterine cervical cancer is reported to be 6.5% after surgery and 26.2% after radiation therapy alone. About half of all

Cervical cancer

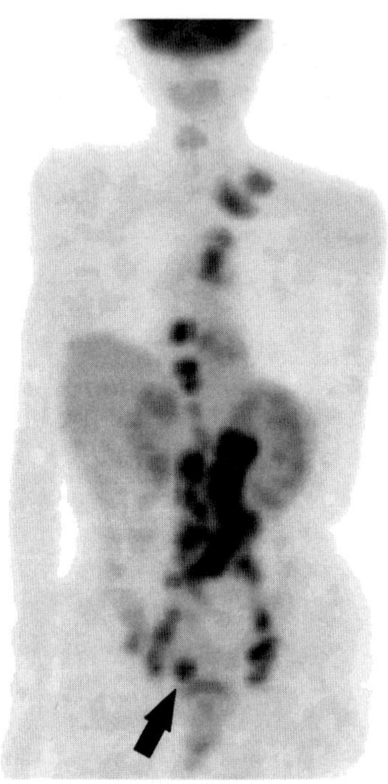

Figure 20.9. Selected coronal PET image of the axial body with ^{18}F-FDG shows multiple metastatic lesions of cervical cancer (*arrow*) in the iliac, para-aortic, mediastinal, and left supraclavicular lymphatic chains.

cases of recurrent uterine cervical cancer are confined to the pelvic cavity, but some cases show metastatic lesions in the lymph nodes, lung, bone, and liver (Fig. 20.12).

Radiologic studies such as intravenous renography, ultrasonography, CT, and MRI are used to detect recurrent cervical cancer. It is difficult, however, for these imagings to differentiate recurrent tumor from postoperative or radiation fibrosis, or to detect metastatic normal-sized lymph nodes and extrapelvic metastases. PET is effective in differentiating recurrence from scar tissue, and, in addition, can be used to obtain whole-body images to detect recurrence that was not clinically suspected (Fig. 20.13).

Park et al[41] reported the accuracy of CT and PET in the diagnosis of recurrent uterine cervical cancer with 36 patients. The sensitivity, specificity, and accuracy of CT were 78%, 83%, and 81%, respectively, while for PET, the corresponding figures were 100%, 94% ($p = .0339$), and 97% ($p = .0244$), respectively. Sun et al[42] reported the sensitivity and specificity of 90% and 100% with FDG-PET in evaluation of recurrent

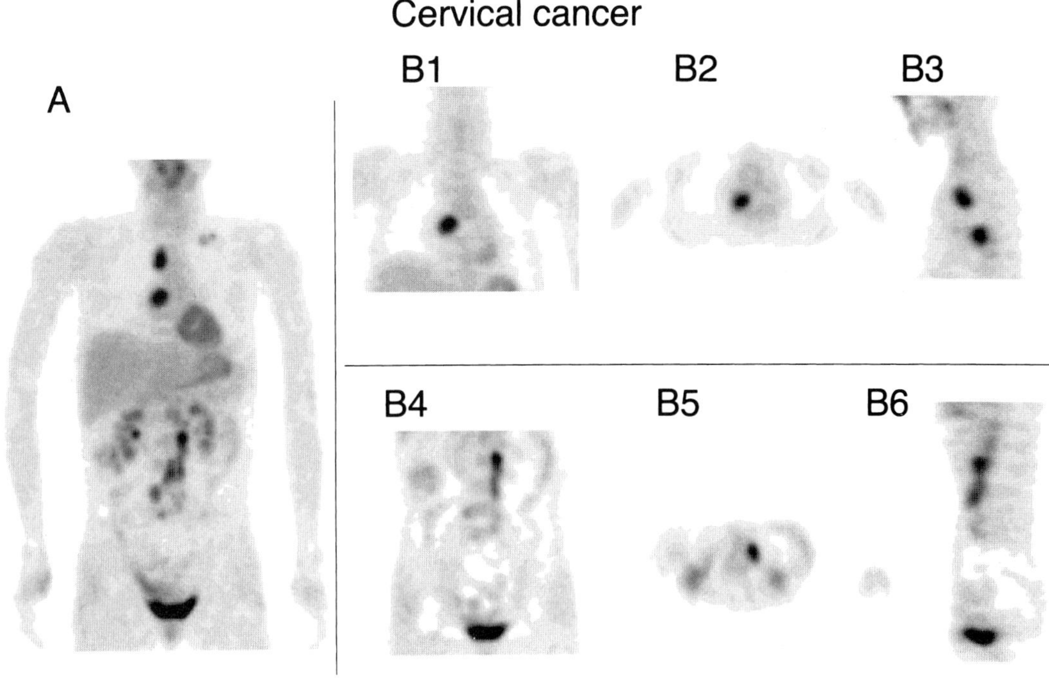

FIGURE 20.10. A: Selected coronal PET image of the axial body with ^{18}F-FDG shows metastatic lesions of cervical cancer in the para-aortic, right paratracheal, right hilar, and left supraclavicular lymphatic chains. B: Selected coronal (B1), axial (B2), and sagittal (B3) images of the chest show a metastatic active lesion in the right hilum. Selected coronal (B4), axial (B5), and sagittal (B6) images of the abdomen show metastatic lesions along the left para-aortic lymph nodes.

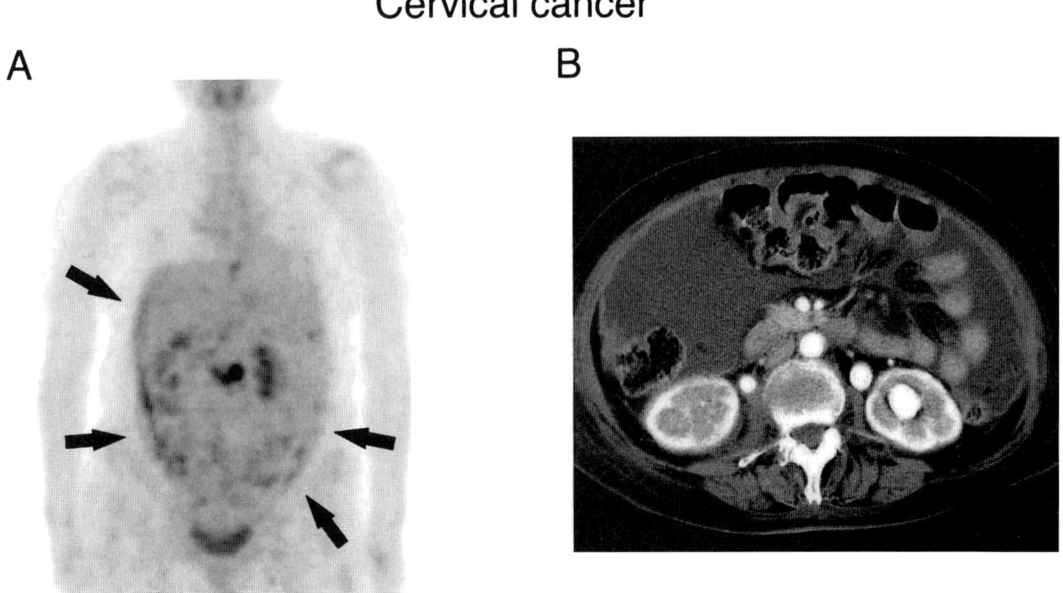

FIGURE 20.11. A: Selected coronal PET image of the axial body with ^{18}F-FDG shows curvilinear increased activity (*arrows*) along the right and left margins of the abdomen due to peritoneal seeding of cervical carcinoma. Note also focal increased activity in the mid-abdomen. B: Axial CT image of the upper abdomen shows ascites and contrast enhancement of the peritoneum as well as periaortic lymph node.

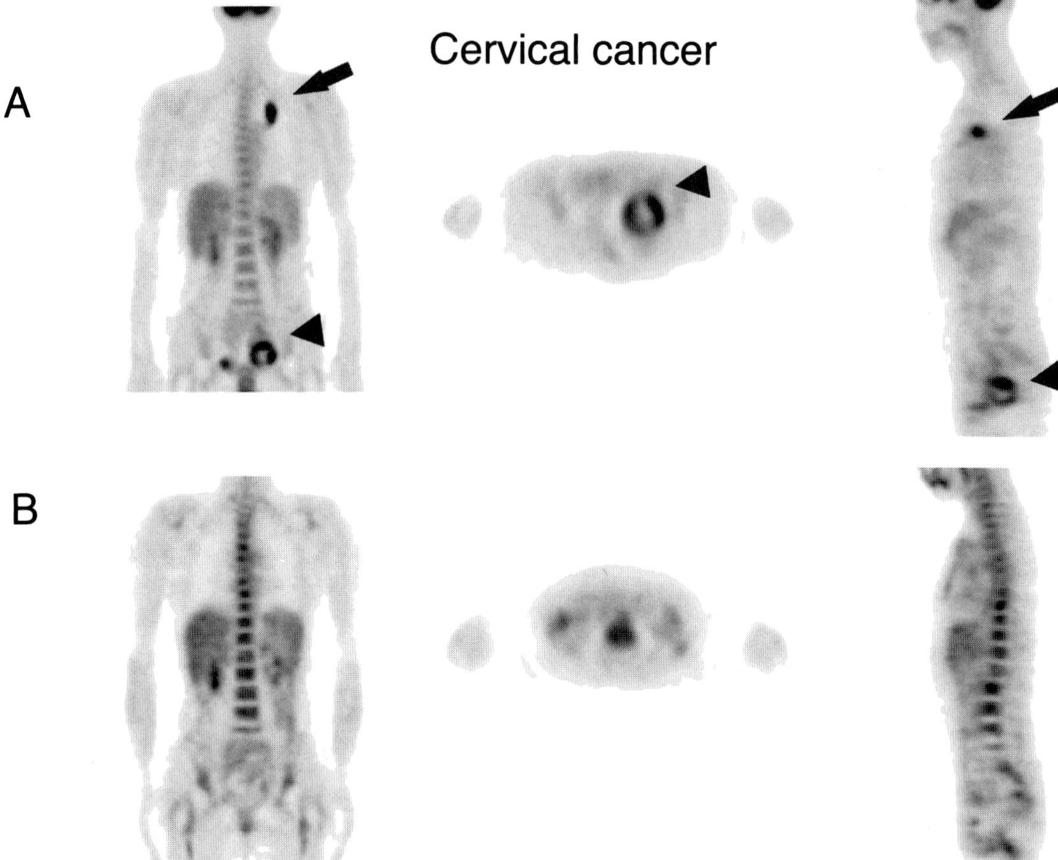

FIGURE 20.12. A: Selected coronal (*left*) and sagittal (*right*) images of the axial body as well as an axial image of the pelvis with ^{18}F-FDG show recurrent cervical cancer with central necrosis (*arrowheads*) as well as metastatic lesions in the left upper lung (*arrows*) and right external iliac lymph nodes. B: Follow-up PET shows no metabolically active lesion after chemotherapy.

ovarian cancer. PET could detect 7.9% of early recurrence in patients with clinically no evidence of disease (NED) status.

Treatment Response

Nakamoto et al[43] reported the high sensitivity of FDG-PET in monitoring the therapeutic response of cervical cancer. In this study FDG-PET scans were performed prior to therapy and at a mean of 4.6 months after radiation in 20 patients with histologically proven uterine cervical cancer who were undergoing "curative" course of radiation. FDG-PET is a sensitive tool for detecting active cervical cancer after radiation therapy. The sensitivity, specificity, and accuracy were 100%, 60%, and 70%, respectively. With regard to the relatively low specificity, it is well known that FDG also accumulates in inflammatory foci, which can lead to false-positive findings.

Although PET would not completely replace the monitoring of tumors using these modalities, this noninvasive technique could come to

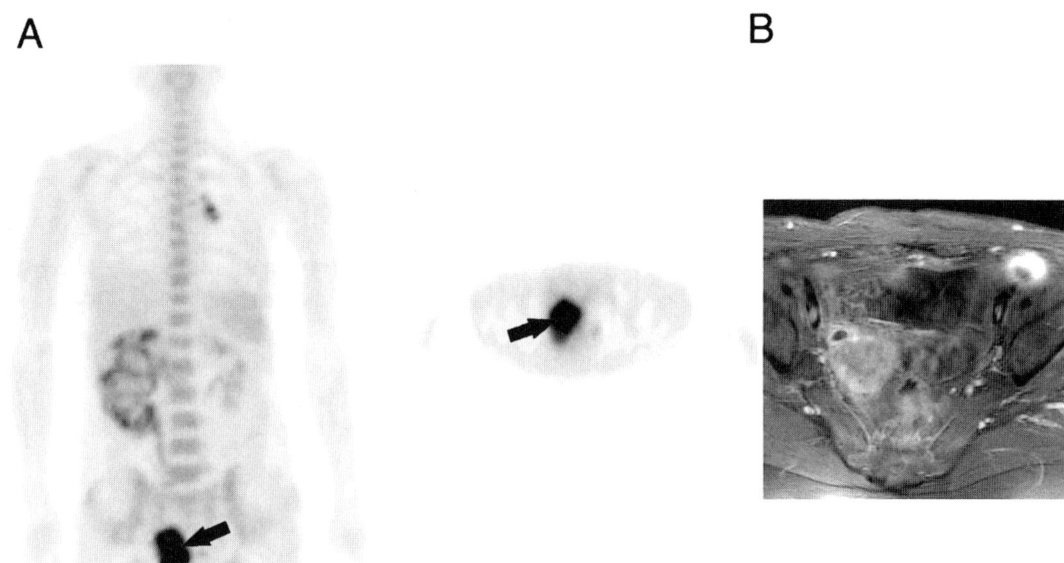

FIGURE 20.13. A: Selected coronal PET image of the axial body with ^{18}F-FDG shows recurrent cervical cancer (*arrows*) and also metastasis in the left hilum. Note right hydronephrosis. Selected axial image of the pelvis (*middle*) shows a focal area of markedly increased activity in the right pelvis. B: Axial T1-weighted MRI of the pelvis with fat suppression shows a contrast-enhanced lesion in the right pelvis. Biopsy revealed a recurrent cervical carcinoma.

have a greater role for screening patients during follow-up due to its high sensitivity.

Prognosis

Grigsby et al[39] reported that the findings on PET are a better predictor of survival than those of CT in patients with carcinoma of the cervix. The 2-year progression-free survival, based solely on para-aortic lymph node status, was 64% in CT-negative and PET-negative patients, 18% in CT-negative and PET-positive patients, and 14% in CT-positive and PET-positive patients ($p < .0001$). A multivariate analysis demonstrated that the most significant prognostic factor for progression-free survival was the presence of positive para-aortic lymph nodes as detected by PET imaging ($p = .025$). Pinkus et al[44] evaluated the prognostic value of FDG-PET in patients with cervical cancer using simple visual analysis of primary tumor characteristics (scoring for heterogeneity, size, shape, and lymph node involvement). For those with a good prognosis, 8% to 10% of patients died while 76% to 85% of them with a poor prognosis died within 2 years. This study extends the value of FDG-PET in cervical cancer patients, powerfully distinguishing patients who have an excellent prognosis from those with a poor prognosis who may require more aggressive initial treatment.

In a study of the prognostic value of SUV on FDG-PET, squamous cell–type uterine cervix cancer with high glucose metabolic activity results in a poor outcome. The survival of the high-peak SUV group (≥13) was worse than that of the low-peak SUV group (<13). Two-year survival was 76.0% and 92.3% for the high- and low-peak SUV groups.[45]

Limitations

Substantially increased uterine vascularity was generally observed in the secretory and menstrual phases by radionuclide imaging. In vivo, FDG uptake could be altered by blood flow, transport, and hexokinase activity; therefore, FDG uptake in a normal uterus could be altered by the phase of the menstrual cycle. Preclinical studies have shown that FDG uptake in the estrogen-stimulated uterus is significantly greater than if no stimulation is present. A case of intrauterine accumulation of FDG during menstruation has been reported.[46]

Other Gynecologic Cancer

Endometrial Cancer

Nakahara et al[47] reported a case of endometrial cancer. FDG-PET revealed heterogeneous and marked accumulation in the endometrium. Belhocine et al[48] reported the feasibility of FDG-PET for detecting early recurrence in endometrial cancer in 14 patients who showed no evidence of disease after treatment. Of the 14 patients, FDG-PET diagnosed two patients as having recurrence. One of these two patients had a PET finding of enlarged hypermetabolic abdominal focus, although her CT was negative. The second patient had a single focus of hypermetabolic activity in the liver and a focal hypodensity in the same location on CT. Therefore, PET may be a useful method in detecting early recurrence in patients with endometrial cancer who showed no evidence of disease on conventional follow-up.

Uterine Sarcoma

FDG-PET was very useful in the diagnosis of sarcoma, even though the SUVs were a little low. Umesaki et al[49] reported on five sarcomas and evaluated the effectiveness of FDG-PET for diagnosis of uterine sarcoma in comparison to other diagnostic methods. PET examinations were 100% positive for the five sarcomas (Figs. 20.14 and 20.15); MRI was 80% positive (four of five cases), and ultrasound was 40% positive (two of five cases). The mean SUV of the sarcomas was 4.5 ± 1.3.

Vulvar Cancer

Cohn et al[50] undertook the prospective pilot study of the performance of FDG as a method for detection of groin metastases from vulvar cancer. Fifteen patients underwent PET prior to exploration of 29 groins. On a patient-by-patient basis, PET had a sensitivity of 80%, specificity

Uterine sarcoma

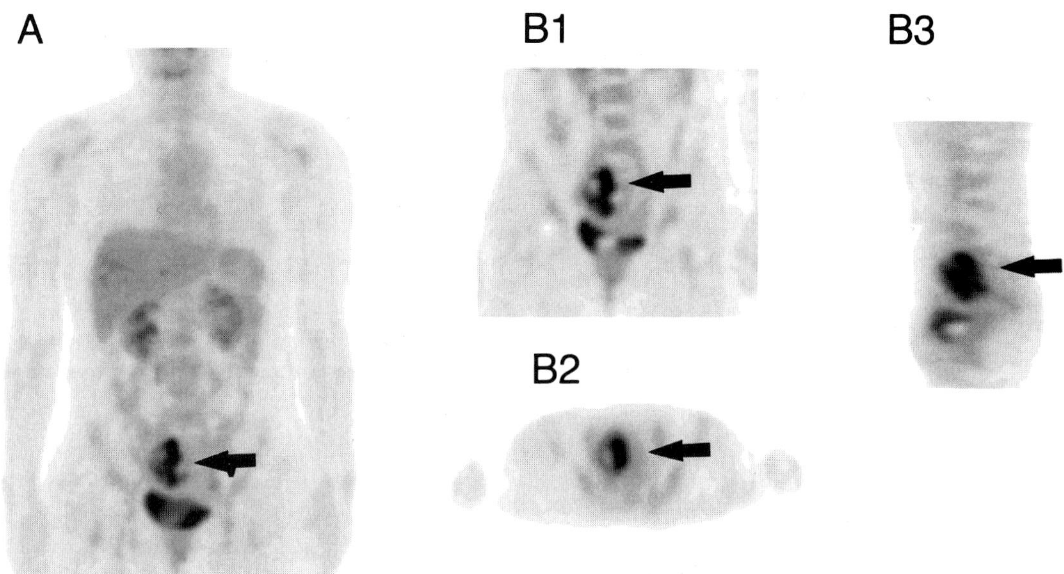

FIGURE 20.14. Selected coronal PET image of the axial body (A) as well as coronal (B1), axial (B2), and sagittal (B3) images of the pelvis show a focal area of irregular increased uptake of ^{18}F-FDG in the right pelvis (*arrows*). Surgery revealed a uterine sarcoma.

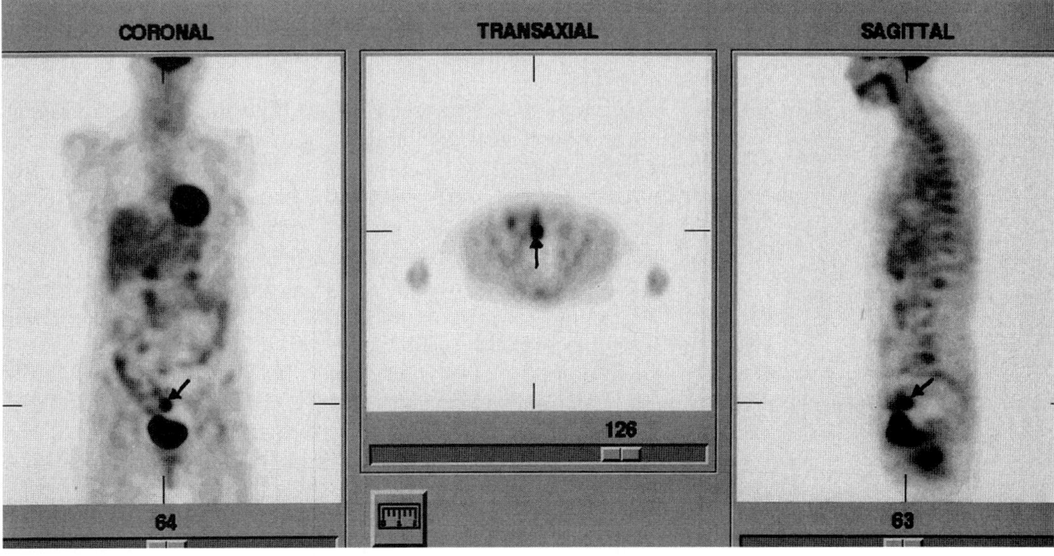

FIGURE 20.15. Selected coronal (*left*) and sagittal (*right*) PET image of the axial body as well as an axial PET image of the pelvis (*middle*) with ^{18}F-FDG show metastatic lesions of uterine sarcoma (*arrow*).

of 90%, positive predictive value of 80%, and negative predictive value of 90% in demonstrating metastases. On a groin-by-groin basis, PET had a sensitivity of 67%, specificity of 95%, positive predictive value of 86%, and negative predictive value of 86%. As the result of this, PET was relatively insensitive in predicting lymph node metastasis, and a negative study is not a reliable surrogate for a pathologically negative groin. However, the high specificity suggests that PET is useful in planning radiation therapy and as an adjunct to lymphatic mapping and sentinel lymph node dissection.

References

1. Soper JT. Radiographic imaging in gynecologic oncology. Clin Obstet Gynecol 2001;44:485–494.
2. Vardi J, Tadros G, Foemmel R, Shebes M. Plasma lipid-associated sialic acid and serum CA125 as indicators of disease status with ovarian cancer. Obstet Gynecol 1989;73:1.
3. Gupta NC, Frank AR, Casey MJ. FDG-PET imaging for post-treatment evaluation of patients with genitourinary malignancies. J Nucl Med 1992; 33:829.
4. Landis SH, Murray T, Bolden S, Wingo PA. Cancer statistics, 1999. CA Cancer J Clin 1999;49:8–31.
5. Chou CY, Chang CH, Yao BL, et al. Color Doppler ultrasonography and serum CA125 in the differentiation of benign and malignant ovarian tumors. J Clin Ultrasound 1994;22:491–496.
6. Krag DN. Clinical utility of immunoscintigraphy in managing ovarian cancer. J Nucl Med 1993;34:545–548.
7. Grab D, Flock F, Stohr I, Nussele K. Classification of asymptomatic adnexal masses by ultrasound, magnetic resonance imaging, and positron emission tomography. Gyncol Oncol 2000;77:454–459.
8. Hubner KF, McDonald TW, Niethammer JG, et al. Assessment of primary and metastatic ovarian cancer by positron emission tomography using 2-[^{18}F]deoxyglucose. Gynecol Oncol 1993;51:197–204.
9. Zimny M, Schroder W, Wolters S, et al. 18F-fluorodeoxyglucose PET in ovarian carcinoma: methodology and preliminary results. Nuklearmedizin 1997;36:228–233.
10. Schroder W, Zimny M, Rudlowski C, et al. The role of 18F-fluoro-deoxyglucose positron emission tomography in diagnosis of ovarian cancer. Int J Cancer Oncol 1999;9:117–122.
11. Römer W, Avril N, Dose J, et al. Metabolische Charakterisierung von Ovarialtumoren mit der Positronen-Emissions-Tomographie und F-18 Fluorodeoxyglukose. Fortschr Rontgenstr 1997;166:62–68.
12. Omura GA, Bradhy MF, Homesley HD, et al. Long-term follow-up and prognostic factor analysis in advanced ovarian carcinoma: the Gynecologic Oncologic Group experience. J Clin Oncol 1991;9:1138–1150.
13. Ozols RF. Chemotherapy of ovarian cancer. In: De Vita VT, Hellman S, Rosenberg SA, eds. Cancer: Principles and Practice of Oncology. Updates. Vol. 2, No. 1. Philidelphia: JB Lippincott, 1988:1–12.
14. Bragg DG, Hricak H. Imaging in gynecologic malignancies. Cancer 1993;71: 1648–1651.
15. Manuel M, Holschneider CH, Williams CM, et al. Correlation of FDG-PET scans with surgicopathologic findings in ovarian cancers. J Nucl Med 2002;43:29.

16. Ak I, Stokkel MPM, Pauwels EKJ. Positron emission tomography with 2-[^{18}F]fluoro-2-deoxy-D-glucose in oncology. Part II. The clinical value in detecting and staging primary tumors. J Cancer Res Clin Oncol 2000;126:560–574.
17. Nakamoto Y, Saga T, Ishimori T, et al. Clinical value of positron emission tomography with FDG for recurrent ovarian cancer. AJR 2001;176:1449–1454.
18. Barter J, Barnes W. Second-look laparotomy. In: Rubin S, Sutton G, eds. Ovarian Cancer. New York: McGraw-Hill, 1993:269–300.
19. Rose PG, Faulhaber P, Miraldi F, et al. Positron emission tomography for evaluating a complete clinical response in patients with ovarian or peritoneal carcinoma: correlation with second-look laparotomy. Gynecol Oncol 2001;82:17–21.
20. Casey MJ, Gupta NC, Muths CK. Experience with positron emission tomography (PET) scans in patients with ovarian cancer. Gynecol Oncol 1994;53:331–338.
21. Zimny M, Siggelkow W, Schroder W, et al. 2-[Fluorine-18]-fluoro-2-deoxy-D-glucose positron emission tomography in the diagnosis of recurrent ovarian cancer. Gynecol Oncol 2001;83:310–315.
22. Chung J-K, Kang SB, Kim MH, et al. The role of 18F-FDG-PET in patients with advanced epithelial ovarian carcinoma as a substitute for second-look operation. J Nucl Med 2002;43:282.
23. Delbeke D, Martin WH. Positron emission tomography imaging in oncology. Radiol Clin North Am 2001;39:883–917.
24. Torizuka T, Nobezawa S, Kanno T, et al. Ovarian cancer recurrence: role of whole-body positron emission tomography using 2-[fluorine-18]-fluoro-2-deoxy-D-glucose. Eur J Nucl Med 2002;29:797–803.
25. Yen R-F, Sun S-S, Shen Y-Y, et al. Whole-body positron emission tomography with ^{18}F-fluoro-2-deoxyglucose for the detection of recurrent ovarian cancer. Anticancer Res 2001;21:3691–3694.
26. Blodgett TM, Meltzer CC, Townsend DW, et al. PET/CT in restaging patients with ovarian carcinoma. J Nucl Med 2002;43:310.
27. Makhija S, Howden N, Edwards R, et al. Positron emission tomography/computed tomography imaging for the recurrent ovarian and fallopian tube carcinoma: a retrospective review. Gynecol Oncol 2002;85:53–58.
28. Smith GT, Hubner KF, McDonald T, et al. Cost analysis of FDG-PET for managing patients with ovarian cancer. Clin Pos Imag 1999;2:63–70.
29. Miraldi F, Vesselle H, Faulhaber PF, et al. Elimination of artifactual accumulation of FDG in PET imaging of colorectal cancer. Clin Nucl Med 1998;23:3–7.
30. Holschneider CH, Manuel M, Williams CM, et al. FDG-PET in ovarian cancer: use of the standardized uptake value (SUV) to differentiate physiological bowel activity from intraperitoneal metastatic tumor. J Nucl Med 2002;43:29.
31. Cook GJR, Maisey MN, Fogelman I. Normal variants, artefacts and interpretative pitfalls in PET imaging with 18-fluoro-2-deoxyglucose and carbon-11 methionine. Eur J Nucl Med 1999;26:1363–1378.
32. Lapela M, Leskinen-Kallio S, Varpula M, et al. Metabolic imaging of ovarian tumors with carbon-11-methionine: a PET study. J Nucl Med 1995;36:2196–2220.
33. Jeong HJ, Chung J-K, Paeng JC, et al. Usefulness of ^{11}C methionine PET in the pelvic region for evaluation of recurrent gynecologic cancer in postoperative state. J Nucl Med 2002;43:283.
34. Eifel PJ, Berek JS, Thigpen JT. Cancer of the cervix, vagina, and vulva. In:

De Vita VT, Hellman S, Rosenberg SA, eds. Cancer: Principles and Practice of Oncology, 5th ed. Philadelphia: Lippincott-Raven, 1997:1433–1478.
35. Morice P, Sabourin JC, Pautier P, et al. Isolated para-aortic node involvement in stage IB/II cervical carcinoma. Eur J Gynaecol Oncol 2000;21: 123–125.
36. Hricak H, Yu KK. Radiology in invasive cervical cancer. AJR 1996;167:1101–1108.
37. Sugawara Y, Eisbruch A, Kosuda S, et al. Evaluation of FDG-PET in patients with cervical cancer. J Nucl Med 1999;40:1125–1131.
38. Rose PG, Adler LP, Rodriguez M, et al. PET for evaluating para-aortic nodal metastasis in locally advanced cervical cancer before surgical staging: a surgicopathologic study. J Clin Oncol 1999;17:41–45.
39. Grigsby PW, Siegel BA, Dehdashti F. Lymph node staging by positron emission tomography in patients with carcinoma of the cervix. J Clin Oncol 2001;19:3745–3749.
40. Reinhardt MJ, Ehritt-Braun C, Vogelgesang D, et al. Metastatic lymph nodes in patients with cervical cancer: detection with MR imaging and FDG-PET. Radiology 2001;218:776–782.
41. Park DH, Kim KH, Park SY, et al. Diagnosis of recurrent uterine cervical cancer: computed tomography versus positron emission tomography. Korean J Radiol 2000;1:51–55.
42. Sun SS, Chen TC, Yen RF, et al. Value of whole-body ^{18}F-fluoro-2-deoxyglucose positron emission tomography in the evaluation of recurrent cervical cancer. Anticancer Res 2001;21:2957–2962.
43. Nakamoto Y, Eisbruch A, Achtyes ED, et al. Prognostic value of positron emission tomography using F-18-fluorodeoxyglucose in patients with cervical cancer undergoing radiotherapy. Gynecol Oncol 2002;84:289–295.
44. Pinkus E, Miller TR, Grigsby PW. Improved prognostic value of FDG-PET in patients with cervical cancer using a simple visual analysis of tumor characteristics. J Nucl Med 2002;43:28.
45. Jang HJ, Lee KH, Kim YH, et al. The role of FDG-PET for predicting prognosis in squamous cell type uterine cervical carcinoma patients. J Nucl Med 2002;43:28.
46. Yasuda S, Ide M, Takagi S, Shohtsu A. Intrauterine accumulation of F-18 FDG during menstruation. Clin Nucl Med 1997;22:793–794.
47. Nakahara T, Fujii H, Ide M, et al. F-18 FDG uptake in endometrial cancer. Clin Nucl Med 2001;26:82–83.
48. Belhocine TZ, Bolle KS, Willems-Foidart J. Usefulness of ^{18}F-FDG-PET in the post-therapy surveillance of endometrial carcinoma. J Nucl Med 2002;43:118–119.
49. Umesaki N, Tanada T, Miyama M, et al. Positron emission tomography 18F-fluorodeoxyglucose of uterine sarcoma: a comparison with magnetic resonance imaging and power Doppler imaging. Gynecol Oncol 2001;80: 372–377.
50. Cohn DE, Dehdashti F, Gibb RK, et al. Prospective evaluation of positron emission tomography for the detection of groin node metastases from vulva cancer. Gynecol Oncol 2002;85:179.

21

Urologic Cancer

Tomio Inoue, Nobukazu Takahashi, and Tetsuya Higuchi

Positron emission tomography (PET) is a unique imaging modality with the capability of studying regional metabolism. ^{18}F-fluorodeoxyglucose (FDG) is the most widely used tracer in the field of PET oncology. The clinical utility of oncology PET using FDG has been proven in the staging and restaging of malignant tumors such as head/neck, lung, breast, and colorectal cancers, as well as malignant lymphoma, and melanoma. In the field of urology, FDG-PET has been evaluated in the relevant malignancies with promising results in certain areas and disappointing results in others. At this stage FDG-PET is capable of visualizing urologic tumors and associated lymph nodes and distal metastatic sites. However, its use is severely limited by the excretion of the most commonly used radioisotope via the urinary tract, making pelvic imaging particularly unrewarding. ^{11}C-choline upregulated in malignant cells has shown potential usefulness in brain, prostate, and esophageal cancers with enhanced synthesis of membrane phospholipids. This chapter discusses the clinical usefulness of oncology PET in the field of urology including renal cell, urinary bladder, and prostate cancer, as well as testicular tumors. We review the related articles of PET oncology in the field of urology.

Renal Cell Carcinoma

FDG is accumulated in some cases with renal cell carcinoma (Fig. 21.1). The accuracy of FDG-PET for staging and management of renal cell carcinoma was reported by Ramdave et al,[1] who investigated 17 patients with known or suspected primary tumors and reported the similar diagnostic accuracy (94%) of CT and FDG-PET. Regarding the diagnostic accuracy of FDG-PET for restaging of renal cell carcinoma, Safei et al[2] found that FDG-PET classified the clinical stage correctly in 32/36 patients with advanced renal cell carcinoma (89%) and was incorrect in 4/36 (11%). The sensitivity and specificity of FDG-PET were 87% and 100%, respectively. In 25 biopsied lesions with 20 malignant lesions and five benign lesions, PET correctly classified 21/25 (84%) (sensitivity 88% and specificity 75%). Poggi et al[3] reported a case

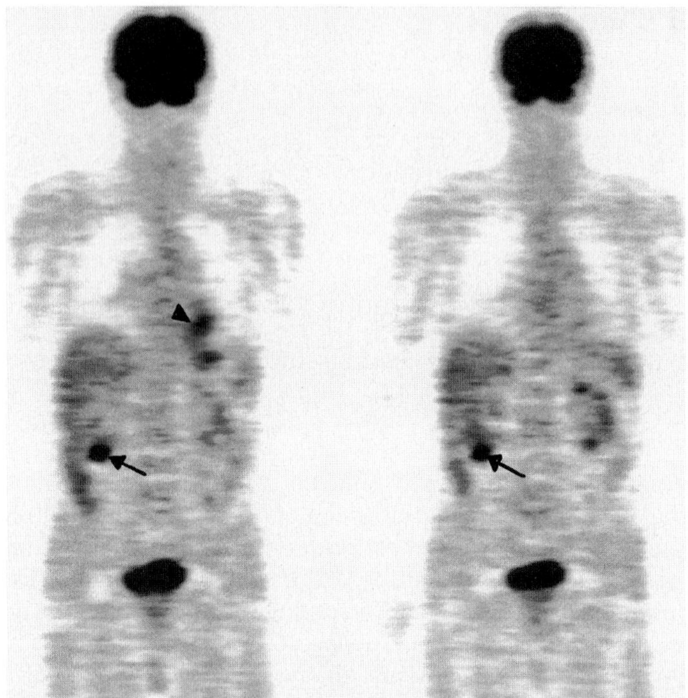

FIGURE 21.1. Selected coronal PET images of the axial body for the evaluation of distal esophageal cancer (*arrowhead*) with ^{18}F-FDG show an unexpected focal area of moderately increased activity in the lower pole of the right kidney, which was pathologically proven as renal cell carcinoma (*arrows*).

of a minimally symptomatic intramedullary spinal cord metastasis, an uncommon and often diagnostically challenging lesion, that was confirmed by PET.

As mentioned above, FDG-PET seems to be useful in characterizing anatomic lesions of unknown significance in patients with renal cell carcinoma. However, we need the clinical results in larger patient numbers to establish the clinical utility of FDG-PET in staging and restaging renal cell carcinoma.

^{11}C-acetate, as a metabolic substrate of beta-oxidation and a precursor of amino acid, fatty acid and sterol, has proved useful in detecting various malignancies. High-quality whole-body images could be obtained by using large doses (20 mCi) of ^{11}C-acetate and a modern PET scanner. PET with ^{11}C-acetate can detect renal cell cancer. The advantages of ^{11}C-acetate are that it is less time-consuming (the whole procedure can be completed within 45 minutes after injection), and it has no hyperglycemic effect and no sink phenomenon due to the high accumulation of radioactive tracer in the urinary tract. The disadvantages are increased uptake in the salivary glands, pancreas, and sometimes the bowels, which may cause either false-positive or false-negative results, and that it is dependent on an on-site cyclotron.

Ureter Cancer

The primary lesions of urinary tract cancer cannot be clearly found by FDG-PET because of the urinary excretion of radioactivity in the urinary tract. However, recurrent or advanced cases of ureter cancer are detected by FDG-PET. The clinical usefulness of FDG-PET in detecting ureter cancer has not been established.

Urinary Bladder Cancer

Irrespective of the staging level being addressed, the available techniques uniformly have limitations, as well as advantages and disadvantages. A common shortcoming of computed tomography (CT) and magnetic resonance imaging (MRI) is a lack of specificity. The specificity of conventional imaging techniques is further compromised by attempts to increase sensitivity. As long as nonspecific anatomic changes are used as discriminating criteria, increases in diagnostic sensitivity may occur at the price of specificity. It is hoped that advances

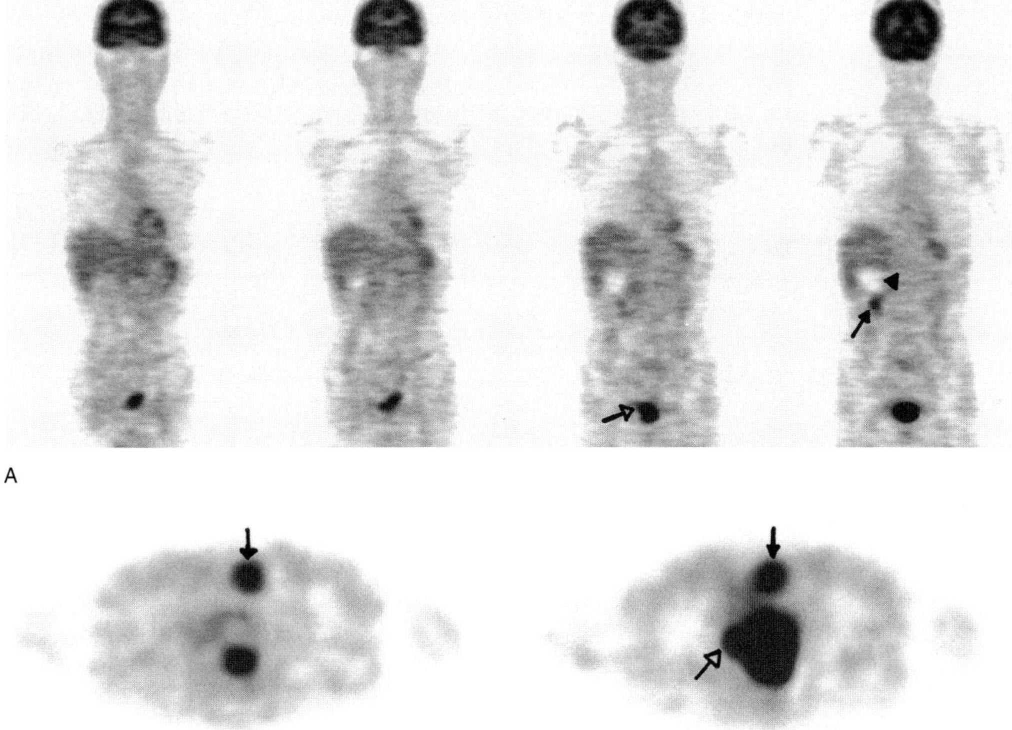

FIGURE 21.2. A: Selected coronal PET images of the axial body with ^{18}F-FDG show questionably irregular activity (*open arrow*) overlying the physiologic activity in the bladder with transitional cell carcinoma. Note the metastatic lesion in the right ureteropelvic junction (*closed arrow*) and photopenia in the right kidney due to hydronephrosis (*arrowhead*). B: Selected axial PET images of the lower pelvis with ^{18}F-FDG show irregular activity along the right wall of the urinary bladder (*open arrow*) with carcinoma and focal increased activity (*closed arrow*) in the superior symphysis pubis due to metastasis.

in PET scanning will overcome the limitations of the currently available techniques (Fig. 21.2). The significance of the limitations of a given imaging modality depends to some degree on whether the modality is being used for clinical decision making or for patient stratification in a clinical trial.[4]

However, the detection of primary lesions of urinary bladder cancer is difficult because it is hampered by the urinary excretion of administered radiopharmaceuticals. From the viewpoint of pharmacokinetics of radiopharmaceuticals, ^{11}C-methionine or ^{11}C-choline is available for detecting primary bladder tumor (Fig. 21.3). It is possible to visualize urinary bladder tumors larger than 1 cm in diameter with PET using ^{11}C-methionine, but the value of the method in the staging of the lesions is not superior to conventional methods.[5]

Lymph node staging with FDG-PET in patients with urinary bladder cancer is valuable in urologic oncology. Heicappell et al[6] used FDG-PET in eight patients with bladder cancer before pelvic lymph node dissection. The results of FDG-PET were then compared to the histology of pelvic lymph nodes obtained at surgery. Lymph node metastases were detected by histopathologic examination in three patients with bladder cancer. At the sites with histologically proven metastases, increased FDG uptake suspicious of metastatic disease was found in two of three patients. These results suggest that FDG-PET may be a valuable diagnostic tool in the staging of pelvic lymph nodes in bladder cancer.

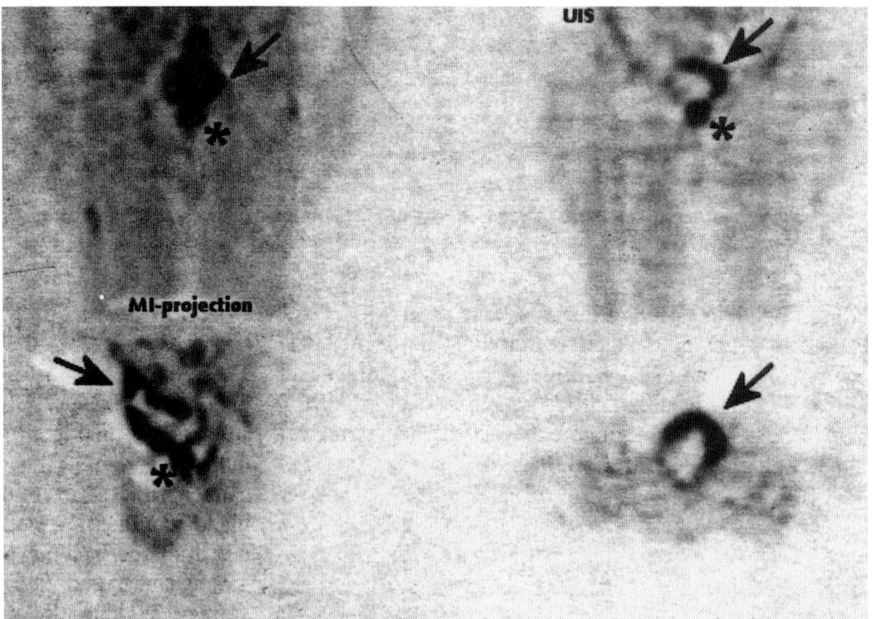

FIGURE 21.3. Selected coronal (*upper row*), sagittal (*lower left*), and transaxial (*lower right*) PET images of the pelvis show markedly increased uptakes of ^{11}C-choline in the bladder wall (*arrows*) with carcinoma and also prostate (*) with tumor invasion. (From Ahlstrom et al,[5] with permission.)

Prostate Cancer

Regarding FDG-PET, prostate cancer poses a diagnostic dilemma for the detection of primary lesions, which may be blocked by the crosstalk from eliminated radioactivity in the urinary bladder. The detectability of FDG-PET for metastatic bone lesions, which are common in prostate cancer, is inferior to that of conventional bone scan.

PET scan with ^{11}C-choline and ^{11}C-acetate can be started at 5 to 10 minutes postinjection (Fig. 21.4). Because there is no elimination of the tracer in the urinary bladder at image data acquisition, the uptake of tracer in the prostate gland can be easily visualized. ^{11}C-choline is a metabolic tracer of phospholipids on the cell membrane; turnover is accelerated in the presence of cell proliferation, such as cancer cells.[7] The uptake of ^{11}C-choline in prostate cancer is higher than that of prostate hypertrophy,[8] but there is some overlap between the tracer uptake in prostate cancer and that in benign disease. PET with ^{11}C-choline is also effective in detecting the metastatic lesions in intrapelvic lymph nodes

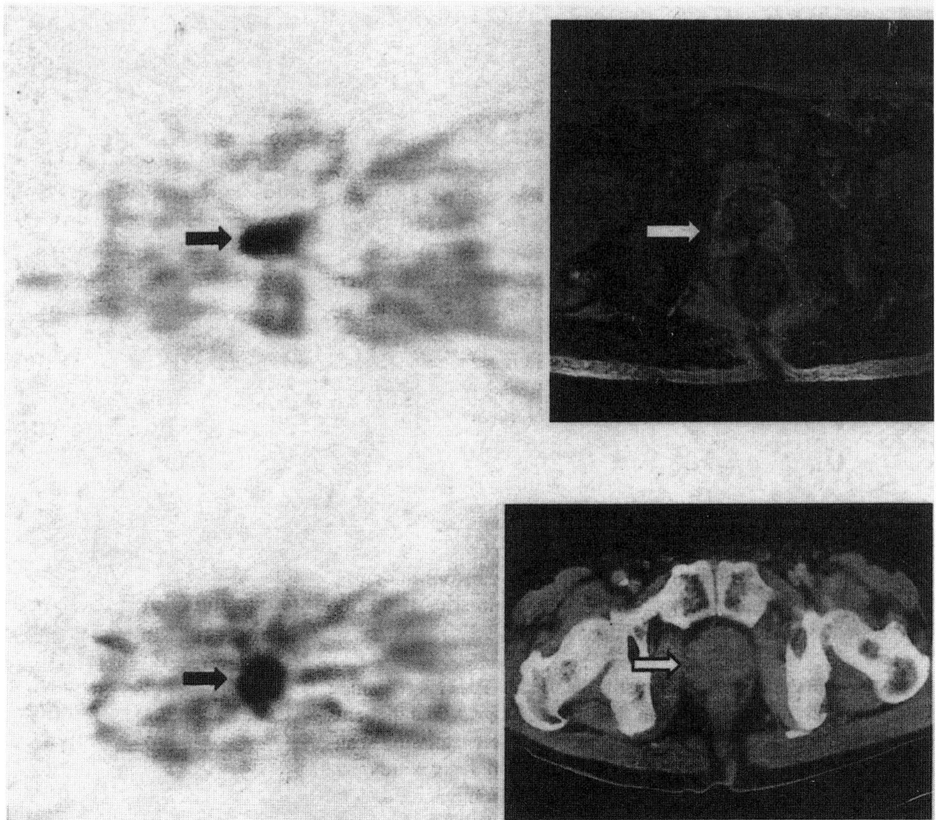

FIGURE 21.4. Selected axial PET images of the lower pelvis with ^{11}C-acetate show increased activity (*black arrows*) in the prostate in patients with benign prostatic hypertrophy (*upper row*) and prostate carcinoma (*lower row*). Note irregular signal intensities in central prostate gland on axial MRI (*upper right*) and slightly enlarged prostate on axial CT (*lower right*). (From Hara et al,[8] with permision.)

(Fig 21.5).[9] However, in some cases, intestinal elimination of ^{11}C-choline hampers the detection of metastatic lesions in intrapelvic and intra-abdominal lymph nodes. Preliminary PET studies on patients with recurrent prostate cancer revealed uptake of ^{18}F-fluorocholine (FCH) in the prostatic bed and also in metastatic lymph nodes (Fig. 21.6).[10]

Testicular Cancer

Testicular cancer is a rare disease, representing 1% of all cancers in males. In the age group between 20 and 40 years, it is the most common cancer in males; 40% to 50% of testicular tumors are seminoma and 50% are nonseminomatous cancers.

There is substantial uptake of FDG into the normal testis, which declines with age. The normal levels of FDG uptake in the testis relative to the patient's age should be considered in the interpretation of FDG scans of the inguinal and lower pelvic regions.[11] In the initial staging of testicular cancer, the clinical utility of FDG-PET has not been estab-

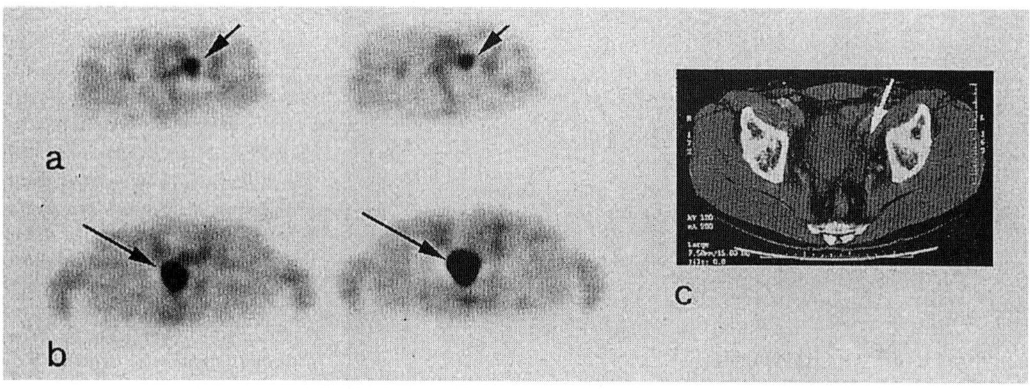

A

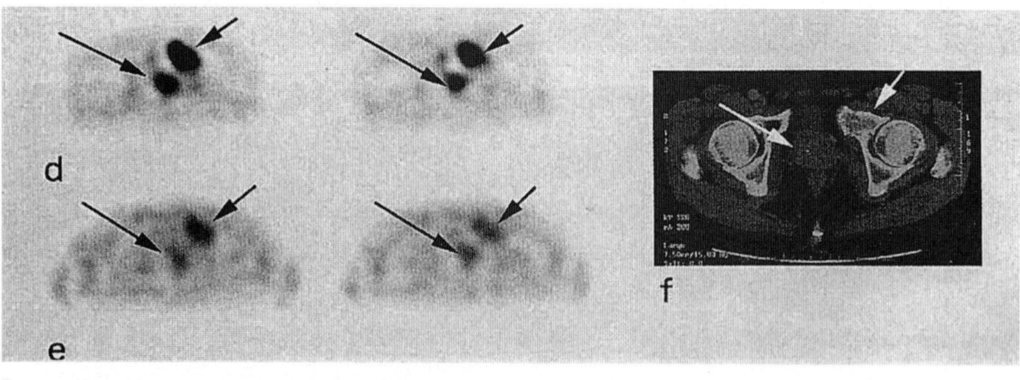

B

Figure 21.5. A: Selected axial PET images of the lower pelvis with ^{11}C-choline show moderately increased activity in the metastatic left external iliac lymph node (*short arrows*) and physiologic bladder activity (*long arrows*). Note small left external iliac lymph node (*arrow*) on the axial CT image (c). B: Axial images of the lower pelvis at the level of prostate show markedly increased uptake of ^{11}C-choline in the prostate carcinoma (*long arrows*) and metastatic lesion in the left pubic bone (*short arrows*), corresponding to abnormalities on the CT image (f). (From Hara et al.[8] with permission.)

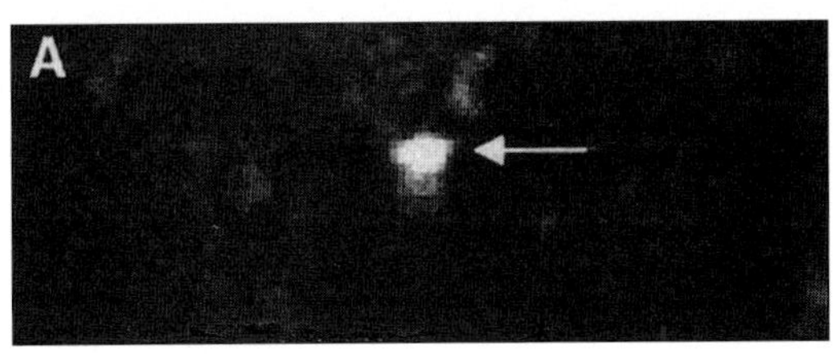

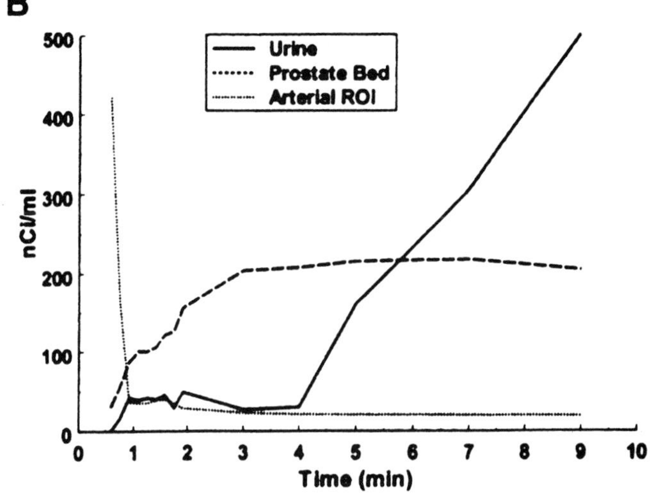

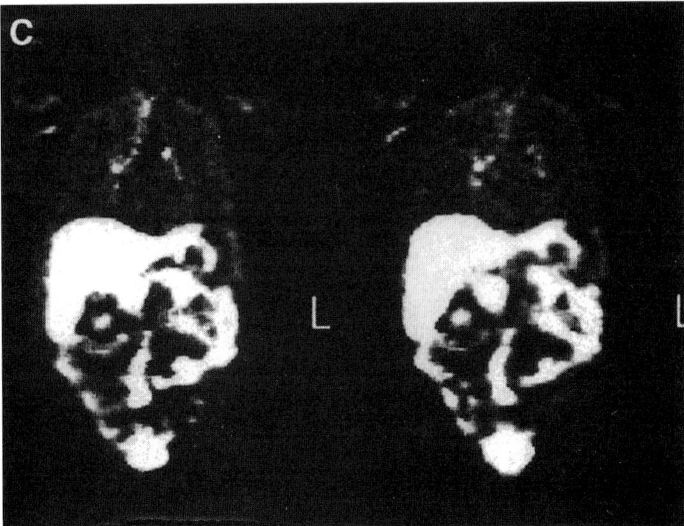

FIGURE 21.6. A: Selected coronal PET image of the lower pelvis shows markedly increased uptake of ^{18}F-FCH (*arrow*) in the recurrent prostate carcinoma. B: Time-activity curve of FCH in the same patient as in A shows very rapid clearance of radioactivity from the iliac artery, rapid uptake of FCH in the prostate bed, and arrival of activity in the bladder at $<$4 minutes after injection. C: Selected coronal images of the axial body show foci of increased FCH uptake in metastatic hilar and para-aortic lymph nodes. ROI, region of interest. (From DeGrado et al,[10] with permission.)

lished. Further data are necessary to determine the role of FDG-PET for the initial staging of germ cell cancer.

In restaging, a negative FDG-PET result predicts fibrotic residual mass in seminomatous germ cell tumors. Moreover, it could be useful in predicting fibrotic residual mass in seminomatous germ cell tumors

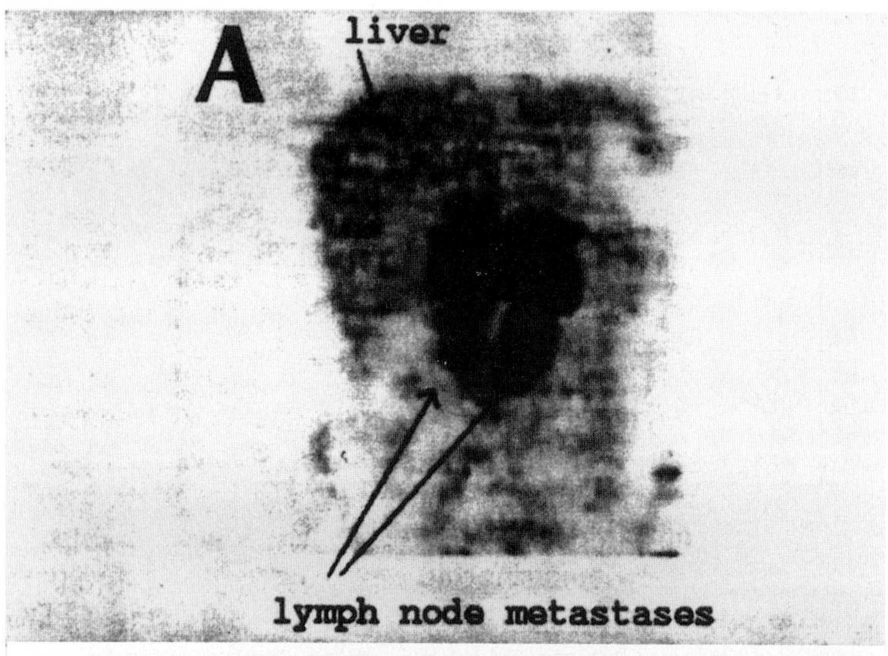

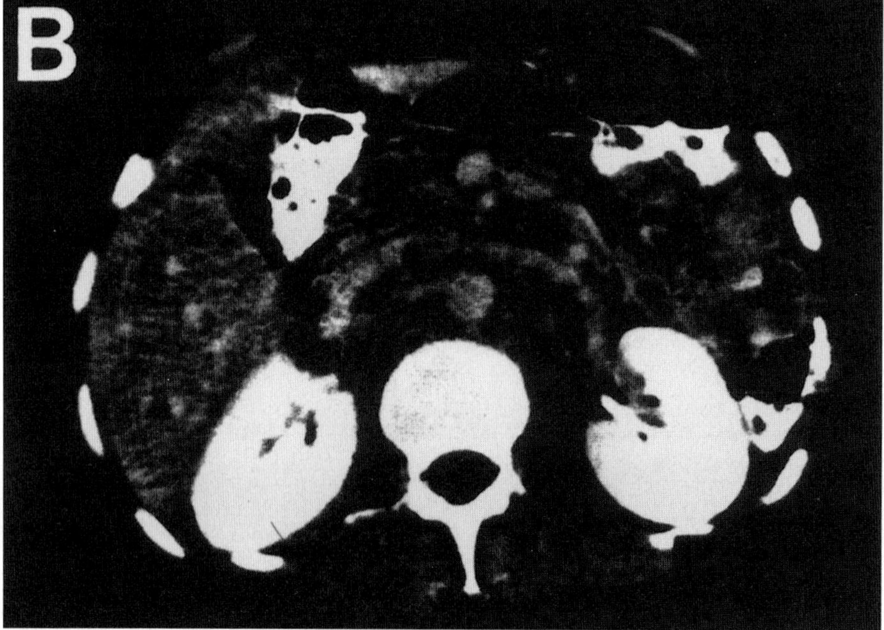

FIGURE 21.7. Selected coronal PET image (A) of the abdomen in a patient with seminoma shows markedly increased uptake of ^{18}F-FDG in multiple retroperitoneal lymph node metastases with a standard uptake value (SUV) of 13.5. Axial CT image (B) of the upper abdomen shows slightly enlarged periaortic lymph node. (From Cremerious et al,[15] with permission.)

in those patients with no teratoma component in their primary tumor.[12] FDG-PET is a clinically useful predictor of a viable tumor in post-chemotherapy residuals of pure seminoma, especially those greater than 3 cm.[13] FDG-PET is superior to CT for the assessment of residual tumor after chemotherapy of germ cell cancer and may thus have an increased effect on patient management (Fig. 21.7). PET must be performed at least 2 weeks after completion of therapy. However, the possibility of false-positive PET findings due to reactive supradiaphragmatic inflammatory processes early after chemotherapy has to be considered.[14,15]

Conclusion

FDG is the most commonly used PET radiopharmaceutical in assessing malignant tumors. However, urinary tract tumor assessment is hampered by the renal elimination of FDG. PET imaging using FDG offers no significant benefits over conventional imaging modalities for renal cell and bladder carcinomas. As a result of the low metabolic activity of prostate cancer, FDG-PET does not differentiate adequately between adenoma and carcinoma, or detect local recurrence after radical prostatectomy with sufficient sensitivity.

PET scan using ^{11}C-choline and ^{11}C-acetate enables us to obtain pelvic images without radioactivity of eliminated tracer in the urinary tract. We can identify the radioactivity of primary lesions in the urinary bladder and prostate. Lymph node staging with FDG-PET, specifically in bladder cancer, has been shown to have a potential clinical benefit. Further studies are required to determine the clinical value of retroperitoneal lymph node staging and recurrent disease detection in germ cell tumors. Encouraging early results have been obtained for the use of serial PET measurements to predict and assess therapy response to chemotherapy, which also may be valuable in urologic oncology. PET undoubtedly is capable of diagnosing malignancy in soft tissue masses or lymph nodes before these changes become apparent on conventional cross-sectional imaging modalities (CT or MRI). Larger studies are required before it can be advocated for clinical use in the field of urology.

References

1. Ramdave S, Thomas GW, Berlangieri SU, et al. Clinical role of F-18 fluorodeoxyglucose positron emission tomography for detection and management of renal cell carcinoma. J Urol 2001;166:825–830.
2. Safei A, Figlin R, Hoh CK, et al. The usefulness of F-18 deoxyglucose whole-body positron emission tomography (PET) for re-staging of renal cell cancer. Clin Nephrol 2002;57:56–62.
3. Poggi MM, Patronas N, Buttman JA, et al. Intramedullary spinal cord metastasis from renal cell carcinoma: detection by positron emission tomography. Clin Nucl Med 2001;26:837–839.
4. See WA, Fuller JR. Staging of advanced bladder cancer. Current concepts and pitfalls. Urol Clin North Am 1992;19:663–683.
5. Ahlstrom H, Malmstrom PU, Letocha H, et al. Positron emission tomography in the diagnosis and staging of urinary bladder cancer. Acta Radiol 1996;37:180–185.

6. Heicappell R, Muller-Mattheis V, Reinhardt M, et al. Staging of pelvic lymph nodes in neoplasms of the bladder and prostate by positron emission tomography with 2-[(18)F]-2-deoxy-D-glucose. Eur Urol 1999;36:582–587.
7. Hara T, Kosaka M, Kishi H. PET imaging of brain tumor with [methyl-^{11}C] choline. J Nucl Med 1997;38:842–847.
8. Hara T, Kosaka N, Kishi H. PET imaging of prostate cancer using carbon-11-choline. J Nucl Med 1998;39:990–995.
9. Inoue T, Oriuchi N, Tomiyoshi K, et al. A shifting landscape: What will be next FDG in PET oncology? Ann Nucl Med 2002;16:1–9.
10. DeGrado TR, Baldwin SW, Wang S, et al. Synthesis and evaluation of F-18 labeled choline analogs as oncologic PET tracers. J Nucl Med 2001;42: 1805–1814.
11. Kosuda S, Fisher S, Kison PV, et al. Uptake of 2-deoxy-2-[18F]fluoro-D-glucose in the normal testis: retrospective PET study and animal experiment. Ann Nucl Med 1997;11:195–199.
12. Spermon JR, De Geus-Oei LF, Kiemeney LA, et al. The role of (18)fluoro-2-deoxyglucose positron emission tomography in initial staging and restaging after chemotherapy for testicular germ cell tumours. Br J Urol Int 2002;89:549–556.
13. De Santis M, Bokemeyer C, Becherer A, et al. Predictive impact of 2-18-fluoro-2-deoxy-D-glucose positron emission tomography for residual post-chemotherapy masses in patients with bulky seminoma. J Clin Oncol 2001; 19:3740–3744.
14. Tsatalpas P, Beuthien-Baumann B, Kropp J, et al. Diagnostic value of F-18 FDG positron emission tomography for detection and treatment control of malignant germ cell tumors. Urol Int 2002;68:157–163.
15. Cremerious U, Effert PJ, Adam G, et al. FDG PET for detection and therapy control of metastatic germ cell tumor. J Nucl Med 1998;39:815–822.

22

Melanoma, Myeloma, and Sarcoma

E. Edmund Kim and Franklin C.L. Wong

Cutaneous melanoma is a readily curable tumor, with 85% of diagnosed patients enjoying long-term survival following simple surgical excision. There has been a steady increase in melanoma incidence over the past century. In the United States, melanoma is diagnosed in at least 54,200 people a year, approximately 15 in 100,000.[1] Disseminated melanoma is a devastating illness with limited effective treatment options, prompting the evolution of efforts designed to identify metastatic disease early and to develop novel biologic therapies. The application of immunotherapy has so far provided benefit to only a small percentage of patients. In the majority of patients with metastatic disease, many of whom are young, the chemotherapy or biologic therapy is unsuccessful.

Melanomas are the most common (70%) primary intraocular malignancy in Caucasians, and they arise from uveal melanocytes residing in the uveal stroma and originating from the neural crest. The precise anatomic origin of ocular melanomas was unspecified in approximately 25% of cases, and 73% of the tumors arose within the globe (mainly from the choroid). Uveal melanoma, like retinitis pigmentosa, may not constitute a single disease but consist of an assortment of maladies with multiple genetic origins that simply culminate in a limited phenotype. In contrast to a phenotype associated with cell death, uveal melanoma is characterized by uncontrolled proliferation. Lymphatic spread has not been demonstrated, as would be expected from the absence of lymphatics in the eye in contrast to cutaneous melanomas. Hematogenous metastasis to the liver is frequent, and plasminogen activator as well as epidermal growth factor may play a role in the occurrence and progression of metastases.

Many aspects of melanoma treatment such as sentinel node dissection, isolated limb perfusion, and cytotoxic or biologic, or both, therapies remain controversial and inconclusive. No lack of effective alternatives has allowed the implementation and evolution of new treatments since no systemic therapy has yet been shown to prolong survival significantly. The identification of tumor rejection antigens recognized by CD4 and CD8 T cells as well as prognostically significant roles of antibody response to melanoma antigens has spawned a renaissance of immunotherapy. Cutaneous and ocular melanomas differ in their systemic symptoms, metastatic patterns, and susceptibility to treatments.

Multiple myeloma is the major plasma cell tumor, which represents a spectrum of diseases characterized by clonal proliferation and accumulation of immunoglobulin-producing cells that are terminally differentiated B cells. The spectrum includes clinically benign conditions such as monoclonal gammopathy of unknown significance (MGUS); indolent conditions such as Waldenström's macroglobulinemia; the more common malignant entity, plasma cell myeloma, a disseminated B-cell malignancy; and a more aggressive form, plasma cell leukemia, with circulating malignant plasma cells in the blood. It is a relatively uncommon malignancy in the U.S. Among hematologic malignancies, it constitutes 10% of tumors and ranks as the second most frequently occurring cancer after non-Hodgkin's lymphoma. Approximately 14,600 new patients will be diagnosed in 2003.[1] Its incidence has slowly increased in the U.S. and increases with advancing age. Clinical manifestations are the results of a variety of pathogenic mechanisms, including cytokine production, effect of the tumor mass itself, deposition of the M protein, suppression of T- and B-cell functions, and occasionally autoimmune disorders.

In the U.S. the incidence of soft tissue sarcoma is approximately 7,800 new cases per year.[1] A little more than 50% of these new patients go on to die of the disease. It is clear that soft tissue sarcoma diagnosed at an early stage is eminently curable by wide en bloc resection, but when diagnosed at the time of extensive local or metastatic disease, it is rarely curable. Soft tissue sarcomas can occur in any site throughout the body. Almost 50% of them appear in the extremities, with two thirds of extremity lesions occurring in the lower limbs, and 30% intraabdominally divided equally between visceral and retroperitoneal lesions. Soft tissue tumors generally are categorized according to the normal tissue they mimic. Although most soft tissues arise from embryonic mesoderm, tumors of the peripheral nervous system (ectoderm), and some tumors of uncertain histogenesis are included as soft tissue tumors that may be benign or malignant. The ratio of benign to malignant tumors is more than 100:1. Unlike carcinomas, sarcomas do not demonstrate in situ changes, nor does it appear that sarcomas originate from benign soft tissue tumors except for malignant peripheral nerve sheath tumor (MPNST) in patients with neurofibromatosis. Sarcomas are characterized by local invasiveness. Lymph node metastases are uncommon, with the exception of selected cell types usually associated with childhood sarcoma. Most sarcomas metastasize hematogenously, and the clinical behavior is determined by anatomic location, grade, and size, rather than by specific histologic pattern.

Malignant tumors arising from the skeletal system are rare. Osteosarcoma and Ewing's sarcoma, the two most common bone tumors, occur mainly during childhood and adolescence. Other mesenchymal (spindle cell) tumors such as malignant fibrous histiocytoma (MFH) are less common. Today, limb-sparing surgery is routine, and adjuvant chemotherapy dramatically increases overall survival.

Diagnosis and Staging

Identification of features that may mark lesions suspicious for melanoma can be simply recalled by using the mnemonic ABCDE: *a*symmetry, *b*orders that are irregular or diffuse, *c*olor variegation, *d*iameter more than 5 mm, and *e*nlargement or *e*volution. Bleeding and ulceration occur in 10% of localized melanomas and 54% of late melanomas, and is a poor prognostic finding. Suspicious lesions with irregular raised surfaces, ulceration, bleeding, variegations, or recent changes in color or size should have a full-thickness excisional biopsy.

The staging of cutaneous melanoma involves segregation by local, regional, or distant disease and strongly correlates with survival. The most important staging information is the Breslow depth, presence of ulceration, and nodal status. Stage I and II designate early (low-risk) and later (intermediate-risk) tumors, respectively. Distant metastases define stage IV disease, whereas regional lymph node metastases (N1 or N3) define stage III disease (Table 22.1).

Asymptomatic patients with T1 lesions do not appear to benefit from any diagnostic imaging. A chest radiograph is obtained in patients with stage IB or greater. Liver function tests, especially lactate dehydrogenase (LDH), and the radiologic tests such as brain magnetic resonance imaging (MRI) and body computed tomography (CT) are indicated in stage III and IV disease or otherwise symptomatic patients. Advances in imaging techniques have improved the ability to identify and localize primary and metastatic melanomas. Lymphoscintigraphy can provide valuable assistance in localizing sentinel lymph node(s) for biopsy, and it is particularly helpful for tumor locations with variable lymphatic drainage. Imagings using technetium (Tc-99m) sestamibi, Tc-99m tetrafosmin, and I 123 iodobenzamide (for melanotic melanomas) show promise, and Tc-99m sestamibi appears a reasonably inexpensive substitute for whole-body positron emission tomography (PET) with ^{18}F-fluorodeoxyglucose (FDG) in staging melanoma.

The diagnosis of choroidal and ciliary body melanomas has reached a high degree of accuracy at eye centers by utilizing clinical examination, ultrasonography, and fluorescein angiography. No biopsy is performed. The most commonly encountered conditions mimicking melanoma include a choroidal nevi, peripheral disciform degeneration, congenital hypertrophy of the retinal pigment epithelium, and choroidal hemangioma. Ocular ultrasonography is more sensitive than MRI or CT for the detection of extraocular extension of choroidal malignant melanoma.[2] Ultrasonography and fluorescein angiography are

TABLE 22.1. Staging of soft tissue sarcoma

Stage	Grade	Tumor	Nodes	Metastasis
I	G1–2	T1A–1B or 2A	N0	M0
II	G1–2	T2B	N0	M0
	G3–4	T1A–1B or 2A	N0	M0
III	G3–4	T2B	N0	M0
IV	Any G	Any T	N0 or N1	M0 or M1

together very useful in patient follow-up. The usefulness of radioactive phosphorus (^{32}P) in determining malignancy remains controversial, and radioimmunoscintigraphy using Tc-99m monoclonal antibodies are still too preliminary to be reliable diagnostic tools.[3] Metastatic workup should be performed with liver enzyme measurement and CT or ultrasonography. Even though it is known that the detection of melanoma cells in blood cannot automatically be taken as a definite sign for the presence of metastatic disease, polymerase chain reaction might help in interpreting the result of conventional markers for metastasis in the future.[4]

As myeloma patients present with a variety of symptoms, the diagnosis of myeloma is quite often delayed. An older patient with unexplained back or bone pain, infection, anemia, or renal insufficiency should be screened for myeloma. The evaluation includes a hemogram, serum and urine protein electrophoresis and immunofixation, quantitative immunoglobulin levels, urinary protein excretion in 24 hours, bone marrow aspiration and biopsy, and complete skeletal radiographic survey. X-ray shows osteopenia in an early phase, and lytic punched out lesions with increasing tumor burden. Bone scans are seldom positive due to the predominant osteolytic activity. Measurement of bone mineral density is useful for the therapeutic response. MRI provides a better assessment of tumor burden, and more than 95% of myeloma patients show MRI abnormalities[5]; one third have focal lesions, and another one third have heterogenous marrow. A focal marrow plasmacytoma can be analyzed through CT-guided fine-needle aspiration allowing cytologic diagnosis. MRI and CT do not readily distinguish between active disease and scar tissue, necrosis, bone fracture, or benign disease. Traditional staging depends heavily on the extent of disease evident on a radiologic bone survey.

The presence of soft tissue sarcoma almost invariably is suggested by the development of a mass. This mass is usually large, often painless, and may be associated by the patient with an episode of injury. The focus of the clinical evaluation is to determine the likelihood of a benign or malignant soft tissue tumor, the involvement of muscular or neurovascular structures, and the ease with which biopsy or subsequent excision can be obtained. Accurate diagnosis requires an adequate and representative biopsy of the tumor, and the tissue must be well fixed and well stained.

The most useful immunohistochemical markers are the intermediate filaments such as keratin and S-100. Cytogenetic analyses reveal clonal chromosome alterations in the majority of sarcomas.[6] The three most common histopathologic subtypes of soft tissue sarcoma are MFH, liposarcoma, and leiomyosarcoma. The most common extremity sarcomas are liposarcoma, MFH, tendosynovial sarcoma, and fibrosarcoma. Most retroperitoneal sarcomas are liposarcomas or leiomyosarcomas. The most frequently encountered chest wall sarcomas are desmoids, liposarcomas, and myogenic sarcomas. Virtually all gastrointestinal sarcomas were previously classified as leiomyosarcomas or leiomyoblastomas. It is now recognized that many gastrointestinal sarcomas do not express markers of myogenic differentiation and are better classified as gastrointestinal stromal tumors (GISTs), or, if they exhibit neural differentiation, gastrointestinal autonomic nerve tumors (GANTs). The pattern of recurrence is intraabdominal, including hepatic metastasis.[7] Leiomyosarcoma is the most common type of genitourinary sarcoma and arises in the bladder, kidney, or prostate. Rhabdomyosarcoma arising in paratesticular tissues is a disease of young men. Approximately 10% to 15% of all sarcomas occur in children. The majority of pediatric patients have small cell sarcomas, including embryonal rhabdomyosarcoma, Ewing's sarcoma, and primitive neuroectodermal tumor. There have been significant changes in the staging of soft tissue sarcoma. The new staging system (Table 22.2) includes both size and depth. Size is a continuous variable, and the decision to divide tumors into less than 5 cm or greater than or equal to 5 cm is arbitrary. Stages IB (low-grade, large superficial tumors) are uncommon, as are stage IIC (high-grade, large superficial tumors). Depth is of less value when incorporated with other prognostic factors such as size. Stage IV disease from lymph node metastasis is rare.

For early recurrence, grade seems predominant, whereas for late recurrence, size assumes a progessively more important role. Whether or not age should be a determinant in a staging system is as yet unclear. It does appear that the early and the late stages of disease are similar in both children and adults, but the intermediate-stage lesions have a better prognosis in children.[8] Site appears to be a significant factor in survival. Patients with retroperitoneal sarcoma can and do die of local recurrence, an uncommon event in extremity lesions. The intraabdominal visceral leiomyosarcomas still maintain a high metastatic rate as the primary cause of death.

Radiographic evaluation combined with the clinical history and histologic examination is necessary for accurate diagnosis of bone sarcoma. A bone tumor is evaluated by five radiographic parameters: anatomic site, border, bone destruction, matrix formation, and periosteal reaction. Benign tumors have round, smooth, well-circumscribed borders without cortical destruction or periosteal reaction. Malignant lesions have irregular, poorly defined margins with bone destruction and wide area of transition with periosteal reaction. The surgical staging system developed by Enneking and colleagues[9] is based on the grade (G), loca-

Table 22.2. The new staging system for soft tissue sarcoma

Stage	Description
IA (G1, T1, M0	Low-grade intracompartmental lesion without metastasis
IB (G1, T2, M0)	Low-grade extracompartmental lesion, without metastasis
IIA (G2, T1, M0):	High-grade intracompartmental lesion without metastasis
IIIA (G1 or G2, T1, M1)	Intracompartmental lesion, any grade, with metastasis
IIIB (G1, or G2, T2, M1)	Extracompartmental lesion, any grade, with metastasis

tion (T), and lymph node involvement as well as metastasis (M). MRI and CT, combined with nuclear bone scans and angiography, allow the physician to develop a three-dimensional construct of the local tumor area before surgery and thereby formulate a detailed surgical approach. MRI is most accurate for determining intraosseous extent of tumor. Angiography is performed only if the primary tumor is in the vicinity of the major vascular structures. CT and MRI are equally accurate in evaluating cortical changes. MRI is superior to CT for detecting muscle involvement in the knee, pelvis, and shoulder.[10]

PET in Melanoma, Myeloma, and Sarcoma

The accurate staging and surveillance of melanoma remain difficult, and a range of conventional structural imaging modalities are often employed in patients with melanoma. Functional imaging using Ga 67 citrate has restricted its regular use to relatively few centers because of its inconvenience of multiple imaging sessions. Ga 67 scanning in melanoma is predicated on the avidity of tumor uptake, most likely mediated by transferring receptor expression. Its utility in the management of patients with malignant melanoma has shown a sensitivity of more than 80% and a specificity of 90%.[11,12] The use of FDG in the management of patients with malignancy has recently been implemented. FDG tumor uptake is related to the nonspecific increase in glucose transporters seen in many malignant processes, and malignant melanoma appears to have a particularly high avidity for this metabolic marker.[13] Comparison of Ga 67 citrate, single photon emission computed tomography (SPECT) and FDG-PET has been made in 121 melanoma patients with high clinical risk of occult metastatic disease.[12] PET correctly identified more disease than Ga 67 SPECT in 14 cases, including three incidental primary tumors, and was true-negative in three further patients with abnormal Ga 67 SPECT. There were six patients with true-positive Ga 67 SPECT in whom FDG-PET was false-negative. FDG-PET provided incremental diagnostic information compared with Ga 67 SPECT in 17/23 patients, while Ga 67 SPECT provided incremental information compared with PET in 6/23 cases ($p = 0.035$). It was concluded that FDG-PET provides incremental and clinically important information in around 10% of patients at a low incremental cost, which, combined with greater patient convenience and lower radiation dosimetry, makes FDG-PET the functional imaging technique of choice for evaluation of suspected metastatic melanoma (Fig. 22.1). Recognition of small-volume disease is a potential limitation of both FDG-PET and Ga 67 SPECT. For deep lesions, the higher spatial resolution of PET may offer a relative advantage.

The efficacy of FDG-PET in the diagnosis of involved lymph node basins was good.[14] Sensitivity was 95% (35/37); specificity, 84% (16/19); accuracy, 91% (51/56); positive predictive value, 92% (35/38); and negative predictive value, 89% (16/18). Metastases were shown histologically in 114 of 657 surgically removed lymph nodes. FDG-PET detected 100% of metastases >10 mm, 83% of metastases 6 to 10 mm, and 23% of metastases ≤5 mm (Fig. 22.2). Morever, FDG-PET had high

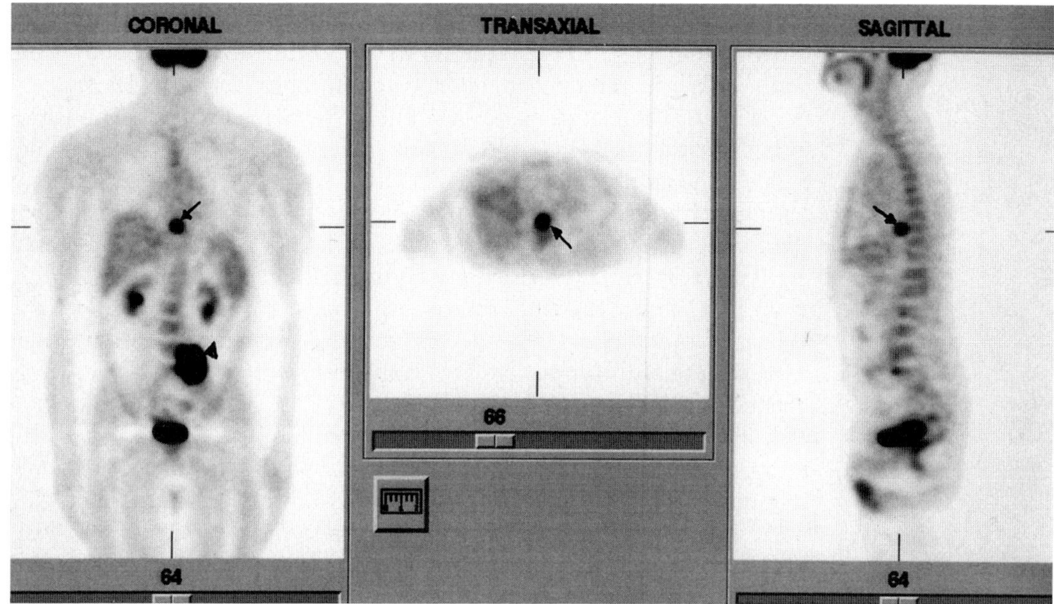

FIGURE 22.1. Selected coronal and sagittal PET images of the axial body as well as an axial image of the lower chest show markedly increased uptake of ^{18}F-FDG in the prevertebral space of lower chest (*arrows*). Ultrasound-guided transesophageal biopsy revealed a metastatic melanoma in para-esophageal lymph node. Note a large metastatic lesion in the left common iliac lymph node (*arrow-head*) on the coronal image.

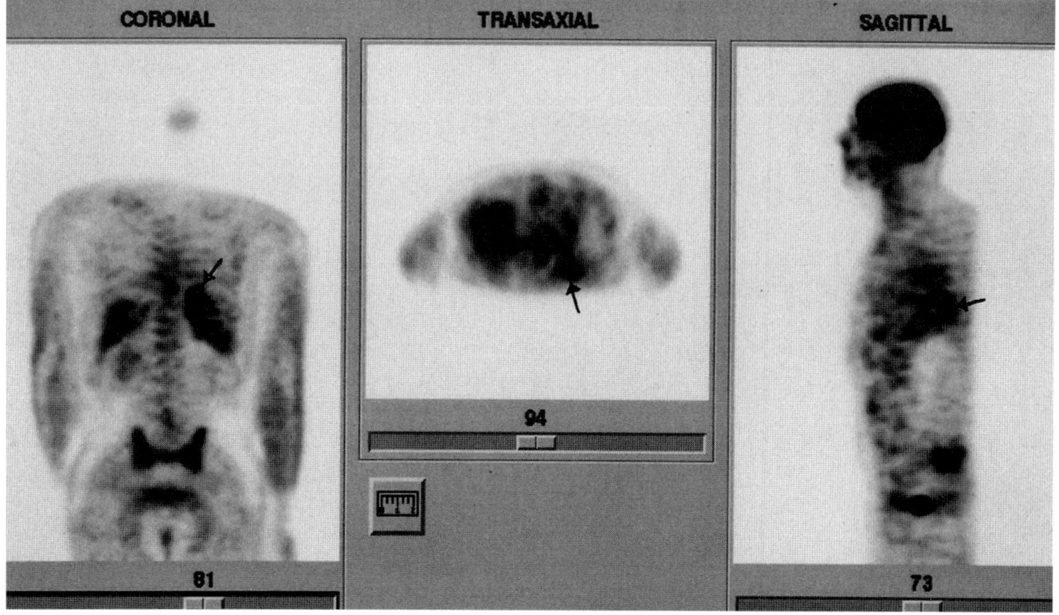

FIGURE 22.2. Selected coronal and sagittal PET images of the axial body as well as an axial image of the lower chest show markedly increased uptake of ^{18}F-FDG in the left lung base posteriorly (*arrows*) with metastatic melanoma.

sensitivity (≥93%) only for metastases with more than 50% lymph node involvement or with capsular infiltration. The sensitivities of whole-body PET and planar coincidence scintigraphy in 55 melanoma patients with 108 lesions were 89% and 18%, respectively.[15] The tumor to background activity contrast was generally lower in planar coincidence scintigraphy than in PET, and the decrease in planar coincidence scintigraphy detection was found in lesions of <22 mm in diameter. Pretreated melanoma lesions can cause diagnostic problems at restaging if the FDG uptake is low and equivalent to the surrounding tissue. Therefore, a new radiopharmaceutical that can provide further information about a lesion is needed. Tyrosine is a well-known amino acid used for melanin formation. It is transported into the cells and transformed to dihydroxyphenylalanine (DOPA). The phenoloxidase is responsible for the complete conversion of DOPA to melanin. 6-[^{18}F]-fluoro-L-dopa (FDOPA) uptake was enhanced in 14 of 22 metastatic lesions (64% sensitivity). FDG uptake was 1.5-fold higher than FDOPA uptake of 18 in 22 metastases from melanoma, whereas FDOPA uptake was 1.5-fold higher than FDG uptake in two patients with hepatic metastases. FDOPA can help to identify viable melanoma metastases in patients with negative FDG findings and thus may help to select patients who would benefit from further treatment.[16]

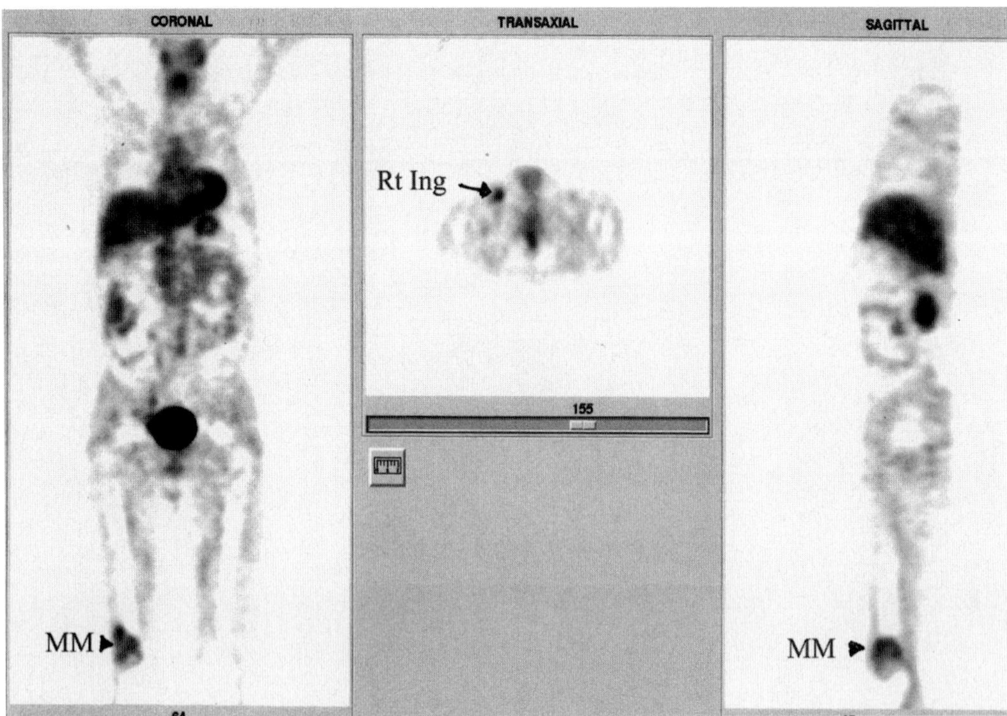

FIGURE 22.3. Selected coronal and sagittal PET images through the right upper leg show irregularly increased uptake of ^{18}F-FDG in the right distal femur (*arrowhead*) with multiple myeloma. Note also small focal increased activity in the right inguinal lymph node (*arrow*) on the axial image due to inflammatory hyperplasia.

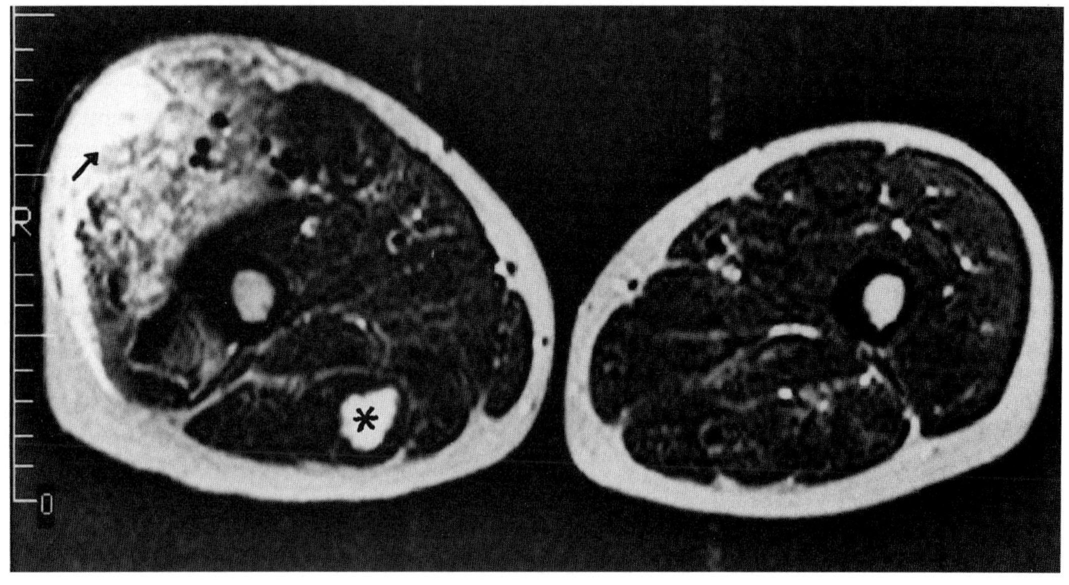

A

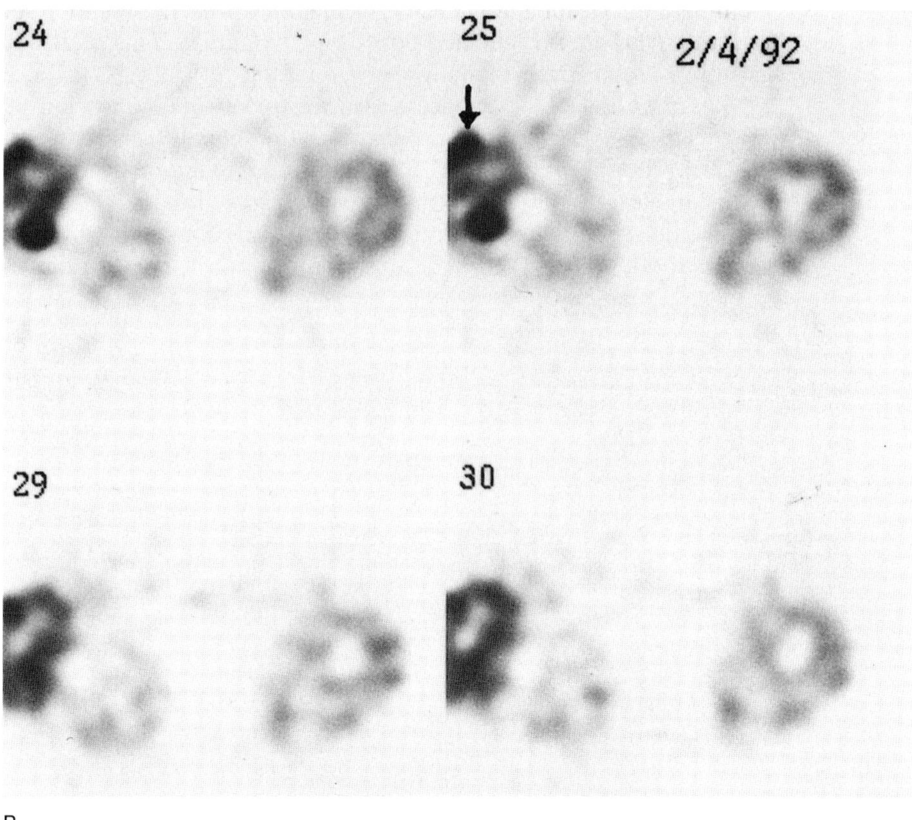

B

FIGURE 22.4. A: Axial T1-weighted axial images of the upper thigh show irregular contrast-enhanced lesion (*arrow*) in the anterior compartment of the left upper thigh with a myxoid liposarcoma. Note a hemorrhagic lesion (*) in the posterior compartment. B: Selected axial PET images of the upper thigh show irregularly increased uptake of ^{18}F-FDG in the liposarcoma (*arrow*).

A reliable whole-body technique with both functional and morphologic information is necessary to identify the extent and activity of multiple myeloma for staging and monitoring treatments. Ninety-eight PET scans using ^{18}F-FDG were obtained in 66 myeloma patients, with 25 patients having two or more scans, and compared with clinical and staging informations including MRI and CT scans.[17] Negative PET findings reliably predicted stable MGUS. Conversely, 16 previously untreated patients with active myeloma all had focal or diffusely positive scan findings; four (25%) had negative full radiologic surveys, and another four had focal extramedullary diseases that were confirmed by biopsy or other imagings. Persistent positive PET findings after therapy predicted early relapse (Fig. 22.3). In 13 (81%) of 16 patients with relapsing myeloma, new sites were identified by PET. PET also was helpful in identifying focal recurrent disease in six patients with nonsecretory or hyposecretory myeloma.

Soft tissue sarcomas are a heterogeneous group of tumors that arise from tissue of mesenchymal origin and are characterized by infiltrative local growth and hematogenous metastases. Morphologic imaging modalities are used for the assessment of tumor location, form, size, infiltration of the surrounding tissue, and presence of satellite metastases. FDG-PET visualized soft tissue sarcomas (Figs. 22.4 and 22.5), indicated the grade of malignancy, and detected local recurrence.[18] The data reported in the literature indicate a high (>90%) sensitivity but a lower (65–88%) specificity in the detection of soft tissue sarcomas (Fig. 22.6). The false-negative results in patients with suspected soft tissue lesions are in low-grade tumors, which have low FDG uptake. False-positive results may be caused by inflammatory lesions, previous irradiation with scar tissue, and fibrolipoma.[19] The standard uptake

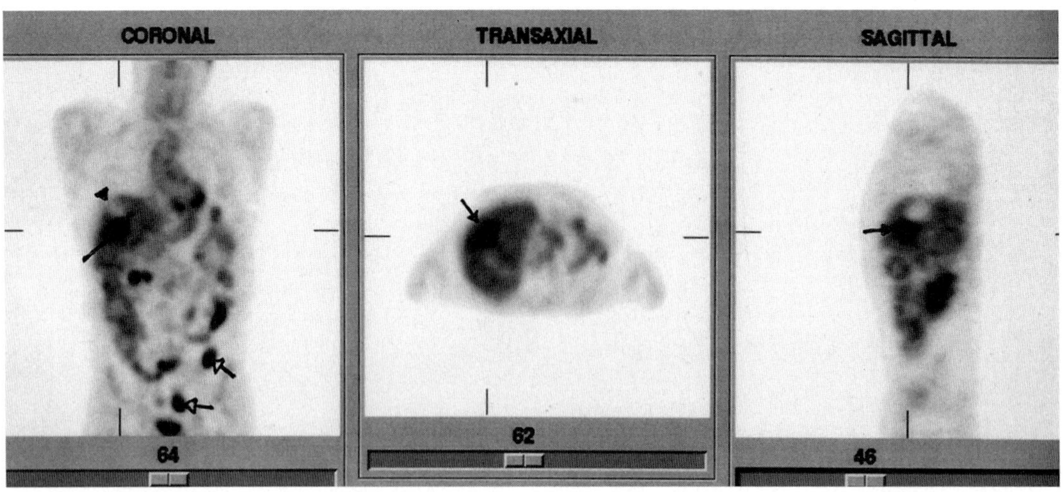

FIGURE 22.5. Selected coronal and sagittal PET images of the axial body as well as an axial image of the upper body show markedly increased uptake of ^{18}F-FDG in the right hepatic lobe (*closed arrows*) with a metastatic gastrointestinal stromal tumor (GIST). Note focal areas of increased activity (*open arrows*) in GIST and focal decreased activity in the right hepatic cyst (*arrowhead*) on the coronal image.

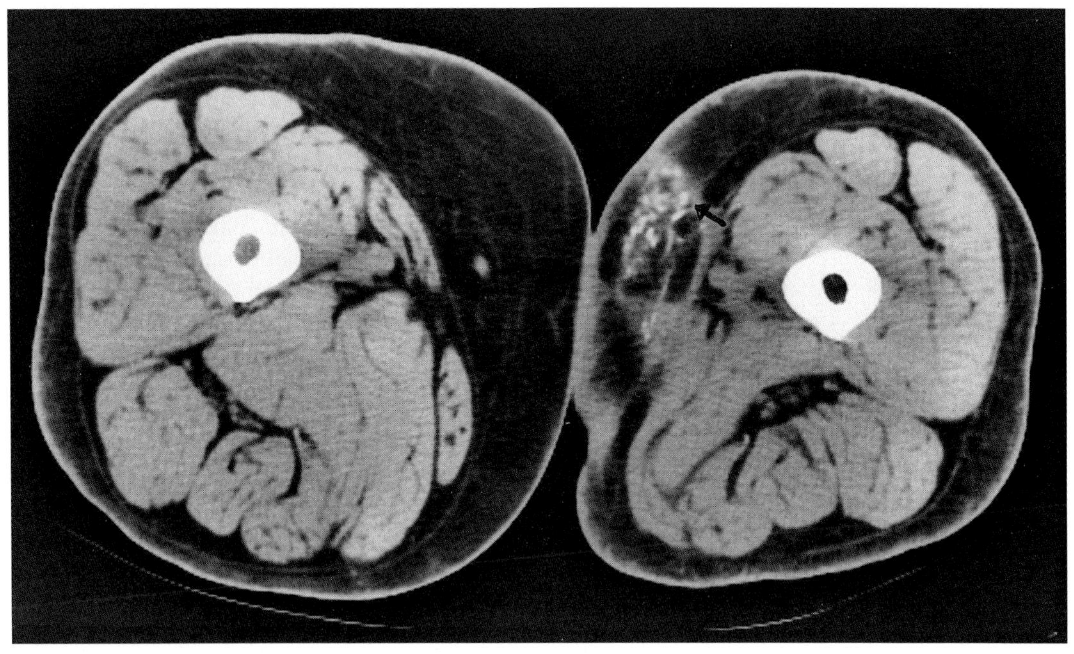

A

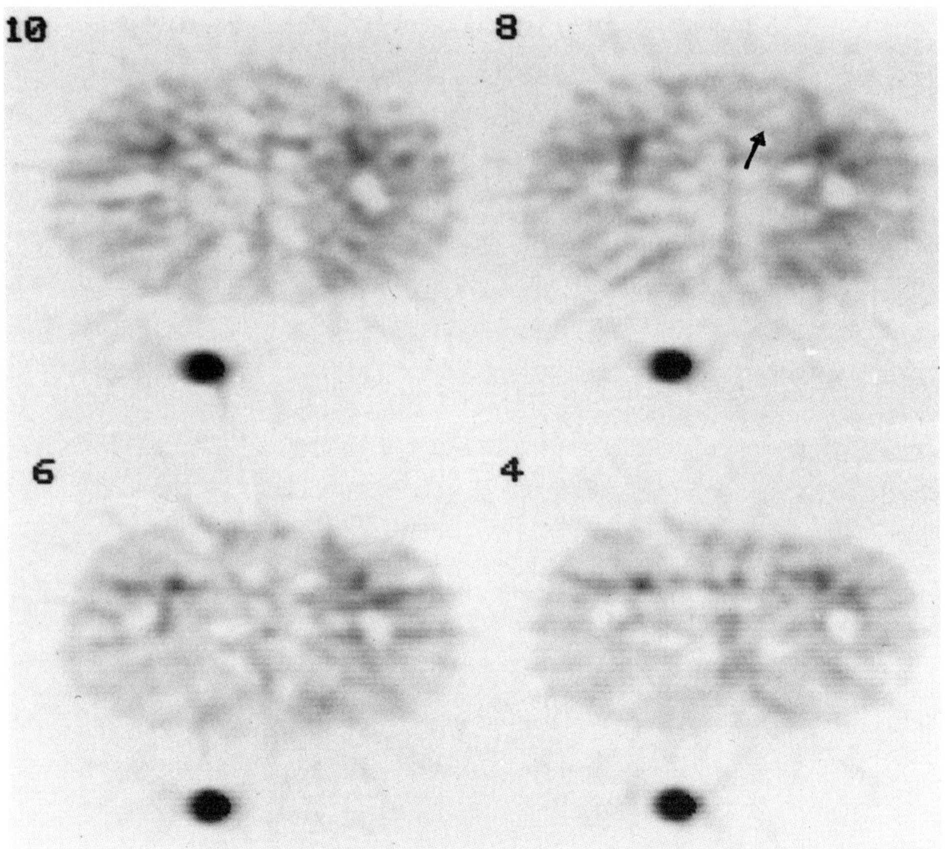

B

FIGURE 22.6. A: Axial CT image of the upper thigh shows a lesion with small multiple calcification (*arrow*) after chemoradiation for synovial sarcoma. B: Selected axial PET images of the upper thigh show no significantly increased uptake of ^{18}F-FDG (*arrow*) in the left upper thigh. Surgery revealed a microscopic residual sarcoma.

value (SUV) has been helpful in the diagnosis of high-grade tumors (Figs. 22.7 and 22.8). The limitation of the SUV is the differentiation of low-grade sarcomas or at least a subset of low-grade soft tissue tumors since sarcomas are histologically heterogeneous. Depending on the histology and phosphorylation, FDG uptake may be different for the various histologic subtypes. The use of several kinetic parameters obtained from the dynamic FDG data provides more information about FDG pharmacokinetics than SUV of a single acquisition. The transport constant k_1 is primarily a parameter for the transport capacity of FDG, and the rate constant k_3 is associated with the phosphorylation rate of the radiopharmaceutical.

The blood volume in a tumor tissue is a parameter that modulates the uptake of the tracer. Therefore, the use of the vascular fraction of a target volume is another parameter that may improve the diagnostic accuracy. Besides compartment analysis, the fractal dimension may help to quantify heterogeneity. All of these parameters may be influenced by the size and shape of a tumor as well as the resolution of imaging system. Pixels at the center of the tumor may have higher values, whereas the values may decrease for pixels located toward the edge of the tumor. However, this effect is generally modulated by the inhomogeneous distribution of FDG within the malignancy because of differences in blood supply, viability, and other factors. The SUV and the fractal dimension seemed to be helpful for the grade II and the grade III classification versus lipoma and scar.[20] According to the data, the FDG turnover in lipomas is more deterministic than in tumors and in scars. Because of large overlap of SUVs between the different grading groups, the comparison of the mean SUV may not be useful in the individual patient. The FDG metabolic rate according to the graphic Patlak method was comparable with the one calculated of the transport

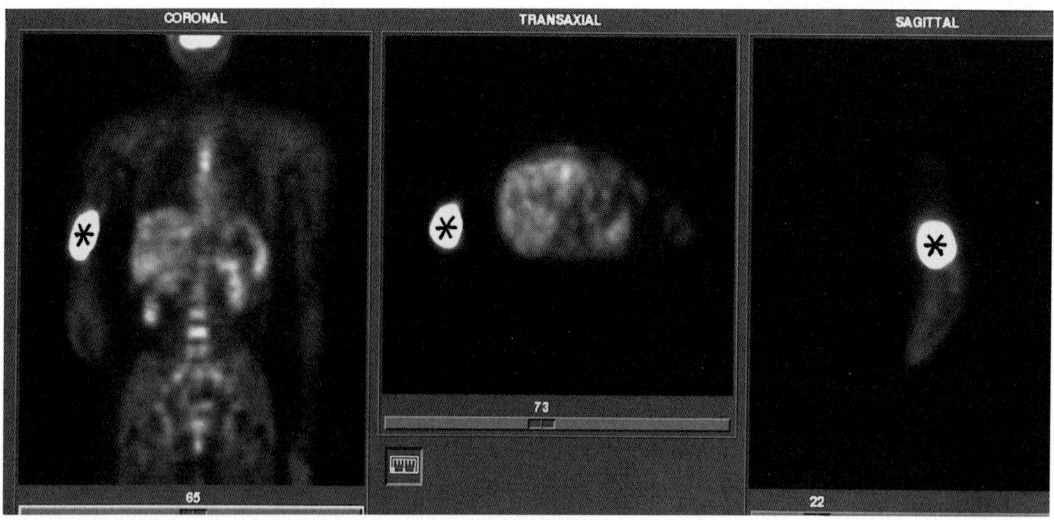

FIGURE 22.7. Selected coronal PET image of the axial body, and axial and sagittal images of the right elbow show markedly increased uptake of ^{18}F-FDG in the osteosarcoma (*).

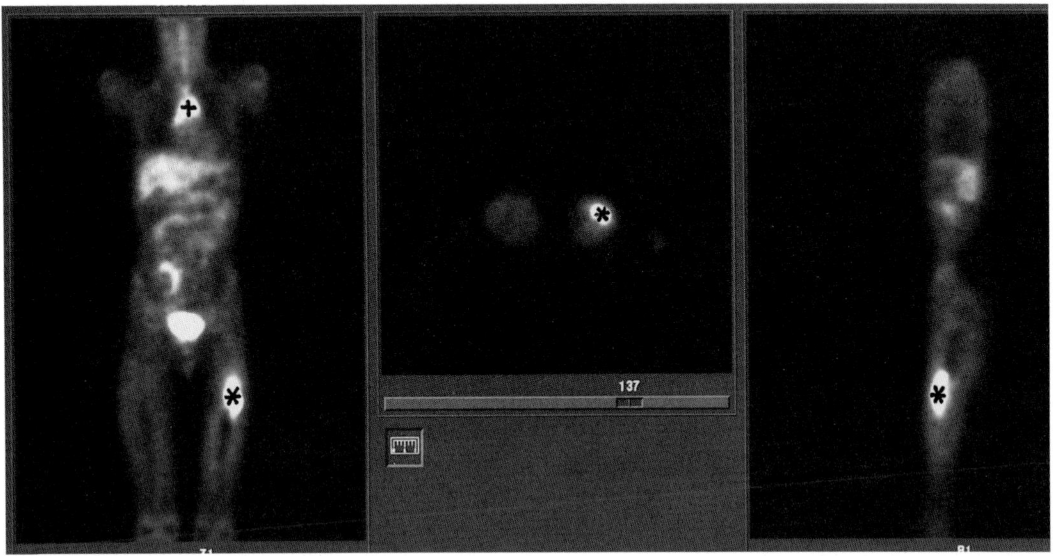

FIGURE 22.8. Selected coronal (*left*) PET image of the axial body, and axial (*middle*) and sagittal images of the left thigh show markedly increased uptake of ^{18}F-FDG in the left proximal femur with Ewing's sarcoma (*). Note also triangular-shaped thymus with markedly increased activity (+).

rates of the two-tissue compartment.[21] The metabolic rate of FDG could distinguish high-grade sarcomas from benign lesions but not low-grade tumors. With 92% accuracy for the prediction of grade III tumors but a low prediction for all other groups when only the SUV was used,[20] the differentiation of inflammatory lesions from tumor tissue, especially grade III tumors, may be a problem. However, an inflammatory

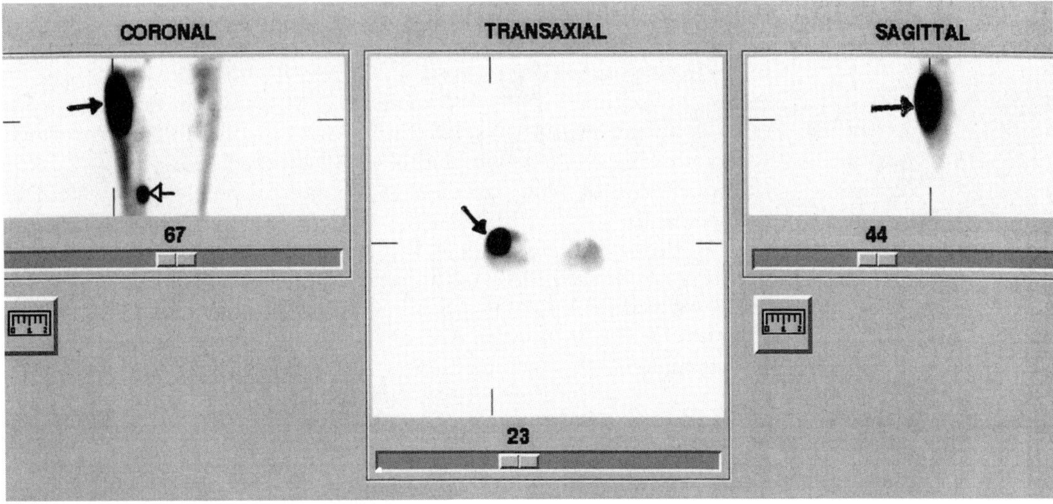

FIGURE 22.9. Selected coronal, sagittal, and axial PET images of the right lower leg show markedly increased uptake of ^{18}F-FDG in the right proximal lower leg with myxoid liposarcoma (*closed arrows*). Note a small abscess (*open arrow*) in the distal right lower leg.

lesion has low prevalence and can often be diagnosed using clinical criteria and laboratory values.

Another problem is the differentiation of scar tissue and tumor recurrence, which is a biologic problem and concerns primarily irradiated patients. Nonspecific repair processes lead to an enhanced FDG (Fig. 22.9) uptake, although radiation therapy usually is performed at least 3 months before FDG-PET. Interestingly, one abscess with high uptake of FDG and enhanced tissue perfusion did not accumulate ^{11}C-aminoisobutyric acid.[22] The amino acids may be advantageous, with clear signal showing only the transport capacity of the tumor and no further metabolic steps.

References

1. Jemal A, Murray T, Samuels A, et al. Cancer Statistics, 2003. CA Cancer J Clin 2003;53:5–26.
2. Scott IU, Murray TG, Randall Hughes J. Evaluation of imaging techniques for detection of extraocular extension of choroidal melanoma. Arch Ophthalmol 1998;116:897–901.
3. Modorati G, Brancato R, Paganelli G, et al. Immunoscintigraphy with three step monoclonal pretargeting technique in diagnosis of uveal melanoma: preliminary results. Br J Ophthalmol 1994;78:19–24.
4. Haynie GD, Shen TT, Gragoudas ES, et al. Flow cytometric analysis of peripheral blood lymphocytes in patients with choroidal melanoma. Am J Opthalmol 1997;124:357–361.
5. Kusumoto S, Jinnai I, Itoh K, et al. Magnetic resonance imaging patterns in patients with multiple myeloma. Br J Hematol 1997;99:649–654.
6. Fletcher J, Kozakewich H, Hoffer F, et al. Diagnostic relevance of clonal chromosome aberrations in malignant soft tissue tumors. N Engl J Med 1991;324:436–441.
7. Conlon K, Casper E, Brennan M. Primary gastrointestinal sarcomas: analysis of prognostic variables. Ann Surg Oncol 1995;2:26–30.
8. LaIuaglia M, Heller G, Ghavimi F, et al. The effect of age at diagnosis on outcome in rhabdomyosarcoma. Cancer 1994;73:109–114.
9. Enneking WF, Spanier SS, Goodman MA. A system for the surgical staging of musculoskeletal sarcoma. Clin Orthop 1980;153:106–109.
10. Bloem JL, Taminian AHM, Euldenink F, et al. Radiologic staging of primary bone sarcoma: MRI, scintigraphy, angiography and CT correlated with pathologic examination. Radiology 1988;169:805–811.
11. Kagan R, Witt T, Bines S, et al. Gallium-67 scanning for malignant melanoma. Cancer 1998;61:272–274.
12. Kaiff V, Hicks RJ, Ware RE, et al. Evaluation of high-risk melanoma: comparison of F-18 FDG PET and high-dose Ga-67 SPECT. Eur J Nucl Med 2002;29:506–515.
13. Tyler DS, Onaitis M, Kherani A, et al. Positron emission tomography scanning in malignant melanoma. Cancer 2000;89:1019–1025.
14. Crippa F, Leutner M, Belli F, et al. Which kinds of lymph node metastases can FDG PET detect? A clinical study in melanoma. J Nucl Med 2000;41: 1491–1494.
15. Steinert HC, Voellmy DR, Trachsel C, et al. Planar coincidence scintigraphy and PET in staging malignant melanoma. J Nucl Med 1998;39:1892–1897.
16. Dimitrakopoulou-Strauss A, Strauss LG, Burger C. Quantitative PET studies in pretreated melanoma patients: a comparison of 6-[F-18] fluoro-L-

dopa with F-18 FDG and O-15 water using compartment and noncompartment analysis. J Nucl Med 2001;42:248–256.
17. Durie BGM, Waxman AD, D'Agnolo A, et al. Whole-body F-18 FDG-PET identifies high-risk myeloma. J Nucl Med 2002;43:1457–1463.
18. Schwarzbach M, Dimitrakopoulou-Strauss A, Willeke F, et al. Clinical value of F-18 FDG-PET imaging in soft tissue sarcomas. Ann Surg 2000; 231:380–386.
19. Strauss LG. F-18 deoxyglucose and false-positive results: a major problem in the diagnostics of oncological patients. Eur J Nucl Med 1996;23:1409–1415.
20. Dimitrakopoulou-Strauss A, Strauss LG, Schwarzbach M, et al. Dynamic F-18 PET-FDG studies in patients with primary and recurrent soft tissue sarcomas: impact on diagnosis and correlation with grading. J Nucl Med 2001;42:713–720.
21. Eary JF, Mankoff DA. Tumor metabolic rates in sarcoma using FDG-PET. J Nucl Med 1998;39:250–254.
22. Schwarzbach M, Wideke F, Dimitrakopoulou-Strauss A, et al. Functional imaging and detection of local recurrence in soft tissue sarcomas by PET. J Nucl Med 1998;39:250–254.

23

Lymphoma

E. Edmund Kim and Franklin C.L. Wong

The term *lymphoma* identifies two distinct groups of tumors: Hodgkin's disease (HD) and non-Hodgkin's lymphoma (NHL). Since the late 1970s, significant progress has been made in the elucidation of the pathogenesis of NHL as a clonal malignant expansion of B or T cells. B lymphocytes are generated in the bone marrow as a result of a multistep differentiation process. On entering the germinal center (GC), B cells activate into centroblasts, proliferate, and mature into centrocytes. Cells that have exited the GC have two fates: differentiation into either plasma cells or memory B cells. Based on the absence or presence of somatic immunoglobulin (Ig) hypermutation, B-cell NHL may be distinguished into two broad histogenetic categories: One derived from pre-GC B cells and devoid of Ig mutations (mantle cell lymphoma, chronic lymphocytic leukemia/small lymphocytic lymphoma), and the other derived from B cells that have transited through the GC and harbor Ig mutations (follicular lymphoma, lymphoplasmacytoid lymphoma, mucosa-associated lymphoid tissue lymphoma, diffuse large cell lymphoma, Burkitt's lymphoma). The pathogenesis of lymphoma represents a multistep process involving the progressive and clonal accumulation of multiple genetic lesions affecting proto-oncogenes and tumor suppressor genes. The genome of lymphoma cells is relatively stable and is characterized by few nonrandom chromosomal abnormalities, commonly represented by chromosomal translocations.

The lymphomas are the third most common childhood malignancy and account for approximately 10% of cancers in children.[1] Approximately two thirds of the lymphomas diagnosed in children are NHL, and the remainder are HD. The three major histologic categories of NHL in children are lymphoblastic, small noncleaved cell (Burkitt's), and large-cell lymphoma. In adults, Burkitt's and lymphoblastic lymphoma are rare, but follicular center cell lymphoma predominates. The age of Hodgkin's incidence is bimodal, with a first peak in adults 20 to 30 years of age and a second peak in late adulthood.

Most patients present with rapidly enlarging neck and mediastinal lymphadenopathy. Cough, wheezing, or shortness of breath and facial swelling are frequent complaints. Other presenting sites include cervical nodes, Waldeyer's ring, cutaneous lesions, bone marrow, and single or multiple bone disease.

In 2002 it was estimated that there would be 60,900 new cases of lymphoma (7000 HD and 53,900 NHL) diagnosed in the United States, and that 25,800 people (1400 HD and 24,400 NHL) would die with this diagnosis.[2] NHL accounts for 5% of new cancers in men and 4% of new cancers in women each year in the U.S., and is responsible for 5% of deaths.[3] The median age at NHL diagnosis was 65 years, and NHL incidence increases with age and peaks in the 80- to 84-year age group. There has been a striking increase in NHL incidence rates over the past four decades, and NHL is more common in males. The overall mortality rate for NHL has decreased significantly in the past 25 years.[4] The 5-year survival rate is approximately 90% for children with early-stage NHL and 70% for those with advanced-stage disease.[4]

The phases of patient management include obtaining an adequate biopsy for an accurate diagnosis, a careful history and physical examination, appropriate laboratory studies, imaging studies, and, possibly, further biopsies to determine the accurate stage and to plan therapy. Treatment choices include no initial therapy, radiotherapy, cytotoxic chemotherapy, a variety of new biologic therapies, and hematopoietic stem cell transplantation.

The purpose of laboratory studies is to aid in determining the prognosis [e.g., lactate dehydrogenase (LDH), β_2-microglobulin, albumin] and identifying abnormalities in other organ systems that might complicate therapy (e.g., renal or hepatic dysfunction). Almost all patients should have a bone marrow aspirate and biopsy performed. Patients with follicular lymphoma have bone marrow involvement approximately 50% of the time, while it is seen in approximately 15% of patients with diffuse large B-cell lymphoma.[5]

Diagnosis and Staging of Lymphoma

The goal of the initial evaluation of a patient with lymphoma is to provide information that allows intelligent planning of therapy, imparting the prognosis to the patient, and making possible comparisons between patients in clinical trials. The studies to accomplish these goals can be aimed at identifying sites of involvement, characteristics of the patient, or characteristics of the lymphoma that predict treatment outcome.

The Ann Arbor staging system was developed for patients with HD and identifies anatomic sites of involvement by lymphoma (Table 23.1).

Table 23.1. Ann Arbor staging system

Stage	Findings
I	Single lymph node region or single extralymphatic organ or site (IE)
II	Two or more lymph node regions on the same side of diaphragm or localized extralymphatic organ or site (IIE)
III	Lymph node regions on both sides of diaphragm or localized extralymphatic organ or site (IIIE) or spleen (IIIS) or both (III SE).
IV	Diffuse one or more extralymphatic organs with or without lymph node involvement

Patients are also subcategorized by the presence of unexplained fevers, night sweats, or weight loss.

Although the chest radiograph is abnormal in less than 50% of patients, identification of hilar or mediastinal adenopathy, parenchymal lesions, or pleural effusions provides an easy method for reevaluation. Computed tomography (CT) can identify both nodal and extranodal sites of involvement for monitoring the response to therapy. Magnetic resonance imaging (MRI) is useful in identifying bone, bone marrow, and central nervous system (CNS) involvement. However, it has not yet been accepted as a substitute for bone marrow biopsy. Nuclear bone scans can sometimes be useful in patients who present with or develop back pain. Gallium scans are more often used as part of the staging evaluation, and they are more likely to be positive in patients with aggressive diffuse large B-cell lymphoma than in more indolent follicular lymphoma (Fig. 23.1). Gallium avidity at midtreatment cycle or at the end of treatment is associated with a much higher relapse rate than seen in patients who have negative results on the gallium scan.[6,7] After patients have received three or four cycles of the planned treatment regimen or at the completion of the entire regimen, reevaluation should be done to determine the response to therapy. Patients who have a complete response are more likely to be cured than patients who have achieved only a partial response. Documenting complete remission is particularly important since salvage treatment such as high-dose therapy and marrow transplantation can sometimes cure disease in patients who fail to respond to initial therapy. In sites of bulky disease, masses do not always completely regress. This does not necessarily mean that patients will have persisting lymphoma. Biopsy under these circumstances can be difficult and is not always accurate. If the patient was known to have a positive gallium or fluorodeoxyglucose (FDG) uptake at the outset of treatment, normal results of that scan, despite a residual mass, raise the possibility that only residual fibrous tissue is present.

Positron emission tomography (PET) offers the unique capability of revealing metabolic activity throughout the body. Increased glucose metabolism is a basic biochemical hallmark of tumor cells, and the glucose analog FDG is transported, phosphorylated, and metabolically trapped in malignant cells.[7,8] L-[methyl-^{11}C] methionine (MET) is another widely used tumor-seeking tracer for PET. Methionine is an essential amino acid needed for protein and polyamine synthesis, and is also involved in transsulfuration and transamination reactions. Furthermore, methionine acts as a precursor for S-adenosyl-methionine, which is the predominant biologic methyl group donor.[9] Methionine metabolism is altered in cancer cells, and the accumulation of MET in malignant tumors is principally caused by its enhanced transport across the plasma membrane of tumor cells. Leskinen-Kallio et al[10] found that MET uptake was increased both in high- and low-grade NHL, whereas FDG was found to be superior to MET in distinguishing high-grade from other grade tumors. Rodriguez et al[11] also concluded that FDG uptake (Figs. 23.2 and 23.3) was associated with malignancy grade, but no relationship was found between MET uptake and malignancy grade.

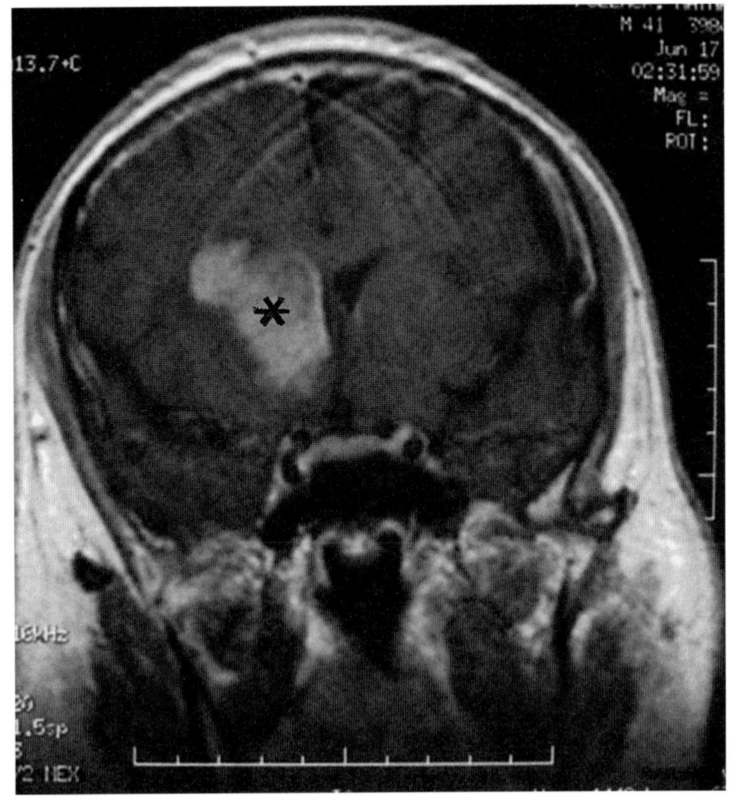

A

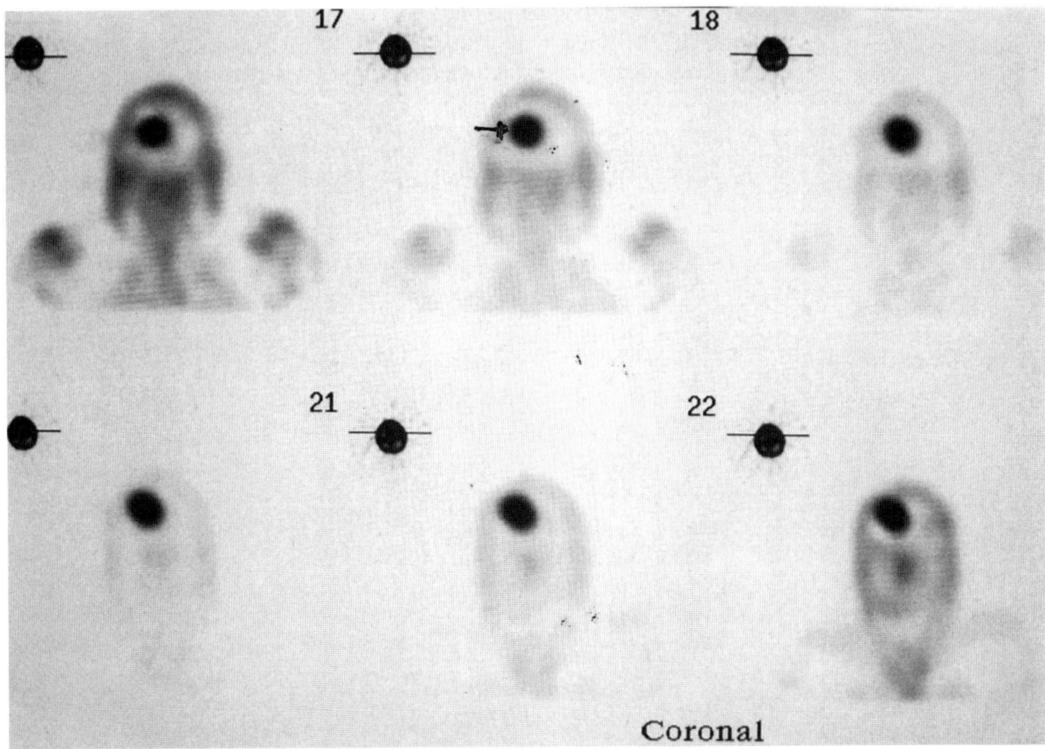

B

FIGURE 23.1. A: Selected T1-weighted coronal MR image of the head shows a contrast-enhanced mass (*) in the right basal ganglia. B: Coronal SPECT images of the head show a marked increased uptake (*arrow*) of Ga 67 citrate in the right basal ganglia with non-Hodgkin's lymphoma.

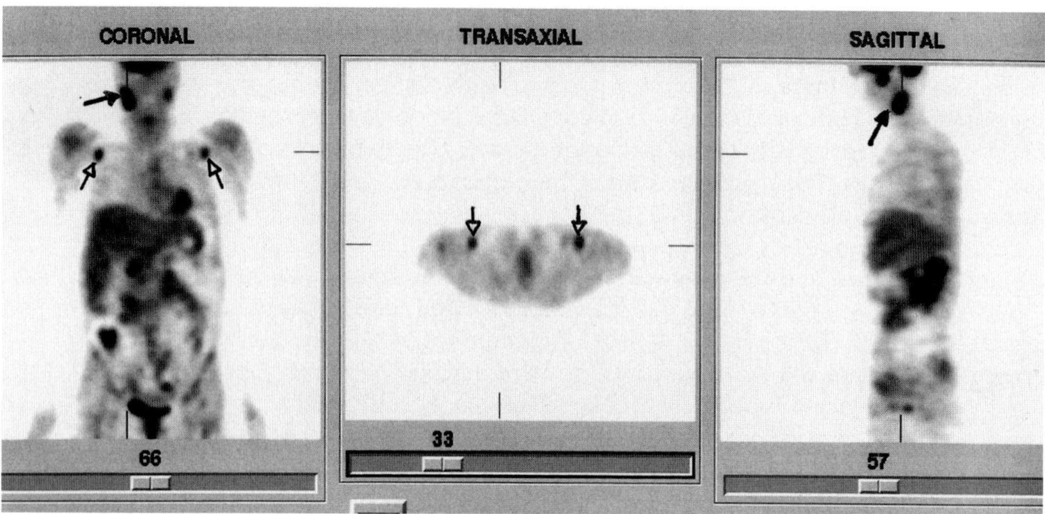

FIGURE 23.2. Selected coronal and sagittal PET images of the axial body as well as axial images of the upper chest show markedly increased uptake of ^{18}F-FDG in the right upper jugular (*closed arrows*) and bilateral axillary (*open arrows*) lymph nodes with lymphoma involvement.

Nodal staging is instrumental but not the only factor defining the treatment strategy for a patient with HD or NHL. The histologic type, presence of B symptoms, such as weight loss, fever or night sweats, age, extent of disease, extranodal manifestations, and serum level of LDH are also important prognostic factors. However, nodal staging is

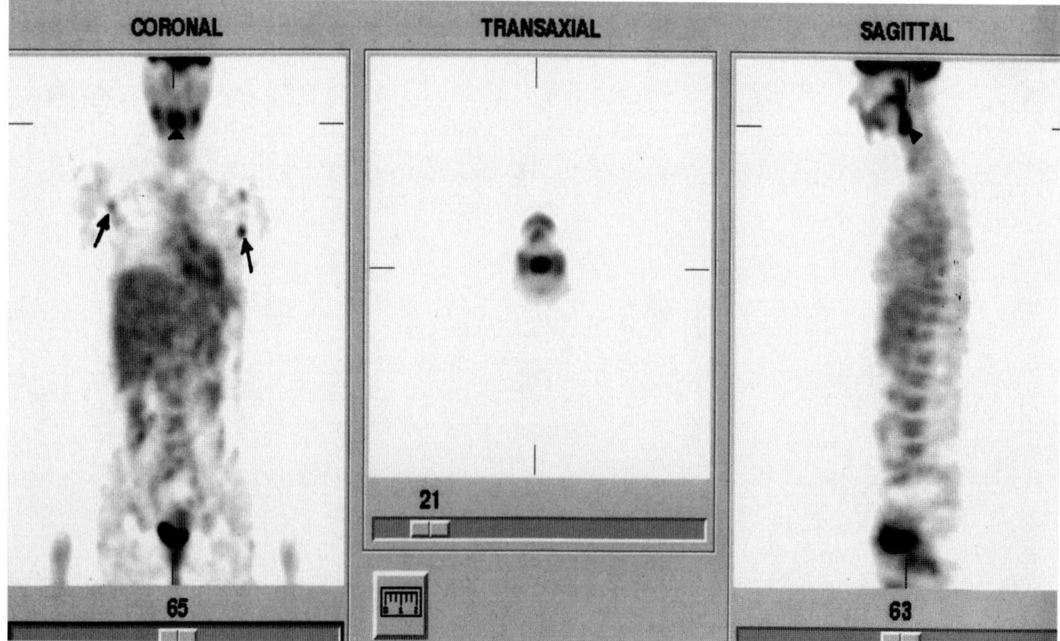

FIGURE 23.3. Selected coronal and sagittal PET images of the axial body in a patient with low-grade lymphoma show slightly increased uptake of ^{18}F-FDG in axillary lymph nodes (*arrows*). Note marked physiologic activity in the lingual tonsil (*arrowhead*).

the major factor differentiating limited from advanced disease. Advanced disease is best managed by aggressive chemotherapy, but involved field radiotherapy, possibly combined with a short course of chemotherapy, is often curative for limited disease. Nodes smaller than 10 mm are usually considered to be free of disease. However, normal-sized nodes may contain tumor cells, whereas enlarged nodes may show only immunoreactive cells.

FDG and MET seemed to accumulate avidly in both high- and low-grade lymphomas, and the total number of discrepant findings in individual lymph node sites (15/178) on CT and PET was similar to those on FDG and MET.[12] The avid physiologic accumulation of MET in liver, pancreas, intestine, and bone marrow concealed a group of pathologic lymph nodes detected by FDG and CT. On the other hand, MET was superior to FDG in detecting mediastinal disease in the patient with diabetes. Not only FDG but also MET is known to accumulate in inflammatory tissue, although MET probably accumulates to a lesser extent.[13] The small size of the lesion is probably the major reason for false-negative findings. The central location together with lack of attenuation correction may have further affected lesion detectability in the paraaortic area. Attenuation correction has not been shown to improve overall sensitivity for tumor detection either with conventional filtered back-projection reconstruction or new iterative reconstruction methods. The advantages of attenuation correction and sophisticated image reconstruction may manifest in easier image interpretation and better anatomic localization. Attenuation correction also makes possible the elimination of reconstruction artifacts and the quantification of tracer uptake. In current clinical practice, the detection of lymphoma in small abdominal nodes may be a problem (Figs. 23.4–23.6). Unfor-

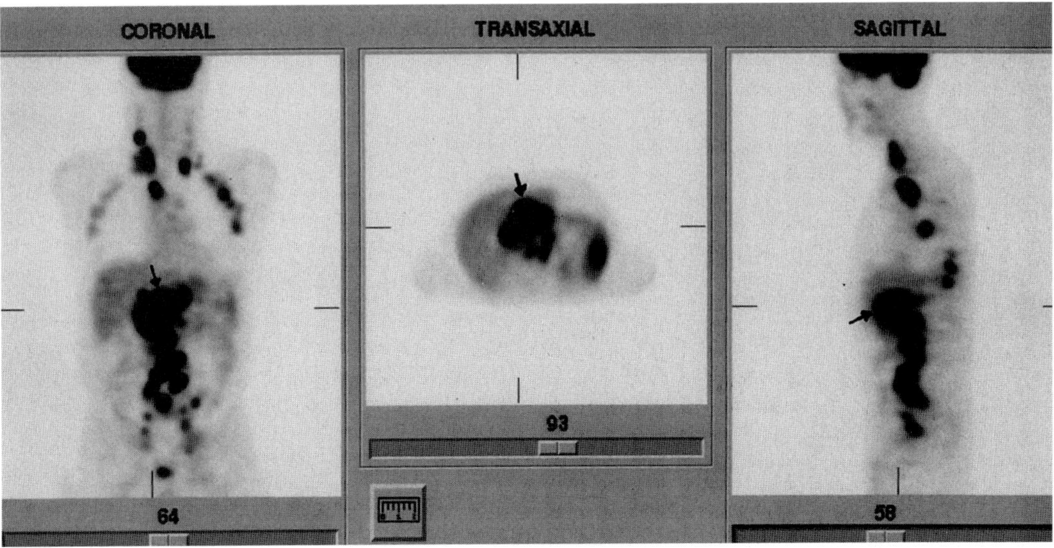

FIGURE 23.4. Selected coronal and sagittal PET images of the axial body and axial image of the upper abdomen show markedly increased uptake of ^{18}F-FDG in periaortic (*arrows*), iliac, right jugular, axillary, and right paratracheal lymph nodes with lymphoma involvement. Note less uptake in right axillary and bilateral external iliac nodes.

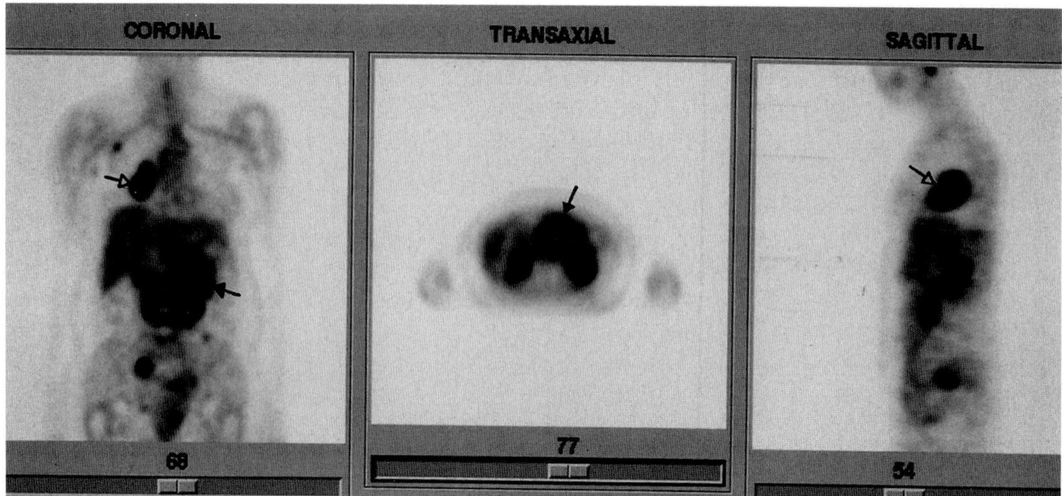

FIGURE 23.5. Selected coronal and sagittal PET images of the axial body and axial image of the upper abdomen show markedly increased uptake of ^{18}F-FDG in periaortic, left mesenteric (*closed arrows*), right iliac, and right axillary lymph nodes with lymphoma involvement. Note also markedly increased activity in the right lower lung lesion (*open arows*).

tunately, the current method for PET does not seem to resolve this challenge completely. Further clinical studies are warranted using combined PET/CT (Fig. 23.7), which has been suggested to be a more useful diagnostic tool than PET alone in cancer patients.[14] Overall, PET seems to show a greater number of positive lesions than does CT, and rigorous histologic verification of all suspected findings in patients

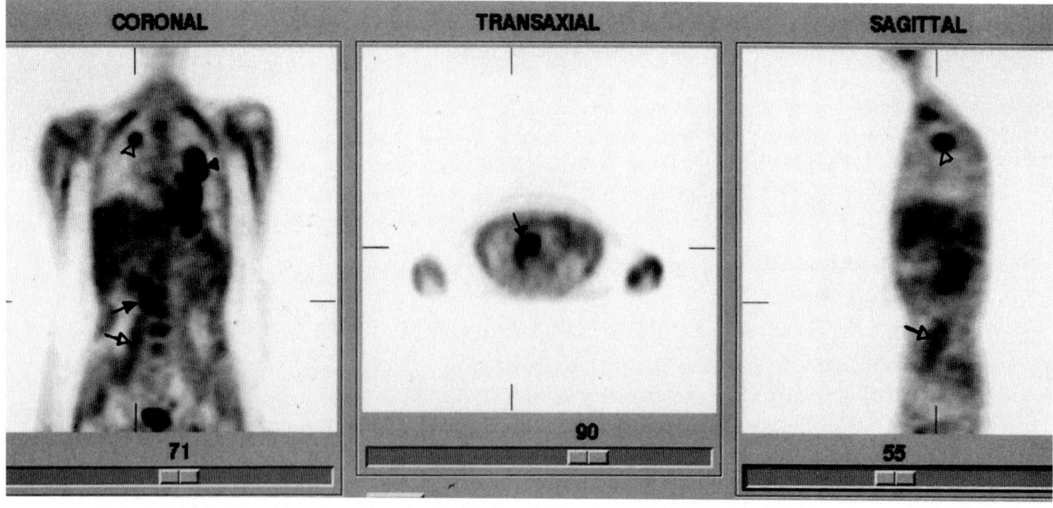

FIGURE 23.6. Selected coronal and sagittal PET images of the axial body and an axial image of the mid-abdomen with ^{18}F-FDG show markedly increased activity in the right para-aortic node (*closed arrows*), and right (*open arrowhead*) and left (*closed arrowhead*) lungs with lymphoma involvement. Note stressed muscles in the neck, upper arms, and right psoas muscle (*open arrows*).

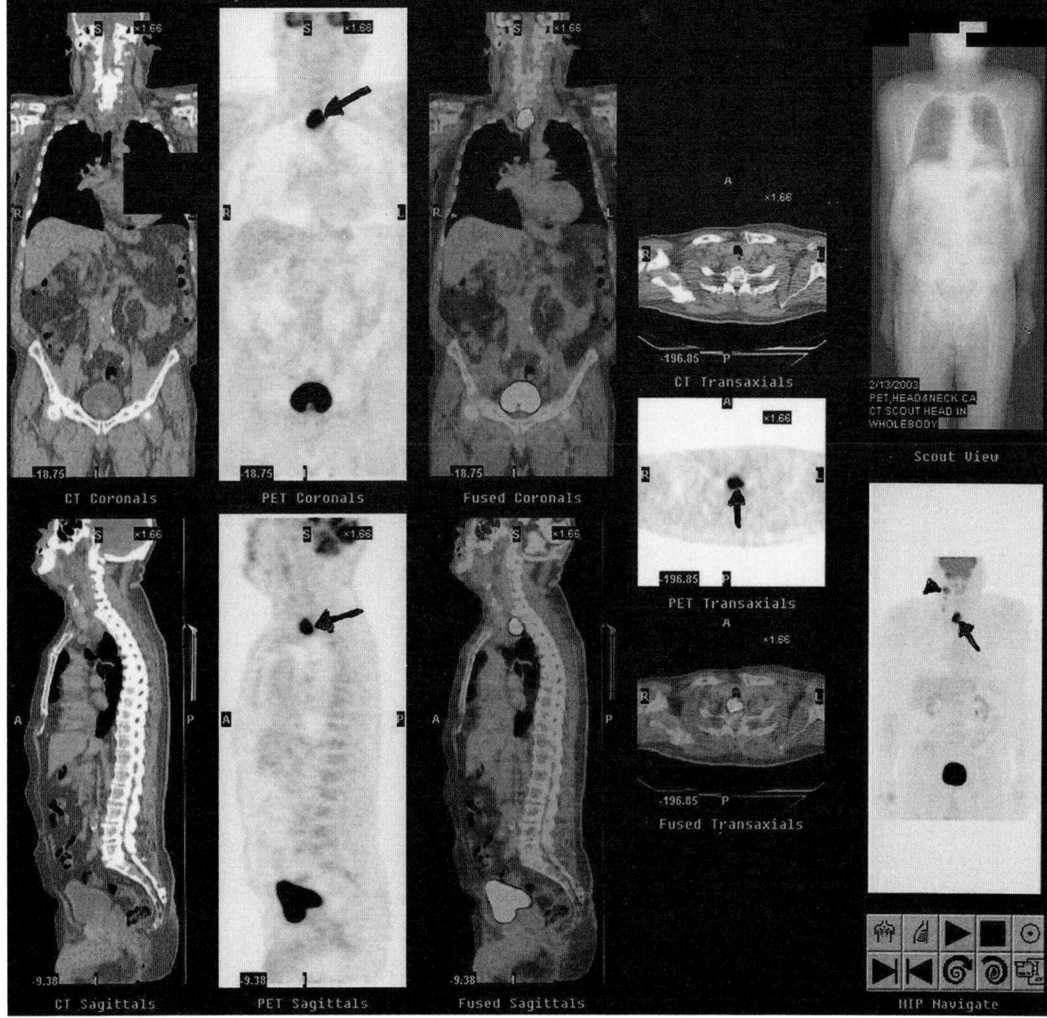

FIGURE 23.7. Selected coronal and sagittal PET/CT images of the axial body as well as axial image of the neck show markedly increased uptake of ^{18}F-FDG in the prevertebral area of the superior mediastinum (*arrows*) due to lymphoma involvement. Note also slightly to moderately increased activity along the right jugular lymphatic chain (*arrowhead*).

with lymphoma is difficult because of possible multiorgan involvement in deeply situated sites.

The bone scan has been used traditionally in the evaluation of bone involvement in lymphoma. Findings are characterized by relatively discrete uptake of tracer, and the sensitivity in detecting bone metastases using diphosphonate molecules results from the early osteoblastic reaction. Osteolytic lesions that are commonly encountered in NHL often escape scintigraphic detection. Radiography is mostly used to exclude false-positive findings on bone scans. Ga 67 scan is of limited usefulness in detecting skeletal involvement of lymphoma. Lymphomatous infiltration of skeletal structures may occur as a result of both hematogenous spread of the disease and direct invasion from adjacent involved tissues. Even localized lymphomatous infiltration of bone marrow is considered evidence of generalized disease, whereas scintigraphic or radiologic findings of an isolated osseous lesion is held to be local disease. FDG-PET (Figs. 23.8 and 23.9) was suitable for identifying osseous involvement in malignant lymphoma with a high positive predictive value and was thereby more sensitive and specific than bone scan.[15] A potential limitation of FDG for assessing malignant osseous lesions may be its physiologic accumulation in bone marrow. In untreated patients, this accumulation is generally quite homogeneous, and is comparatively low with standard uptake value (SUV) levels of 0.7 to 1.3. On the other hand, in areas of lymphomatous involvement, despite large differences depending on the degree of malignancy, FDG uptake is high with SUVs of 3.5 to 31.0 (median 8.5) (Fig. 23.10).[15,16]

Human immunodeficiency virus (HIV) is neutrotrophic and is involved in the pathogenesis of several of the neurologic syndromes, including HIV encephalopathy and progressive dementia. The CNS may also be involved with opportunistic infections or malignancies associated with progressive immunosuppression. The opportunistic infection that most commonly involves the CNS in patients with acquired immune deficiency syndrome (AIDS) is *Toxoplasma gondi*. This infection

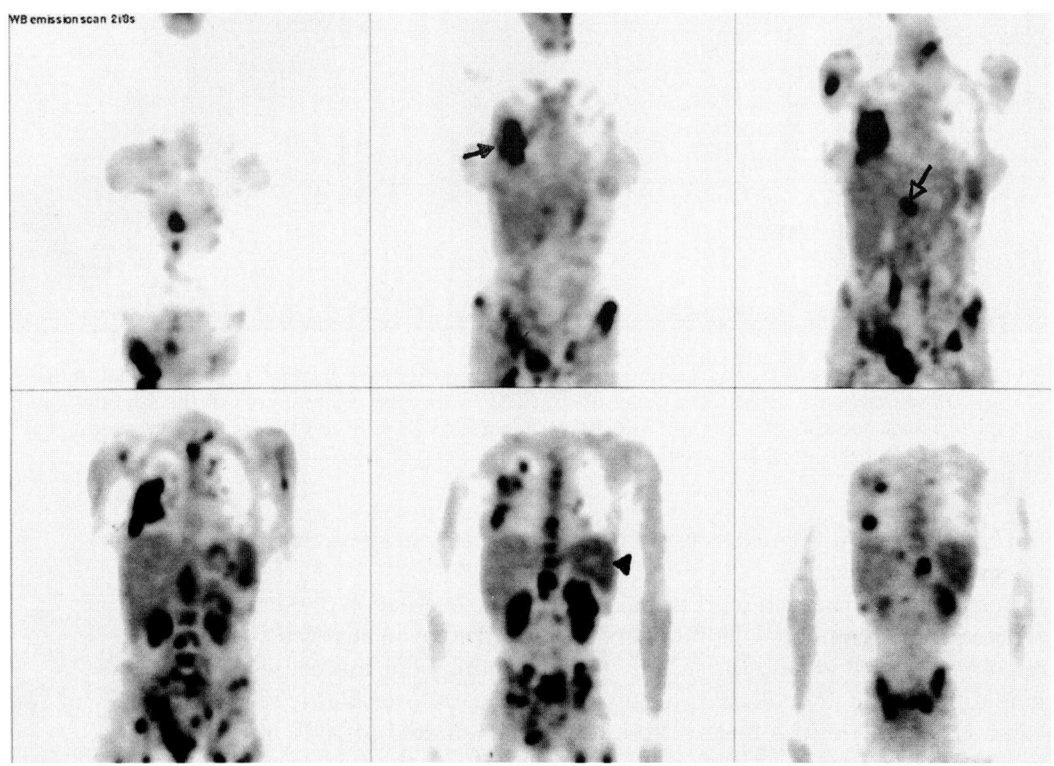

FIGURE 23.8. Coronal PET images of the axial body with ^{18}F-FDG show numerous focal areas of markedly increased activity in the right lung (*closed arrow*), upper periaortic node (*open arrow*), and multiple vertebrae, pelvic bones, bilateral proximal humeri and femurs due to lymphoma involvement. Note also diffusely increased activity in the spleen (*arrowhead*).

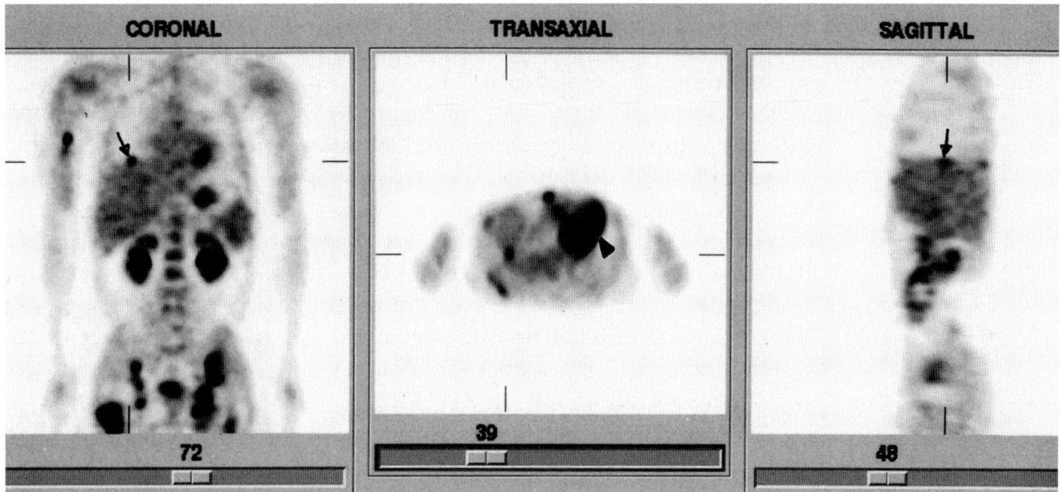

FIGURE 23.9. Selected coronal and sagittal PET images of the axial body and an axial image of the lower abdomen with ^{18}F-FDG show multiple focal areas of markedly increased activity in pelvic bones, proximal femurs, right humerus, and right lung base (*arrows*) with lymphoma involvement. Note also left lower mesenteric lesion (*arrowhead*).

may produce a diffuse meningoencephalitis or cause focal lesions. Imaging studies such as CT and MRI are used to detect treatable complications of HIV infection such as toxoplasmosis or lymphoma and may often reveal focal or multifocal ring-enhanced lesions. However, without histopathologic confirmation, a specific diagnosis may be dif-

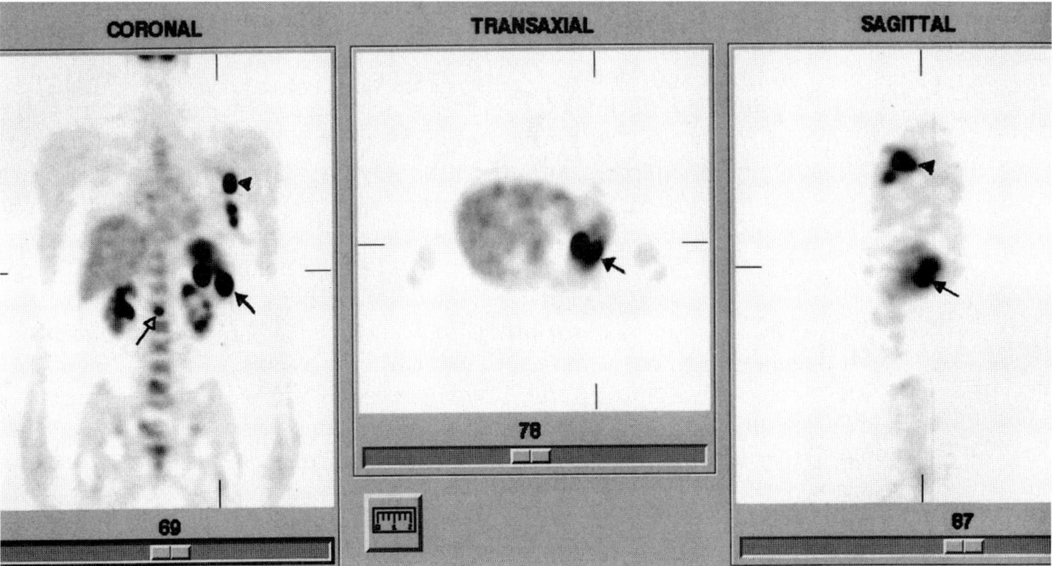

FIGURE 23.10. Selected coronal and sagittal PET images of the axial body and an axial image of the upper abdomen show markedly increased uptake of ^{18}F-FDG in the spleen (*closed arrows*), L1 vertebral body (*open arrow*), and left axillary nodes (*arrowheads*).

ficult. It is not possible to differentiate CNS lymphoma from toxoplasmosis in the HIV-infected individual on the basis of CT or MRI findings due to the similarity in the appearance of the lesions. FDG-PET was able to accurately differentiate between a malignant (lymphoma) and nonmalignant etiology for the CNS lesions.[17] Both qualitative visual inspection of the images as well as semiquantitative analysis using count density ratios revealed similar results. It was concluded that FDG-PET may be useful in the management of AIDS patients with CNS lesions since high FDG uptake most likely represents a malignant process that should be biopsied for confirmation rather than treated presumptively as infectious.

Assessment of Lymphoma Therapy Using ^{18}F-FDG-PET

Accurate evaluation of therapeutic response is of vital importance in the management of lymphoma patients.[18] The main end point of chemotherapy is the achievement of complete remission, which is associated with a longer progression-free survival and potential cure than is partial remission. The definition of complete remission is usually based on anatomic imagings that may be unable to differentiate viable tumor from posttreatment changes such as scarring or fibrosis. Residual abnormalities that occur after therapy are usually considered to represent persistent lymphoma; however, only a maximum of 10% to 20% of residual masses was reported to be positive for lymphoma at the completion of treatment.[19] Thus, there was no difference in the CT-documented response rates and the size of residual masses between patients who experience disease relapse and those who remain disease free.[20] CT does not consistently distinguish between dividing tumor cells and posttherapy fibrosis. Patients with aggressive NHL have positive CT findings in approximately 50% of cases after chemotherapy, and long-term follow-up shows that only 50% or fewer of those with positive CT findings have disease relapse or other evidence of residual tumor.[21] CT is a poor predictor of clinical outcome after treatment of aggressive NHL, and a posttherapy CT scan positive for NHL does not indicate that the time to progression for that patient will be significantly different from that for a patient with normal CT findings.[20] Although MRI provides better morphologic details than does CT when contrast material is not used, the low sensitivity rate (45%) showed that MRI was not ideal for predicting outcome.[22] Ga 67 scan has also been reported to be an independent predictor of outcome after one to two cycles of chemotherapy.[21] Nevertheless, Ga 67 scan is less efficacious than ^{18}F-FDG-PET for intraabdominal tumors, and may be less sensitive in detecting disease in some instances of aggressive lymphoma or HD.[23]

Over the past few years, a large body of evidence has confirmed the potential role of ^{18}F-FDG-PET, including both dedicated and coincidence PET systems, in the monitoring of lymphomas.[24] Although a change in ^{18}F-FDG uptake at multiple early times during chemotherapy has been described, this change was only marginally predictive of outcome.[25] The response to neoadjuvant chemotherapy has been characterized as one of the most important prognostic factors. It has been recently found that ^{18}F-FDG-PET has a high prognostic value for evaluation of therapy as early as after one cycle of chemotherapy in aggressive NHL and HD.[26] After the completion of chemotherapy, although there was a statistically significant difference between patients with ^{18}F-FDG-PET–negative findings and patients with ^{18}F-FDG-PET–positive findings, ^{18}F-FDG-PET results were not as good a predictor of long-term outcome. ^{18}F-FDG-PET findings after the completion of chemotherapy yielded a significantly lower sensitivity and negative predictive value than did findings after the first cycle. Resolution of therapy-induced anatomic changes on CT or MRI usually lags behind tumor cell mortality.

Various reports have shown the effectiveness of ^{18}F-FDG-PET in the posttreatment evaluation of lymphomas. ^{18}F-FDG-PET was found to be superior to Ga 67 scan in accurately detecting disease sites in aggressive NHL and HD, with a sensitivity of 100% and 80.3%, respectively.[23] Furthermore, ^{18}F-FDG-PET scans have a higher diagnostic and prognostic value than CT scans in the posttreatment evaluation of lymphomas.[27] Thus, ^{18}F-FDG-PET has become the most helpful noninvasive modality in differentiating tumor recurrence from fibrosis when CT scans show a residual mass.[26] Positive ^{18}F-FDG-PET results after one cycle of chemotherapy reflect the metabolic activity of potentially resistant clones that, although responding to chemotherapy, do so more slowly than do those homogeneously sensitive tumor cells. Negative ^{18}F-FDG-PET results after the first cycle were highly suggestive of long-term remission, whereas negative results after the completion of chemotherapy were less accurate. ^{18}F-FDG-PET after the first cycle of chemotherapy remains far more predictive of outcome than later ^{18}F-FDG-PET.

I 131 anti-B1 (CD 20) radioimmunotherapy (RIT) has been recognized as a promising approach for treatment of NHL. It is sometimes difficult to differentiate posttherapeutic scar tissue from viable residual tissue on CT scan, potentially leading to incorrect management of patients. Baseline tumor glucose metabolism (SUV) did not predict the response of NHL to treatment, and SUV at 1 to 2 months after RIT correlated well with the ultimate best response of NHL to RIT. The decreases in SUV in responders were almost parallel to the decreases in tumor size measured by CT.[28] Metabolic changes with radiation therapy appear to be more gradual than those after chemotherapy.

Conclusion

Three principal opportunities for FDG-PET (Fig. 23.11) to optimize the management of Hodgkin's disease and non-Hodgkin's lymphoma can be defined: in improving the accuracy of initial staging, in defining response to treatment, and in refining follow-up after completion of treatment. In low-grade lymphoma, FDG-PET appears to be of less value, frequently failing to demonstrate disease seen on conventional imag-

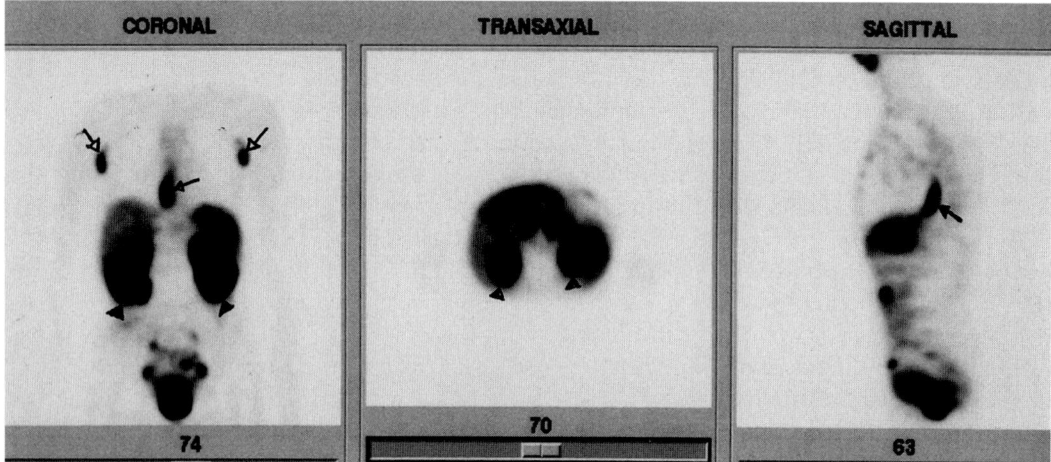

FIGURE 23.11. Selected coronal and sagittal PET images of the axial body and an axial image of the upper abdomen with ^{18}F-FDG show markedly increased activity in the distal esophagus (*closed arrows*), axillary lymph nodes (*open arrows*), and kidneys (*arrowheads*) with lymphoma involvement.

ing.[29] Functional imaging with FDG-PET may have an important role in the management of lymphoma, enabling more precise and accurate tailoring of treatment to the patient's true disease status both at presentation and subsequently during and after completion of first-line treatment.

References

1. Sandlund JT, Downing JR, Crist WM. Non-Hodgkin's lymphoma in childhood. N Engl J Med 1996;334:1238–1241.
2. Jemal A, Thomas A, Murray T, et al. Cancer statistics. CA Cancer J Clin 2002;52:23–47.
3. Newton R, Ferlay J, Beral V, et al. The epidemiology of non-Hodgkin's lymphoma: comparison of nodal and extra-nodal sites. Int J Cancer 1997; 72:923–927.
4. Glass AG, Karnell LH, Menck HR. The National Cancer Data Base report on non-Hodgkin's lymphoma. Cancer 1997;80:2311–2320.
5. Weisenburger D. The International Lymphoma Study Group Classification of non-Hodgkin's lymphoma: pathology findings from a large multicenter study. Mod Pathol 1997;10:136A.
6. Larcos G, Farlow DC, Antico VF, et al. The role of high dose Ga-67 scintigraphy in staging untreated patients with lymphoma. Aust NZ J Med 1994; 24:5–8.
7. Tatsumi M, Kitayama H, Sugahara H, et al. Whole-body hybrid PET with F-18 FDG in the staging of non-Hodgkin's lymphoma. J Nucl Med 2001;42:601–608.
8. Carr R, Barrington S, Madam B, et al. Detection of lymphoma in bone marrow by whole-body positron emission tomography. Blood 1998;91:3340–3346.

9. Finkelstein JD, Martin JJ. Methionine metabolism in mammals. J Biol Chem 1986;26:1582–1587.
10. Leskinen-Kallio S, Ruotsalainem U, Nägren K, et al. Uptake of C-11 methionine and fluorodeoxyglucose in non-Hodgkin's lymphoma: a PET study. J Nucl Med 1991;32:1211–1218.
11. Rodriguez M, Rehn S, Ahlström H, et al. Predicting malignancy grade with PET in non-Hodgkin's lymphoma. J Nucl Med 1995;36:1790–1796.
12. Sutinen E, Jyrkiö S, Varpula M, et al. Nodal staging of lymphoma with whole-body PET: comparison of C-11 methionine and FDG. J Nucl Med 2000;41:1980–1988.
13. Kubota R, Kubota K, Yamada S, et al. Methionine uptake by tumor tissue: a microautoradiographic comparison with FDG. J Nucl Med 1995;36:484–492.
14. Charion M, Beyer T, Kinahan PE, et al. Whole-body FDG PET and CT imaging of malignancies using a combined PET/CT scanner. J Nucl Med 1999;40:256.
15. Moog F, Kotzerke J, Reske SN. FDG-PET can replace bone scintigraphy in primary staging of malignant lymphoma. J Nucl Med 1999;40:1407–1413.
16. Lapela M, Leskinen-Kallio S, Minn H, et al. Increased glucose metabolism in untreated non-Hodgkin's lymphoma: a study with PET and F-18 FDG. Blood 1995;9:3522–3527.
17. Hoffman JM, Waskin HA, Schifter T, et al. FDG-PET in differentiating lymphoma from nonmalignant central nervous system lesions in patients with AIDS. J Nucl Med 1993;34:567–575.
18. DeVita VT, Cannelos GP. The lymphomas. Semin Hematol 1999;36:84–94.
19. Surbone A, Longo DL, DeVita VL, et al. Residual abdominal masses in aggressive non-Hodgkin's lymphoma after combination chemotherapy; significance and management. J Clin Oncol 1988;6:1832–1837.
20. Janicek M, Kaplan W, Neuberg D, et al. Early re-staging gallium scans predict outcome in poor prognosis patients with aggressive non-Hodgkin's lymphoma treated with high-dose CHOP chemotherapy. J Clin Oncol 1997; 15:1631–1637.
21. Front D, Bar-Shalom R, Mor M, et al. Aggressive non-Hodgkin's lymphoma: early prediction of outcome with Ga-67 scintigraphy. Radiology 2000;214:253–257.
22. Hill M, Cunningham D, MacVicar D, et al. Role of magnetic resonance imaging in predicting relapse in residual masses after treatment of lymphoma. J Clin Oncol 1993;11:2273–2278.
23. Kostakoglu L, Leonard JP, Coleman M, et al. Comparison of F-18 fluorodeoxyglucose PET and Ga-67 scintigraphy in evaluation of lymphoma. J Clin Oncol 2000;19:10a.
24. Mikhaeel NG, Timothy AR, Hain SF, O'Doherty MJ. F-18 FDG PET for the assessment of residual masses on CT following treatment of lymphomas. Ann Oncol 2000;11:147–150.
25. Romer W, Hanauske A, Ziegler S, et al. Positron emission tomography in non-Hodgkin's lymphoma: assessment of chemotherapy with fluorodeoxyglucose. Blood 1998;91:4464–4471.
26. Kostakoglu L, Coleman M, Leonard JP, et al. PET predicts prognosis after 1 cycle of chemotherapy in aggressive lymphoma and Hodgkin's disease. J Nucl Med 2002;43:1018–1027.
27. Jerusalem G, Beguin Y, Fassotte MF, et al. Whole-body PET using F-18 FDG for post-treatment evaluation in Hodgkin's disease and non-Hodgkin's lymphoma has higher diagnostic and prognostic value than classical CT scan imaging. Blood 1999;94:429–433.

28. Torizuka T, Zasadny KR, Kison PV, et al. Metabolic response of non-Hodgkin's lymphoma to I-131 anti-B1 radioimmunotherapy: evaluation with FDG PET. J Nucl Med 2000;41:999–1005.
29. Hoskin PJ. FDG PET in the management of lymphoma: a clinical perspective. Eur J Nucl Med 2002;29:449–451.

Index